AF866026

HANDBOOK OF PEDIATRIC CARDIOLOGY

Brent Alexander

ALLIED
HEALTH
PRESS

Handbook of Pediatric Cardiology

Author: **Brent Alexander**

Allied Health Press
4164 Lakeshore Road
Burlington ON L7L 1A4
Canada
www.alliedhealthpress.com
Email: orders@arclereducation.com

© 2026 Allied Health Press
ISBN: 978-1-77956-823-6

This book contains information obtained from highly regarded resources. Reprinted material sources are indicated and copyright remains with the original owners. Copyright for images and other graphics remains with the original owners as indicated. A Wide variety of references are listed. Reasonable efforts have been made to publish reliable data. Authors or Editors or Publishers are not responsible for the accuracy of the information in the published chapters or consequences of their use. The publisher assumes no responsibility for any damage or grievance to the persons or property arising out of the use of any materials, instructions, methods or thoughts in the book. The authors or editors and the publisher have attempted to trace the copyright holders of all material reproduced in this publication and apologize to copyright holders if permission has not been obtained. If any copyright holder has not been acknowledged, please write to us so we may rectify.

General Disclaimer:
This book is a summation of information from different sources and encompasses a wide range of medical conditions, the latest therapy methods, principals and techniques that are used in current practice, at the time of publication. This book offers general information with educational purposes, it is not to be applied or relied on for any diagnostic or treatment purposes. Please do not use the data/matter as a substitute for professional diagnosis and treatment. Please consult your healthcare provider or a licensed physician before making any healthcare queries or treatment choices. The medical information and research findings presented in this book are for educational purposes only and should not be used for the treatment of specific individual patients, as individual cases may vary. The author(s), editors(s) and publisher cannot be held accountable and make no guarantees that the information provided in this book will apply to each and individual patient. This book is meant to serve as a basic guideline and other relevant literature sources should be used for more specific information. This text can be a vital resource for students, trainees, and practitioners, covering essential topics. This book encompasses a wide range of medical conditions and the latest therapy options used in current practice. Through the utilization of many different medical studies this book provides the basics of different medical conditions, which can be used as a basic guide from where medical students, trainees and practitioners can extract necessary information. Further, some of the books have graphic images to explain anatomy for medical/educational purposes only. Hence, the book is intended for students or teachers/staff or individuals with a mature outlook looking to learn or enhance their knowledge.

Notice: Registered trademark of products or corporate names are used only for explanation and identification without intent of infringement.

Allied Health Press publishes wide variety of books and eBooks. For more information about Allied Health Press and its products, visit our website at www.alliedhealthpress.com

ABOUT THE AUTHOR

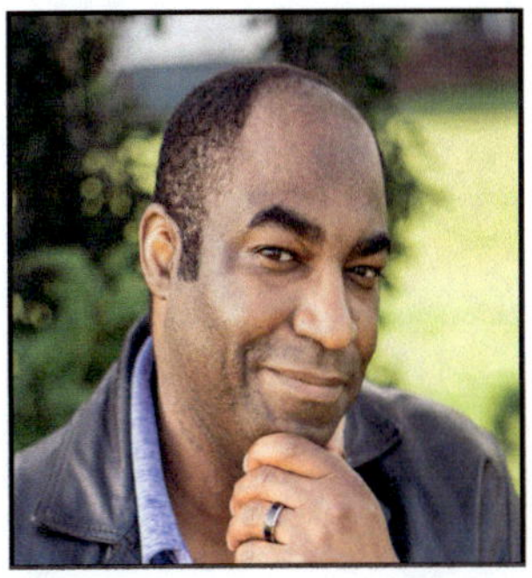

Brent Alexander is a dedicated, senior level, healthcare and life science advisor with over 14 years of medical research and healthcare consulting experience. He is skilled in strategic thinking, data analysis & interpretation, project management, and building relationships. Brent has effectively planned, executed, and evaluated several major medical research projects for organizations such as Suncor Energy Inc., Calgary Flames Hockey Organization, and Own the Podium. Brent has an intrinsic love for science and has expanded on this through gaining academic accolades in maternal/child health and perinatal physiology, as well as in the chronobiological and physiological principles of sleep medicine. Since completing a Masters degree in Medical Science, Brent has previously managed a role as the Clinical Research Coordinator at the Centre for Sleep and Human Performance, a College of Physicians and Surgeons of Alberta, and American Academy of Sleep Medicine accredited sleep centre in Calgary, Alberta. Currently, he holds two positions within Alberta Health Services Brent is the Senior Advisor for Public Health, Calgary Zone, providing integration of technology and quality improvement alignment with the clinical operations of immunization and public health programs. He is also a Tissue Specialist with the Southern Alberta Tissue Program where he uses his laboratory experience to expertly assist in the surgical recovery, processing, preservation and distribution of donor tissues that are used for banking, transplantation, and research procedures help improve the quality of life for Albertans. Brent is also an accomplished writer and editor. He has authored and co-authored several abstracts and peer reviewed articles on fever & pregnancy, jet lag & travel fatigue management in elite athletes, and sleep & long-term athletic development (LTAD). In his down time, Brent enjoys staying active through sports and enjoying the outdoors with his wife and son.

Brief Table of Contents

Detailed Table of Contents

CHAPTER 5

Echocardiography in Pediatrics 139

CHAPTER 6

Congenital Heart Diseases – Acyanotic 171

CHAPTER 10

CHAPTER 11

LIST OF FIGURES

PREFACE

Cardiovascular disease in children is a unique and frequently complicated category of illnesses that necessitates early detection, nuanced diagnosis, and individualized treatment. In contrast to the field of cardiology in adults, pediatric cardiology involves a developmental approach, wherein the anatomical and physiological transitions from fetal development to adolescence must be meticulously addressed. Clinical manifestation of cardiac illness in children varies greatly and often bears a resemblance to other illnesses in children, demanding an assessment skill integrating pediatric and cardiologic knowledge. Also, the advancement in the diagnostic methods and therapy approaches has changed outcomes over the last decades but enduring problems persist in early detection, accurate interpretation of symptoms, and the delivery of proper care in their age category.

Understanding heart disease in children involves more than diagnosing structural or functional defects; it involves understanding the dynamic physiological adaptation accompanying growth and maturation. From the fetal period (when the heart operates in a unique circulatory mode) to postnatal transitional changes and the shifting of cardiac output demands through childhood, the cardiovascular system is continuously being remodeled. Pediatric cardiology is thus not a static specialty—it demands sensitivity to the evolving norms of clinical practice, technical innovation, and the psychosocial dimensions of the care of children and their families.

The author of *Essentials of Pediatric Cardiology* has intended to give students, residents, and clinicians a good and pragmatic foundation in the understanding of pediatric cardiac disease. The book has been composed on best evidence-based guidelines and is meant to serve both as a teaching resource as well as a clinical guide. The book integrates theoretical fundamentals with practical advice, condensing fundamental principles, diagnostic strategy, and management recommendations into one comprehensive manual that is equally relevant to frequent and uncommon cardiac conditions in children. Clarity of clinical decision, ready access to technical information, and logical order are given top priority for study and bedside reference.

Chapter 1 establishes an overall view of pediatric cardiology, laying the groundwork for why it is important to value cardiac physiology and presentation of disease across various pediatric ages. Chapter 2 deals with fetal circulation and transitional events at birth, outlining critical information about etiology of congenital heart defects and the physiological changes of the neonatal period. Chapter 3 focuses on the clinical method of assessing a child with suspected heart disease – highlighting the salient signs, symptoms, and physical findings in infancy and childhood.

Chapter 4 outlines the diagnostic tools used in pediatric cardiology (i.e., electrocardiography, chest X-ray, and advanced imaging tools like cardiac MRI and CT) in terms of indications and interpretation. Chapter 5 is the emphasis on pediatric echocardiography, the sine qua non of non-invasive cardiac imaging, and discusses its role in non-complex and complex cases. Chapter 6 discusses acyanotic congenital heart defects, such as atrial and ventricular septal defects, patent ductus arteriosus, and aortic coarctation, along with pathophysiology, clinical presentation, and management descriptions.

Chapter 7 deals with cyanotic congenital heart disease, including tetralogy of Fallot, great arteries transposition, and truncus arteriosus – presenting a structured approach to diagnosis, stabilization, and surgical planning. Chapter 8 deals with acquired heart disease of childhood (including rheumatic fever, Kawasaki disease, and myocarditis) relating clinical presentation to causative mechanisms and therapeutic options. Chapter 9 addresses pediatric heart failure (explaining etiologies ranging from structural abnormalities to cardiomyopathies) and summarizing evaluation, medical management, and support.

Chapter 10 presents pediatric arrhythmias from benign to life-threatening and their detection by ECG and treatment with pharmacologic and procedural interventions. Chapter 11 presents cardiomyopathies of the child, including dilated, hypertrophic, and restrictive cardiomyopathies, along with diagnostic signs and newer therapies. Chapter 12 presents hypertension in the child and adolescent (an emerging problem in modern pediatrics) covering its etiology, risk factors, diagnostic thresholds, and treatment protocols.

Chapter 13 introduces interventional pediatric cardiology, including catheter-based interventions like device closure, balloon angioplasty, and valvuloplasty, with emphasis on indications, techniques, and results. Chapter 14 discusses cardiac emergencies in the child, such as shock, tamponade, and acute arrhythmias, and provides recommendations on prompt recognition and treatment in the acute care setting. Chapter 15 is concluded with a discussion of pediatric cardiac surgery, including preoperative assessment, surgical repair of common defects, and postoperative care issues.

This book is aimed at a prolonged readership that includes undergraduate and postgraduate students of medicine, pediatric residents, pediatricians, cardiology fellows, and pediatric cardiac unit nursing staff. It is also helpful for new practitioners seeking an organized idea of pediatric heart diseases and experienced practitioners seeking a concise reference in the clinic. The text is structured for the convenience of study and clinical use, making it an ideal guide for academic study and patient practice alike.

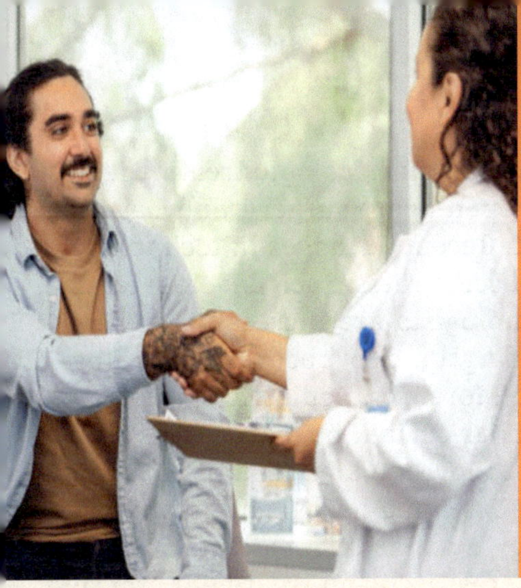

Chapter 1

INTRODUCTION TO PEDIATRIC CARDIOLOGY

Contents

Introduction

Pediatric cardiology is specialized medicine that focuses on the diagnosis and treatment of congenital and acquired cardiovascular disorders in children. Children have physiological differences when compared to adults. Due to these differences, the specialty requires understanding these differences in order to treat cardiovascular diseases. Conditions like congenital heart defects, which affect approximately 1 in every 100 infants, require early detection and intervention. Early diagnosis (typically by means of high-technology imaging modalities like echocardiography) is also significant in defining the appropriate management course for these children. Pediatrics are also assisted by a team of experts when offering complete care, and every child will be given proper treatment to address his or her own specific medical, developmental, and psychological needs. In addition to congenital disease, pediatric cardiology includes acquired illnesses such as myocarditis or arrhythmias that can complicate a child's condition. Some pediatric patients can also have heart disease as a direct result of underlying systemic illness such as diabetes or autoimmune illness. Therapies range from pharmacologic treatment to advanced interventions such as catheter-based interventions or open-heart surgery and have a profound effect on outcome and quality of life in the young patient. Recent advances in technology and medical procedures have improved surgical and intervention success rates. Such developments facilitate a mechanism of preventive care wherein pediatric cardiologists are increasingly using techniques that assist in minimizing invasiveness while maximizing quicker recovery, allowing the children to return to their normal lives in a shorter duration. Moreover, pediatric cardiology also places significant emphasis on long-term follow-up of patients as certain heart ailments may lead to late complications or be lifelong requiring care. Long-term follow-up is important as it can detect possible issues early on before it becomes severe, ensuring extended health and happiness even after childhood. With the inclusion of cutting-edge technology, such as telemedicine, follow-up treatment has changed to be more convenient for families. Also, research and treatment ethical guidelines for child patients emphasize informed consent and family involvement in making health care decisions. With further advancement, the field of pediatric cardiology is poised to enhance not merely survival, but the overall quality of life among children with cardiac illness, and to be a quantum leap in the science of medicine.

Definition and Scope of Pediatric Cardiology

Pediatric cardiology is the diagnosis, treatment, and management of congenital and acquired heart disease in children, ranging from infancy to adolescence. Pediatric cardiologists are trained specialists who have expertise in the cardiology of younger patients. This is a developmentally and structurally different population from adults; therefore, pediatric cardiology needs to incorporate knowledge of the physiological differences as well as the psychosocial considerations that influence the health of the child.

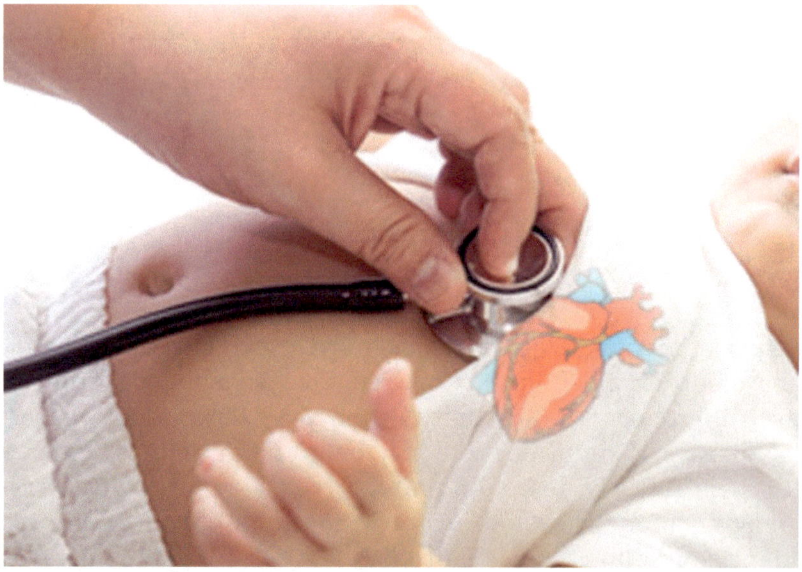

Figure 1.1. Pediatric cardiology.

Source: https://www.kailashhealthcare.com/Content/images/thumb/paediatric-cardiology.jpg.

The most common disorder treated is congenital heart defects, which may be corrected through surgery or long-term medical management. In addition, acquired cardiovascular diseases such as cardiomyopathy and myocarditis also come under the category of pediatric cardiology, reflecting the specialties extensive scope and relevance to long-term cardiovascular health in children. Most recently, the specialty has developed with increasingly more focus being laid on transitional care, an awareness of the chronicity of heart disease. When adolescents are being transitioned from pediatric to adult care, continuity of care becomes important in a bid to avert negative changes in health status, particularly in those with chronic illnesses. Based on research, successful transitions entail individualized models that incorporate the developmental needs of adolescent patients and their families and facilitate collaboration between pediatric and adult providers (Bagnall et al., 2013) (Figure 1.1).

Pediatric cardiology not only addresses immediate patient needs but also establishes systems to allow long-term effects on health. As a result, progressive transition programs have been established with the goal of bridging the gap between pediatric and adult health. These programs recognize continuation of care is essential to optimal well-being and making the unique process of developing the young patient population possible. Besides, the specialty of pediatric cardiology has relevance in the domain of preventive care and early intervention methods. As communicators and educators, pediatric cardiologists become important for the identification of risk factors contributing to cardiovascular disease in adulthood. Lifestyle modification, for example, in the form of promoting appropriate diet and regular exercise among children with high risk for obesity-induced cardiac disease is included in such a preventive approach. Furthermore, advances in technology have revolutionized the diagnosis and management of cardiac disease, leading to better results in children. Techniques such as echocardiography and cardiac MRI have improved the imaging and evaluation of cardiac disease to generate reliable information for when intervention should be performed. By investigation and collaboration among the healthcare professionals, pediatric cardiology continues to evolve, hence children receive complete cardiovascular care along their growth journey (Adi et al., 2009).

Importance of Specialized Care for Children

Pediatric cardiology is one of those subspecialties whose importance cannot be overstated. Children with congenital heart disease represent unique clinical challenges that are very different from what is encountered in adults with similar diseases. These demand a very large knowledge base of the physiological differences between children and adults, ranging from developmental concerns to differences in disease presentation and progression. Pediatric cardiologists are well positioned to address these details, offering personalized treatment plans incorporating not just the medical management of cardiac disease but also the psychosocial variables affecting young patients as well as their families. Specialist care of all this is required to optimize outcomes because children might depend on long-term plans incorporating feedback from an interdisciplinary team including pediatricians, surgeons, and dietitians among many more. This collective experience enhances the quality of care and enhances communication with families struggling with complicated treatment options. Economic factors also emphasize the need for upgraded pediatric cardiac care. Throughout most of the world, therapy is often very expensive for families struggling with a congenital heart disease (CHD) diagnosis in a child. More families are forced to make difficult decisions on how to redirect meager resources, as procedure expenses can be significantly greater than their yearly incomes. Consider India, for example – studies revealed that the median expense of surgery and admission stood at INR 201,898, which is comparable to the annual income of the affected families and therefore reflects the financial burden of accessing necessary medical treatment. This financial strain highlights the importance of creating affordable, specialized pediatric cardiac care services that minimize the financial strain on families while enabling children to receive the life-saving care they require. In the absence of affordable options and insurance coverage for pediatric cardiac disease, there are far too many families trapped in a debt and despair cycle, exacerbating the already difficult circumstances. Furthermore, education and awareness of the integrated care systems are required in order to improve the prognosis of children with congenital heart defects. Specialist pediatric cardiac centers possess infrastructure that enables early diagnosis, preventive screening, and timely intervention, significantly improving the outcome of patients. As an example, the strategies of care are not only limited to surgical intervention but also continuous monitoring for associated comorbidities that are commonly seen with CHD, such as developmental delay or nutritional deficiencies. Evidence is found that children under intensive, specialized management practices have improved survival and quality of life. As clinical guidelines have highlighted, pediatricians play a key role in recognizing and addressing such children's all-round needs so that they get holistic care throughout the treatment process. Coordinated care programs for specialties optimize the effectiveness of the treatment in general and address the multi-faceted health problems of children with cardiac conditions, ensuring the brighter future of these vulnerable patients.

Historical Development of the Field

Historical background of pediatric cardiology can be traced to the diagnosis and awareness of congenital heart disease in children. In the early 20th century, understanding of such illnesses was rudimentary, primarily due to lack of diagnostic methods and effective treatment modalities. Notably, the introduction of electrocardiography in the 1930s and echocardiography in the 1950s significantly altered the specialty. These technologies facilitated the more precise diagnosis of heart disease, making theories a reality of medical practice. The development of these diagnostic tools co-occurred with growing awareness of the prevalence of congenital heart disease, stimulating advances both in medical and surgical management. This was the beginning of a more specialized treatment of pediatric patients, as medical specialists began to address the unique anatomical and physiological differences of children from adults and thus opened the door for pediatric cardiology as a specialty. With advancements in pediatric cardiology, further advancements in surgical techniques were crucial for better outcomes in children with defects of the heart. The 1940s and 1950s saw the beginning of cardiac surgery, with milestone procedures such as the Blalock-Taussig shunt, which provided a solution for cyanotic heart disease. This milestone operation was a groundbreaking step in the line of treatment – making what was otherwise untreatable, treatable. Moreover, these developments went hand in hand with the establishment of specialized centers for pediatric cardiology, which could offer surgical as well as medical care for the treatment of congenital heart disease. The collaboration between cardiologists and surgeons encouraged treatment protocols, emphasizing the importance of multidisciplinary care to enhance patient outcomes. Notably, the following decades integrated advances in anesthesia and perioperative care, along with even more progressing pediatric cardiac surgeries, and initiatives focused on safety and efficacy and encouraging further advancement in pediatric cardiology as a subspecialty. The integration of genetics into pediatrics over the past few years has introduced new knowledge on congenital heart disease. With the advent of genetic screening, clinicians are now able to identify children at risk of genetic syndromes with their attendant heart defects and act early to develop customized treatment plans. Research into the genetic etiology of the majority of pediatric cardiovascular diseases has increased significantly, accelerated by collaboration among clinicians, geneticists, and scientists. Such an interdisciplinarity is the tip of the technology in pediatric cardiology, putting genetics and traditional medical practice together. In addition, technological advances in telemedicine have also had a revolutionary impact, enhancing specialized care for distant populations, especially during difficult periods like the COVID-19 pandemic. The history of pediatric cardiology exhibits a trend of progressive innovation, underscored by the need for continuous investigation and transitioning to accommodate novel problems and progressive concepts within the field of cardiovascular therapy as discussed within current literature regarding telemedicine and practice guidelines (Bernard et al., 2011; Rashid et al., 2020).

1.1. Anatomy of the Pediatric Heart

Pediatric cardiac anatomy contains significant departures from the anatomy of adult hearts, which demonstrate the unique physiological demands of the developing child. Each structural component, beginning with the chambers and extending through the valves, is integral to the healthy function of the heart. In infants and young children, these anatomical idiosyncrasies provide flexibility that supports accommodations to their unique metabolic needs. As an example, the considerably larger size of the right atrium and ventricle compared to their left-sided counterparts is one of the typical pediatric heart morphologies. This spatial arrangement is essential for maintaining correct blood flow dynamics, especially due to the presence of persistent fetal shunts (e.g., the foramen ovale and ductus arteriosus) to allow optimal oxygenation and perfusion early in life. It is essential to understand these anatomical features to diagnose CHD, which is common among pediatric patients. CHD is a wide variety of anatomical anomalies, from the simple defects in the form of ventricular septal defects (VSD) to complex conditions such as hypoplastic left heart syndrome. The diversity of variations in cardiac anatomy demands sufficient information regarding normal and abnormal heart anatomy so that the decision of management can be rendered effectively. In pursuit of this, advanced imaging techniques, like echocardiography and magnetic resonance imaging, are pivotal in the visualization of cardiac morphology (Figure 1.2).

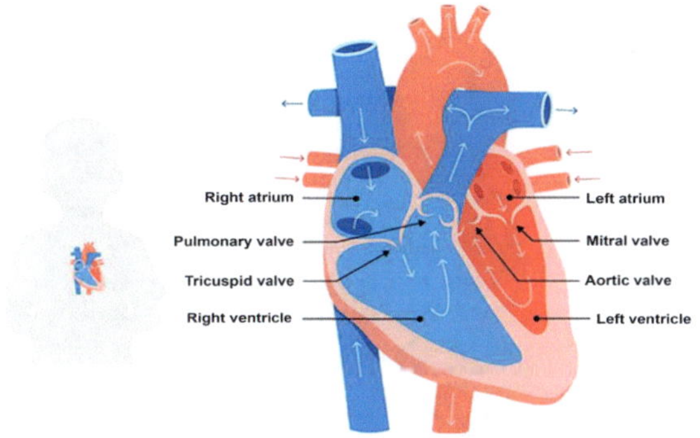

Figure 1.2. Understanding pediatric heart.

Source: https://www.ohsu.edu/sites/default/files/2020-12/01-Heart-anatomy-blood-flow-600px.jpg.

New technologies are also transforming the way clinicians practice pediatric cardiology. For instance, 3D-printed models have proven to enhance the comprehension of intricate anatomical relationships and surgical precision as well as preoperative surgical planning in

CHD patients (Sun, 2023). The inclusion of 3D printing technology within pediatric cardiology is a leap toward augmented advancement of medical education and clinical practice. Of note, studies show that the use of 3D-printed models greatly enhances the understanding of complex cardiac anatomy among various levels of healthcare providers, including students and fellows. For instance, participants showed a significant enhancement in understanding crisscross heart anatomy upon being instructed through 3D models as opposed to traditional imaging methods (Valverde et al., 2021). This improvement in understanding highlights the significance of such models to fill the gap between theoretical education and practical application in clinical settings. The general occurrence of high rates of satisfaction among the trainees further shows the successful impact of 3D printing on medical training – which suggests an exciting future where such technology can greatly improve the learning environment for pediatric cardiology professionals (Figure 1.3).

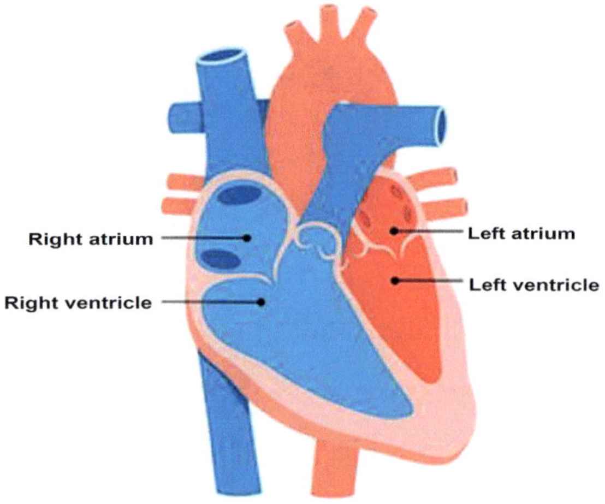

Figure 1.3. The heart's chambers.

Source: https://www.ohsu.edu/doernbecher/understanding-pediatric-heart-conditions.

1.1.1. Differences Between Adult and Pediatric Heart Anatomy

Anatomical variations between the pediatric and adult heart are significant and reflect various physiological functions required for each population. In children, the heart is in proportion to the body compared to adults and is required for adequate cardiac output to meet the increased metabolic requirements of infancy and childhood. For instance, neonates possess a higher heart rate that helps in their cardiac output, a demand because of their underdeveloped circulatory system.

Also, the left and right ventricles of the child heart are nearer in size to one another compared to adults, with the left ventricle predominating. This is because of the manner in which the right ventricle bears a more vital role in fetal circulation, through the ductus arteriosus (before birth); this region of the heart is a witness to the capacity of the heart to make physiological adaptations throughout development. Another noteworthy difference in adult and infant heart anatomy is the presence of fetal structures that increasingly atrophy as the child matures. Major structures such as the foramen ovale and ductus arteriosus allow bypassing of blood past the non-working fetal lungs. These structures close after birth as a manifestation of significant alteration in cardiovascular dynamics with lung circulation as the dominant factor. The ductus arteriosus actually closes specifically during the first weeks of life, forming the ligamentum arteriosum. Non-closure of this duct causes congenital heart disease that will require treatment, once again highlighting the importance of these anatomical changes in pediatric cardiology. An understanding of these changes is imperative to make an accurate diagnosis and manage children with cardiac abnormalities (Figure 1.4).

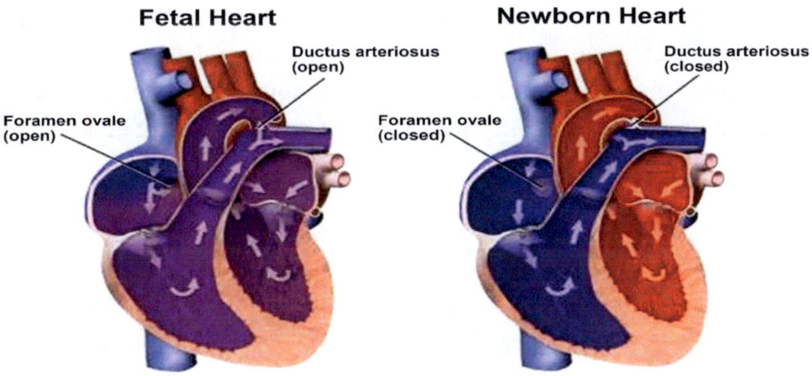

Figure 1.4. Changes that occur to the heart following birth.

Source: https://teachmesurgery.com/cardiothoracic-surgery/general-principles/foetal-vs-adult-circulation/.

Moreover, alterations in the pediatric conduction system of the hearts are also typical as compared to adults. A young patient's sinoatrial (SA) node is comparatively larger than an adult's and the atrioventricular (AV) node is positioned differently, which can be accountable for differences in the heart rate and rhythm stability. Resting higher heart rates are present in pediatric patients, which are usually between 100 and 160 beats per minute, which is proportionate to their increased metabolic activities. Furthermore, development of such systems occurs with increasing age, and this can result in transient arrhythmias during periods of enhanced growth. Pediatric cardiologists therefore not only have to identify these differences in anatomy but also appreciate their functional counterparts in clinical practice, as required in recent guidelines providing advice on the management of children with cardiovascular disease (Eric et al., 2022; Lorusso et al., 2021).

1.1.2. Common Congenital Heart Defects

It is vital that pediatric cardiologists are familiar with the majority of frequent congenital heart defects (CHDs) as they have a significant influence on the health and development of the affected children. Ventricular septal defect (VSD) is the most frequent one among these CHDs and constitutes a significant percentage of infant congenital heart conditions.

The defect occurs due to an abnormal opening between the heart's chambers, the ventricular septum in this instance. In research conducted in the Pediatric Cardiology Department of Combined Military Hospital, Dhaka, it was observed that majority of the patients with VSD present with the symptoms of dyspnea, cough, and feeding difficulty, leading to early presentation. Findings of the research highlight the importance of timely and correct echocardiographic assessment to determine treatment strategies, be it medical management, device closure, or surgery (Sarker et al., 2024) (Figure 1.5). Genetic considerations are also of prime significance in the occurrence of congenital heart disease. There has been evidence in recent years of a strong association of specific genetic syndromes with the formation of CHD. A variety of genetic disorders can lead to structural abnormalities of the cardiovascular system, with some congenital defects being inevitably linked with particular defects in genes. The identification of such associations helps in enhanced diagnostic plans and enables early intervention techniques for the affected children. Identification is vital since not only does it assist in the identification of heart defects, but it also promotes the understanding of more complex genetic conditions in pediatric patients. With a profound knowledge of the genetic underpinning, medical practitioners can develop comprehensive treatment plans that address both the cardiac and systemic impacts of such syndromes (Selska et al., 2024).

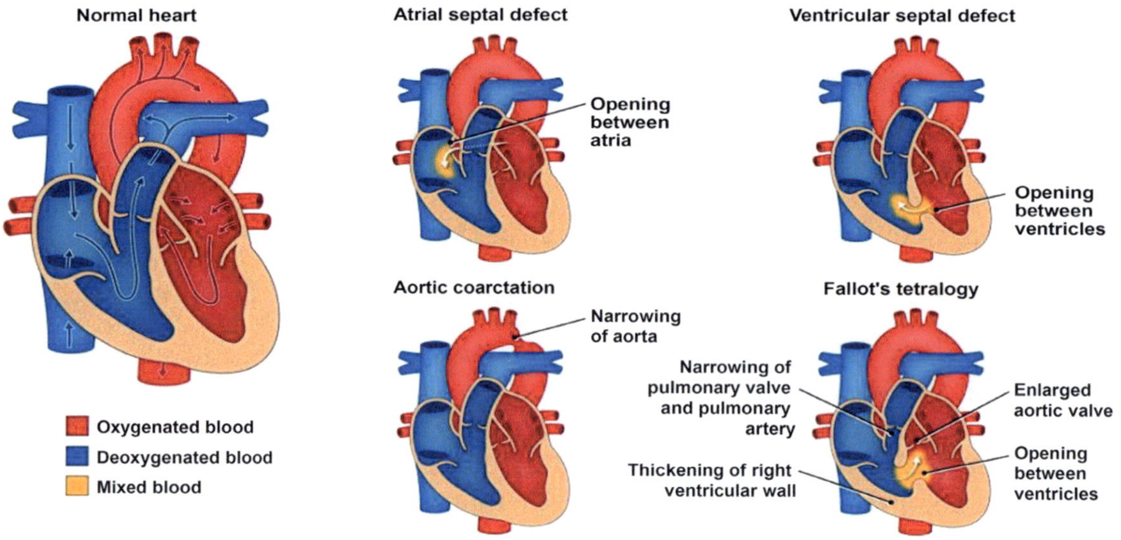

Figure 1.5. Common congenital heart defects (CHDs).

Source: https://cdn-assets-eu.frontify.com/s3/frontify-enterprise-files-eu/eyJwYXRoIjoiaWhoLWhlYWx0aGNhcmUtYmVyaGFkXC9hY2NvdW50c1wvYzNcLzQwMDA2MjRcL3Byb2plY3RzXC8yM DlcL2Fzc2V0c1wv MzdcLzM2MjE4XC84Y WU0O DNkOGM5MWJiZjU4OGIxNDQ2ZTc 3ZDhlMjBmMC0xNjU2Mzg0MTAyLmp wZyJ9:ihh-healthcare-berhad:7PqeWGhXqoP_k3n33hwoVU3d1TNuW Lihi3TpRuYC5E4?format=webp.

In conclusion, congenital heart anomalies are still a multisided and complex problem in pediatric cardiology that requires an interdisciplinary approach taking into consideration anatomical as well as genetic aspects. Knowledge of prevalent defects such as VSD, and even their modes of clinical presentation, informs medical professionals on the best interventions that assist in altering patient outcomes. Additionally, the relationship between genetic abnormalities and congenital heart defects states the significance of continued studies in these fields with emphasis on early diagnosis and treatment regimens. As pediatric cardiology continues to advance, there is an expectation that early detection will lead to better quality of life and reduced mortality in children who are diagnosed with these heart defects (Sarker et al., 2024; Selska et al., 2024).

1.1.3. Developmental Stages of the Heart in Children

The heart undergoes significant developmental changes at important points in infancy and childhood, making its investigation critical for the discipline of pediatric cardiology. Development of the heart begins early in embryonic development (i.e., with the differentiation of mesodermal cells into cardiac progenitor cells by the third week of gestation). The cells migrate and become organized and subsequently give rise to a tubular structure, which later folds and separates into the four chambers of the heart. This intricate remodeling is responsive to environmental and genetic factors, influencing global morphology and function of the heart. Pathological remodeling of the neonatal heart may lead to congenital heart malformations – a disorder that can alter the trajectory of cardiovascular disease in children and requires early diagnosis for effective treatment. During childhood, the heart persists in remodeling through repeated physiological adaptations susceptible to growth and increased metabolic burden. Infants also have a higher heart rate than adults and older children, and this reflects their lower cardiovascular capacity. Heart function and structure are altered during growth; the chambers increase in volume, and the myocardium thickens to support the body's increasing energetic needs. The vascular level also demonstrates adaptations including vascular resistance changes and blood flow patterns (Figure 1.6).

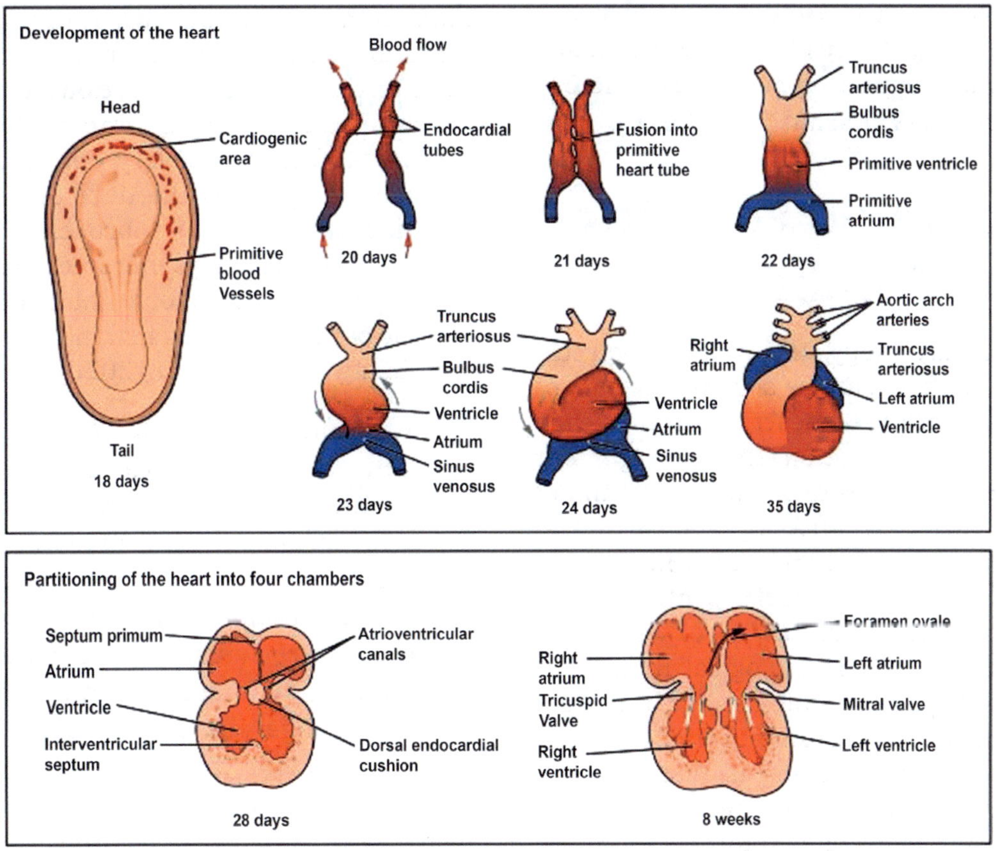

Figure 1.6. This diagram outlines the embryological development of the human heart during the first eight weeks and the subsequent formation of the four heart chambers.

Source: https://courses.lumenlearning.com/suny-ap2/chapter/development-of-the-heart/.

Having an insight into these advancing developments is crucial for pediatric cardiologists and pediatricians since it is essential to differentiate between normal physiological growth and potential pathological conditions that might need to be treated or more closely monitored. Lastly, knowledge about the range of cardiac development is significant because it enables recognition of children's cardiovascular conditions that can occur at a variety of ages, ranging from congenital anomaly at birth through acquired heart disease presented in childhood subsequently. The incidence of cardiovascular diseases, including strokes in children, has been seen to depend significantly on age and medical conditions, necessitating careful clinical evaluation and additional research in the field. Pediatric stroke incidence rates annually range from 3 to 25 per 100,000 children, while newborns have a notably higher risk ratio at 1 in 4000 live births, which highlights the imperative of early detection and prevention interventions in pediatric cardiology (Donna et al., 2019; Rashid et al., 2020).

1.2. Common Pediatric Cardiac Conditions

In pediatric cardiology, the range of typical cardiac ailments includes a constellation of congenital and acquired heart conditions, each with its own presentation and management problem. CHD continues to be the most common problem in this area, affecting almost one in every 100 live births. Forms of CHD include atrial septal defects, ventricular septal defects, and patent ductus arteriosus, all of which can lead to considerable physiological impact on oxygen supply and overall cardiac function. Early identification through screening and accurate diagnostic imaging is important in order to have proper intervention ranging from pharmacological management to surgical repair in acute conditions. The unpredictability and sophistication of such congenital abnormalities necessitate a sophisticated understanding of developmental, anatomical, and hemodynamic issues during continued pediatric care, gaining insight into the need to manage the patients throughout life. Apart from congenital disease, pediatric cardiology must also deal with numerous acquired cardiac diseases, which may present as a consequence of infection, autoimmune diseases, or genetic syndromes. One of the most pressing issues of the current times is multisystem inflammatory syndrome in children (MIS-C), a disease linked with the SARS-CoV-2 virus that is characterized by the extreme inflammation and cardiac presentation. Treatment is clinical, encompassing acute cardiogenic shock and arrhythmias recognition, for which a multidisciplinary approach is recommended for optimal outcomes. Successful treatment regimens often include immunotherapy and supportive care, particularly targeting cardiac function stabilization. As the relationship between infectious diseases and cardiac health becomes more obvious both in the post-infection recovery period and during the acute stage, it is the duty of cardiologists to come up with new approaches to address these newly emerging syndromes while striving for continuity of care for established pediatric cardiac conditions, thus making overall patient well-being (Lauren et al., 2020).

Yet another extremely prevalent condition encountered in pediatric cardiology is an arrhythmia, which may present as bradycardia or tachycardia in the involved pediatric patient. In such an instance, conditions like congenital complete atrioventricular block (CCAVB) once more reflect the absolute need for early diagnosis and management to avoid dangerous cardiac events. Patients with CCAVB, for instance, typically require pacemaker implantation to sustain adequate heart rates and avert complications due to possible bradycardia. The process of making decisions regarding the application of cardiac implantable electronic devices reflects a call for shared decision-making with families in order to ascertain patient-centered care. In addition, as our knowledge of genetic susceptibility to different cardiac arrhythmias increases, early screening and monitoring regimens have been added to routine practice, enabling improved individualized interventions that respond to the changing needs of the pediatric population (Michael et al., 2022).

1.2.1. Congenital Heart Disease

Congenital heart disease (CHD) is a critical area in pediatric cardiology encompassing a broad range of structural heart defects that are present at birth. Such defects may be of mild nature requiring minimal or no treatment or serious malformations requiring multiple surgeries. The prevalence of CHD has increased, resulting in more patients living into adulthood, and the medical community has therefore highlighted long-term care management beyond infancy. At adulthood, these patients have specific challenges that include the control of arrhythmias produced by both the congenital lesions themselves and the resulting treatment to correct them. The complexity of such cases demands detailed knowledge of the cardiac anatomy and physiology implicated, thus necessitating the administration of specialized care throughout the lifetime of a patient (Michael et al., 2021). CHD patients in the pediatric population have been blessed with extraordinary developments in technologies and therapeutic modalities to treat arrhythmias.

Pharmacological therapy, catheter ablation techniques, and the use of cardiac implantable electronic devices have revolutionized the therapy of such patients. Catheter ablation, in specific, has become popular as an acceptable form of treatment for arrhythmia, leveraging enhanced mapping technology and techniques allowing safer and more effective treatments. This technological innovation allows practitioners to adjust treatment strategies in accordance with the specific anatomical and physiological challenges created by each patient's condition. In addition, the increasing use of device therapies highlights the critical importance rhythm management plays in improving the overall quality of life and clinical outcomes for CHD patients (Michael et al., 2021) (Figure 1.7).

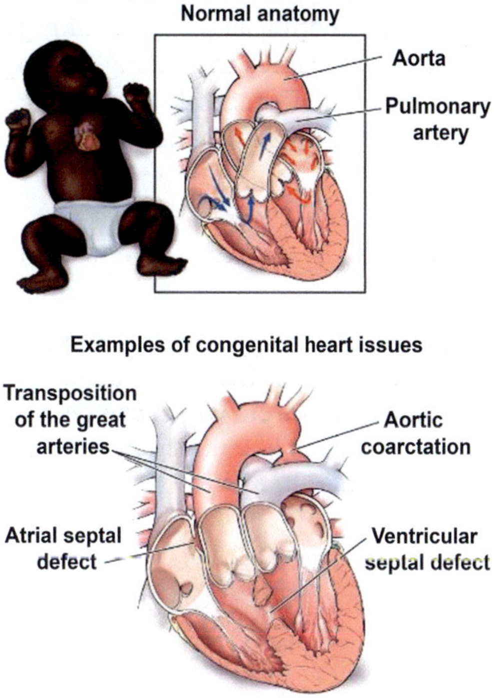

Figure 1.7. Congenital heart disease (present at birth) can affect many different parts of your heart. It can be mild or severe.

Source: https://my.clevelandclinic.org/-/scassets/images/org/health/articles/congenital-heart-disease.jpg.

Pediatric patients with CHD entering adulthood, often require a multidisciplinary team effort with numerous medical specialties working together due to the intricacies of their condition. A team that includes pediatric cardiologists, adult cardiologists, electrophysiologists, and other appropriate healthcare professionals can offer a cohesive plan individually suited to each patient's needs. This encounter is critical not only for cardiac arrhythmia evaluation and management but also for management of other aspects of care, including psychological support and lifestyle change education. Understanding the natural history of CHD and long-term complications is needed to guide treatment and improve prognosis. As concern for such issues continues to be disseminated across healthcare networks, the emphasis on providing patient-centered care becomes increasingly recognized as a cornerstone of successful management for individuals with congenital heart disease (Hern et al., 2018).

1.2.2. Acquired Heart Conditions in Children

The pediatric cardiology scenario also continues to recognize the significance of acquired heart disease among children, which can be caused by a variety of reasons like infection, malnutrition, and autoimmune illness.

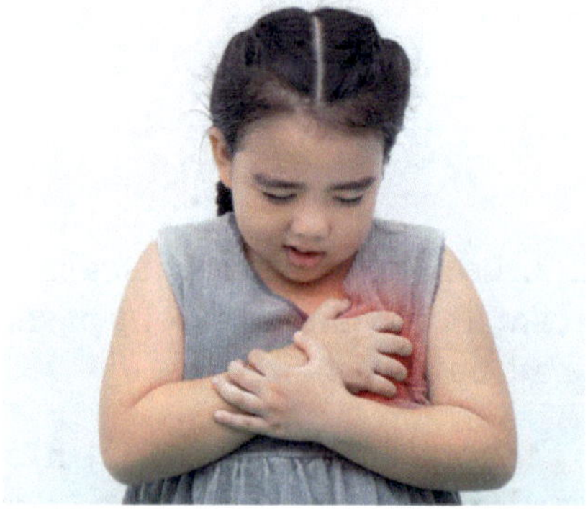

Figure 1.8. Acquired heart diseases.

Source: https://external-content.duckduckgo.com/iu/?u=https%3A%2F%2Fwww.drravindersinghrao.com%2Fwp-content%2Fuploads%2F2022%2F06%2FHeart-Disease-in-Children-Symptoms-Causes-Treatment.jpg&f=1&nofb=1&ipt=85f99886d14101c78f90a97b46499e1082cba08aded1b1f5253d50939bfcb28b.

Among these, viral infections like COVID-19 have been the leading causes of cardiac illness among children. SARS-CoV-2 virus has not only shown human-to-human transmission but has also been associated with severe lung injury and cardiac injury in children, illustrating the multi-dimensional impact of such infections on general health. Although most pediatric COVID-19 presents with mild illness, the potential for severe cardiac injury makes it crucial to carefully observe and understand underlying cardiac pathologies. As the COVID-19 experience keeps developing, it is important to evaluate its impact on children with a pre-existing cardiac condition, once more emphasizing the role of acquired cardiac conditions in pediatric cardiology (Tan et al., 2020) (Figure 1.8).

Acquired cardiac disease can also have non-infectious etiologies, such as inflammatory processes and congenital processes that occur over a period of time. Pediatric stroke is a classic example (albeit one typically discussed only in the adult) although increasingly one to be recognized in the pediatric population. Pediatric stroke can be ischemic or hemorrhagic and is related to a number of risk factors, some of which are congenital heart disease and coagulopathies. The incidence of stroke is remarkably high, ranging from 3 to 25 in 100,000 children, and newborns have a high-risk ratio in particular. A good understanding of the pathophysiology of these strokes is important in order to diagnose them at the right time and intervene, as any delay can lead to significant morbidity. As pediatric cardiologists transition to address conditions beyond congenital defects, the need for robust methodologies to diagnose and address acquired heart conditions becomes a priority in clinical treatment (Donna et al., 2019). Furthermore, an acute distinction between acquired heart conditions and congenital heart conditions is essential when identifying treatment approaches and outcomes. While congenital heart disease typically requires surgical intervention, acquired heart disease may be more manageable by medical therapy or lifestyle modification. This difference in treatment itself highly ghts the necessity for personalized treatment in pediatric cardiology. Proper care for such issues is best managed through a mix of specialties such as pediatric cardiologists, dietitians, and rehabilitation specialists to avert risk factors and create optimal cardiac health. Furthermore, prevention efforts on public health levels to reduce the occurrence of infection, improve nutrition, and promote heart health education are essential. In understanding the nuances of acquired heart disease, the field of pediatric cardiology can work towards better outcomes in children and families impacted.

1.2.3. Risk Factors and Prevalence of Pediatric Cardiac Issues

The incidence of pediatric cardiac abnormalities is a significant public health problem that must be extensively studied and comprehended. Congenital heart anomalies (CHAs) are the most common type of pediatric cardiac abnormalities, affecting approximately 1 in every 100 live births. Several risk factors have been identified among this group, and maternal medical conditions such as diabetes, hypertension, and obesity may predispose infants to cardiac anomalies. Moreover, environmental factors, such as exposure of the mother to certain drugs or substances during pregnancy, also play an important role in causing the high prevalence of such defects. An early diagnosis and treatment demand a firm working alliance among obstetricians, cardiologists, and pediatricians, with appropriate diagnoses being provided timely interventions to enhance outcomes, as well as to enhance quality of life for involved families. Other than congenital diseases, there are also acquired cardiac conditions that are increasingly gaining importance among children, particularly in the context of viral infections. Recent COVID-19 has revealed shocking correlations between SARS-CoV-2 infection and the development of acute myocardial injury in children. Specifically, multisystem inflammatory syndrome in children (MIS-C) is a severe post-infectious illness that can cause cardiac complications like myocarditis and injury to the coronary arteries. Studies indicate that children with MIS-C will have widespread cardiac involvement, where immediate and specialized care needs to be provided to avoid deterioration. Continuing research on the long-term COVID-19 implications for pediatric cardiology is essential to provide insights for future prevention policies and managing risks due to viral infections, as highlighted in the broader health context influenced by emerging pathogens (Nakra et al., 2020). The interaction of genetic predisposing forces and environmental factors also plays a key role in the risk profile of pediatric cardiovascular diseases. Genetic syndromes such as Down syndrome, Turner syndrome, and Marfan syndrome are highly associated with congenital heart malformations. These genetic syndromes reflect the necessity to screen at-risk populations and establish specialized medical interventions. Lifestyle behaviors such as physical inactivity, poor diet, and obesity also increasingly manifest in the pediatric population, driving the burden of acquired cardiac diseases such as hypertension and dyslipidemia. With the increase in knowledge about these risks, healthcare professionals are encouraged to embrace preventive practices and educational programs that allow children to have assistance from their families in building better lifestyle habits, which ultimately reduce the incidence of pediatric cardiac diseases among populations (Campbell et al., 2020).

1.3. Diagnostic Techniques in Pediatric Cardiology

In pediatric cardiology, minimizing radiation exposure during diagnostic testing has become an important focus, especially as a result of long-term risks from ionizing radiation. Recent advances in imaging technology have worked toward solving this problem, particularly during interventional procedures such as atrial septal defect (ASD) closures. A study demonstrated that with a protocol (which prioritizes low radiological exposure reduction regardless of weight) significant radiation dose reduction was possible without compromising imaging quality. This is a significant departure from traditional body weight-based strategies, and it indicates that new methods have the potential to enhance patient safety without sacrificing diagnostic efficacy. The findings offer a compelling case for revising existing pediatric interventional cardiology guidelines to prioritize radiation dose management in everyday practice (Pilati, 2024). Additionally, application of new echocardiographic techniques, namely left atrial (LA) strain analysis, emerged as an emerging non-invasive tool to assess cardiac function in children. This method has been found to be more sensitive than the conventional indicators, which allow for early identification of myocardial deformation, diastolic failure, and other cardiac abnormalities. Recent studies identify the prognostic significance of LA strain parameters in a range of pediatric cardiac diseases, such as cardiomyopathy and multisystem inflammatory syndrome complications. This emerging branch of pediatric cardiology emphasizes the need for individualized diagnostic approaches that are responsive to the unique physiology of children and infants, providing invaluable information to clinical handling by practitioners. Incorporation of LA strain assessment in routine clinical practice has the potential to drastically improve monitoring and therapeutic strategies for kids (Begić et al., 2023). With the constant evolving improvements in pediatric cardiology, more emphasis needs to be laid on creating a comprehensive array of diagnostic techniques. Cross-talk between newer imaging modalities and traditional methods ensures enhanced, comprehensive insight into congenital and acquired heart disease in children. Continued investigation into new approaches, such as the integration of LA strain analysis with other echocardiographic indices, may enhance diagnostic sensitivity and facilitate intervention earlier. Besides, there is also a need for coordination among cardiologists, radiologists, and pediatricians in order to effectively implement these advances within the clinic. This cross-functional working will not only improve diagnostic techniques but also make them accessible and beneficial for every child, ultimately translating into improved quality of care for pediatric cardiology (Begić et al., 2023; Pilati, 2024).

1.3.1. Role of Echocardiography

Echocardiography is a mainstay in pediatric cardiology diagnosis assessment, particularly in the identification and evaluation of CHD. As CHDs are one of the most prevalent congenital defects, occurring in approximately 4–10 of every 1000 live births, its application becomes critical in early identification and management. This non-invasive imaging technique allows doctors to take real-time pictures of the heart and monitor its structure, function, and dynamics of blood flow without subjecting the children to radiation risks associated with the use of ionizing radiation. Through visualization of conditions such as pulmonary stenosis and ventricular septal defects, echocardiography contributes to decision-making by facilitating timely interventions essential for improving health outcomes in children with cardiovascular conditions (N/A, 2023). In addition to its essential role in diagnosis, echocardiography supports ongoing monitoring and assessment for children undergoing treatment for cardiovascular conditions. As the child's body grows and matures, heart function dynamics can be altered drastically; thus, regular echocardiographic monitoring is critical. Clinicians are able to evaluate the efficacy of interventions, either medical or surgical, and modify treatment plans accordingly by performing such monitoring. Of special interest is that with the incorporation of advanced echocardiographic modalities, such as Doppler imaging and three-dimensional echocardiography, the ability to measure blood flow has improved, cardiac mechanics has been better evaluated, and complex anatomic structures have been better visualized. Thus, the potential to get long-term comprehensive assessments secures echocardiography's position as an important role in long-term management for pediatric cardiology patients (N/A, 2023) (Figure 1.9).

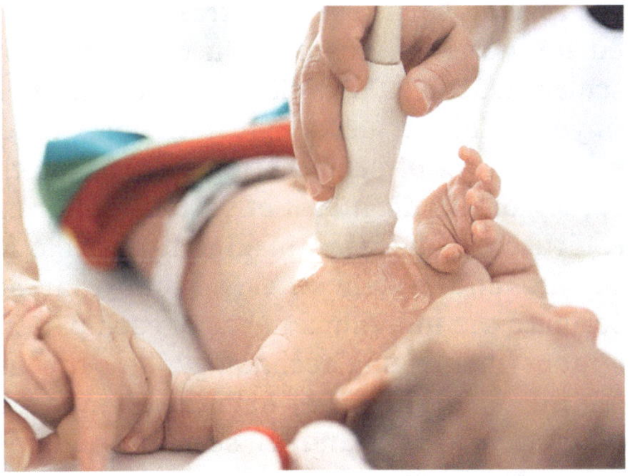

Figure 1.9. Pediatric echocardiography.

Source: https://storage.googleapis.com/jacksonh/1/Pediatric_Echocardiography-Advanced-Imaging.jpg.

In addition, the technological innovation in echocardiography has been important in expanding its applications in pediatric cardiology. Echocardiography's combination with other imaging modalities, such as computed tomography and nuclear imaging, provides a comprehensive assessment of cardiac structure and function, complementing the existing information with echocardiography, which plays an important role in determining the approach to treating challenging cases. For instance, while echocardiography is very effective in identifying the majority of congenital defects, the shear complementarity of nuclear imaging to evaluate myocardial perfusion and viability can allow for more subtle information about cardiovascular health. While the terrain of pediatric cardiology continues to change, that of echocardiography is at least a cornerstone, forming the foundation for both diagnosis and therapy, with a promise of the best care and better prognosis for children with heart diseases.

1.3.2. Importance of Electrocardiograms (ECGs)

The electrocardiogram, or ECG, is an important diagnostic imaging study in pediatric cardiology that provides crucial information regarding the electrical activity of the heart. It cannot be overstated since it enables physicians to identify arrhythmias, congenital heart disease, and other cardiac abnormalities that may be present from birth or that develop during childhood. Familiarity with typical electrocardiographic patterns observed in children and infants compared with adults is paramount to interpretation. Pediatric ECGs are quite different from one another in waveform morphology and rate, and therefore, it is important for doctors to be skilled at recognizing these differences. With the inclusion of ECG interpretation in routine examinations, healthcare professionals can respond with interventions in a timely fashion that are needed to improve patient outcomes as well as prevent potential complications in pediatric populations. Furthermore, ECGs play an integral role in the long-term management of children with diagnosed cardiac diseases. Routine electrocardiography is an essential component of monitoring disease progression and assessing the efficacy of treatment protocols in patients being monitored for congenital heart disease or structural abnormalities. Adherence to evidence-based guidance, such as that suggested by Levitov et al. (2016), enables improved application of ECGs in children's facilities. These guidelines specify when and under what conditions ECGs must be performed, allowing for detection of potential conditions that could lead to severe consequences at an early point. Individualized monitoring with ECGs can also be used to determine the effects of drugs and other interventions on individual patients, informing a customized strategy to each child's cardiac well-being (Figure 1.10).

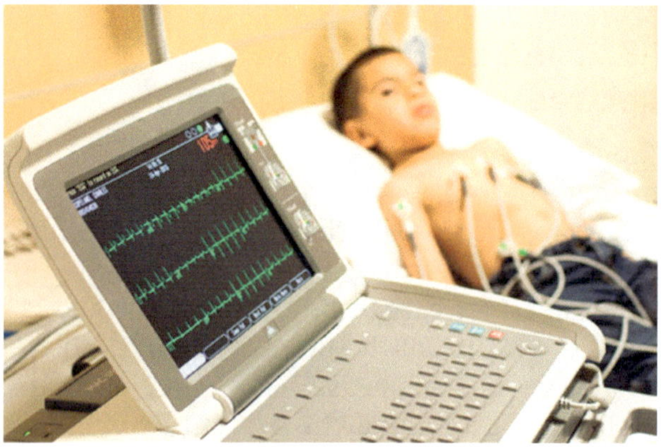

Figure 1.10. Pediatric electrocardiograms (ECG).

Source: https://choc.org/wp-content/uploads/2015/04/Electrocardiogram.jpg.

Second, advancing technologies in ECG monitoring, like portable ECG devices, have revolutionized pediatric cardiology with enhanced convenience and accessibility. The technologies facilitate continuous monitoring in outpatients, allowing families and clinicians to detect abnormal rhythms in time. As cited in various studies reviewed by Richard et al. (2015), the integration of new ECG modalities enhances the detection of silent arrhythmias, particularly among vulnerable populations. Remotely monitorable ability not only contributes to better clinical management but also reassures parents about the health of their child. The applicability of ECGs thus transcends direct diagnosis in terms of being crucially significant in the ongoing management that occurs and in enabling collaborative pediatric cardiology.

1.3.3. Advanced Imaging Techniques (MRI, CT Scans)

In pediatric cardiology, advanced imaging modalities such as Magnetic Resonance Imaging (MRI) and Computed Tomography (CT) scans have emerged as indispensable diagnostic and planning tools for precise diagnosis and treatment. The ability of the modalities to obtain high-resolution cross-sectional anatomy of cardiac morphology allows clinicians to image congenital heart defects and associated anatomical abnormalities. MRI, in particular, has superior soft tissue contrast that can be used for better discrimination of cardiac and vascular structures, as well as the measurement of myocardial perfusion and function. Hence, the integration of such methods enhances the accuracy of the diagnosis of various children's cardiovascular diseases, making it possible for adequate and timely interventions that are tailored to the individual needs of each patient. Upgrades in imaging technology, like the use of artificial intelligence, have also improved the function of MRI and CT scans in pediatric cardiology (Figure 1.11).

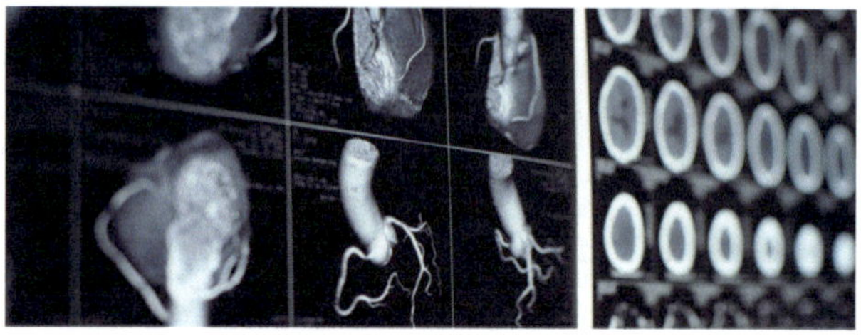

Figure 1.11. Pediatric cardiac CT scan.

Source: https://ajronline.org/cms/10.2214/AJR.19.22745/asset/images/large/12_19_22745_09d.jpeg.

Computer algorithms driven by artificial intelligence read medical images with unparalleled accuracy, reducing the potential for diagnostic errors and expediting the interpretive process. Machine learning techniques have been found through prior studies to take a primary role in computerized analysis of cardiac imaging, enabling more efficient diagnostic workflows that are critical within emergent clinical settings. As introduced by Nia et al. (2023), such technologies are adjuncts to more than traditional practice; they are a paradigm-based approach for decision-making in medical practice, with the result of enabling better-quality evaluations that guide the management of pediatric cardiovascular conditions overall. The implications of newer imaging techniques extend beyond diagnosis, with fundamental impacts on therapy paradigms for pediatric cardiology. The ACC/AHA 2022 Guideline for Aortic Disease Diagnosis and Management concentrates on the use of comprehensive imaging as a guide that directs clinicians from one stage of treatment to the next depending on the severity of the disease (Eric et al., 2022). With accurate description of the aortic anatomy by means of MRI and CT scans, clinicians are well able to give informed opinions concerning intervention while monitoring the disease over time. This kind of multidisciplinary imaging approach is required for long-term care to ensure that pediatric patients receive proper and tailored care that best addresses their individualized cardiovascular profiles.

1.4. Treatment Options for Pediatric Cardiac Patients

In pediatric cardiology, there are as many treatment approaches for patients with cardiac disease as there are for the diseases they address. Treatment is typically initiated with medical therapy in the form of drugs such as beta-blockers, ACE inhibitors, and diuretics, which play a key role in maintaining cardiac output and fluid status. These drug therapies are required, particularly in cardiomyopathies or congenital heart disease, in which deranged heart function needs to be constantly and immediately treated. For instance, neonates with structural heart disease may require preoperative initial therapies to stabilize their conditions before they are operated on. This basis of care not only strives to enhance patients quality of life but also prepares them for more aggressive procedures as appropriate – an adaptive approach that respects both short- and long-term results. Surgical therapy is a cornerstone to management of the majority of pediatric cardiac illness, particularly congenital heart malformations such as ventricular septal defects, atrial septal defects, and tetralogy of Fallot. Surgical interventions typically range from minimal invasiveness to the complex open-heart surgeries, depending on the patient's individualized anatomical and physiological problems. Ongoing advancements in surgical techniques, coupled with progress in postoperative management, have considerably reduced children's heart surgery morbidity. Also, the timing of surgical intervention matters; pediatric cardiologists attempt to perform corrective surgeries during ideal periods of growth in an effort to prevent complications and stimulate healthier patterns of development. Ongoing communication between pediatricians, cardiologists, and cardiac surgeons is necessary so that each patient has uniquely customized treatment plans that address their respective conditions comprehensively. In the past few years, minimally invasive interventions such as catheter-based procedures and extracorporeal membrane oxygenation (ECMO) have increased in the treatment of children with cardiac abnormalities. Catheter-based methods, such as balloon atrial septostomy or defects closure through a transcatheter approach, have significant advantages, such as reduced recovery and hospitalization time compared with traditional surgery. In addition, ECMO is a bridging life-support for critically ill patients, providing oxygenation and circulatory assistance while allowing the lungs and heart some time to recover from severe failure. Technological and technical advancements, including advances in ECMO systems, have facilitated their safety and performance in pediatric patients, allowing caretakers more effectively to manage complicated cases. As treatment paradigms change, the use of novel and traditional methods is a combination that enables pediatric cardiologists to maximize care and enhance outcomes in different settings (Lorusso et al., 2021; Marilyn et al., 2022).

1.4.1. Medical Management and Pharmacotherapy

Effective medical therapy and pharmacology play important roles in pediatric cardiology to manage the cardiac diseases prevalent in the pediatric population.

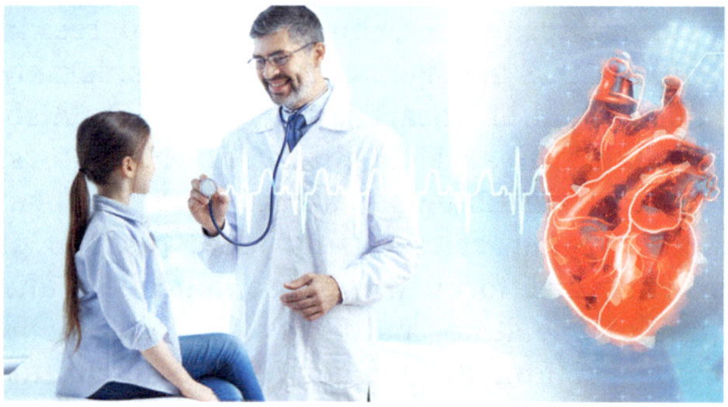

Figure 1.12. Effective medical management.

Source: https://english-blog.s3.amazonaws.com/uploads/2023/06/Pediatric-Cardiology-Hospitals.jpg.

The initial approach depends upon recombinant therapy and prophylactic interventions aimed at symptom control and improvement of the quality of life. Careful monitoring of the clinical condition of the pediatric patients allows individualized therapeutic interventions that may include the use of diuretics, antihypertensive drugs, or anticoagulants depending on the etiological diagnosis. For instance, patients with congenital heart disease can be treated with pharmacotherapy to achieve appropriate hemodynamic stability as well as to optimize cardiac output. Co-treatment by pediatric cardiologists, family physicians, and pharmacists ensures the delivery of appropriate drugs in a safe dose, and intimate monitoring of potential drug interactions, particularly in view of the intricate metabolic patterns of a developing child's body (Figure 1.12).

Management strategies may also encompass a variety of pharmacotherapy for long-term care and prevention of complications. For children with conditions including hypertension or heart failure, proper drugs are critical in preventing progression of cardiovascular conditions. The American College of Cardiology emphasizes the role of carefully monitored medical therapy of patients with aortic disease, with particular emphasis on patient-specific treatment regimens based on patient-specific data and severity of disease. With advances in pediatric pharmacology, pharmacotherapy for children is an ever-expanding body of literature on the use of new medications, particularly in cases where older medications have been less effective. This paradigm shift demands that healthcare providers remain abreast of evolving clinical practice guidelines to optimize care in a spectrum of pediatric cardiac presentations, and address comorbid conditions that complicate therapy. Moreover, the input of ongoing research into medical management and new pharmacotherapies cannot be overstated. Ongoing studies continually redefine what is known about treating pediatric cardiac diseases and enhancing outcomes. Ongoing research into genetic susceptibility and biomarkers in pediatric cardiology is of crucial significance to future management strategies. Knowledge from current literature might determine therapeutic targets of new potential that are of particular effectiveness at the initial phases of cardiac disease, thereby improving prognosis and quality of life for these children. Results from studies on the management of aortic disease highlight the intervention of both medical therapy and surgical intervention within a balanced treatment protocol, providing children with holistic and efficient treatment in their developing years (Eric et al., 2022). As future studies focus on more detailed disciplines, it is expected that medical management and pharmacotherapy will further improve, leading to improved approaches and results in pediatric cardiology (Vieta et al., 2018).

1.4.2. Surgical Interventions and Procedures

Pediatric cardiovascular surgery is a key component in the treatment of CHD and the establishment of long-term health status in affected children. Technological advances in surgical techniques, including cardiac operations and catheter-based interventions, have significantly increased survival in CHD children. The advances, albeit life-saving, are also now recognized to have increased the patient population that will come with complications of repaired and unrepaired conditions. This complex interaction necessitates careful preoperative evaluation to establish the risks of surgical management, particularly given that the mortality and complication rates in noncardiac surgery have been found to be high among such patients. Surgical intervention of congenital heart disease, therefore, necessitates a rigorous framework that entails multidisciplinary interaction among cardiologists, surgeons, and anesthesiologists to enhance patient outcomes during surgery (Viviane et al., 2022). The anesthesiologist's contribution to pediatric cardiac surgery cannot be overstated, particularly because it has become a special subspecialty over the past eight decades. The call for specialty training is delineated by evidence that a significant proportion of pediatric cardiac anesthesiologists have not received formal fellowship training. This disparity highlights an increasing challenge to maintaining a pace with increasing demand for surgical procedures due to improved survival rates for congenital heart disease. Anesthesiologists play critical roles, not only within the operating room but also in the cardiac catheterization suite and in noncardiac procedures in these patients. Survey data shows that pediatric cardiac anesthesiologists spend considerable portions of their time in the clinic on cardiac and noncardiac procedures, reinforcing the compelling need for this exceptionally specialized skill set to enhance surgical effectiveness and safety (Viviane et al., 2022) (Figure 1.13).

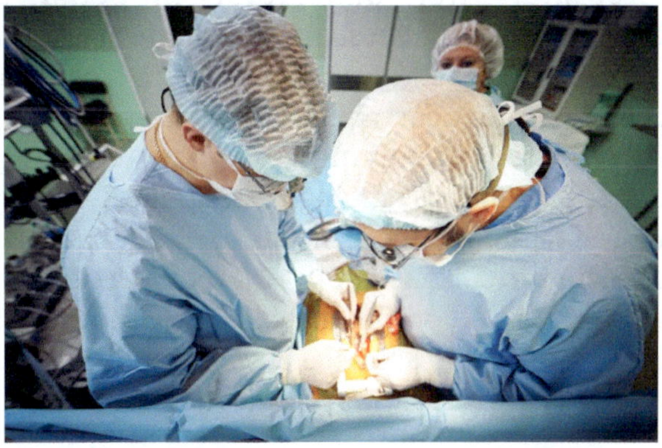

Figure 1.13. Pediatric cardiac surgery.

Source: https://i0.wp.com/childhearthealth.com/wp-content/uploads/2018/02/Congenital-Heart-Disorder-CHD-10.png?resize=1024%2C683&ssl=1.

Further, with increasing survival rates and increasing numbers of congenital heart disease, the evolution of pediatric cardiology will require continuous attempts to upgrade skill sets of healthcare providers involved in surgical care. This shift towards increased complexity of patients will require building of multi-dimensional tools for risk prediction for addressing the needs of targeted subsets of patients for diverse levels of severity of congenital heart disease. These developments are important to guide clinical decision-making and optimize perioperative care. Perioperative care providers must periodically educate and train themselves to meet the complex needs of this patient population. Emphasizing the need for ongoing research into surgical outcomes will ultimately result in an evidence-based practice in pediatric cardiac care so that surgical interventions not only maximize short-term survival but also long-term health and quality of life in pediatric patients (Viviane et al., 2022).

1.4.3. Role of Cardiac Rehabilitation

The role of cardiac rehabilitation (CR) is increasingly well understood in pediatric cardiology as a necessary component of the course of recovery in children with acquired or congenital heart disease. CR is a holistic intervention involving exercise training, education, and psychological support, exactly tailored to the particular needs of young patients. Following a cardiac event, the comprehensive rehabilitation program can help improve physical function, enhance overall quality of life, and reduce recurrence of cardiovascular disease. Of particular significance, exercise training is a cornerstone of CR since it will improve endurance, enhance heart muscle strength, and help integrate healthy habits into daily living activities in children. This prospective approach not only facilitates recovery on an emotional level but also underlies a lifestyle that promotes the continued upkeep of health among cardiac patients, setting a good foundation for their long-term health (Makita et al., 2022). Perhaps most critical of the components of effective cardiac rehabilitation is the multidisciplinary team charged with creating and implementing customized treatment plans. Pediatric cardiologists, dietitians, physical therapists, and psychologists collaborate to offer a combined method of care. In younger patients, it is also desirable to include families in the rehabilitation, as parental contribution can contribute significantly to a child's motivational and compliance factors in regard to exercise programs and lifestyle modifications. Progress review on a regular basis and treatment modification as needed is crucial in order to address any emerging health complications and promote physical and psychological health. This consolidated model addresses not only immediate rehabilitation needs but also long-term health priorities, negating risk associated with physical inactivity and mental tension commonly observed in children patients with cardiac ailments (Jarosław et al., 2022). In conclusion, cardiac rehabilitation is a vital aspect of treating pediatric patients with heart diseases. As a structured program aiming for exercise, education, and psychological counseling, CR makes it easier to regain everyday activities in gradual patterns, setting the stage for enhanced quality of life. The significance of early rehabilitation intervention should not be overstated enough, as it is a significant component to promote resilience and autonomy in young patients. Moreover, ongoing support from healthcare providers, peers and the child's family ensures that the benefits of rehabilitation are carried over outside the clinical setting, including practices that work inside the child's daily life. Lastly, embracing the CR role in pediatric cardiology is crucial for maximizing short-term improvements in health as well as ensuring a promising journey toward healthier lives for children with heart disease (Makita et al., 2022).

1.5. Impact of Pediatric Cardiac Conditions on Families

The impact of pediatric cardiac disease on families extends far beyond clinical diagnosis, influencing emotional, financial, and social dimensions of family life. Parents experience tremendous stress in dealing with the complexities of their child's illness, having a tendency to generate higher levels of anxiety and concerns about the child's future. The uncertainty that is associated with acute health events, medical interventions, and possible long-term sequelae creates a challenging landscape upon which families must work. Furthermore, the psychosocial burden can be magnified through isolation, particularly if families are stigmatized or feel they have no support from their communities. The psychosociality of caregiving requires acknowledgement and affirmation by healthcare workers to enable families to cope with this life-changing occurrence, ensuring emotional well-being along with physical health (Laura et al., 2022). The financial aspects also have a significant influence on the lives of pediatric cardiac disease-affected families. The costs of hospitalization, medication, and routine outpatient care can be prohibitive for most families, particularly those without comprehensive health insurance. Aggregated with potential loss of income from caregiving, these financial costs can lead to excessive stress and strain on family relationships. Families also frequently report difficulties in being able to work while managing the child's complex health care. Unavailability to quality, consistent medical care can potentially perpetuate this financial strain as households must contend with the problem solving of arranging specialist appointments and gaining access to needed treatments. This demands advocacy and structural reform that secures families affected by pediatric cardiac disease appropriate care and access to resources from the healthcare system (Tuczy et al., 2021). The social effect of infant cardiac disease is wide-ranging and not limited to the immediate family, but also to the overall social networks. Families do socially isolate, limiting their activity to avoid the stress of explaining to others their child's special situation. This withdrawal can create a cycle of isolation, as siblings and parents increasingly feel disconnected from relatives and friends who are not fully aware of the difficulties they are experiencing. Siblings themselves can even develop their own emotional and social difficulties, overshadowed by the demands of their brother or sister. In this respect, it is critical that the family unit be considered in the broader sense, promoting support systems and processes that are appropriate for the needs of all persons involved. With the support of family counseling as well as support groups, the healthcare system plays a critical role in the prevention of social distress arising from pediatric cardiac disease, which promotes family resilience (Laura et al., 2022).

1.5.1. Emotional and Psychological Effects on Parents and Siblings

The psychological and emotional effect on parents given a pediatric cardiology diagnosis is significant and potentially enduring. Parents become acute about their anxiety and stress, added to that uncertainty which envelops their child's life-threatening illness. The efficacy of an acceptance and commitment therapy-based intervention designed to decrease posttraumatic stress symptoms (PTSS) in parents of children with serious diseases like congenital heart disease was investigated. This randomized clinical trial revealed intervention group members had a notable reduction in PTSS compared to control groups. The emotional burden that comes with parents not only affects their well-being but can also be observed influencing the healing of their child due to the interdependent composition of family relations within the context of health care (Muscara et al., 2020). Therefore, understanding and coping with these emotional problems are critical aspects of pediatric cardiology care. Siblings of CHD children also have important emotional and psychological issues. Research indicates that the siblings are likely to undergo extensive life transitions and emotional distress that are not necessarily well addressed in the health system. A literature review revealed that siblings of children with chronic conditions like

CHD experience adverse consequences that cross various areas of their life and impact their emotional development and interactions with family members. Lack of special interventions for such siblings may result in neglect or resentment, which significantly impacts their mental health. This absence of understanding and intervention regarding the special needs of siblings concerns because interventions can eliminate negative effects and enhance resilience within the family (Parker et al., 2020) (Figure 1.14).

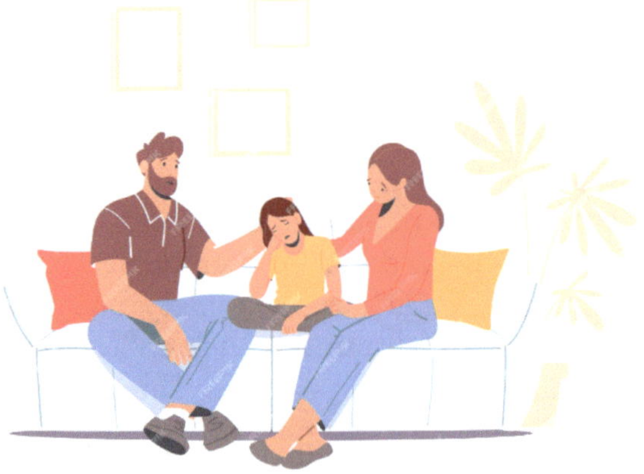

Figure 1.14. Emotional effects on parents with a pediatric cardiology diagnosis.

Source: https://external-content.duckduckgo.com/iu/?u=https%3A%2F%2Fimg.freepik.com%2Fpremium-vector%2Ffather-mother-comforting-upset-kid-loving-parents-support-child-daughter-with-sad-emotions-dull-face-sit-sofa-with-mom-dad-family-characters-cartoon-people-vector-illustration_1016-10723.jpg%3Fw%3D2000&f=1&nofb=1&ipt=4e1c585e61a72cb50e650783a2f1493ecd37af7185feb9b5930591a6b8efb927.

Recognition of the emotional landscape of siblings is also imperative in holistic pediatric cardiology. To achieve holistic patient and family care, health systems must prioritize emotional and psychological guidance of parents and siblings of children with heart disease. Integrative therapy programs for parents and sibling education may better alleviate stress and improve more harmonious family dynamics. Furthermore, increased awareness and education of medical practitioners towards the significance of such emotional factors can help towards enhanced overall efficiency in pediatric cardiac care. Upon identification of the psychological impacts that the family goes through, interventions could be developed not only to treat the child – but also to treat the entire family system. This shift toward a family-centered model of care is required to create resilience and enhance the overall quality of life in families with the complexity of pediatric cardiology (Muscara et al., 2020; Parker et al., 2020).

1.5.2. Financial Implications of Treatment

The financial cost of treatment in pediatric cardiology is multifaceted, encompassing direct healthcare costs, potential long-term economic effects, and total effect on healthcare systems and families. Patients with CHDs can require extensive medical interventions comprising of surgeries, outpatient sessions, and follow-ups. All these therapies tend to be characterized by high cost through specialized care and the need for advanced medical technology. According to recent studies, the initial surgical intervention for severe heart defects may cost over tens of thousands of dollars without considering subsequent treatment and therapies that may be needed throughout the life of the child. Such financial outlay could impose significant strain on families (particularly those without adequate insurance coverage or financial support) making it worthwhile to ensure proper resource management and financial planning in pediatric cardiology (Marilyn et al., 2022). In addition to direct cost of treatment, there is also needed to consider long-term financial issues. Children with serious cardiac ailments may end up having life-long ailments that require regular medical attention, drugs, and secondary ailments. For example, many patients may develop other diseases such as arrhythmias or heart failure and therefore need treatments that may be long and costly. In addition, these longer treatment courses have the potential to result in lost work productivity among parents who may be forced to take a leave of absence from employment due to care needs.

This impacts family income and alters family dynamics, with resultant psychological implications further complicating the pediatric cardiology financial situation (Eldridge et al., 2016). Seeking to understand the comprehensive costs of cardiac care is thus vital to policy formulation as well as the development of supportive healthcare infrastructures. It is critical that healthcare system stakeholders, including policymakers, clinicians, and funding support agencies, work together to address these financial implications. Strategies such as insurance reform, greater access to financial counseling, and enhanced support services can mitigate some of the burden on families of children with cardiac disease. Furthermore, preventative care programs (intended to reduce the incidence of CHDs) can be cost-effective to the health system through avoiding the need for expensive and extensive interventions. Early detection and early treatment can also go a long way towards improving outcomes while reducing pediatric cardiac management costs. Generally, an active and responsible approach is very important in the control of treatment costs in pediatric cardiology (Marilyn et al., 2022).

1.5.3. Support Systems and Resources Available

The world of pediatric cardiology is complemented by an extensive group of support systems and services designed to assist healthcare professionals, patients, and their relatives. In the center of this framework stand multi-disciplinary teams of pediatric cardiologists, surgeons, nurses, and social workers. These teams provide full care by addressing not just the medical needs of pediatric patients but also emotional and psychological well-being of families. Increasing access to care is important, especially in resource-limited regions, where prevalence for heart disease is high. Telemedicine-incentivizing policies and outreach programs can increase awareness and encourage early diagnosis, hence leading to better outcomes for children with congenital heart defects. It also enables research work and allows treatment effects and patient experiences to be monitored, ultimately to supply inputs into best practice in pediatric cardiology and other support materials that can be offered. In addition to clinical resources, support systems from families also play a considerable role in the health care experience of pediatric cardiology patients. The American Heart Association and other in-town foundations offer free information, including educational material, support groups, and assistance with finances for families who are dealing with medical bills associated with treatment. The sites are a meeting ground for parents and caregivers to network and share, building a support network which eliminates isolation and fear. Furthermore, connecting families to social services can offer counseling on the complexity of healthcare, school, and financial assistance systems so that children can obtain holistic care to meet their individual needs. It is crucial that the clinical community works together with these organizations to facilitate synergy, to maximize resources, and to ensure optimal patient care and family support. Looking towards the future of pediatric cardiology, we have to remain sensitive to the requirement for continuous extension and enhancement of systems of aid and resources (Figure 1.15).

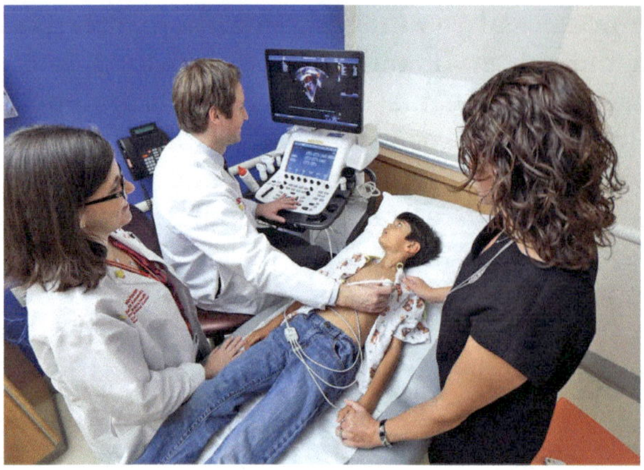

Figure 1.15. The support systems and resources designed to assist healthcare professionals, patients, and their families.

Source: https://external-content.duckduckgo.com/iu/?u=https%3A%2F%2Fcardioped.ro%2Fwp-content%2Fuploads%2F2022%2F07%2Ff4a4c6_ff7d98e49dfd40f39f5a3ebc52ff60b8_mv2.jpg&f=1&nofb=1&ipt=719b83cfe144848a41708796df35cb9169a115aa538a3fed2d5c496e10f6ec1a.

Emphasis on professional training for health professionals improves their capacity to deliver quality care. Training programs in communication skills can often be able to empower practitioners to communicate better with families, keeping them educated and reassured throughout the treatment process. At the same time, enhancing mentorship among health professionals can be able to promote sharing of experience and knowledge and eventually enhance the practice of pediatric cardiology nationwide. Legislative lobbying in an effort to increase funding and support is also vital, particularly for public health programs in prevention of congenital heart defects and other cardiac conditions in children. Collaboration among medical, educational, and legislative groups interdisciplinary will provide stronger support structures vital for dissemination of information and resources to set a better future for children with cardiac issues.

1.6. Advances in Pediatric Cardiology

Pediatric cardiology has witnessed a revolutionary transformation, with tremendous gains in the prognosis of children with congenital and acquired heart diseases. Perhaps one of the most significant changes has been the evolution of extracorporeal membrane oxygenation (ECMO), which has revolutionized the management of pediatric cardiac failure. The use of ECMO has been growing, driven by development in cannulation technology and pump and oxygenator technology, as highlighted in current medical literature (Lorusso et al., 2021). ECMO is a life-support intervention that can also be employed as a bridge to recovery or heart transplantation, particularly for severe cardiogenic shock.

With advances in pediatric cardiologists' skills of patient selection and case management, the ability to provide timely and proper circulatory support has become increasingly effective, hence reducing the risk of morbidity and mortality due to serious cardiac disease in children. Additionally, ongoing research into genetics is profoundly changing our understanding of CHD. During the time since the most recent American Heart Association statement in 2007, the use of high-level genomic techniques has revealed immense information regarding the etiology of CHD, expanding diagnostic potential for pediatric cardiologists. Identification of genetic mutations and copy number variations enlightens the pathology of isolated and syndromic heart defects and improves the prognosis for involved patients (Pierpont et al., 2018). This new knowledge facilitates individualized therapeutic strategies based on individual genetic profiles, thus enhancing pediatric medicine's contribution to the personalization of medicine. By integrating genetic testing into the realm of everyday clinical practice, pediatric cardiologists are able to advise families more effectively regarding risk factors, counseling, and possible interventions, thus improving management of these complex diseases. In addition to genetic advances, novel imaging techniques and interventional methods have transformed the landscape of pediatric cardiology. Echocardiography (once restrictive in its use), has been improved with the inclusion of three-dimensional imaging, which offers improved visualization of cardiac anatomy and function. This capability is priceless in accurate diagnosis and preoperative planning for patients with serious heart defects in children. Advances in catheter-based therapies, such as transcatheter aortic valve replacement and balloon angioplasty, minimize open-heart surgery to its lowest requirements, significantly decreasing recovery time and risks. These technologies not only improve survival rates but the quality of life for child patients as well. These developments, despite their individual isolated nuances, collectively signify the ever-evolving nature of pediatric cardiology and the necessity of further research and technological advancement to drive patient improvement (Figure 1.16).

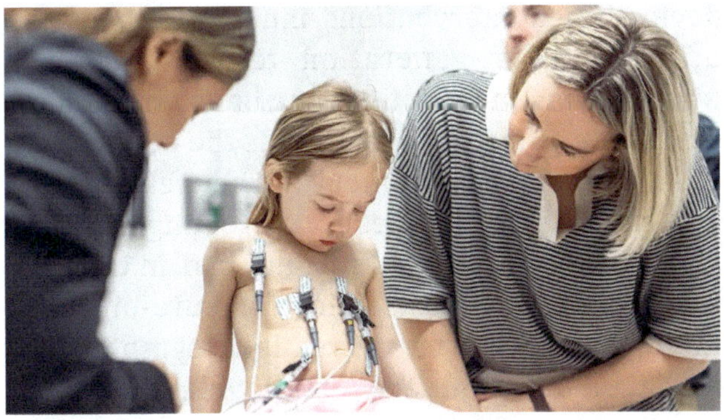

Figure 1.16. Advances in pediatric cardiology.

Source: https://assets.clevelandclinic.org/transform/LargeFeatureImage/cd530911-a56e-44f4-845f-57cde37eab29/CCC_6010660_05-02-25_1462_AMO.

1.6.1. Innovations in Surgical Techniques

Surgical advancements are a cornerstone of advancement in pediatric cardiology, particularly in the management of congenital heart disease. With pediatric surgeons working day and night towards improved patient outcomes, they have invested all their resources into developing new surgical techniques, leading to transformative leaps such as with minimally invasive surgery. These surgical procedures, which can involve smaller cuts and lesser physical trauma, have transformed the process of children facing surgery. Indeed, this is particularly significant, as pediatric patients present uniquely anatomical issues. Altering surgical procedures, including the use of robot assistance and improved imaging, allows the surgeon to be more accurate and flexible with fewer complications and recovery periods in comparison to the existing benchmark of open-heart surgery. By embracing new surgergical practices, pediatric cardiology maximizes immediate treatment and supports an overall trend towards patient-centered treatment. The Ross procedure stands out among the spectrum of surgical interventions in pediatric cardiology, providing a beneficial alternative for the replacement of the aortic valve in young patients. Although it has been relegated to class IIb recommendations by prominent cardiology organizations, recent evidence brings its advantages into focus. Studies have identified that the Ross procedure is associated with improved long-term survival and fewer valve-related complications compared to conventional alternatives and therefore presents a preferable choice in specialist centers. The procedure, in which the abnormal valve is replaced by the patient's own pulmonary valve, is not only an evolution in surgical skills but also in patient criteria for selection. Additionally, recent advances in surgery, including new imaging technologies and tissue engineering applications, also aid in the success of the Ross procedure, paving the way for broader acceptance and use in all pediatric cardiac clinics (Galzerano et al., 2024). Despite the unquestionable advances realized in surgical practices, the specialty of pediatric cardiology still contends with gaps in high-level evidence to aid in their practice to the best possible extent. As noted in recent literature, less than a quarter of the research conducted in this area achieves the standard of randomized controlled trials, which are crucial in the provision of strong evidence-based practice. Lack of high-level trials inhibits understanding the long-term outcomes of newer surgical developments. Whereas improvement in surgery such as ductal stenting and the use of hybrid approaches has been adopted with haste, these are often accompanied by insufficient testing through controlled studies (Yadav et al., 2023). The paradox highlighted the imperative of combined effort towards enhancing research practices in pediatric cardiology, highlighted by multicenter collaboration towards the production of high-quality data that can substantively impact surgical decision-making and maximize patient care outcome in pediatric populations.

1.6.2. Development of New Medications and Therapies

The development of new treatment drugs in pediatric cardiology is an active and important research activity, particularly in the treatment of congenital and acquired heart disease in children. Traditional drugs have been based largely on adult dosing – a factor that has that has created a significant challenge to solve, considering the variation in pharmacokinetic and pharmacodynamic characteristics observed in children; hence, there has been a pressing requirement for drug formulation tailored to pediatric patients. Existing initiatives have focused on clinical trials to explore both the safety and effectiveness of new pharmacological drugs designed specifically for use in pediatrics, thereby ensuring optimal therapeutic outcomes. As such, the inclusion of pediatric considerations in drug development processes is now becoming the norm, an effort that helps in arresting risks associated with off-label use as well as maximizing personalized care in this vulnerable group (Michael et al., 2021). Cardiac implantable electronic device (CIED) therapies are also emerging alongside advances in medication in pediatric cardiology. These devices, including pacemakers and implantable cardioverter-defibrillators, provide vital solutions to the treatment of arrhythmias and bradycardia in children. However, as the technologies advance, so should the technology of CIEDs in order to accommodate the particular anatomical and physiological characteristics of the pediatric patient. Protocols have emerged to address the implantation and management of such devices specifically in this age group since usual adult-centered protocols would not always work to be effective. To that end, expert consensus statements have been established upon which the indication, optimization, and follow-up evaluation should be designed as specifically tailored protocols. These recommendations highlight the importance of developing therapies specific to the specific needs of children, particularly long-term management and outcomes (Siripanthong et al., 2020). In addition to traditional pharmacotherapy and device-based interventions, innovative therapies utilizing latest-generation technologies are transforming the practice of pediatric cardiology. Gene therapy, for example, holds the potential to be a gigantic advancement in the treatment of inherited heart diseases by correcting intrinsic genetic defects. These strategies can, in the long term, open up possibilities for cure-oriented therapies that replace conventional symptomatic management. Similarly, employment of stem cell therapy and tissue engineering has bright prospects to address cardiac repair and regeneration in children. These medications are being vigorously explored to assess their viability and effectiveness in clinical settings. As such advances continue to evolve, interdisciplinary collaboration among researchers, clinicians, and regulators becomes necessary to efficiently translate laboratory research into clinical practice. This kind of collaborative work drives the field forward, enabling new drugs and therapies to be innovative and readily translatable to improve pediatric cardiac care (Michael et al., 2021).

1.6.3. Research Trends and Future Directions in the Field

In pediatric cardiology, expansive trends in research are being revealed with improving methodology and technology. Artificial intelligence (AI) and machine learning are redefining the diagnostic process and treatment algorithms, and by extension, a paradigm shift is taking place on how congenital and acquired heart disease is addressed. Future research is being directed towards personalized medicine, wherein genetic profiling has a central role in tailoring the treatment process for children. The application of generative artificial intelligence (GAI) in educational systems is a new era, enabling future practitioners to have the latest tools for interpreting complex cardiac congenital heart diseases. This platform facilitates interprofessional collaboration among clinicians, educators, and researchers coming together to develop holistic training programs and fusing the existing state of AI technology and pediatric cardiology (Bahroun et al., 2023). Moreover, the use of advanced technologies, such as 3D printing, is going to transform preoperative planning and surgical education in pediatric cardiology. By creating patient-specific models of cardiac morphology, 3D printing facilitates more effective simulation of surgery, which will enhance surgical outcomes and reduce adverse effects of advanced procedures. This growing trend in research emphasizes the importance of utilizing advanced technologies to facilitate better pre-procedural planning and simulation of complicated procedures. Also important is multidisciplinary collaboration among professionals in refining these technologies to ensure they are assimilated into practice. The exploration of these methodological enhancements, and the ethical considerations of utilizing these sophisticated devices, is an investment in raising patient outcome and care to higher levels within pediatric cardiology (Jarosław et al., 2022). The research agenda in pediatric cardiology in the future will have the potential to involve more emphasis on outcome research that assesses long-term impacts of novel interventions. As telemedicine and remote monitoring continue to develop technologically, researchers are turning their attention not only to short-term postoperative conditions but to the patient's quality of life longitudinally. This is a broader focus that incorporates the psychological and development aspects that accompany having cardiac disease. Stakeholder engagement (that of patients and families) will be central to shaping research agendas attuned to the interests of the pediatric populace. Through the promotion of longitudinal studies and the development of patient-focused care models, the practice of pediatric cardiology will be significantly enhanced, reflecting a commitment to holistic, balanced care for younger patients presenting with cardiac conditions (Bahroun et al., 2023).

SUMMARY

The work of pediatric cardiology is an interactive balance of advanced practice and fundamental research aimed at fulfilling the unique cardiovascular well-being demands of children. Although advances in diagnostic technology and in treatment modalities are transforming ever more quickly, practitioners are becoming increasingly skilled in caring for a broad variety of acquired and congenital heart ailments. Demand for specialized attention focused on the younger patient is of utmost concern, given their varying physiological constitution and problem of growth. Ongoing research ensures evidence-based clinical practice and that any new treatment modality is effective and safe for children. Therefore, there is a requirement for an integrated approach in education, research, and clinical practice to improve outcomes for this age group. Moreover, the guarantee of equal access to pediatric cardiac care is increasingly being viewed as a foundational element of the field. Children living in disadvantaged neighborhoods or from diverse socioeconomic backgrounds often have limited capacity for successful diagnosis and treatment. The ethical implications of these disparities highlight the need for system changes in medicine to allow all children to be subjected to timely and appropriate treatment. Healthcare providers, policymakers, and stakeholders in communities can collaborate to help optimize resource allocation and awareness. With the combination of public health interventions and community outreach programs, the pediatric cardiology community can achieve significant steps toward equity in pediatric heart health outcomes and access to healthcare. Lastly, the future of pediatric cardiology is rosy, not only with clinical advancement, but also with the creation of rigorous training programs centered on the subtle complexities of cardiovascular care in children. It takes a multilateral effort to form the next generation of pediatric cardiologists in terms of robust clinical training, access to state-of-the-art research, and solid understanding of the psychosocial dynamics of cardiac disease in kids. Furthermore, increased emphasis on pilot studies and feasibility trials, supported by statements such as the CONSORT statement, will enhance quality research in this area, with an immediate positive effect on pediatric cardiac practice. Each one of these measures, along with the others, plays a part in providing a better reply to the issues evolving in pediatric cardiology (Eldridge et al., 2016; N/A, 2017).

In pediatric cardiology, prevention and management of post-transplant complications, and indeed post-transplant lymphoproliferative disorders (PTLD), are an overarching concern. Observations have indicated that antiviral prophylaxis reduces the incidence of EBV viremia in close association with PTLD following solid organ transplantation. A meta-analysis demonstrated considerable reduction in risk (RR 0.69, 95% CI 0.54 to 0.88) in recipients who underwent antiviral drugs. Furthermore, the same research identified pediatric patients, which had a significant reduction in PTLD risk (RR 0.58, 95% CI 0.43 to 0.79), noting the specific need within the group. These findings emphasize the significance of personalized therapeutic strategies in pediatric cardiology for the relief of severe transplant solid organ complications and for enabling better long-term results for such high-risk patients as they continue along their clinical trajectories. Another of the essential points of debate in pediatric cardiology relates to successful communication dynamics associated with transitions of care, namely handoffs between care providers. Standardized handoff curricula have helped maximize the safety and quality of patient care. Penn State Health investigated the benefits of standardized handoff communications and recommended incorporating verbal in addition to written modes as well as multidisciplinary team involvement. The study demonstrated there to be significant gains in several measure of evaluation following implementation, proposing several resident physician's handoff skills improved measurably over time. This evidence speaks strongly in favor of using systematic mechanisms of handovers, being both well-suited to communicating and potentially preventing avoidable patient harm in pediatric settings where clinical acuity and the need for precise information transfer are paramount. Finally, the relationship between infection complications and therapeutic approaches to treating children in pediatric cardiology cannot be overstressed. The therapeutic approaches developed from studies committed to the treatment of children with post-transplant complications are fundamental discoveries. For instance, though antiviral prophylaxis use is promising in reducing PTLD incidences, efficacy is lost in high-risk groups, particularly with adults (RR 0.88, 95% CI 0.64 to 1.21). This implies the need for additional research to more effectively fine-tune treatment regimens by age and risk stratification. And constant scrutiny of handoff practice, as in the above-referenced study, reminds us of the unparalleled criticality of interaction and communication in pediatric cardiology. Together, these discussions underscore the requirements of multigeneric clinical care which incorporates preventive measures as well as effective communication among caregivers in the treatment of pediatric cardiology patients.

CLOSER LOOK

PEDIATRIC CARDIOVASCULAR DEVELOPMENT

Pediatric cardiovascular development is the highly complex process through which the heart and vessels evolve, mature, and accommodate from fetal life into childhood. It begins early in embryogenesis and continues well into late adolescence, involving intricate morphologic changes and physiologic accommodation required for life after the womb (Figure 1.17).

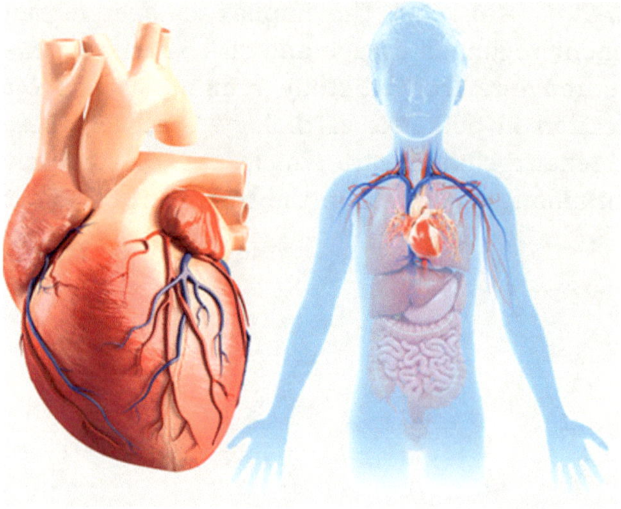

Figure 1.17. Anatomical illustration of the human heart and its placement within the circulatory system, highlighting the major blood vessels and organs involved in systemic and pulmonary circulation.

Source: https://dm3omg1n1n7zx.cloudfront.net/rcni/static/journals/ncyp/aop/ncyp.2020.e1245/tile/ncyp.2020.e1245_abs.jpg.

The heart is the first working organ to develop in the embryo. A primitive heart tube forms in the third week of gestation and begins to contract and pump blood by the end of the fourth week. The tube then loops, divides, and forms a four-chambered heart. Concurrently, the vascular system starts to develop to allow oxygen and nutrient delivery via the placenta. Fetal circulation is not the same as in the postnatal life; it incorporates shunts like foramen ovale and ductus arteriosus that bypass the lungs, which are non-functional during fetal life.

At birth, the transition from fetal to neonatal circulation is dramatic. The initial inspiratory effort of the newborn opens up the lungs and lowers pulmonary vascular resistance, which augments pulmonary artery blood flow. The elevated left atrial pressure causes functional closure of the foramen ovale. In contrast, high oxygen tension and changes in prostaglandin levels cause the ductus arteriosus to shut down and become fully constricted. This marks the beginning of an independent pulmonary circulation, a milestone in cardiovascular development.

In infancy and early childhood, the heart also grows over size and function. While following birth cardiac myocytes do not grow in number to much, their size and complexity of intracellular structures increase, which enhances the contractile efficiency of the heart over time. The very high heart rate at birth (about 120–160 beats/min) decreases with age and, with a rise in systemic vascular resistance, blood pressure increases.

Vascular system development also continues into childhood. Veins and arteries dilate and elongate to encase the growing body, and vessel walls become thicker to resist rising pressures. The autonomic nervous system also develops, fine-tuning the regulation of heart rate and vessel tone. These developments ensure oxygen and nutrients are efficiently delivered to tissues during periods of greatest growth.

Developmental disturbances of the cardiovascular system can lead to congenital heart defects (CHDs), the most common type of birth defect. CHDs may affect septation, valve formation, or development of large vessels and may have significant impact on cardiac function. Prenatal detection by screening or by neonatal echocardiogram and early medical or surgical treatment are critical to improving the prognosis for affected children.

References

1. Adi, Y., Carter, Y., Doug, M., et al. (2009). Transition to adult services for children and young people with palliative care needs: A systematic review. https://core.ac.uk/download/44454.pdf (accessed on 15th July 2025).
2. Alexander, L., Frankel, H. L., Blaivas, M., Kirkpatrick, A. W., Su, E., Evans, D. P., Summerfield, D. T., et al. (2016). Guidelines for the appropriate use of bedside general and cardiac ultrasonography in the evaluation of critically ill patients—Part II: Cardiac ultrasonography. *Critical Care Medicine, 44*, 1206–1227. https://doi.org/10.1097/ccm.0000000000001847 (accessed on 15th July 2025).
3. Bagnall, A., Day, R., & Kime, N. H. (2013). Systematic review of transition models for young people with long-term conditions: A report for NHS Diabetes. https://core.ac.uk/download/29018738.pdf (accessed on 15th July 2025).
4. Bahroun, Z., Anane, C., Ahmed, V., & Zacca, A. (2023). Transforming education: A comprehensive review of generative artificial intelligence in educational settings through bibliometric and content analysis. *Sustainability, 15*, 12983–12983. https://doi.org/10.3390/su151712983 (accessed on 15th July 2025).
5. Bashshur, R. L., Doarn, C. R., Frenk, J., Kvedar, J. C., & Woolliscroft, J. O. (2020). Telemedicine and the COVID-19 pandemic, lessons for the future. *Telemedicine Journal and e-Health, 26*, 571–573. https://doi.org/10.1089/tmj.2020.29040.rb (accessed on 15th July 2025).
6. Begić, Z., Djukic, M., Begić, E., Aziri, B., Mladenović, Z., Iglica, A., Šabanović-Bajramović, N., et al. (2023). Left atrial strain analysis in the realm of pediatric cardiology: Advantages and implications. *Technology and Health Care, 32*, 1255–1272. https://www.semanticscholar.org/paper/03c3f2d6ceaf4879db3aa9d0b7efd908bcdf1737 (accessed on 15th July 2025).
7. Bull, M. J., Trotter, T. L., Santoro, S. L., Christensen, C. K., & Grout, R. W. (2022). Health supervision for children and adolescents with Down syndrome. *Pediatrics, 149*. https://doi.org/10.1542/peds.2022-057010 (accessed on 15th July 2025).
8. Campbell, C., & Kahwash, R. (2020). Will complement inhibition be the new target in treating COVID-19–related systemic thrombosis? *Circulation, 141*, 1739–1741. https://doi.org/10.1161/circulationaha.120.047419 (accessed on 15th July 2025).
9. Eldridge, S., Chan, C., Campbell, M. J., Bond, C., Hopewell, S., Thabane, L., & Lancaster, G. (2016). CONSORT 2010 statement: Extension to randomized pilot and feasibility trials. *BMJ*. https://doi.org/10.1136/bmj.i5239 (accessed on 15th July 2025).
10. Faisal, N. V., Handa, A., & Ramakrishnan, S. (2024). Pediatric cardiac procedures in India: Who bears the cost? *Annals of Pediatric Cardiology, 17*, 1–12. https://doi.org/10.4103/apc.apc_67_24 (accessed on 15th July 2025).
11. Ferriero, D. M., Fullerton, H. J., Bernard, T. J., Billinghurst, L., Daniels, S. R., DeBaun, M. R., deVeber, G., et al. (2019). Management of stroke in neonates and children: A scientific statement from the American Heart Association/American Stroke Association. *Stroke, 50*. https://doi.org/10.1161/str.0000000000000183 (accessed on 15th July 2025).
12. Galzerano, D., Kholaif, N., Al Amro, B., Al Admawi, M., Eltayeb, A., Alshammari, A., Di Salvo, G., et al. (2024). The Ross procedure: Imaging, outcomes and future directions in aortic valve

replacement. *Journal of Clinical Medicine, 13*, 630–630. https://doi.org/10.3390/jcm13020630 (accessed on 15th July 2025).

13. Gersh, B. J., Maron, B. J., Bonow, R. O., Dearani, J. A., Fifer, M. A., Link, M. S., Naidu, S. S., et al. (2011). 2011 ACCF/AHA guideline for the diagnosis and treatment of hypertrophic cardiomyopathy. *Journal of Thoracic and Cardiovascular Surgery, 142*, e153–e203. https://doi.org/10.1016/j.jtcvs.2011.10.020 (accessed on 15th July 2025).

14. Ghaffar Nia, N., Kaplanoğlu, E., & Nasab, A. (2023). Evaluation of artificial intelligence techniques in disease diagnosis and prediction. *Discover Artificial Intelligence, 3*. https://doi.org/10.1007/s44163-023-00049-5 (accessed on 15th July 2025).

15. Henderson, L. A., Canna, S., Friedman, K. G., Gorelik, M., Lapidus, S., Bassiri, H., Behrens, E. M., et al. (2020). American College of Rheumatology clinical guidance for multisystem inflammatory syndrome in children associated with SARS–CoV-2 and hyperinflammation in pediatric COVID-19: Version 1. *Arthritis & Rheumatology, 72*, 1791–1805. https://doi.org/10.1002/art.41454 (accessed on 15th July 2025).

16. Hernández-Madrid, A., Paul, T., Abrams, D. J., Aziz, P. F., Blom, N. A., Chen, J., Chessa, M., et al. (2018). Arrhythmias in congenital heart disease: A position paper of the European Heart Rhythm Association (EHRA), Association for European Pediatric and Congenital Cardiology (AEPC), and the European Society of Cardiology (ESC) Working Group on Grown-up Congenital Heart Disease, endorsed by HRS, PACES, APHRS, and SOLAECE. *EP Europace, 20*, 1719–1753. https://doi.org/10.1093/europace/eux380 (accessed on 15th July 2025).

17. Isselbacher, E. M., Preventza, O., Black, J. H., Augoustides, J., Beck, A. W., Bolen, M. A., Braverman, A. C., et al. (2022). 2022 ACC/AHA guideline for the diagnosis and management of aortic disease: A report of the American Heart Association/American College of Cardiology Joint Committee on Clinical Practice Guidelines. *Circulation, 146*. https://doi.org/10.1161/cir.0000000000001106 (accessed on 15th July 2025).

18. Lorusso, R., Shekar, K., MacLaren, G., Schmidt, M., Pellegrino, V., Meyns, B., Haft, J. W., et al. (2021). ELSO interim guidelines for Veno arterial extracorporeal membrane oxygenation in adult cardiac patients. *ASAIO Journal, 67*, 827–844. https://doi.org/10.1097/mat.0000000000001510 (accessed on 15th July 2025).

19. Makita, S., Yasu, T., Akashi, Y. J., Adachi, H., Izawa, H., Ishihara, S., Iso, Y., et al. (2022). JCS/JACR 2021 guideline on rehabilitation in patients with cardiovascular disease. *Circulation Journal, 87*, 155–235. https://doi.org/10.1253/circj.cj-22-0234 (accessed on 15th July 2025).

20. Malone, L. A., Morrow, A. K., Chen, Y., Curtis, D., de Ferranti, S. D., Desai, M., Fleming, T. K., et al. (2022). Multi-disciplinary collaborative consensus guidance statement on the assessment and treatment of postacute sequelae of SARS-CoV-2 infection (PASC) in children and adolescents. *PM&R, 14*, 1241–1269. https://doi.org/10.1002/pmrj.12890 (accessed on 15th July 2025).

21. Meyer-Szary, J., Luis, M. S., Mikulski, S., Patel, A., Schulz, F., Tretiakow, D., Fercho, J., et al. (2022). The role of 3D printing in planning complex medical procedures and training of medical professionals—Cross-sectional multispecialty review. *International Journal of Environmental Research and Public Health, 19*, 3331–3331. https://doi.org/10.3390/ijerph19063331 (accessed on 15th July 2025).

22. Moghadamnia, M., Delroba, K., Heidari, S., Rezaie, Z., & Dashti-Khavidaki, S. (2025). Impact of antiviral prophylaxis on EBV viremia and posttransplant lymphoproliferative disorders in

solid organ transplant recipients: A systematic review and meta-analysis. *Virology Journal, 22*. https://www.semanticscholar.org/paper/558ef4a6921ec2590e05be86ea089f85c8b4d466 (accessed on 15th July 2025).

23. Muscara, F., McCarthy, M., Rayner, M., Nicholson, J. M., Dimovski, A., McMillan, L., Hearps, S., et al. (2020). Effect of a videoconference-based online group intervention for traumatic stress in parents of children with life-threatening illness. *JAMA Network Open, 3*, e208507–e208507. https://doi.org/10.1001/jamanetworkopen.2020.8507 (accessed on 15th July 2025).
24. Nakra, N., Blumberg, D. A., Herrera-Guerra, A., & Lakshminrusimha, S. (2020). Multi-system inflammatory syndrome in children (MIS-C) following SARS-CoV-2 infection: Review of clinical presentation, hypothetical pathogenesis, and proposed management. *Children, 7*, 69–69. https://doi.org/10.3390/children7070069 (accessed on 15th July 2025).
25. Nasr, V. G., Markham, L. W., Clay, M. A., DiNardo, J. A., Faraoni, D., Gottlieb-Sen, D., Miller-Hance, W. C., et al. (2022). Perioperative considerations for pediatric patients with congenital heart disease presenting for noncardiac procedures: A scientific statement from the American Heart Association. *Circulation: Cardiovascular Quality and Outcomes, 16*. https://doi.org/10.1161/hcq.0000000000000113 (accessed on 15th July 2025).
26. Nasr, V. G., Staffa, S. J., Vener, D. F., Huang, S., Brown, M. L., Twite, M., Miller-Hance, W. C., et al. (2022). The practice of pediatric cardiac anesthesiology in the United States. *Anesthesia & Analgesia, 134*, 532–539. https://doi.org/10.1213/ane.0000000000005859 (accessed on 15th July 2025).
27. Page, R. L., Joglar, J. A., Caldwell, M. A., Calkins, H., Conti, J. B., Deal, B. J., Estes, N. A. M., et al. (2015). 2015 ACC/AHA/HRS guideline for the management of adult patients with supraventricular tachycardia. *Circulation, 133*. https://doi.org/10.1161/cir.0000000000000311 (accessed on 15th July 2025).
28. Parker, R., Houghton, S., Bichard, E., & McKeever, S. (2020). Impact of congenital heart disease on siblings: A review. *Journal of Child Health Care, 24*, 297–316. https://doi.org/10.1177/1367493520914738 (accessed on 15th July 2025).
29. Pierpont, M. E., Brueckner, M., Chung, W. K., Garg, V., Lacro, R. V., McGuire, A. L., Mital, S., et al. (2018). Genetic basis for congenital heart disease: Revisited: A scientific statement from the American Heart Association. *Circulation, 138*. https://doi.org/10.1161/cir.0000000000000606 (accessed on 15th July 2025).
30. Pilati, M. (2024). The importance of weight-based protocols and reduction of frame rates in ASD percutaneous closure. *Clinical Radiology and Imaging Journal*. https://www.semanticscholar.org/paper/90f0ffaeb05245b93735db87b7bec7b86eafe814 (accessed on 15th July 2025).
31. Ramakrishnan, S. (2023). Being a young pediatric cardiologist in India: Aspirations versus reality. *Annals of Pediatric Cardiology, 16*, 163–167. https://doi.org/10.4103/apc.apc_127_23 (accessed on 15th July 2025).
32. Rao, P., Khalpey, Z., Smith, R. G., Burkhoff, D., & Kociol, R. D. (2018). Venoarterial extracorporeal membrane oxygenation for cardiogenic shock and cardiac arrest. *Circulation: Heart Failure, 11*. https://doi.org/10.1161/circheartfailure.118.004905 (accessed on 15th July 2025).
33. Reilly, D., Shandilya, S., Streater, B., Aprile, B. M., & Aprile, J. M. (2024). Improving and sustaining resident physician handover. *Cureus, 16*. https://www.semanticscholar.org/paper/0e230c6ab1e31679145b155e26648f8ddedda8aa (accessed on 15th July 2025).

34. Sarker, M. F. R., Moniruzzaman, M., Bhuiyan, M. N. I., & Khan, M. A. A. (2024). Clinical presentation, echocardiographic findings, treatment options available for ventricular septal defect in children: A study in a tertiary care military hospital. *Journal of Armed Forces Medical College, Bangladesh*. https://www.semanticscholar.org/paper/47742c62c3b53dbf2dc0052d83dc578031b217f1 (accessed on 15th July 2025).

35. Selska, Z., & Vasylkova, I. V. (2024). Children with gene defects are a risk group for the development of abnormalities of the cardiovascular system. *Ukrainian Journal of Perinatology and Pediatrics*. https://www.semanticscholar.org/paper/8c5ae9f9bd395a3a7787606b90e660919fa92d5e (accessed on 15th July 2025).

36. Silka, M. J., Shah, M. J., Avari Silva, J. N., Balaji, S., Beach, C. M., Benjamin, M. N., Berul, C. I., et al. (2021). 2021 PACES expert consensus statement on the indications and management of cardiovascular implantable electronic devices in pediatric patients: Executive summary. *Heart Rhythm, 18*, 1925–1950. https://doi.org/10.1016/j.hrthm.2021.07.051 (accessed on 15th July 2025).

37. Silka, M. J., Shah, M. J., Avari Silva, J. N., Balaji, S., Beach, C. M., Benjamin, M. N., Berul, C. I., et al. (2022). 2021 PACES expert consensus statement on the indications and management of cardiovascular implantable electronic devices in pediatric patients. *Annals of Pediatric Cardiology, 15*, 323–346. https://doi.org/10.4103/0974-2069.361245 (accessed on 15th July 2025).

38. Siripanthong, B., Nazarian, S., Muser, D., Deo, R., Santangeli, P., Khanji, M. Y., Cooper, L. T., et al. (2020). Recognizing COVID-19–related myocarditis: The possible pathophysiology and proposed guideline for diagnosis and management. *Heart Rhythm, 17*, 1463–1471. https://doi.org/10.1016/j.hrthm.2020.05.001 (accessed on 15th July 2025).

39. Sun, Z. (2023). Patient-specific 3D-printed models in pediatric congenital heart disease. *Children, 10*, 319–319. https://doi.org/10.3390/children10020319 (accessed on 15th July 2025).

40. Tan, W., & Aboulhosn, J. (2020). The cardiovascular burden of coronavirus disease 2019 (COVID-19) with a focus on congenital heart disease. *International Journal of Cardiology, 309*, 70–77. https://doi.org/10.1016/j.ijcard.2020.03.063 (accessed on 15th July 2025).

41. Tuczyńska, M., Matthews-Kozanecka, M., & Baum, E. (2021). Accessibility to non-COVID health services in the world during the COVID-19 pandemic: Review. *Frontiers in Public Health, 9*. https://doi.org/10.3389/fpubh.2021.760795 (accessed on 15th July 2025).

42. Valverde, I., Gómez, G., Byrne, N., Anwar, S., Silva Cerpa, M. A., Martín Talavera, M., Pushparajah, K., et al. (2021). Criss-cross heart three-dimensional printed models in medical education: A multicenter study on their value as a supporting tool to conventional imaging. *Anatomical Sciences Education, 15*, 719–730. https://doi.org/10.1002/ase.2105 (accessed on 15th July 2025).

43. Venet, M., Friedberg, M., Mertens, L., Baranger, J., Jalal, Z., Tlili, G., & Villemain, O. (2022). Nuclear imaging in pediatric cardiology: Principles and applications. *Frontiers in Pediatrics, 10*. https://www.semanticscholar.org/paper/b7d0b170d900809f9ba6d341c065f423f32ac4e6 (accessed on 15th July 2025).

44. Vieta, E., Salagre, E., Grande, Í., Carvalho, A. F., Fernandes, B. S., Berk, M., Birmaher, B., et al. (2018). Early intervention in bipolar disorder. *American Journal of Psychiatry, 175*, 411–426. https://doi.org/10.1176/appi.ajp.2017.17090972 (accessed on 15th July 2025).

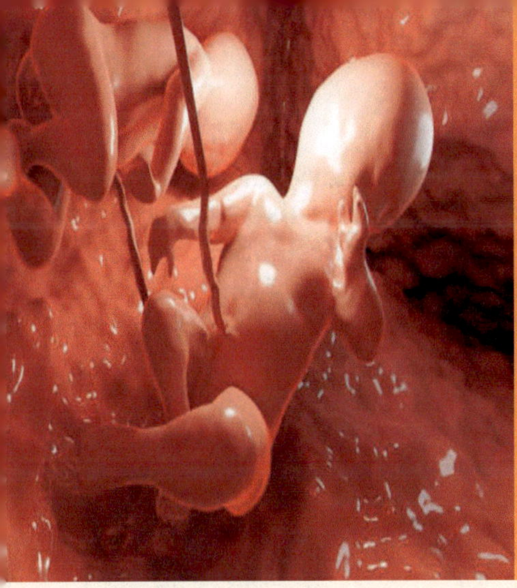

Chapter 2
FETAL CIRCULATION AND TRANSITION AT BIRTH

Contents

Introduction

The fetal circulation phenomenon is a complex and fascinating component of human biology that appears during pregnancy to support the growing fetus. Within a fetal setting, the fetus relies on a sophisticated circulatory system that functions in a different way compared to postnatal circulation. Oxygen and nutrients are basically supplied at this time through the placenta, whose main role is gas exchange, preventing the lungs from exerting themselves until birth. This unique circulatory pattern is made up of several key components that involve the umbilical cord, the ductus venosus, foramen ovale, and ductus arteriosus. It is necessary to grasp this physiological setup in order to realize how the transition is achieved at birth – a time when the circulatory system fundamentally changes to accommodate life outside the uterus, and readies itself for regular respiratory and circulatory function. At birth, this change from fetal to postnatal circulation is marked by a sequence of basic physiological alterations. The instant that the umbilical cord is clamped and cut, the fetus is abruptly severed from the placenta, and the lungs are compelled to begin their primary function of gas exchange. This process triggers a cascade of events including closure of shunts like the foramen ovale and ductus arteriosus to facilitate transition towards single-sided lung circulation of blood. Notably, these changes in anatomy are crucial for the neonate to begin breathing on his or her own because they enable oxygenated blood to be circumvented from the lungs and directly enter systemic circulation. Such identification of intricate changes can provide significant information about possible complications during this time that will impact the health of the newborn in the long term. The implications of fetal circulation and transition at delivery extend beyond the short-term physiological adaptations; they pose deep issues for clinical management and neonatal care. Adaptive failures during transition can lead to various diseases, such as persistent pulmonary hypertension, thereby highlighting that medical professionals must possess adequate knowledge about these processes. In addition, advances in neonatal monitoring as well as management of birth complication ensure healthy deliveries in newborns. Recent research stresses the value of early intervention and specialized care considering prenatal and postnatal factors such as maternal health and environmental context. As research continues to explore the subtleties of fetal circulation, growing knowledge can inform clinical guidelines and improve strategies for avoiding the issues encountered at transition at birth, with the consequent influence on infant long-term health outcomes (Alengebawy et al., 2021; Hou et al., 2022).

Definition of Fetal Circulation

Fetal circulation represents an independent physiological system that occurs during the prenatal period, acting as a mediator in the delivery of oxygen and nutrients from the maternal environment to the developing fetus. It is quite different from that in a postnatal subject, largely based on the fact that the fetus receives its source of oxygen through placental circulation rather than pulmonary respiration. The blood is oxygenated through the placenta, whose maternal blood approaches the fetal blood vessels to allow for exchange of gases. This bypass of the lungs is crucial for fetal survival as the lungs are not yet functional within the fetus.

The organs integral to the process include the umbilical cord, by which the fetus is supplied with blood from the placenta, and three primary shunts: the ductus venosus, foramen ovale, and ductus arteriosus, all of which facilitate good circulation of blood and pressure during development. Through this unique system of circulation, the fetus maintains a high level of shunting blood, which is needed because of the incapacities of its developing organ systems. More specifically, the foramen ovale permits blood to pass directly from the right atrium to the left atrium, circumventing the non-functioning lungs. The ductus arteriosus, also links the pulmonary artery to the aorta, permitting the majority of the blood to bypass the lungs. While this is happening, the ductus venosus allows some of the blood from the umbilical vein to go to the inferior vena cava, so oxygen-rich blood can get to the heart and then the brain. The combination of these adaptations ensures that the fetal organs are adequately oxygenated and nourished even when mature respiratory mechanisms are lacking. However, this transient system also sets the stage for the potential for birth complications – that is, in the preterm infant, who will inevitably struggle with the sudden shift to normal circulatory patterns, as emphasized by the stringent need for strict regulation of conditions of hypocirculation in such individuals (Yin, 2018) (Figure 2.1).

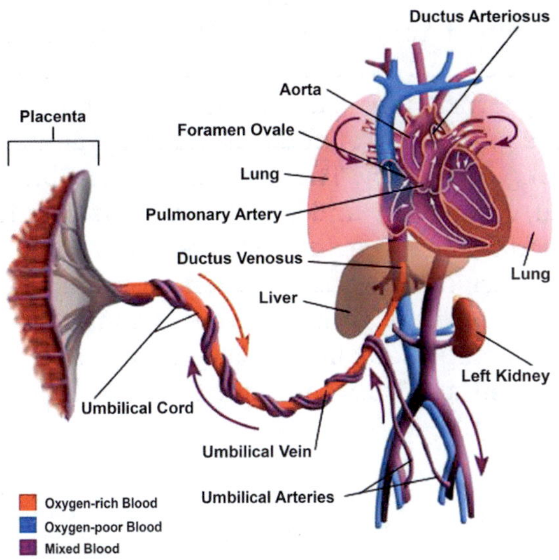

Figure 2.1. The fetal circulatory system work.

Source: https://api.kramesstaywell.com/Content/ebd5aa86-5c85-4a95-a92a-a524015ce556/ucr-images-v1/Images/illustration-of-fetal-blood-flow-or-circulation-281867.

In neonatal transition during birth, fetal to neonatal transition involves drastic physiological changes upon the initiation of newborn breathing. The transition demands shunt closure that has characterized fetal circulation. For instance, foramen ovale tends to close within minutes or hours after birth as left atrial pressure rises, effectively separating the systemic and pulmonary circulations. In contrast, the ductus arteriosus naturally closes early in life, shunting blood to the lungs for oxygenation.

The changes are critical; failure to have the changes done effectively results in circulatory issues becoming extremely likely. This is particularly the case with preterm infants, who are bound to develop severe issues at this time, potentially leading to hypotension and impaired perfusion (Greisen et al., 2016). Therefore, fetal circulation and the ensuing conversion at birth are not merely significant for theoretical understanding but also essential in clinical practice, particularly in neonatal care.

Importance of Understanding Fetal Circulation

Fetal circulation must be understood not only for obstetric practice but also to provide insight into potential pregnancy and childbirth complications. Fetal circulation is different from adult circulation in that it relies on the placenta for oxygenation and nutrient delivery – the basis of fetal growth. Understanding blood perfusion across structures such as the ductus arteriosus and foramen ovale allows medical practitioners to anticipate and manage conditions such as congenital heart disease or pulmonary hypertension that may occur after the process of adaptation to postnatal life has been commenced. Such understanding is also imperative in managing high-risk pregnancies where abnormalities such as pre-eclampsia or gestational diabetes may compromise placental function, leading to decreased fetal perfusion and fetal growth restriction. A good appreciation of fetal circulation can therefore enhance prenatal care and optimize maternal and infant outcomes, making it central to contemporary obstetric practice. Secondly, understanding of fetal circulation is fundamental for the appreciation of how maternal complications affect fetal health. Pre-eclampsia (both early and late onset) is a condition that severely compromises placental blood supply, which in turn affects fetal circulation. Abnormal placentation has been found through studies to be a significant cause of early onset pre-eclampsia and systemic complications that can devastate fetal growth. Given that the role of the placenta is the core of fetal circulation, anything that affects it can lead to disastrous consequences such as intrauterine growth restriction or even stillbirth. Therefore, an extensive understanding of maternal health complications and their influence on fetal circulation provides health professionals with tools to actively control and counteract potential risks, ultimately assuring fetal health under critical phases of development (Graham et al., 2019). Furthermore, an understanding of fetal circulation paves the way for healthcare professionals to intervene in good time and efficiently. In light of the fact that diseases like gestational diabetes mellitus (GDM) have such extremely high incidences and have such major repercussions for the child and mother alike, understanding fetal circulation intricacies is imperative. GDM is associated with increased insulin resistance and can lead to fetal hyperglycemia, affecting circulation and resulting in macrosomia and perinatal complications. The interface between maternal metabolic health and fetal circulation emphasizes the necessity of early intervention and screening mechanisms to prevent poor outcomes. In this context, an integrated model that incorporates fetal circulation and maternal health facilitates clinicians in creating patient-centric care plans that ensure maximum fetal growth while addressing underlying maternal pathologies (Jasmine et al., 2018). This integrated model is essential in promoting perinatal outcomes and developing maternal-fetal medicine.

2.1. Anatomy of Fetal Circulation

An understanding of fetal circulation anatomy is key to understanding how the developing fetus supports its physiological needs within the uterine setting. In postnatal circulation, fetal circulation exists in a unique configuration to optimize the pick-up of oxygen and nutrient supplies from the placenta. The two principal structures of this circulatory system are the umbilical vein, which carries oxygenated blood from the placenta to the fetus, and the umbilical arteries, which carry deoxygenated blood back to the placenta. Principal shunts (such as the ductus venosus) allow blood to bypass the liver, directly sending a large portion of this oxygen-rich blood to the heart. These adaptations ensure critical nutrients are delivered to tissues that grow rapidly in an effective way, indicating the significance of fetal circulatory anatomy during pregnancy. The heart is responsible for fetal circulation and has specific anatomical structures that provide effective blood flow. The right atrium also has an essential relationship with the left atrium via the foramen ovale, an opening that allows the passage of blood preferentially from the right to the left side of the heart.

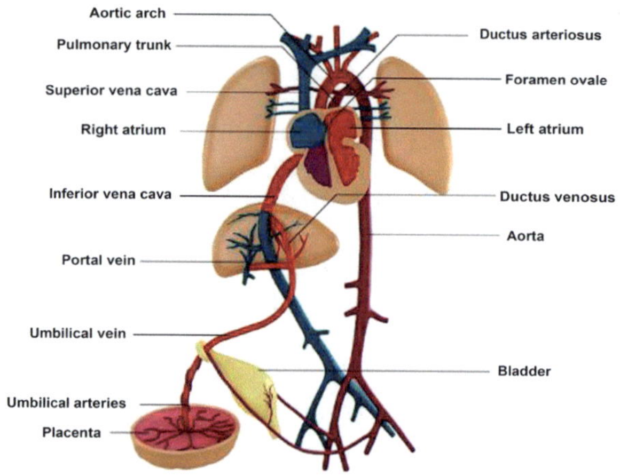

Figure 2.2. Fetal circulation anatomy.

Source: https://upload.medbullets.com/topic/103011/images/fetal_cir_v5_(1).jpg.

This shunt bypasses the non-functional lungs since the fetus uses placental respiration rather than pulmonary function. The pulmonary artery is also associated with the aorta via the ductus arteriosus, a shunt that bypasses the lungs. Concurrently, these shunts create a system in which less than 10% of cardiac output is going to the lungs, keeping most of the oxygenated blood available for delivery to vital organs. These mechanisms illustrate the remarkable ability of the fetal heart to accommodate the new conditions of prenatal life (Figure 2.2).

With impending birth, the transition from fetal to neonatal circulation is one requiring massive physiological change, which in turn requires an understanding of the anatomy involved. With birth, closure of various shunts that have maintained fetal circulation begins. With commencement of respiration, increased pulmonary blood flow closes off the ductus arteriosus, which typically occurs in the first few days after birth. Concurrently, the foramen ovale closes since left atrial pressure is now higher than the right atrium, thus separating the systemic and pulmonary circulations. These changes are necessary to develop an efficient stand-alone circulatory system that caters to the newborns oxygenation needs through the lungs. Understanding these changes not only points to the complexity of fetal anatomy but also outlines important transitional changes that allow for postnatal survival, illustrating the intricate relationship between function and structure at this period of intense development.

2.1.1. Key Structures Involved in Fetal Circulation

Fetal circulation is maintained by the presence of a variety of significant structures that ensure efficient transmission of oxygen and nutrients from the mother to the developing fetus. Central to the system is the placenta, an interface between fetal and maternal blood supplies. Through the presence of a network of maternal and fetal blood vessels, the placenta ensures exchange of gases, nutrients, and waste.

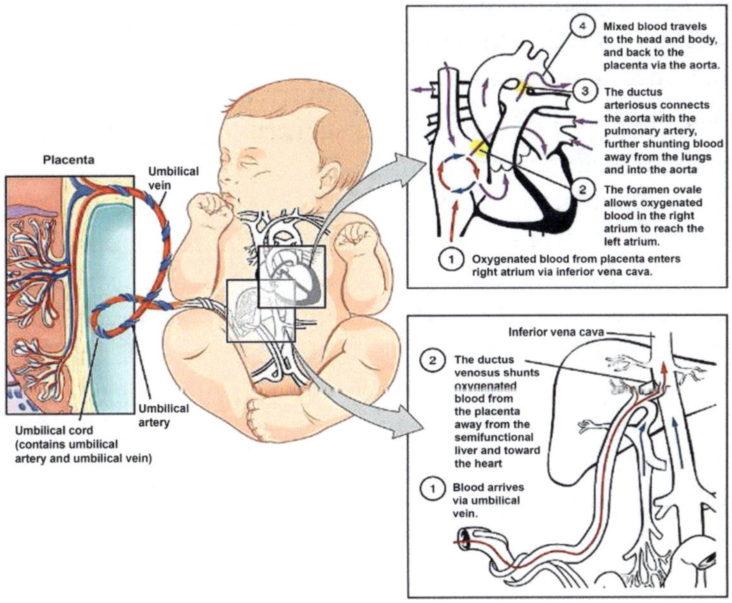

Figure 2.3. The fetal circulatory system includes three shunts to divert blood from undeveloped and partially functioning organs, as well as the blood supply to and from the placenta.

Source: https://en.wikipedia.org/wiki/File:2916_Fetal_Circulatory_System-02.jpg.

The umbilical cord, made up of two umbilical arteries and one umbilical vein, is the conduit through which oxygenated blood is directed from the placenta to the fetus, and deoxygenated blood is directed back to the placenta for expulsion. Strikingly, the placenta also produces hormones essential for pregnancy upkeep and lactation preparation, noting its multifaceted role in fetal development and maternal health (Casarotto et al., 2024). Besides, other shunts also have critical functions in fetal circulation, ensuring that blood does not circulate through non-functioning pulmonary and hepatic circuits. The foramen ovale allows a passageway under which the blood will move directly from the right atrium to the left atrium, effectively bypassing the lungs, which are still non-functional and underdeveloped in gas exchange. Conversely, the ductus arteriosus connects the pulmonary artery and the aorta to let blood flow around the lungs and into systemic circulation. The ductus venosus benefits the liver in the same way by providing most of the umbilical vein's oxygenated blood directly into the inferior vena cava. These modifications are essential to optimize blood flow and oxygen delivery to vital organs throughout fetal growth, ultimately preparing the fetus for successful adaptation after birth (Zhang et al., 2023) (Figure 2.3).

As the fetus proceeds to birth, the intricate circuitry of circulatory mechanisms needs to be refined for the adaptation from fetal to neonatal circulation. Upon birth, when the sudden pressure and oxygen level change, these shunts close, and blood starts flowing through the now-functional lungs and liver. The foramen ovale closes to prevent right-to-left shunting of blood, and the ductus arteriosus constricts and eventually becomes ligamentous. The ductus venosus also closes, leading to complete reliance on the liver to metabolize nutrients. This dramatic transformation is necessary to begin independent breathing and oxygenated circulatory supply effectively throughout the newborns body, reflective of the dynamic fetal circulation process and physiological adaptation at birth (Casarotto et al., 2024; Zhang et al., 2023).

2.1.2. Role of the Placenta in Nutrient and Gas Exchange

The placenta is a central organ in fetal circulation, primarily tasked with transferring nutrients and gases from the maternal to fetal circulations. The placenta serves both as a barrier and middleman, allowing necessary components to pass in from the mother to fetus simultaneously with removing waste products for removal. This connection of fetal circulation to maternal blood is achieved through a network of subtle structure and function within the placenta, like specialized trophoblast cells, which optimize the efficiency of nutrient transfer.

The fetal circulation, according to this, is suited to operate in the best possible manner in the low oxygen pressure of the uterus. Thus, the placental role of controlling the transfer of essential nutrients like glucose and amino acids is significant in promoting fetal development and growth. Besides its function as a site of nutrient transfer, the placenta is responsible for controlling gas exchange, that is, the exchange of oxygen and carbon dioxide levels. The unique structure of the placenta allows space for an immense surface area to facilitate these exchanges, raising the fetus chances for survival under the relatively low oxygen levels of the uterus.

Oxygen-rich blood from the mother is carried near fetal blood without becoming directly mixed, so oxygen enters into the fetal circulation and carbon dioxide leaves. It is especially important that this mechanism provides a high level of oxygen saturation in fetal circulation, required for ensuring maximal levels of this vital gas to the growing organs. Combined, these processes turn the placenta into a key component of fetal physiology, adapting to the needs of the organism at the developmental stage (Figure 2.4).

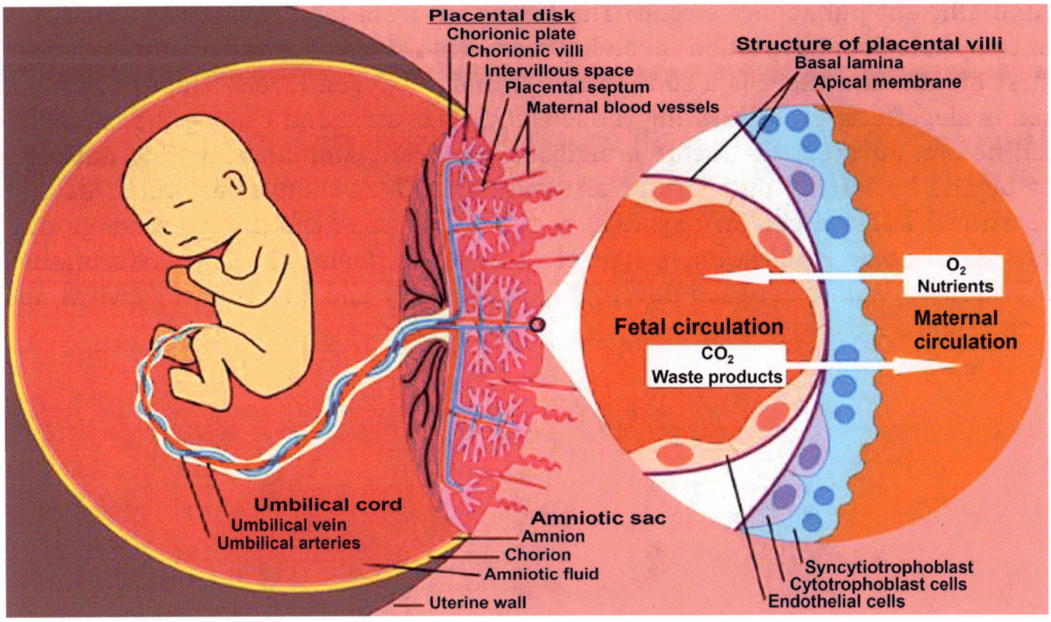

Figure 2.4. Illustration of the placental barrier that separates between fetal and maternal circulations in the human placenta.

Source: https://www.researchgate.net/figure/llustration-of-the-placental-barrier-that-separates-between-fetal-and-maternal_fig1_257837399.

The placenta does not just facilitate gas and nutrient exchange, but also has a protective as well as an immunological role. It ensures semiallogeneic fetus tolerance and minimizes the risk of maternal immune response that results in compromising the pregnancy. Immunological tolerance is crucial because it enables the fetus to develop without rejection by the mother's immune system. The placenta also serves as an immune barrier to any potential pathogens, providing a measure of defense against vertical transmission of infection. This diversified role highlights the placenta's function in fetal health and development, with the provision of necessary conditions for effective adaptation to extrauterine life. As the growing fetus prepares to enter the outside world, the efficient functioning of the placenta becomes more crucial, readying itself for the radical changes that await it outside the uterus (Stephanie et al., 2019; Tan et al., 2019).

2.1.3. Differences Between Fetal and Adult Circulatory Systems

The adult and fetal cardiovascular systems are dramatically different only because the two systems exist in different physiological environments that they themselves sustain. Fetal life depends largely on the placenta for the transport of oxygen and nutrients, which makes it possible for there to be an alternative path that can circumvent the non-ventilated lungs. Instead of being distributed via the pulmonary arteries into the lungs, the blood is shunted through pathways such as the foramen ovale and ductus arteriosus. This unique setup allows for blending of oxygenated and oxygen-deficient blood, tolerable in consideration of fetal reliance on maternal circulation. This fetal circulation also allows for shunting of blood supply to vital organs like the brain while saving energy and resources, basically unlike the adult circulatory system that functions through a complete and efficient pulmonary circuit. The transition from fetal to adult circulation at birth is a significant physiological adaptation involving many significant alterations. Upon birth, the infant takes its first breath, and there is a sudden rise in blood oxygen levels. This results in closure of the foramen ovale, effectively separating the left and right atria and closing the right-to-left shunt that existed before. Further, the ductus arteriosus constricts and closes within subsequent days, closing the bypass between pulmonary artery and aorta. Such changes are required to formulate a fully operational adult circulatory system, which supports efficient gas exchange and delivery of nutrients via alveolar respiration in lieu of placental diffusion. Such transformatory changes indicate the subtle dynamic between developmental biology and short-term survival needs at the time of birth (Figure 2.5).

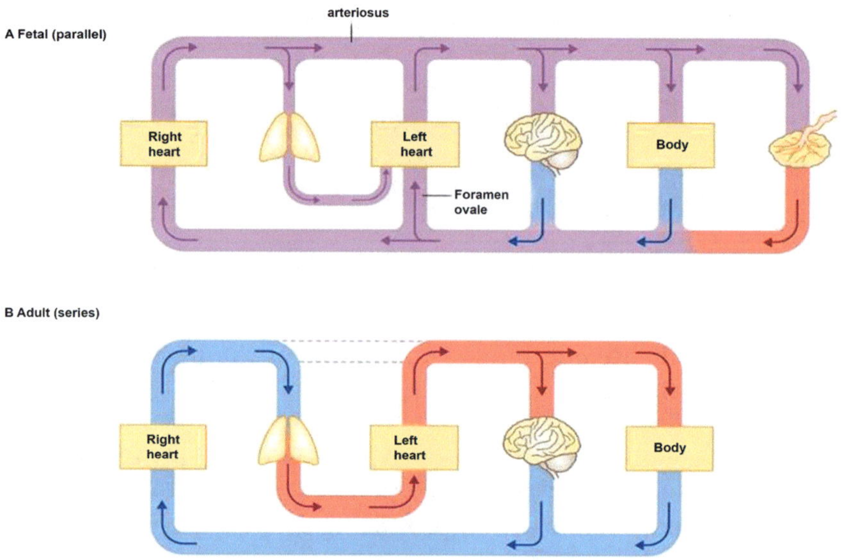

Figure 2.5. Comparison of fetal and adult circulatory systems.

Source: https://www.grepmed.com/images/4878/peds-circulation-anatomy-fetal-cardiology#google_vignette.

The immune system's function in the process also should be considered since it contributes significantly to the adaptation of the newborn to the change in the environment, as in usual immunological adaptation during pregnancy. The maternal immune system adapts to tolerate the allogeneic fetus, perhaps through counter-expressing systemic resilience in the newborn upon birth. Exploring these immunological processes can potentially lead to understanding how mother health influences fetal and newborn outcomes. For example, disruptions to this transition can lead to vulnerabilities in immune function and therefore increase susceptibility to infection in early life. When the infant begins to formulate its immune profile, the foundation laid during fetal development continues to influence health outcomes, demonstrating the interfacing between immunological and circulatory systems, and affirming the need for comprehensive maternal-fetal health considerations as described in the literature (Abu-Raya et al., 2020; Peng et al., 2022).

2.2. Blood Flow Pathways in Fetal Circulation

Fetal circulatory pathways are characterized by specialized patterns of blood flow to address the needs of the developing fetus. Due to the dependance on the maternal bloodstream, circulation during fetal life is designed to function in a state of minimal oxygenation. The key structures involved in this function are the placenta, umbilical vessels, and shunts such as the ductus arteriosus and foramen ovale. Blood is returned from the placenta through the umbilical vein, carrying oxygenated blood to the fetus, through the ductus venosus into the inferior vena cava. This is a typical example of a well-engineered system, with oxygenated blood managing to reach the vital organs (e.g., the brain and the heart) central to fetal development during pregnancy. As fetal development continues, deoxygenated blood is returned to the placenta through divergent pathways. Most of the fetal blood passes through the right atrium to the right ventricle; but a significant proportion passes through the foramen ovale and directly enters the left atrium. This is due to the pressure gradients that provide a bypass for the oxygen-rich blood to enter the systemic circulation without passing through the pulmonary circuit, which is not yet well developed. In addition, the ductus arteriosus connects the pulmonary artery to the descending aorta, allowing further diversion of blood from the lungs. The complexity of this circulation is crucial, as it maintains fetal development and becomes ready for the transition of postnatal circulation at birth. During birth, fetal circulation undergoes significant alterations to maintain life outside the mother. As the infant takes its first breath, the lungs expand and pulmonary resistance decreases, initiating changes in the hemodynamics of blood flow. The effect is that the foramen ovale begins to close when left atrial pressure rises, closing the window that had been shunting blood away from the pulmonary circuit. The ductus arteriosus also constricts because of increased oxygen levels, contributing to diversion of blood flow to the working lungs for oxygenation. The development of the structural changes within both the vessels and the heart defines the termination of fetal existence and the initiation of independent respiration, thereby ending a crucial phase in the process of development characterized by complex adaptations along blood flow pathways that highlight the outstanding complexity of fetal circulation and its change at birth.

2.2.1. The Role of the Umbilical Vein

The umbilical vein plays a significant role as the principal vessel to transfer oxygenated blood from the placenta to the fetus. It plays a vital role in maintaining fetal growth and development through the supply of required oxygen and nutrients needed for cellular metabolism. As the main constituent of fetal circulation, the umbilical vein is unique in carrying oxygen-rich blood in contrast to most veins in the adult circulatory system. When entering the fetus, oxygenated blood passes into the liver via the ductus venosus to facilitate proper distribution of nutrients and fetal homeostasis. The ability of the umbilical vein to provide vital resources is critical in the prenatal life, particularly in situations such as fetal growth restriction, where oxygen and nutrient demands become imperative to survival (Bava et al., 2019). Transitions from fetal to neonatal life come with a radical physiological adaptation, whereby the umbilical vein also closes and becomes redundant shortly after birth. During delivery, the transition is facilitated by the pre-existing mechanical and physiological changes (e.g., clamping of the umbilical cord) which effectively cease the blood circulation from the placenta. The transition also serves the purpose of allowing initiation of neonatal circulation independently because the infant is now completely reliant on its own respiratory action for oxygen introduction into the bloodstream. Curiously enough, cord clamping timing has dramatic impacts on the infants circulatory stability. The current guideline to clamp the umbilical cord immediately for non-vigorous infants illustrates the subtleties involved with postnatal care, since immediate cord clamping may bring cardioprotective benefits at this vulnerable period (Bava et al., 2019) (Figure 2.6).

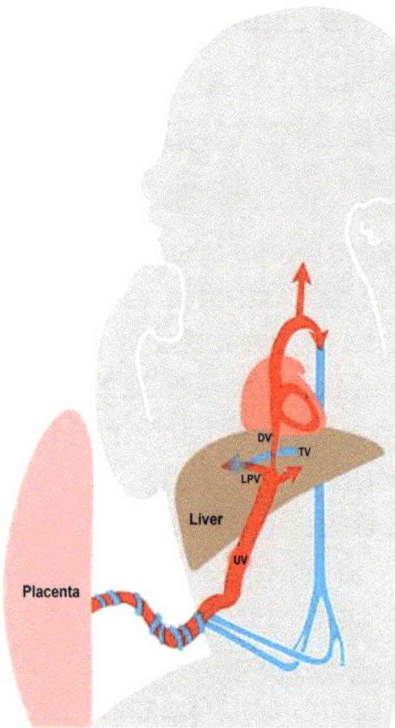

Figure 2.6. The fetal umbilical venous circulation schematic: well-oxygenated and nutrient-rich blood (red) from the placenta reaches the fetus through the umbilical vein (UV). This blood is distributed either to the fetal liver (arrows within the liver) or shunted through the ductus venosus (DV) to supply the heart and brain. The portal vein (PV) carries low-oxygenated blood (blue) from the visceral organs and blends with the umbilical blood from the left portal branch (LPV) to supply the right liver lobe.

Source: https://www.researchgate.net/figure/The-fetal-umbilical-venous-circulation-schematic-Well-oxygenated-and-nutrient-rich-blood_fig1_353938247.

In addition, the activity and health of the umbilical vein can directly impact infant outcomes. Studies have indicated that fetal growth restriction is associated with alterations in umbilical vein endothelial function, as reflected by increased levels of nitric oxide production. Endothelial dysfunction not only impacts placental perfusion but may impair the child's cardiovascular health in adulthood. The umbilical vein's response to pregnancy-related stressors is both an adaptive process in ensuring circulation and a possible risk factor for future health difficulties. As such, understanding the role played by the umbilical vein in fetal development and how it changes at birth is important, since it sheds light on determinants of neonatal health and long-term cardiovascular health (Begliuomini et al., 2012).

2.2.2. The Function of the Ductus Venosus

During fetal circulation, the ductus venosus plays a crucial role in directing oxygenated blood from the placenta to the fetal heart. This single vascular pathway plays a crucial role in maintaining efficiency within the fetal circulatory system, particularly in light of the limited function of direct gas exchange in the lungs intrauterinely. Blood from the placenta via the umbilical vein is shunted through the ductus venosus, effectively circumventing the liver and allowing much of this oxygen-rich blood directly into the inferior vena cava. This mechanism allows for maximum brain and visceral organ perfusion during a naturally constrained supply time, thereby allowing for a venue of efficient fetal development and growth (Melamed et al., 2021). The physiological significance of the ductus venosus is more than just shunting blood; it is a critical adaptation that allows for fetal tolerance in an environment of hypoxia. The single anatomical site of the ductus venosus facilitates fetal optimization of placental oxygenation. Because the fetal lungs are not viable until birth, effective flow of blood through the ductus venosus is of top priority. It is important to appreciate that disturbances in such structure can result in impaired hemodynamics; FGR can directly impact its function, threatening overall fetal viability. Research into such physiological adaptation reinforce the importance of the ductus venosus in assisting the transition towards independent life from placental life (Tan et al., 2019).

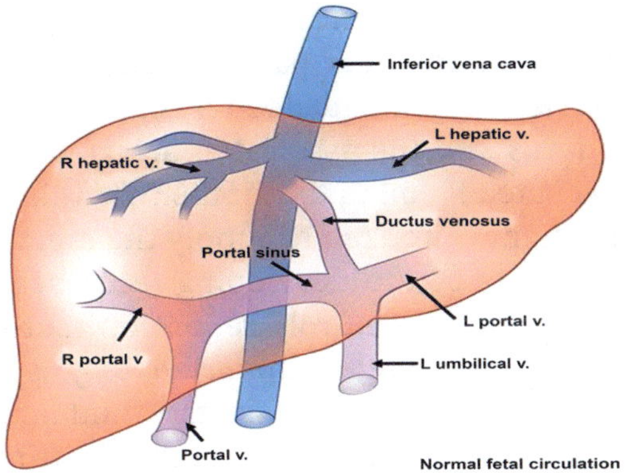

Figure 2.7. In fetal circulation, oxygenated and nutrient-rich blood from the placenta travels to the fetus via the umbilical vein. A portion of this blood bypasses the liver through the ductus venosus, merging with deoxygenated blood in the inferior vena cava (IVC).

Source: https://journals.sagepub.com/doi/10.1177/10935266231211760.

With impending delivery, the ductus venosus and its role of interest come in the setting of the complicated hemodynamic changes which characterize the shift to neonatal circulation. At the time of delivery, cues of the extrauterine world initiate the physiological changes, of which closure of fetal shunts is one aspect. Functional closure of the ductus venosus is typically accomplished several hours after birth, redirecting flow across the liver and establishing an adult-type hepatic portal circulation. This is a necessary adaptation to satisfy the metabolic demand of the neonate, which must cope with new challenges such as thermoregulation and independent respiration. It is during these transitional dynamics that the importance of the ductus venosus in fetal growth is revealed to be vital in making the newborn capable of surviving in its initial adaptation from life inside the uterus (Melamed et al., 2021) (Figure 2.7).

2.2.3. The Significance of the Foramen Ovale

The foramen ovale, a life-saving shunt for fetal circulation, permits efficient flow of oxygen-rich blood from the right atrium to the left atrium by circumventing the non-pulmonary fetal lungs. Its significance lies in its role in ensuring hemodynamic stability during crucial phases of development. During pregnancy, up to 30% of blood flowing towards the lungs is shunted via the foramen ovale in a bid to make sure that the oxygenated blood gained from the placenta is maximized to be distributed around the body. When the neonate transitions from fetal to postnatal existence, shunt closure in this area is absolutely crucial immediately; otherwise, it may result in significant circulatory adaptations, such as reliance on the ductus arteriosus, which may be responsible for gaining conditions like patent ductus arteriosus (PDA) or overcirculation of the lungs – both of which have adverse effects on respiratory and systemic well-being (Laere et al., 2018). As the infant is exposed to life outside the womb, physiological reactions associated with breathing lead to the functional closure of the foramen ovale. The increase in left atrial pressure due to inflation of the lungs leads to apposition of the septum primum against the septum secundum and closure of the foramen ovale. This rapid adaptation plays an important role in establishing normal postnatal circulation, directing blood properly through the lungs for gas exchange. This closure failure can manifest in the clinical environment with patients cyanosed or otherwise presenting with respiratory complications, contributing to neonatal morbidity. The evolution of neonatal monitoring, including the use of echocardiography, allows patency of the foramen ovale to be determined, and intervention can thus be responded to early enough to avoid attached risk and enable normal transition (Emily et al., 2017). The foramen ovale is also of significant clinical significance due to its failure to close in some individuals, known as a patent foramen ovale (PFO) (Figure 2.8).

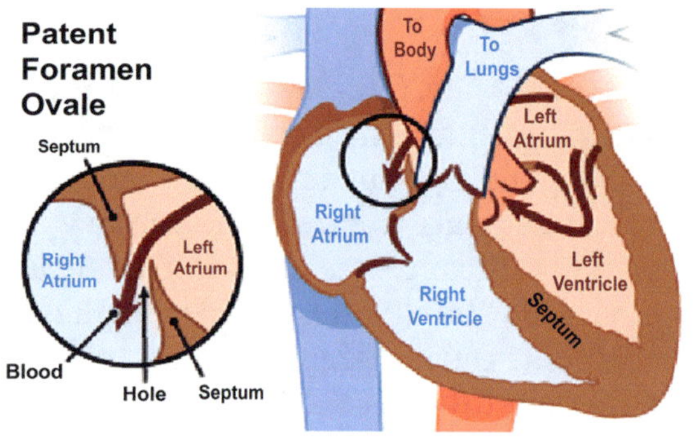

Figure 2.8. Patent foramen ovale (PFO).

Source: https://kidshealth.org/content/dam/patientinstructions/en/images/PFO_415x259_enIL.png.

While the majority of individuals with a PFO are asymptomatic, its ability to lead to embolic disorders and altitude illness guarantees that clinical suspicion is warranted. Present research into the consequences of a PFO is still ongoing, particularly in individuals with a history of cardiovascular disease. Because the foramen ovale is such a critical factor in fetal pliability and ensuing cardiovascular health, an understanding of its dynamics is not only educational regarding neonatal treatment but also predictive of long-term health (Laere et al., 2018). Ultimately, the significance of the foramen ovale extends beyond its role in fetal circulation; it speaks to the complexity of cardiovascular adaptation and the need for ongoing research and clinical acumen (Laere et al., 2018).

2.3. Oxygenation and Nutrient Supply

In the intricate mechanism of fetal growth, mechanisms of oxygenation and delivery of nutrients are important. The placenta is the primary maternal-fetal interface and holds the key to the opening of the vascular routes for the passage of vital substances such as oxygen and glucose to the developing fetus. The fetal circulation, with its typical features—such as the umbilical cord containing two arteries and a vein—facilitates this passage. The umbilical vein carries oxygenated blood from the placenta to the fetus and the associated arteries return deoxygenated blood to the mother. This singular arrangement is utilized to supply the metabolic requirements of the developing fetus because its oxygenation is entirely reliant on maternal circulation. It is therefore important to grasp this dynamic relationship so that the fundamental concepts of fetal circulation and transition at birth can be appreciated. The transition from fetal to neonatal circulation signifies the most drastic changes in oxygenation and nutrient delivery. The neonate, upon birth, must suddenly adapt to a condition where placental provision is now a thing of the past. Foramen ovale and ductus arteriosus closure signals this transition, redirecting blood flow into the lungs for the very first time. Increased blood flow to the lungs is vital for oxygenation since the newborn's lungs become the primary site of gas exchange. This process is not only a structural accommodation; it also involves complex biochemical processes that must be precisely controlled so that the level of oxygenation of the blood is in the best possible condition for the demands of life outside the womb. Any disruption during this transition can lead to complications, emphasizing the significance of proper regulatory mechanisms in fetal and neonatal circulation. Furthermore, placental health has a significant impact on the effectiveness of oxygen and nutrient exchange, which is explained in conditions such as pre-eclampsia. This condition, which is more common in first-time pregnancy, can disrupt normal placentation and cause suboptimal oxygenation and delivery of nutrients to the fetus, which can lead to prospective growth restriction and other complications. Understanding the nuances of placental function and its vascular physiology is crucial. As recent research indicates, investigating intersections between placental formation and mother's health may unlock novel approaches to anticipating and treating diseases such as pre-eclampsia, ultimately leading to better outcomes for both mother and baby (Graham et al., 2019). This convergence of mother's health and fetal health reflects the vast implications of fetal circulation and transitions at birth on long-term health outcomes.

2.3.1. Mechanisms of Oxygen Transfer from Mother to Fetus

The placenta is the key to the processes of mother-fetus oxygen transfer, supporting effective exchange of gases essential for fetal growth. It acts as a barrier and a conduit through which the oxygen diffuses in a selective process while, at the same time, carbon dioxide is washed out of the fetal circulation. Maternal blood pervades the intervillous spaces of the placenta, oxygen passing from maternal erythrocytes to fetal blood vessels. High affinity of fetal hemoglobin for oxygen compared to adult hemoglobin ensures that even relatively low levels of oxygen in maternal blood are adequate to nourish the fetus. This is specialized physiology that is essential in sustaining the metabolic needs of the growing fetus, particularly as it approaches the time of birth and needs increased oxygen for organ maturation and growth. The structure of the placentas is also specially designed to ensure optimal gas exchange through a colossal surface area and a thin trophoblast cell membrane. The proximity of fetal and maternal blood, with only a thin layer of placental tissue in between, enhances the efficiency of oxygen exchange. The surface area of the placenta is increased to accommodate the growing oxygen requirement as fetal growth progresses. Furthermore, the placental circulation is low-resistance, facilitating blood flow and consequently oxygen delivery. Any deviation in placental structure or function is capable of inhibiting this vital process and leading to complications. These limitations direct the need for right placental health to facilitate effective oxygen delivery and resultant fetal health. An understanding of the intricacies of oxygen transfer mechanisms gives insight into various obstetric complications, including the role of preterm birth and other conditions that can lead to interference in placental function. Infections such as intra-amniotic infection and interference with maternal-fetal tolerance can significantly impact oxygen exchange. For instance, infection and inflammation can lead to preterm labor, resulting in a chain of issues for fetal oxygenation (Romero et al., 2014) (Figure 2.9).

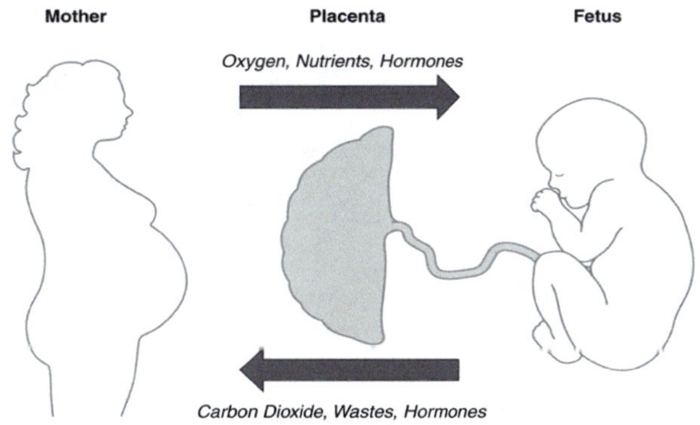

Figure 2.9. The placenta plays a pivotal role in the mechanisms of oxygen transfer from mother to fetus.

Source: https://static.cambridge.org/binary/version/id/urn:cambridge.org:id:binary:20200413035534776-0236:9781108163705:19480fig5_1.png?pub-status=live.

In addition, comprehension of the placenta as an active interface necessitates continued research into the ways that maternal health deficiencies would influence fetal oxygenation and development. Acceptance of such complexities highlights the need for clinical interventions centered on maternal and fetal health in terms of optimizing outcomes for both. By elucidating these mechanisms, clinicians and researchers can further develop means of controlling and mitigating risks of defective fetal oxygenation.

2.3.2. Nutrient Transport Processes in Fetal Circulation

Transportation in fetal circulation is a complex process that delivers the developing fetus with an adequate supply for growth and development. It is also facilitated mainly by the placenta, which serves as the interface between maternal and fetal blood. Trophoblasts, the specialized placental cells, play a vital role in the transfer of nutrients by infiltrating and restructuring the mother's uterine vasculature to provide for good circulation. Placental development structurally is necessary as it provides for selective permeability that brings necessary nutrients such as glucose, amino acids, and fatty acids through while simultaneously keeping out dangerous substances.

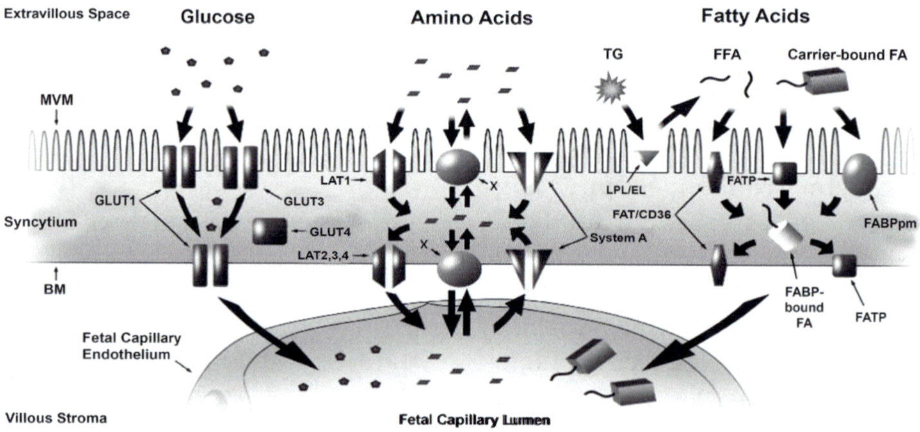

Figure 2.10. Nutrient transport across the placenta, featuring the SCTB and the fetal endothelium, and the location of key proteins involved in macronutrient (glucose, amino acids, fatty acids) transport at the MVM and BM.

Source: https://www.mdpi.com/ijms/ijms-15-16153/article_deploy/html/images/ijms-15-16153-g001.png.

Understanding of these mechanisms is not only critical to an understanding of normal fetal development but also to an understanding of the impact of interference with nutrient transport leading to complications of pregnancy and development disorders later in life. The placenta, besides providing crucial nutrient transport, actively regulates the mechanism of waste removal from fetal circulation. Removal of metabolic waste and gases such as carbon dioxide is by a process of diffusion, based on the concentration gradient between maternal and fetal blood. This function is vital, since fetal lungs are non-functional prior to birth, and there therefore must be the efficiency of placental gas exchange. As shown, maternal blood contains a high concentration of oxygen and a low concentration of carbon dioxide, creating the ideal situation for oxygen diffusion across into fetal circulation and carbon dioxide removal. The intricate organization of the placental interface, with trophoblastic cells delivering hemostasis and repelling maternal immune attack, highlights the high-level physiological adaptation required for these occurrences (Figure 2.10).

This flexibility underscores the placenta's role in fetal homeostasis and adapting its growth in a highly regulated manner (Maltepe et al., 2015). Recent studies have shed light on the intricate interactions between maternal nutrition and fetal metabolic programming by placental nutrient transfer mechanisms. Understanding trophoblast function and how they adapt to varying maternal nutrient delivery is important for fetal well-being. Nutrient transport changes can lead to conditions like intrauterine growth restriction (IUGR) or obesity in later adulthood, showing the importance of appropriate maternal nutrition during pregnancy. Further, recent studies also analyze the accumulation of toxic substances like heavy metals and pesticides in the placenta that can compromise these transport mechanisms for nutrients (Alengebawy et al., 2021). The implications of the findings themselves transcend the realm of prenatal development because they add to the broader argument about public health and the need for environmental protection measures in order to protect both fetal and maternal health during pregnancy.

2.3.3. Impact of Maternal Health on Fetal Oxygenation

The health of the mother has profound impacts on fetal oxygenation, an important consideration in prenatal development and overall fetal well-being. Pregnancy hypertension, diabetes, and respiratory disease all have immediate impacts on the efficiency with which oxygen is transferred from mother to fetus. Poor maternal health can lead to compromised placental function and therefore the reduced supply of oxygen and nutrition necessary for optimal fetal development.

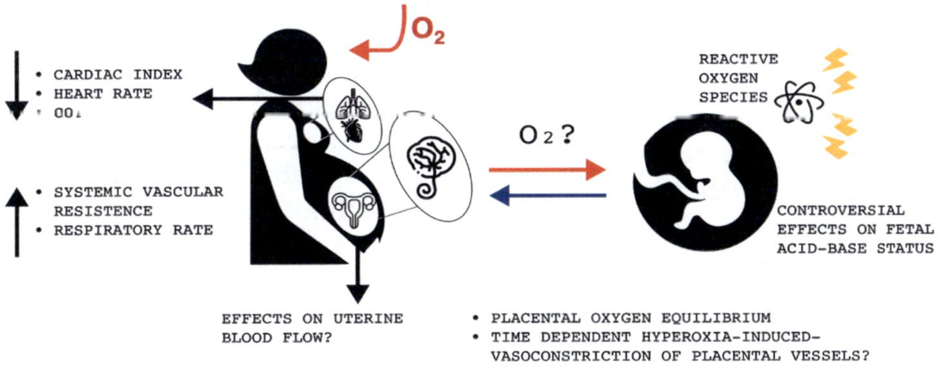

Figure 2.11. Effects of exogenous oxygen administration to normoxic pregnant women during labor.

Source: https://external-content.duckduckgo.com/iu/?u=https%3A%2F%2Fwww.mdpi.com%2Fchildren%2Fchildren-10-01420%2Farticle_deploy%2Fhtml%2Fimages%2Fchildren-10-01420-g001.png&f=1&nofb=1&ipt=8e4fb82f1c8c8b2a628c4336d14c98f75828a0a89cc8e5abd2ac81cfb9e2ef10.

This condition creates a hypoxic environment that can impede normal growth, leading to such complications as intrauterine growth restriction (IUGR), which is typically accompanied by many long-term health issues for the infant. Since the placenta exists as a barrier as well as a conduit of oxygen, maternal health has an important part in ensuring the fetus receives adequate oxygenation required for proper growth during pregnancy. In addition to the mechanical limitations related to maternal health, chemical considerations also have a crucial role to play in fetal oxygenation. For example, high maternal levels of carbon dioxide or decreased oxygen saturation may alter fetal hemodynamics and exacerbate any pre-existing hypoxic condition. Disturbances of metabolism such as these cause delays not only to the fetus during gestation but even for adaptation to life outside the uterus upon birth. Research indicates that the fine balance between fetal oxygenation and maternal well-being determines the structural and functional alterations the fetal cardiovascular system must adapt to (Tan et al., 2019) (Figure 2.11).

If the fetal environment is disrupted, these adaptations (critical to the transition from fetal to neonatal circulation) may be negatively affected. This once again underlines the requirement of robust maternal health in order to support a successful transition to life outside the uterus. Understanding the contribution of maternal health to fetal oxygenation is especially relevant given the heterogeneity of pregnancy complications. For instance, preeclampsia or gestational diabetes conditions worsen present ailments, leading to severe oxygen deficiencies in the infant. These are not only challenges for immediate adaptation at birth but also can predispose the child to future chronic disease (Hedi et al., 2021). While the body adapts the necessary cardiovascular changes to support extrauterine life, compromised fetal oxygenation can result in abnormal cardiac remodeling and enduring cardiovascular adversity. Thus, optimizing maternal health preconception and during pregnancy is critical to maximize fetal oxygenation and to facilitate an easier transition at birth, which in turn translates to improved health in mothers and their children.

2.4. Hormonal Regulation of Fetal Circulation

Hormonal control of fetal circulation is a dynamic and multifaceted process that provides the fetus-to-be with adequate oxygenation and nutrition and, simultaneously, prepares for transition into extrauterine life. Prostaglandins and catecholamines are among the principal hormones to modulate vascular resistance and blood flow within this unique circulatory system. During pregnancy, prostaglandins maintain the patency of the ductus arteriosus, a significant vessel connecting the pulmonary artery with the aorta, which allows blood to bypass the non-pulmonary fetal lungs. This process not only optimizes oxygenation to vital organs but also illustrates the intricate coordination of hormonal messages that fine-tune vascular reflexes in order to meet enlarging demands of an expanding fetus. The second change at birth is an accurate transition in these hormonal levels to enable fetal shunts to close and normal circulation after birth to start. Moreover, maternal hormones cannot be underrated in fetal circulation. Insulin and cortisol hormones, for example, not only influence maternal metabolism but play an immense role in fetal growth, such as circulatory adaptation. For instance, gestational diabetes mellitus (GDM) can impact the hormonal environment such that there is an increased risk of fetal macrosomia and subsequent complications during delivery due to hyper-delivery of nutrients (Jasmine et al., 2018). The fetus' hormonal interaction plays a critical role in ensuring appropriate growth and development of the cardiac chambers and the vasculature. Any disruption of such hormonal regulation can bring about irreversible effects on fetal outcomes, which might lead to chronicity in mother and child. Thus, understanding these endocrine effects is essential in maintaining optimal maternal-fetal health throughout pregnancy. When fetal to neonatal circulation changes, hormonal adjustment is critical to ensure successful adaptation. For example, placental flow decrease at birth leads to a premature prostaglandin level decline, which is responsible for functional closure of the ductus arteriosus. Meanwhile, an elevation of circulating catecholamines allows for transition from fetal to postnatal circulation via increased heart contractility and systemic vascular resistance (Douglas et al., 2016). This hormonal regulation is responsible for the direction of blood to the liver and lungs for maximal gas exchange and metabolic handling during the newborn period. Coordination and timing of these hormonal changes are critical, and delay or dysfunction can result in failure to transition with resultant neonatal complications. Therefore, a detailed appreciation of hormonal control in fetal circulation provides important information about normal physiology as well as potential pathological events at birth.

2.4.1. Role of Hormones in Fetal Development

Hormonal function in fetal development is vital in ensuring a smooth transition to birth. The hormone is a messenger responsible for coordinating physiological changes in favor of the mother and developing fetus as well. In fetal gestation, some of the hormones like human chorionic gonadotropin (hCG) maintain the corpus luteum active, hence sustaining progesterone secretion, which is instrumental in sustaining pregnancy and inhibiting uterine contractions. In addition, hormones such as estrogen and progesterone permit the preparation of the mother's body for birth and the development of fetal organs and systems, including the cardiovascular system. The subtle equilibrium of such hormones not only sustains the environment of the fetus but also prepares the mother's physiology for the impending delivery, demonstrating the complexity of hormonal interaction at this period of growth need.

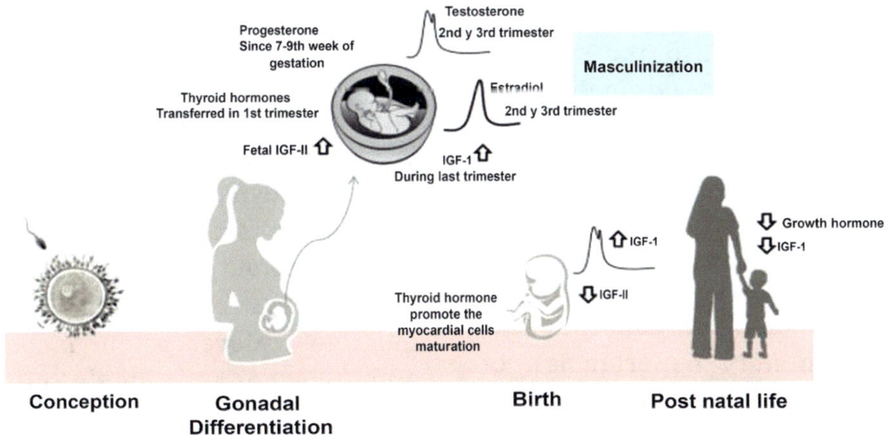

Figure 2.12. Role of hormones during gestation and early development.

Source: https://media.springernature.com/lw685/springer-static/image/chp%3A10.1007%2F978-3-031-32554-0_2/MediaObjects/480145_1_En_2_Fig3_HTML.png.

Furthermore, placental hormones function to regulate maternal metabolism and maximize nutrient transfer to the fetus. Insulin resistance in the mother is provoked by hormones like prolactin and placental lactogen, which may seem counterintuitive but is vital in ensuring glucose delivery to the growing fetus. This pathway is particularly relevant to gestational diabetes mellitus (GDM) where the balance of these hormones may be upset, and there could be detrimental effects on both mother and child. The evidence currently points to the derangements in placentation and subsequent changes in hormones being at the core of pre-eclampsia pathogenesis, as a condition manifesting as hypertension and proteinuria (Graham et al., 2019) (Figure 2.12).

Understanding the hormonal milieu of pregnancy can provide some information regarding potential therapeutic interventions that would reduce concomitant complications, and therefore their significance to fetal growth as well as maternal health. With birth transition, hormones facilitate deep physiological transformations necessary for independent life. Cortisol from fetal adrenal glands triggers breathing by fetal lungs by promoting the production of surfactant that reduces surface tension within the alveoli. Also, the surge of catecholamines during delivery aids in diverting fetal from placental to pulmonary respiration.

This transition is achieved through ductus arteriosus and foramen ovale closure that is mediated by hormonal changes and environmental stimuli. Dysregulation of these processes may result in consequences like persistent pulmonary hypertension of the newborn. Hence, the proper timing and interaction of hormones not only control fetal growth but also orchestrate the crucial transition to postnatal life, illustrating their supremacy in fetal health and best birthing outcome (Jasmine et al., 2018).

2.4.2. Influence of Maternal Hormones on Fetal Circulation

The intricate interaction among maternal hormones and fetal circulation is a significant factor in modulating the changing fetal environment. Pregnancy progesterone and estrogen tightly control a broad spectrum of physiological events essential for fetal development and growth. These maternal hormones regulate vascular adaptation so the placenta can effectively facilitate mother-fetal exchange of nutrients and oxygen. Specifically, progesterone is known to play a role of inducing vasodilation that helps increase blood supply to the uterus and hence the placental perfusion. Oxygenation and nutrition at this time are critical to the maintenance of proper function of fetal organs and systems, including the circulatory system itself that sets the stage for the transition at birth.

The influence of maternal hormones is not limited to the mere regulation of blood flow; they have a direct impact on fetal circulatory dynamics as well. Alteration in hormonal levels can influence the equilibrium in the fetal heart and great vessels, facilitating adaptation as the fetus prepares itself for birth. For instance, elevated maternal blood levels of estrogen are accompanied by enhanced production of nitric oxide, a potent vasodilator that regulates systemic vascular resistance and triggers preferential blood flow to central fetal organs. Such hemodynamic changes are most important because they are used to regulate blood pressure and cardiac output in the fetus's circulation. As pregnancy advances, the interactions between these fetal development maternal hormones and pregnant femme's circulating fetal systems become increasingly more intricate, demonstrating the function of hormones in prenatal growth (Figure 2.13).

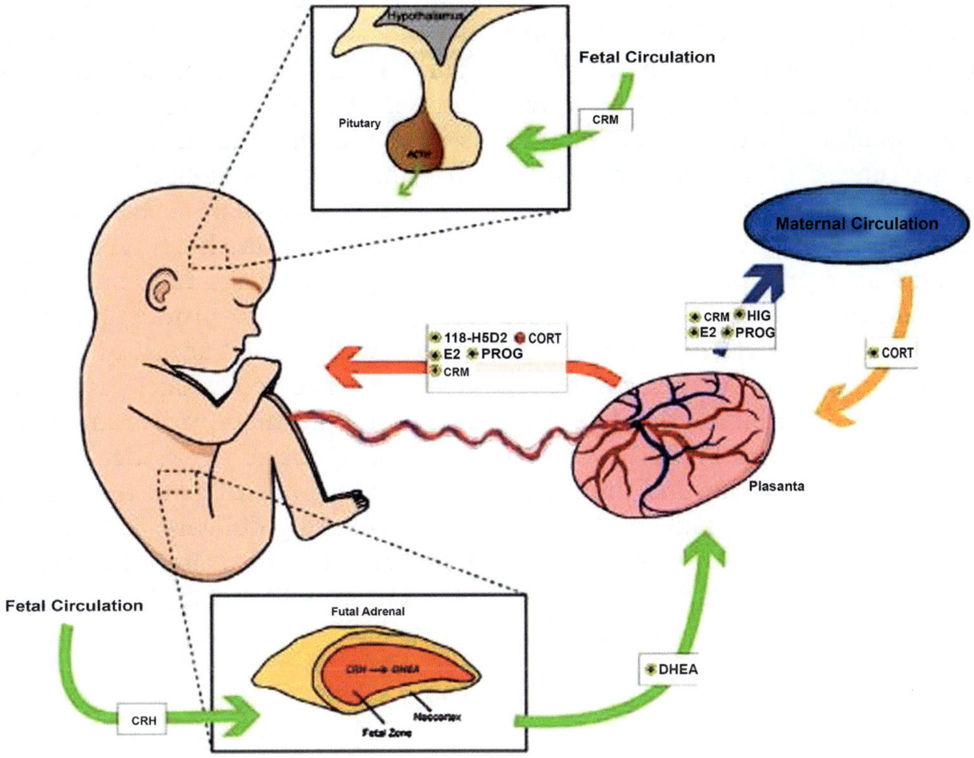

Figure 2.13. Representation of the third-trimester fetus and the hormone flux from the placenta to fetal circulation (red arrow), placenta to maternal circulation (blue arrow), and reciprocal exchanges (orange arrow).

Source: https://www.researchgate.net/publication/334684102_The_Third_Trimester_Human_Fetus_may_be_Protected_from_Prenatal_Stress_and_Programmed_Adult_Mental_Illness.

Additionally, maternal stress and resulting hormone levels may also direct fetal circulatory parameters and results. Elevated cortisol levels, most often due to chronic stress, have been shown to have detrimental effects on fetal growth and preterm birth, as viewed in several studies. This chronic increase in stress hormones imparts additional complexity to fetal circulation by the potential increase of allostatic load on the mother, with direct effect on fetal heart rate and vascular resistance. Uncovering such complex mechanisms provides an opportunity for intervention; as a prime example, monitoring maternal stress and profiling maternal hormones can lead to specific approaches that minimize threats of adverse pregnancy outcomes (Granger et al., 2014; McCreary et al., 2015). Thus, maternal hormones shape fetal circulation not only in a normal state but also adaptively respond to pregnancy pathophysiology stressors.

2.4.3. Changes in Hormone Levels at Birth

Childbirth results in a profound hormonal shift which plays a crucial role in fetal to neonatal circulation transition. Prior to birth, the placenta releases a set of hormones including human placental lactogen and progesterone that support pregnancy and prepare the fetus for birth.

Nevertheless, after giving birth, the supply of these hormones from the mother comes down very quickly and plasma levels lower. This abrupt change in the levels of hormones alerts the newborns organs of adaptation to the outside world. For instance, a reduction in progesterone levels is credited with stimulating the drive to breathe in the newborn to allow for the initiation of proper lung function. As the neonate takes its first breaths, the inflow of oxygen into the lungs causes the release of catecholamines, further enhancing the redistribution of blood flow from the placental circuit and autonomous systemic circulation. Apart from progesterone, some other significant hormonal changes are seen as cortisol levels (which are generally high in the fetus at term) also drop precipitously at birth. This fall triggers a cascade of metabolic responses, including gluconeogenesis and lipolysis that are required for energy production in the newborn. Glucose metabolism is particularly important since the newborn must adjust quickly to the end of the placental glucose supply. Furthermore, changes in hormone levels, such as increased insulin sensitivity immediately after birth, stimulate the uptake of glucose, thereby prevent hypoglycemia—a normal danger to infants after birth. These mechanisms emphasize the critical role of hormonal transitions in the perinatal phase and the importance of such transitions to the short-term health outcomes of the infant. Additionally, the hormonal milieu during delivery continues to influence the long-term health outcomes of the neonate. Experiments demonstrate that abrupt changes in hormone concentration, particularly relating to stress and growth factors, have long-term effects on an infant's metabolic profile (Figure 2.14).

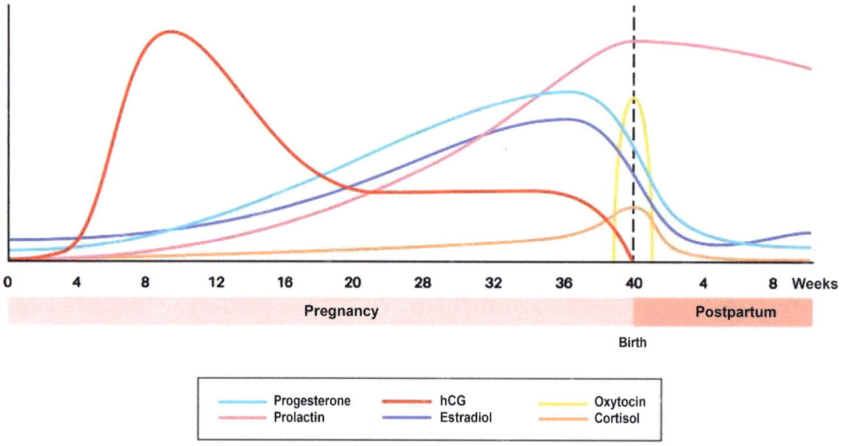

Figure 2.14. Levels of hormones in pregnancy.

Source: https://external-content.duckduckgo.com/iu/?u=https%3A%2F%2Fimg.freepik.com%2Fpremium-vector%2Flevels-hormones-pregnancy-hcg-prolactin-cortisol-estradiol-progesterone-oxytocin-woman-body-female-hormones-changes-chart-from-first-weeks-birth-postpartum-vector_206049-7690.jpg%3Fw%3D1800&f=1&nofb=1&ipt=7b9206baf4a19438e518a98a54980d6a5af10d34fa3cfa3931addaf95bf81821.

For example, maternal disease gestational diabetes mellitus (GDM) is able to induce altered hormone patterns, predisposing infants to metabolic disease during adult life, such as obesity and type 2 diabetes. Similarly, hormonal alterations in diseases such as pre-eclampsia are able to influence fetal growth, leading to short- and long-term morbidity. As the science continues to uncover the mechanics of these hormonal interactions, particularly as they relate to their effects on the health of neonates, it is increasingly important to see how abnormal levels of maternal or placental hormones can result in detrimental effects for the neonate, as supported by current research within the field (Graham et al., 2019; Jasmine et al., 2018).

2.5. Transition from Fetal to Neonatal Circulation

Transition from fetal to neonatal circulation is a critical process occurring at the time of birth, involving significant physiological alterations. During fetal life in the uterus, a fetus relies on placental circulation, diverting oxygenated blood from the umbilical vein without passing through the lungs and liver through shunts such as the ductus arteriosus and foramen ovale. By birth, however, the need for these shunts diminishes as the infant begins to take in air and generate its own circulation. Initial aeration of lungs largely increases pulmonary blood flow (PBF), the onset of such a vital transition. Rapid lung aeration thus becomes pivotal in order for the newborn to begin pulmonary gas exchange necessary for survival outside the uterus. The pathologies during this transition may manifest in the modes of hemodynamic instability, and such problems become neonatal care concerns with the necessity of immediate monitoring and intervention (Sehgal et al., 2021). One of the most frequent complications that arise due to inadequate transition is pulmonary arterial hypertension of the neonate (PAHN), which can be a result of gestational chronic hypoxia. Failure to adjust to the respiratory needs of postuterine life can lead to increased pulmonary vascular resistance and pulmonary arterial remodeling. As evidenced by research, fetal hypoxia, intrauterine growth restriction, and other adverse prenatal conditions contribute significantly to neonatal respiratory distress and complications. Discovery of the underlying mechanisms by which these conditions impact the transition is imperative for their targeted medical management. From the investigation of various animal models, and sheep in particular, scientists were capable of gaining valuable insights about the complex interaction between prenatal factors and neonatal cardiorespiratory outcomes, and advance the field's knowledge about PAHN and its significance on neonatal health (Gonz et al., 2020) (Figure 2.15).

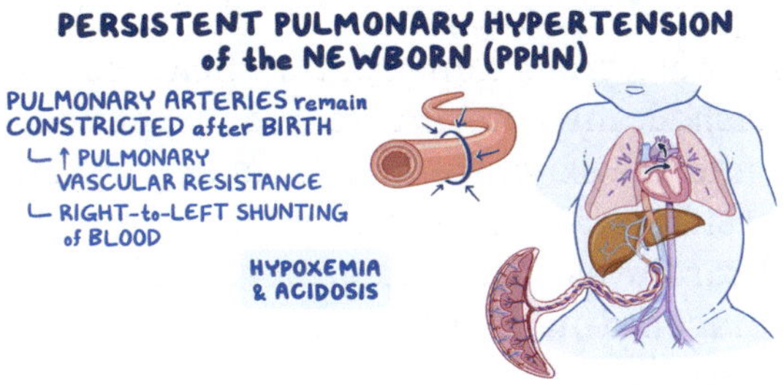

Figure 2.15. Pulmonary hypertension of the newborn (PPHN).

Source: https://external-content.duckduckgo.com/iu/?u=https%3A%2F%2Fosmose-it.s3.amazonaws.com%2Fc8oMVmigRauOjl9mEOAPEiIpRnet0UWF%2F_.jpg&f=1&nofb=1&ipt=483e62d7dfb0a8a38b5bffc70c6989f509b2f1b270bd4dd41e16cbb7aad6030b.

In addition, effective transition management plays an essential role in neonatal outcomes, particularly in complicated cases by pathological conditions or birth interventions. Timing and mode of umbilical cord clamping are important since delayed clamping has been identified to increase blood volume and stabilize neonatal hemodynamics. Physiological cord clamping may have the capability to support optimal transition through the delivery of blood to the lungs, and the development of normal pulmonary perfusion. Contemporary neonatal assessment techniques, including the application of targeted echocardiography, also provide valuable information regarding post-delivery cardiovascular status. By using advanced monitoring techniques, clinicians can individualize therapies according to the personalized requirements of each infant and hence develop enhanced outcomes in high-risk patients with hypoxic-ischemic injury or associated complications (Sehgal et al., 2021).

2.5.1. Immediate Changes at Birth

The moment of birth is characterized by an interposed transitional period, in which a baby must transition from a sheltered, well-nourished intrauterine to the challenges of extrauterine existence. Such a sudden transition necessitates a dramatic reorganization of the fetal cardiovascular system, specifically geared to placenta-dependent life. The neonate, at birth, experiences an acute increase in systemic oxygenation, with subsequent closure of ductal shunts that had shunted blood from the lungs. The foramen ovale and ductus arteriosus, essential fetal circulation structures, begin to close, making room for pulmonary circulation to develop. In itself, this is normally a smooth process, however this can present unique challenges in some instances, such as transposition of the great arteries. In such cases, the newborn will develop significant complications, to which immediate intervention should be offered in a bid to stabilize oxygen and maintain circulation (Jesse et al., 2024). Besides the cardiovascular adaptations, the brain also undergoes a sophisticated series of changes throughout this process. The perinatal window represents one of dynamic transitions in brain structure and function evoked by the need for rapid adaptation to an external environment. Evidence indicates that neurodevelopmental trajectories show a mix of discontinuity and continuity throughout the course of newborns across the crossing of the birth barrier. For example, some of the characteristics of the brain, including total white matter and gray matter volume, show consistent growth patterns, whereas extra-cerebrospinal fluid volume and ventricular volume show abrupt change. It is important to appreciate these6 neurodevelopmental changes because they may be linked with later cognitive and physiological consequences. Recognition of the significance of such acute adaptations underscores a requirement for comprehensive neonatal care, with an equal focus on circulatory health and best neurodevelopment (Mihailov et al., 2024). The acute adaptations of birth are not only physiological and neurodevelopmental; they also have far-reaching implications for clinical handling of the newborn. Doctors must be prepared to manage complications of the complexities of this transition, such as persistent pulmonary hypertension of the newborn (PPHN). In situations like transposition of the great arteries, in which the circulatory adaptation places an infant at risk of catastrophic hemodynamic instability, early detection and management become essential. Treatment interventions typically include non-invasive ventilation and pharmacologic therapy to maintain ductal patency. It is essential to monitor such infants closely in the initial hours of birth since early intervention is very effective in optimizing outcomes and reducing the risk for long-term complications. Therefore, comprehension of multi-aspectual causality of changes at birth is essential for clinicians to optimize neonatal health and development (Jesse et al., 2024).

2.5.2. Closure of Fetal Shunts

The closure of fetal shunts is an imperative component of the fetal to neonatal transition. During fetal life, the ductus arteriosus (DA) and the foramen ovale (FO) enable the shunting of the non-pumping fetal lungs so that oxygenated blood from the placenta can perfuse vital organs effectively. The DA shunts blood from the pulmonary artery to the aorta directly, while the FO allows blood from the right atrium to flow into the left atrium without passing through pulmonary circulation whatsoever. During birth, the closure of placental circulation and the onset of lung ventilation impose significant pressure changes in the cardiovascular system. These alterations cause the physiological closure of the DA and FO, remodeling fetal circulation to supply the respiratory needs of the newborn, ensuring proper oxygenation through the lungs as the umbilical cord has been obstructed and the placenta is no longer used (Souza et al., 2023). The processes behind the closure of these shunts can be explained and clarify potential complications when this physiological response does not occur as expected. For instance, if the DA persists into life, patent ductus arteriosus (PDA), it will create significant hemodynamic changes, such that there will be an abnormal shunt of blood from the aorta into the pulmonary artery. This not only impairs systemic oxygenation but also increases the workload of the left ventricle, which will cause left ventricular hypertrophy and pulmonary hypertension if neglected. Recognition of these complications is necessary to inform early intervention. Murmurs on physical examination, as part of clinical presentation, may need additional assessment with echocardiography to assess the size of the shunt and cardiac function effects (Souza et al., 2023). Early intervention for PDA needs to be initiated to avoid chronic sequelae of persistent fetal shunting patterns (Figure 2.16).

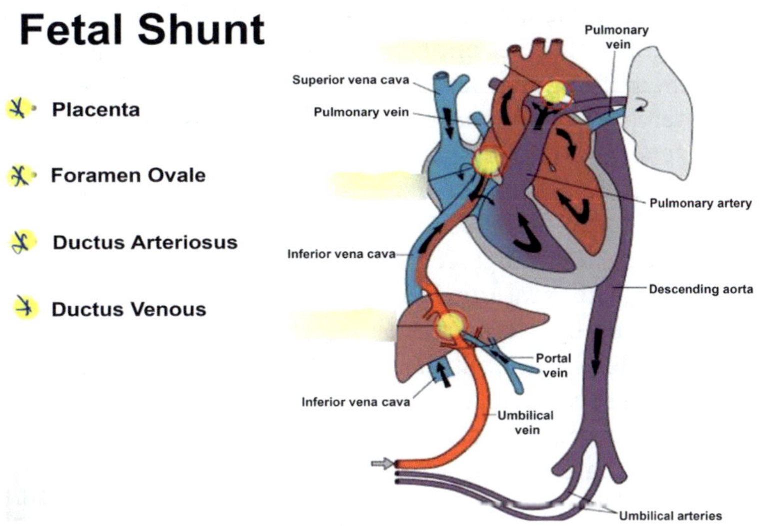

Figure 2.16. Fetal shunts.

Source: https://external-content.duckduckgo.com/iu/?u=https%3A%2F%2Fo.quizlet.com%2FgKXmP3HvvqQrHcBZTwKT4A_b.png&f=1&nofb=1&ipt=435eac01943344bd9b92921320cc40ab3cb1f0fec9fc1cda3f574432af4a895d.

The mode and timing of shunt closure are also influenced by various perinatal factors, which need to be known about neonatal care guidelines. Recent controversy regarding delayed cord clamping (DCC) has educated us regarding its role in the regulation of fetal-neonatal transition. DCC supports increased blood volume in the neonate, which is perhaps able to enhance transitional hemodynamics by giving a good access perfusion to important organs and reducing the frequency of complications due to premature fetal shunt closure. This is particularly applicable to preterm infants, who may have immature cardiopulmonary circuitry. By adjusting the clamping of the umbilical cord, healthcare providers aim to facilitate more seamless cardiovascular adaptation, thus avoiding pathologies such as PDA and subsequent cardiovascular distress, improving the outlook for vulnerable newborns (Robinson et al., 2022).

2.5.3. Establishment of Independent Neonatal Circulation

Accomplishment of independent neonatal circulation is a critical turning point in the physiology of a newborn. In fetal development, the fetal circulatory system relies on the placenta for oxygen and nutrients, with oxygenated blood supplied from the mother through the umbilical vein. At birth, however, this reliance ends abruptly, necessitating immediate adjustments in the cardiovascular system of the neonate. Transition itself involves several key changes, primarily the obliteration of fetal shunts such as the foramen ovale and ductus arteriosus that direct blood flow through the lungs for the first time. Additionally, these adaptations in circulatory pattern are facilitated by increased systemic vascular resistance following umbilical cord clamping, affecting pressure gradients and a premium being placed on effective pulmonary circulation to oxygenate the blood. The physiological process by which neonates can respire and oxygenate independently is highly coordinated physiologically, with initiation brought about by the act of birth itself. When the new baby takes its first respiration, immense negative intrathoracic pressure is generated, allowing air into the lungs. This air intake drains fetal lung fluid, which must be expelled in order that effective gas exchange can occur. Clearance of lung fluid is an important factor in determining the manner in which retention leads to respiratory distress in preterm infants who may not effectively utilize catecholamine-mediated mechanisms of absorption of lung interstitial fluid. Consequently, lung fluid clearance dynamics determine the onset of functional neonatal respiration (Hemananda, 2020). In addition, delayed cord clamping following birth can impact the establishment of independent circulation. Delayed cord clamping (DCC), allowing continued placental blood flow for a brief period following birth, has been demonstrated to enhance neonatal outcome through promotion of optimal transfusion and iron storage maximization, necessary for brain development. Maximal fetal-maternal gas exchange is developed during this time, enabling neonates to maintain some oxygenation while switching over to independent air-breathing physiology. The evidence indicates that DCC is particularly beneficial in extremely preterm infants by improving hemodynamic stability and reducing the risk of complications such as anemia and respiratory distress. However, a careful clinical judgment is necessary as contraindications of DCC exist and need to be evaluated to ensure the safety of both mother and neonate (Govindaswami et al., 2020).

2.6. Complications in Fetal Circulation

Complications of fetal circulation are crucial because they can lead to undesirable outcomes in both the postnatal and perinatal periods. The specialized physiology of fetal life (with the dependence on placental circulation) enables special adaptation within the cardiovascular system. Such adaptations prove troublesome if they fail to properly resolve during transition at birth. For instance, conditions like PDA arise when the ductus arteriosus fails to close, resulting in aberrant patterns of blood flow which can stress the neonatal heart and lungs. Such conditions have the potential to become catastrophic complications if they go unchecked, pointing to the importance of close monitoring and management during this phase of transition from fetal to independent circulation. The fetal circulation problems are compounded if preterm birth is experienced. Preterm infants are particularly susceptible to instability of their cardiovascular system from poorly developed adaptations that would otherwise facilitate a safe transition at birth. Research indicates that preterm infants are more likely to experience the complications of hemodynamic instability and persistent fetal patterns of circulation, which have important short-term and long-term prognoses. The physiological variations of preterm neonates necessitate special approaches to adopt in their care, remembering that their cardiovascular system may not react with the same effective transition as full-term neonates. It is a period of intricate hemodynamics where interventions to manage conditions like PDA are necessary, remembering that even a delay results in increased morbidity and long-term effects. Echocardiographic investigations have yielded important information regarding the incidence of ductal patency in neonates, outlining complications that can occur in fetal circulation. Results from the Copenhagen Baby Heart Study indicate that roughly 36% of full-term neonates have an open ductus arteriosus upon birth, decreasing remarkably to as little as 0.6% by day seven. This early closure serves to underscore the normal physiological sequence that is to occur, as well as the fact that a large proportion of neonates are vulnerable to ductal complications in the first instance. This finding emphasizes the need for vigilant cardiac assessment in the initial week of life, since preclosure can result in serious effects, including compromised pulmonary circulation and cardiac failure. Transition from fetal to neonatal thus represents an important window of opportunity, in which knowledge regarding complications in fetal circulation can guide enhanced healthcare policy and intervention among vulnerable groups to more favorable outcomes for vulnerable infants (Mariager et al., 2023; Robyn et al., 2023).

2.6.1. Congenital Heart Defects

Congenital heart defects, or CHDs, are a critical part of fetal circulation and the birth transition. CHDs are abnormalities in heart development during gestation that lead to various complications in the newborn. The complexity of fetal circulation, which is distinct from postnatal circulation, underscores the necessity for understanding how defects alter the blood flow dynamics. During intrauterine life, oxygen supply through shunts such as the ductus arteriosus and foramen ovale is supplemented, circumventing malfunctioning lungs. Any defects in these mechanisms can result in calamitous effects such as hypoxia or heart failure upon birth. The intricacies of CHDs emphasize the urgency of early detection and treatment to counteract the risk factors, illustrating how the prenatal cardiovascular development influences neonatal health as a whole. The transition from fetal to postnatal circulation is a critical juncture closely connected with congenital heart defects. During birth, the closure of the shunt like the ductus arteriosus should be triggered, directing blood to the pulmonary capillaries to make oxygenation easier. When CHDs are present, this may not be so smooth though. Tetralogy of Fallot or septal defects in the ventricles may result in poor pulmonary circulation, and therefore oxygenating the blood may be hard. The physical adjustments required during birthplace severe stress on CHD infants, which could be in the shape of compromised breathing, cyanosis, or somnolence. Understanding these transitions and their impacts on newborns with congenital conditions represents an essential requirement for clinical practitioners to enable timely intervention towards fostering cardiovascular stability and health in the newborns. Congenital heart defect treatment requires concerted effort that is not only surgical in scope but also requires continued follow-up of patients as well as readjustment of treatment regimens. Treatment protocol development reflects the acknowledgment of the unique challenges presented by pediatric cardiac disease, particularly with regard to the developments of research. One of the central features of care is aligning practice with guidelines established by regulatory bodies like the American College of Cardiology and American Heart Association, which publish evidence-based guidelines for best patient outcomes. The guidelines address the nuances of diagnosing and managing CHDs, such as shared decision-making and patient engagement to tailor interventions based on individual circumstances. Finally, thorough understanding and application of these recommendations are necessary in order to give maximum care to congenital heart-defective infants, as they go through the critical transition from fetal to postnatal life (Erika et al., 2018; Stout et al., 2018).

2.6.2. Placental Insufficiency

Placental insufficiency is one of the principal etiologic factors for adverse conditions in fetal circulation and transition at birth. Placental insufficiency is when the placenta is unable to supply an adequate amount of oxygen and nutrients to the developing fetus, resulting in conditions such as fetal growth restriction (FGR). The fetus relies on the placenta for necessary nutrients, so any disruption in placental function can hinder normal development and growth. Inadequate placental perfusion may result in hypoxia, wherein the fetus remains inadequately oxygenated and entirely disrupts its mechanism for adaptation during the newborn transition to postnatal life. This critical interaction underscores the lifeline role of placentas in the preservation of fetal health, since FGR and associated pathologies can complicate delivery and transition even more, underlining the critical implications of placental insufficiency on fetal physiology. The sophisticated biological processes of fetal transition during birth highlight the significance of placental insufficiency. Abnormal placentation results in hypoxia that can initiate a cascade of inflammatory events, further exacerbating the transition process from fetal to neonatal circulation. Diseases such as chorioamnionitis, inflammation of fetal membranes, have been associated with serious circulatory disorders during birth. Research has established that the cytokine interleukin (IL)-1 is pivotal in this inflammation, and it is responsible for exacerbating complications of placental insufficiency, such as poor transition outcomes. Inflammatory pathway interventions might help in countering issues resulting from dysfunctional placenta, as an indication of the necessity for a thorough understanding of the mechanisms involved in order to improve care processes and outcomes of the affected newborns, particularly in preterm babies, whose vulnerability is considerably increased (Josephine et al., 2023) (Figure 2.17).

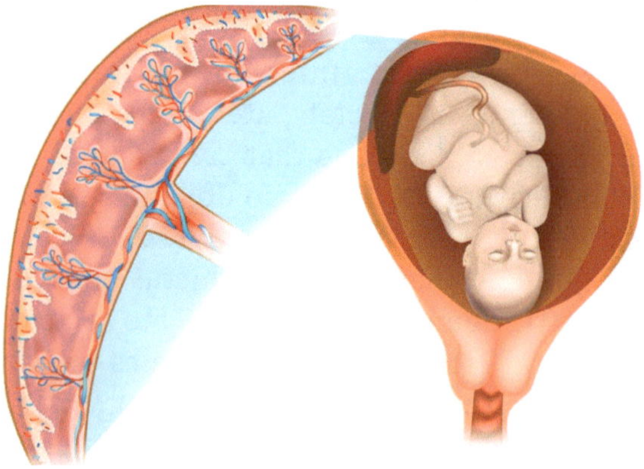

Figure 2.17. Placental insufficiency.

Source: https://cdn.apollohospitals.com/health-library-prod/2022/08/shutterstock_1277952880-Converted.jpg.

Moreover, a plan for managing placental insufficiency needs to take into account its long-term effects on the circulatory health and developmental potential of an affected infant. Individuals with issues in their placentas can expect a variety of chronic problems-from cardiovascular disease complications to increased susceptibility to adult-onset metabolic disease. To investigate the relationship between early life conditions linked with placental insufficiency and how they are expressed later on is most crucial in order to devise targeted interventional studies. Indeed, current developments in neonatal therapy and intervention science are promising to reverse the impact of placental insufficiency. This can involve the optimization of screening devices for the high-risk pregnancies, implementation of preventive interventions, and seeking therapeutic interventions that can enhance the health of the fetus to facilitate delivery at birth with ease, hence relieving the related diseases of early life hinging on placental insufficiency (Hedi et al., 2021).

2.6.3. Impact of Maternal Conditions on Fetal Circulation

Maternal effects on fetal circulation are a critical area of research, with hypertensive disorders of pregnancy (HDP) being a prime example. HDP can significantly modify placental blood flow, thus affecting fetal oxygenation and nutrient delivery. High blood pressure that develops during pregnancy puts the mother and fetus at risk and leads to adverse outcomes like fetal growth restriction and preterm birth. Optimal management of HDP is essential to prevent such risks since this has a direct effect on fetal circulation and general pregnancy outcomes. Such studies as are referenced by Kwun et al. (2024) show the potential of digital health interventions in optimizing blood pressure control throughout pregnancy, showing how technology acts as an agent of change in enhancing maternal-fetal health through enhanced engagement and monitoring approaches. Therefore, management of maternal conditions with new care has the ability to stimulate preferable changes in fetal circulation. Complications during motherhood may lead to a deviation from normal fetal circulation to pathologic conditions. Preterm labor (which occurs prior to the 37th week of gestation) is very dangerous to the infant since the development of effective circulatory transition becomes more complex. Maternal chorioamnionitis and fetal growth restriction are well-established preterm conditions, both of which can potentially severely jeopardize the process necessary to secure successful neonatal circulation. This is mediated through inflammatory processes that can potentially interfere with normal adaptation processes necessary to secure optimal physiological change following birth, as posited by Josephine et al. (2023). These are not only complications that impact neonatal outcomes within the acute time period but also predispose infants to long-term health issues, making it critical that maternal care be managed to ensure proper fetal circulation during critical periods of gestation. Ascertaining factors impacting maternal health, particularly inflammatory reactions, is a fundamental point in the study of fetal circulation. An environment of conditions such as chorioamnionitis or FGR initiates a cascade of inflammatory cytokines, effectively compromising fetal adaptations to the intrapartum environment. Maternal inflammation and fetal circulation interaction can lead to impaired transitions at birth and result in states of hypoxia or reduced perfusion. Current research also shows that modulation of inflammatory mediators like interleukin-1 can amplify circulatory transitions in neonates with involvement, tailoring therapy to the specific challenges presented by maternal disease (Josephine et al., 2023). If prevention and treatment approaches are geared towards maternal health, clinicians can maximize fetal health and have circulatory transitions at birth as smooth as possible, thus providing healthier newborn outcomes.

SUMMARY

In combining fetal circulatory dynamics with the critical transition that occurs at birth, it is evident that understanding these processes is at the center of optimizing neonatal outcomes. Transient transition from a fetal to an independent circulatory system is a critical mechanism of physiological adaptation in neonates. With their shift from placental oxygenation and nutrition delivery, the role of each cardiovascular structure—particularly the right ventricle and its relationship to the pulmonary and systemic circulations—only becomes increasingly important. The case of infants born with congenital illness, including pulmonary valve abnormalities, underscores the necessity for early diagnosis and intervention, as described in existing studies involving prenatal diagnosis and treatment protocols (Xie et al., 2024). The evolving comprehension of fetal and neonatal cardiac performance will continue to gain our understanding of these transitions. Furthermore, the introduction of novel echocardiographic approaches offers incomparable information regarding the hemodynamic changes that accompany and occur after birth. Traditional approaches alone are insufficient to properly discern subtle changes in ventricular geometry and function, particularly in structurally abnormal fetuses. Quantitative measurement of stroke volume and cardiac output has recorded tremendous differences between fetal and postnatal systemic right ventricles and indicated the need for intensive monitoring and tailor-made interventions among these high-risk populations (Brett et al., 2024). Such a policy signals a focus on multidisciplinary care among obstetricians, neonatologists, and pediatric cardiologists with a focus towards aggressive management of high-risk neonates. Lastly, the transition at birth is much more than a physiological event but instead a complex process requiring complete understanding of fetal cardiovascular development. Future studies should focus on refinement of diagnostic methods and treatment strategies that consider the specific needs of the patients. It is also important to maintain collaboration among different healthcare multidisciplinary professionals as it is heightened efforts to advance knowledge in this area. The practice of tailored management strategies according to the in-depth assessment of fetal conditions is the foundation for the opportunity for increased prognosis, thereby warranting continued innovation in fetal and neonatal health practice (Brett et al., 2024).

Fetal circulation study reveals astounding physiological changes, allowing development to occur and providing in-utero fetus oxygenation required for nourishment. These changes occur through specialized tissues such as the placenta, umbilical cord, and some vessels, allowing oxygen and nutrient delivery from mother to fetus and waste product removal to be effective. Of special interest are the primary shunts, including the ductus venosus, foramen ovale, and ductus arteriosus, that play significant roles in guiding blood flow in the fetal circulation. In circumventing the unavailable-to-the-fetus pulmonary circuit, the shunts allow for the delivery of oxygenated blood to essential organs, such as the brain and heart, thereby allowing for optimal fetal development and growth. This fine-tuned balance emphasizes the role of fetal adaptations in making the transition to independent postnatal life, which is based on the immediate physiological adaptation during birth (Hedi et al., 2021). Birth transition describes a remarkable transformation of circulatory patterns, in which the newborn must successfully establish an effective pulmonary circulation. During the first breath, lung inflation has an immediate effect on intrathoracic pressure, resulting in the closure of the ductus arteriosus and foramen ovale that were critical for fetal circulation. This closure redirects flow of blood to the lungs for oxygenation, establishing normal adult-type circulation. Furthermore, cessation of placental circulation results in contraction of the umbilical artery and veins, adding further strength to the alteration of blood flow patterns. These critical physiological changes ensure that the newborn is capable of sustaining independent life outside the womb. Understanding these mechanisms plays a vital role in detecting any potential complications during and after delivery, which arise due to incomplete or abnormal changes in circulatory function (Griselda et al., 2020). Successful fetal to neonatal circulation is not just crucial for survival but also determinantal to overall health outcomes. Complications due to the failure of the big structures to close or transform properly can lead to a variety of neonatal disorders, such as patent ductus arteriosus or pulmonary hypertension. Clinically speaking, it is necessary that healthcare professionals oversee and enable this transition, particularly for preterm or at-risk infants. Advances in neonatal medicine—such as better respiratory support and intervention—are needed to manage these complications appropriately. By focusing on fetal circulation nuances and physiological variations that take place at birth, healthcare personnel can better prepare for early postnatal treatment, which ultimately improves newborns. Subsequent studies on these processes will likely offer further explanations, enabling us to more comprehensively understand fetal and neonatal condition in different groups and clinical settings (Hedi et al., 2021).

CLOSER LOOK

PHYSIOLOGY OF TRANSITIONAL CIRCULATION

Transitional circulation is the period when fetal circulation transitions to neonatal phenotype. This occurs a few minutes after birth with clamping of the umbilical cord and aeration of the lungs following the first few breaths. Physiological adaptation post-birth is a complex process with numerous adaptive changes happening at the same time in a variety of organs. The most critical are the respiratory and cardiovascular systems. Two factors immediately at birth determine whether the new baby is going to make a successful transition or not.

After clamping of the cord, systemic vascular resistance increases, lungs become aerated, and fetal shunts close functionally; the order of changes described in Figure 2.18 allows for transition from fetal to neonatal circulation.

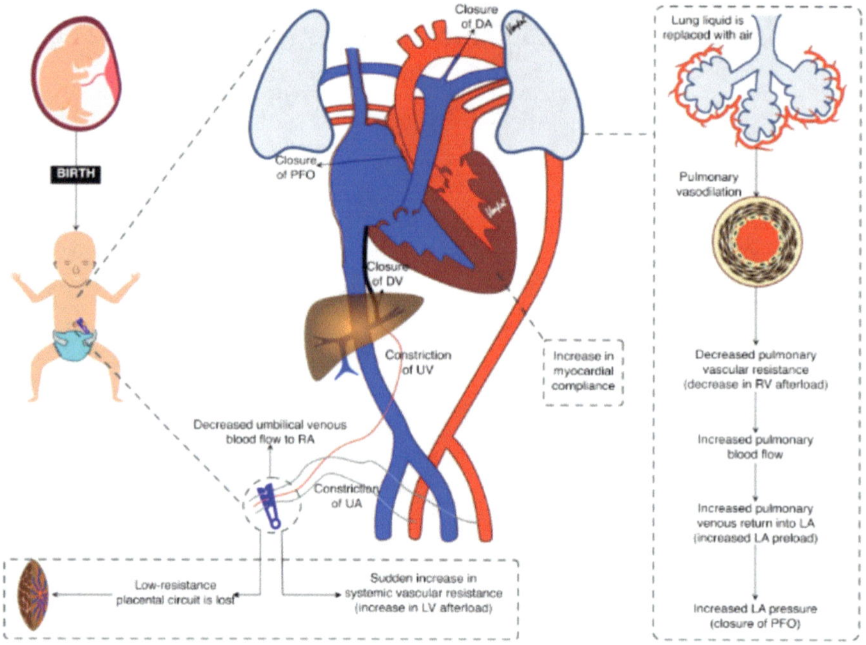

Figure 2.18. Diagram illustrating the physiological changes in the cardiovascular and pulmonary systems at birth, including closure of fetal shunts (ductus arteriosus, ductus venosus, and foramen ovale) and initiation of pulmonary circulation.

Source: https://encrypted-tbn0.gstatic.com/images?q=tbn:ANd9GcQYN5yOGa51Li4Joj7NhfzWhNq1Zni657GkzQ&s.

First, air displaces lung fluid at the start of air breathing. Despite the mechanism not appearing to be clear, air inflation of the lung is a strong pulmonary vasodilator. In a paper by Lang et al., it was clear that an increase in total pulmonary blood flow (PBF) due to partial lung aeration can be mediated by a vagal reflex. This leads to an abrupt drop PVR and an abrupt and notable increase

(~30 fold) in PBF. When PVR abruptly declines below SVR, shunting through the DA becomes reversed (left-to-right) allowing LV output to feed into PBF. Additional deoxygenated blood is thus pumped to the lung for oxygenation by this mechanism. Pulmonary veins carry oxygenated blood back from the lungs to the left atrium, thereby adding the contribution of the lungs to LV preload, and lungs being the sole source of preload.

Second, with cord clamping, umbilical venous blood flow via ductus venosus and foramen ovale decreases and consequently preload arriving at the left ventricle via the left atrium decreases. Clamping of the umbilical artery also obliterates the low-resistance placental circuit leaving the neonatal left ventricle to perceive an abrupt increase in SVR (increase in LV afterload), leading to an abrupt "step-like" increase in arterial blood pressure and upper body blood flow.

To understand what happens in the transition and how the changes occur, one must first be aware of fetal cardiovascular structure and function.

References

1. Abu-Raya, B., Michalski, C., Sadarangani, M., & Lavoie, P. M. (2020). Maternal immunological adaptation during normal pregnancy. *Frontiers in Immunology, 11*. https://doi.org/10.3389/fimmu.2020.575197 (accessed on 15th July 2025).
2. Alengebawy, A., Abdelkhalek, S. T., Qureshi, S. R., & Wang, M. Q. (2021). Heavy metals and pesticides toxicity in agricultural soil and plants: Ecological risks and human health implications. *Toxics, 9*, 42–42. https://doi.org/10.3390/toxics9030042 (accessed on 15th July 2025).
3. Ander, S. E., Diamond, M., & Coyne, C. B. (2019). Immune responses at the maternal-fetal interface. *Science Immunology, 4*. https://doi.org/10.1126/sciimmunol.aat6114 (accessed on 15th July 2025).
4. Bava, S., Katheria, A. C., Lakshminrusimha, S., et al. (2019). Placental transfusion for asphyxiated infants. https://core.ac.uk/download/323071671.pdf (accessed on 15th July 2025).
5. Begliuomini, S., Boldrini, A., Casarosa, E., et al. (2012). Compensatory feta-placental upregulation of the nitric oxide system during fetal growth restriction. https://core.ac.uk/download/224999362.pdf (accessed on 15th July 2025).
6. Burton, G. J., Redman, C. W. G., Roberts, J. M., & Moffett, A. (2019). Pre-eclampsia: Pathophysiology and clinical implications. *BMJ*. https://doi.org/10.1136/bmj.l2381 (accessed on 15th July 2025).
7. Cabral-Pacheco, G. A., Garza-Veloz, I., Castruita-De la Rosa, C., Ramirez-Acuña, J. M., Perez-Romero, B. A., Guerrero-Rodriguez, J. F., Martínez-Avila, N., et al. (2020). The roles of matrix metalloproteinases and their inhibitors in human diseases. *International Journal of Molecular Sciences, 21*, 9739–9739. https://doi.org/10.3390/ijms21249739 (accessed on 15th July 2025).
8. Casarotto, L., Jones, H. N., Chavatte-Palmer, P., Laporta, J., Peñagaricano, F., Ouellet, V., Bromfield, J., et al. (2024). Late gestation heat stress alters placental structure and function in multiparous dairy cows. *Journal of Dairy Science*. https://www.semanticscholar.org/paper/6793df15f2698eaef5ebe330046efdf4824a3e44 (accessed on 15th July 2025).
9. Claahsen-van der Grinten, H. L., Speiser, P., Ahmed, S. F., Arlt, W., Auchus, R. J., Falhammar, H., Flück, C. E., et al. (2021). Congenital adrenal hyperplasia—Current insights in pathophysiology, diagnostics, and management. *Endocrine Reviews, 43*, 91–159. https://doi.org/10.1210/endrev/bnab016 (accessed on 15th July 2025).
10. Dudley, A. C., & Griffioen, A. W. (2023). Pathological angiogenesis: Mechanisms and therapeutic strategies. *Angiogenesis, 26*, 313–347. https://doi.org/10.1007/s10456-023-09876-7 (accessed on 15th July 2025).
11. González-Candia, A., Candia, A. A., Ebensperger, G., Reyes, R. V., Llanos, A. J., & Herrera, E. A. (2020). The newborn sheep translational model for pulmonary arterial hypertension of the neonate at high altitude. *Journal of Developmental Origins of Health and Disease, 11*, 452–463. https://doi.org/10.1017/s2040174420000616 (accessed on 15th July 2025).
12. Govindaswami, B., Nudelman, M., Jegatheesan, P., & Song, D. (2020). A narrative review of delaying cord clamping 2020—Who, what, when, where, why and how? *[Volume 3]*, 25–25. https://www.semanticscholar.org/paper/9257cdab22ceec9a3aeafd7b98c076ce19dbb3ed (accessed on 15th July 2025).

13. Granger, D. A., & Voegtline, K. M. (2014). Dispatches from the interface of salivary bioscience and neonatal research. https://core.ac.uk/download/287624205.pdf (accessed on 15th July 2025).

14. Greisen, G., Andresen, B., Plomgaard, A. M., & Hyttel-Sorensen, S. (2016). Cerebral oximetry in preterm infants: An agenda for research with a clear clinical goal. *Neurophotonics, 3.* https://www.semanticscholar.org/paper/837d4db2a1abe6e6db924bb570131bad8c51fb3b (accessed on 15th July 2025).

15. Hou, K., Wu, Z. X., Chen, X. Y., Wang, J. Q., Zhang, D., Xiao, C., Zhu, D., et al. (2022). Microbiota in health and diseases. *Signal Transduction and Targeted Therapy, 7.* https://doi.org/10.1038/s41392-022-00974-4 (accessed on 15th July 2025).

16. Krzyszczyk, P., Schloss, R., Palmer, A. F., & Berthiaume, F. (2018). The role of macrophages in acute and chronic wound healing and interventions to promote pro-wound healing phenotypes. *Frontiers in Physiology, 9.* https://doi.org/10.3389/fphys.2018.00419 (accessed on 15th July 2025).

17. Kwun, J., Choi, J., Yoon, Y., Choi, H. M., Park, J. Y., Kim, H. J., Lee, M. J., et al. (2024). Prospective validation of a mobile health application for blood pressure management in patients with hypertensive disorders of pregnancy: Study protocol for a randomized controlled trial. *Trials, 25.* https://www.semanticscholar.org/paper/78e09530a1924142b6dc495f4b15d6faf38c7cf7 (accessed on 15th July 2025).

18. Maltepe, E., & Fisher, S. J. (2015). Placenta: The forgotten organ. *Annual Review of Cell and Developmental Biology, 31,* 523–552. https://doi.org/10.1146/annurev-cellbio-100814-125620 (accessed on 15th July 2025).

19. Mariager, A. F., Hammeken, A., Malham, M., Raja, A., Sellmer, A., Skjellerup, S. L., Raja, R., et al. (2023). Age-related prevalence of open ductus arteriosus in full-term newborns. *Neonatology, 120,* 527–531. https://www.semanticscholar.org/paper/84ad86c753c9eba74764eda7e55a4bab1b413437 (accessed on 15th July 2025).

20. May, R. W., Maso Talou, G. M., Clark, A., Mynard, J., Smolich, J., Blanco, P., Müller, L. O., et al. (2023). From fetus to neonate: A review of cardiovascular modeling in early life. *WIREs Mechanisms of Disease.* https://www.semanticscholar.org/paper/cc676185700de04d8f327d6512dd556d151a6bee (accessed on 15th July 2025).

21. McCreary, J. K., Metz, G. A. S., Ng, J. W. Y., et al. (2015). Allostatic load and preterm birth. https://core.ac.uk/download/74559442.pdf (accessed on 15th July 2025).

22. Melamed, N., Baschat, A., Yinon, Y., Athanasiadis, A., Mecacci, F., Figueras, F., Berghella, V., et al. (2021). FIGO (International Federation of Gynecology and Obstetrics) initiative on fetal growth: Best practice advice for screening, diagnosis, and management of fetal growth restriction. *International Journal of Gynecology & Obstetrics, 152,* 3–57. https://doi.org/10.1002/ijgo.13522 (accessed on 15th July 2025).

23. Meyers, B. A., Bhattacharya, S., Brindise, M. C., Loke, Y., Payne, R. M., & Vlachos, P. (2024). Fetal and neonatal echocardiographic analysis of biomechanical alterations for the systemic right ventricle heart. *PLOS ONE, 19.* https://www.semanticscholar.org/paper/71e62108e1f4224406865478f8a95d9217e2ec4d (accessed on 15th July 2025).

24. Mihailov, A., Pron, A., Lefèvre, J., Deruelle, C., Desnous, B., Bretelle, F., Manchon, A., et al. (2024). Normative models combining fetal and postnatal MRI data to characterize neurodevelopmental

trajectories during the transition from in- to ex-utero. *bioRxiv*. https://www.semanticscholar.org/paper/edd6cd255648244741aebef9a8c600a8fcdb982c (accessed on 15th July 2025).

25. Muniraman, H. K. (2020). Fetal lung fluid: Not the same as amniotic fluid. *Pediatric Pulmonology, 56*. https://www.semanticscholar.org/paper/450b2c9e7716be44ed71b58c300bf8149169b169 (accessed on 15th July 2025).

26. Owen, J. C., Garrick, S. P., Peterson, B., Berger, P., Nold, M., Sehgal, A., & Nold-Petry, C. (2023). The role of interleukin-1 in perinatal inflammation and its impact on transitional circulation. *Frontiers in Pediatrics, 11*. https://www.semanticscholar.org/paper/302084d6ad100e5865e460f8205e5f62397b72dd (accessed on 15th July 2025).

27. Partridge, E. A., Davey, M. G., Hornick, M. A., McGovern, P. E., Mejaddam, A. Y., Vrecenak, J. D., Mesas Burgos, C., et al. (2017). An extra-uterine system to physiologically support the extreme premature lamb. *Nature Communications, 8*. https://doi.org/10.1038/ncomms15112 (accessed on 15th July 2025).

28. Peng, X., Cheng, L., You, Y., Tang, C., Ren, B., Li, Y., Xu, X., et al. (2022). Oral microbiota in human systematic diseases. *International Journal of Oral Science, 14*. https://doi.org/10.1038/s41368-022-00163-7 (accessed on 15th July 2025).

29. Pérez-Muñoz, M. E., Arrieta, M. C., Ramer-Tait, A. E., & Walter, J. (2017). A critical assessment of the "sterile womb" and "in utero colonization" hypotheses: Implications for research on the pioneer infant microbiome. *Microbiome, 5*. https://doi.org/10.1186/s40168-017-0268-4 (accessed on 15th July 2025).

30. Plows, J. F., Stanley, J. L., Baker, P. N., Reynolds, C. M., & Vickers, M. H. (2018). The pathophysiology of gestational diabetes mellitus. *International Journal of Molecular Sciences, 19*, 3342–3342. https://doi.org/10.3390/ijms19113342 (accessed on 15th July 2025).

31. Robinson, J. L., & Darby, J. (2022). Something worth waiting for: Is delayed cord clamping always beneficial? *The Journal of Physiology, 600*. https://www.semanticscholar.org/paper/5908e1d81294e0ef95da18579e86bf4266b105b3 (accessed on 15th July 2025).

32. Romero, R., Dey, S. K., & Fisher, S. J. (2014). Preterm labor: One syndrome, many causes. *Science, 345*, 760–765. https://doi.org/10.1126/science.1251816 (accessed on 15th July 2025).

33. Rosenfield, R. L., & Ehrmann, D. A. (2016). The pathogenesis of polycystic ovary syndrome (PCOS): The hypothesis of PCOS as functional ovarian hyperandrogenism revisited. *Endocrine Reviews, 37*, 467–520. https://doi.org/10.1210/er.2015-1104 (accessed on 15th July 2025).

34. Rosenzweig, E. B., Abman, S. H., Adatia, I., Beghetti, M., Bonnet, D., Haworth, S. G., Ivy, D. D., et al. (2018). Pediatric pulmonary arterial hypertension: Updates on definition, classification, diagnostics and management. *European Respiratory Journal, 53*, 1801916–1801916. https://doi.org/10.1183/13993003.01916-2018 (accessed on 15th July 2025).

35. Ross, D. S., Burch, H. B., Cooper, D. S., Greenlee, M. C., Laurberg, P., Maia, A. L., Rivkees, S. A., et al. (2016). 2016 American Thyroid Association guidelines for diagnosis and management of hyperthyroidism and other causes of thyrotoxicosis. *Thyroid, 26*, 1343–1421. https://doi.org/10.1089/thy.2016.0229 (accessed on 15th July 2025).

36. Sehgal, A., Allison, B. J., Miller, S., Polglase, G. R., McNamara, P. J., & Hooper, S. B. (2021). Impact of acute and chronic hypoxia-ischemia on the transitional circulation. *Pediatrics, 147*. https://doi.org/10.1542/peds.2020-016972 (accessed on 15th July 2025).

37. Shapouri Moghaddam, A., Mohammadian Haftcheshmeh, S., Vazini, H., Taghadosi, M., Esmaeili, S. A., Mardani, F., Seifi, B., et al. (2018). Macrophage plasticity, polarization, and function in health and disease. *Journal of Cellular Physiology, 233*, 6425–6440. https://doi.org/10.1002/jcp.26429 (accessed on 15th July 2025).

38. Souza, G. R., Barreto do Amaral, A., Busch, S., & Martignoni, F. V. (2023). Natural history of a disease: Patent ductus arteriosus diagnosed on an elderly woman. *Cureus, 15*. https://www.semanticscholar.org/paper/32bbd4c4c0104afcb628619e9b60ab331b6cf5e2 (accessed on 15th July 2025).

39. Stout, K., Daniels, C. J., Aboulhosn, J., Bozkurt, B., Broberg, C. S., Colman, J. M., Crumb, S. R., et al. (2018). 2018 AHA/ACC guideline for the management of adults with congenital heart disease: A report of the American College of Cardiology/American Heart Association Task Force on Clinical Practice Guidelines. *Circulation, 139*. https://doi.org/10.1161/cir.0000000000000603 (accessed on 15th July 2025).

40. Tan, C., & Lewandowski, A. J. (2019). The transitional heart: From early embryonic and fetal development to neonatal life. *Fetal Diagnosis and Therapy, 47*, 373–386. https://doi.org/10.1159/000501906 (accessed on 15th July 2025).

41. Van Laere, D., Van Overmeire, B., Gupta, S., El-Khuffash, A., Savoia, M., McNamara, P. J., Schwarz, C. E., et al. (2018). Application of neonatologist performed echocardiography in the assessment of a patent ductus arteriosus. *Pediatric Research, 84*, 46–56. https://doi.org/10.1038/s41390-018-0077-x (accessed on 15th July 2025).

42. Weeda, J. A., te Pas, A. T., Haak, M. C., Blom, N. A., & van der Palen, R. L. (2024). Fetal-to-neonatal transition of an infant with transposition of the great arteries and intact ventricular septum: A case report. *Biomedicine Hub, 10*, 1–7. https://www.semanticscholar.org/paper/0d98949dd5fbab34ebf40aa0934ef348b28ef773 (accessed on 15th July 2025).

43. Xie, J., Yin, X., Pei, Q., Yan, L., Zhang, L., Liu, J., Zhang, H., et al. (2024). Integrated management and prognosis analysis of 30 cases of fetal pulmonary valve abnormalities during pregnancy and perinatal period: A retrospective study. *Translational Pediatrics, 13*, 1560–1570. https://www.semanticscholar.org/paper/42b2841528e012b83f9925861811d9e817d1124c (accessed on 15th July 2025).

44. Yin, J. (2018). Diagnosis and management of hypotension in premature infants at early postnatal stage. *International Journal of Pediatrics, 45*, 509–513. https://www.semanticscholar.org/paper/cfaca630455863d95692e2f9a162a92825c77404 (accessed on 15th July 2025).

45. Zhang, J., Ouyang, Z., Xia, L., Wang, Q., Zheng, F., Xu, K., Xing, Y., et al. (2023). Dynamic chromatin landscape encodes programs for perinatal transition of cardiomyocytes. *Cell Death Discovery, 9*. https://www.semanticscholar.org/paper/72b4b1a8e85cfbbe248fd08f20c21849e318d3c2 (accessed on 15th July 2025).

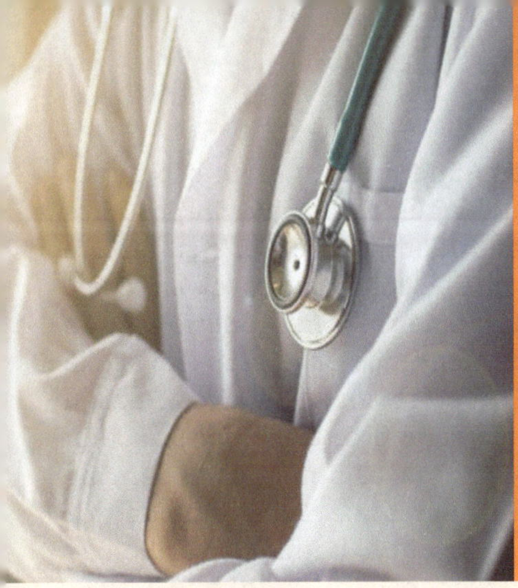

Chapter 3

CLINICAL ASSESSMENT IN PEDIATRIC CARDIOLOGY

Contents

Introduction

Pediatric cardiology is a critical specialty for promotion of cardiovascular health in children and necessitates an extensive clinical assessment to identify congenital or acquired heart disease. Clinical assessments tend to be multimodal in nature, beginning with meticulous patient history taking and physical examinations that serve as the basis for understanding the individualized cardiovascular picture in pediatric patients. Apart from these initial evaluations, advanced examinations such as echocardiograms and electrocardiograms allow for the detection of cardiovascular abnormalities that may otherwise be unapparent. Healthcare providers need to take special notice of emerging trends, particularly as hypertension during childhood becomes increasingly common, an issue featured in recent research attempting to develop a definition of childhood hypertension as well as its long-term implications (Lurbe et al., 2016). Hence, the introduction of pediatric cardiology must highlight the importance of meticulous clinical assessments as being the core to the enhancement of patient outcomes. Moreover, the integration of the latest recommendations and guidelines into practice is necessary to optimize assessments in pediatric cardiology. The new guidelines give importance to the urgent need for accurate measurement of blood pressure and identification of risk factors for hypertension in teenagers as a growing concern for the cardiovascular status of children. Clinicians should attempt to view it holistically and include environmental and genetic factors that could influence the cardiovascular profile of a child. This strategy not only helps to make clinical assessment more accurate but also helps families and doctors make evidence-based decisions regarding cardiovascular risk management. Increasing awareness of the significance of cardiovascular well-being among youth may initiate public policy responses aimed at enhancing screening and preventive interventions, establishing a preventive rather than reactive model for the care of child heart health (Lurbe et al., 2016). Other than hypertension, pediatric cardiology is also affected by the increasing complexities of the long-term prognosis of childhood cancer treatment, which yet again underscores incorporating fertility preservation into the evaluation of patients. The intersection of pediatric oncology and cardiology requires specialists to work together and guarantee the welfare of the afflicted children beyond short-term cardiological concerns. By placing more emphasis on the integration of fertility preservation in clinical assessment, pediatric cardiologists can uphold a multi-dimensional strategy for dealing with children's current and future health. This preventative initiative keeps important components of health from being overlooked, allowing comprehensive assessments that consider the overall pediatric patient needs. Overall, these allied fields highlight that successful clinical assessments are integral to pediatric cardiology, ultimately leading to better quality of life and health outcomes among children.

Definition of Pediatric Cardiology

Pediatric cardiology is an important subspecialty of the overall study of cardiology that deals specifically with the diagnosis and management of heart disease in infants, children, and adolescents. The specialty includes a broad spectrum of acquired and congenital heart diseases, which requires a universal knowledge base to provide appropriate care for the special physiological and growth considerations in this younger patient population. The importance of pediatric cardiology lies in its purpose to not only cure existing conditions but also to avoid ensuing complications, hence improving the long-term health status of such children. Through this, pediatric cardiologists must be skilled in both medical and surgical interventions specifically for children and offer a sympathetic understanding of the intricate interplay of congenital anomalies and external conditions and psychosocial influences on young patients and families. The discipline of pediatric cardiology is itself multidisciplinary, extending into its clinical evaluation strategies that are critical to accurate diagnosis and treatment. This evaluative process is generally thorough patient history, physical exam, and advanced diagnostic studies such as echocardiography, electrocardiogram (ECG), and cardiac catheterization. Because of the variability in cardiac form and function that exists from birth through adolescence, pediatric cardiologists are required to utilize specialized assessment tools and techniques different from those of adult cardiology. This advanced strategy ensures that unique characteristics of child patients are considered, thereby ensuring the highest accuracy of diagnoses and effectiveness of subsequent therapeutic interventions. Further, ongoing advancements in diagnostic technology and clinical trials have significant impacts on the clinical evaluation context in pediatric cardiology, ensuring better outcomes in patients. Moreover, interprofessional teamwork is a hallmark of excellent pediatric cardiology, a reflection of the need for multidisciplinary care. Pediatric cardiologists often work with other clinical providers including pediatricians, cardiac surgeons, nurses, and social workers, to develop individualized care plans based on each child's specific needs. This collaborative effort not only increases the extent of patient care but also includes various perspectives that can enhance the effectiveness of treatment and family support. Problems such as communication breakdowns and emotional stressors are problems that can affect both families and patients; therefore, being in a position to handle such problems effectively is critical. The incorporation of evidence-based interventions grounded in solid guidelines, as mandated in the CONSORT statement, may facilitate the process of evaluation, in that therapeutic approaches are at the same time scientifically valid and morally acceptable (Eldridge et al., 2016). Essentially, the definition of pediatric cardiology itself involves not only the clinical management of heart disease in children but also the seeking of continually improving care for patients through shared, innovative practice.

Importance of Clinical Assessment

Clinical assessment is at the heart of pediatric cardiology because it informs diagnosis and subsequent management strategies that are tailored to a single child's needs. Cardiac symptoms in children create a necessity for clinicians to use both comprehensive history taking and careful physical assessment to identify underlying pathologies. Once more, comprehensive clinical assessments permit identification of trivial signs that are easily overlooked, including altered heart sounds or abnormalities of peripheral perfusion. Because pediatric patients often present subtly, unlike adults, it is important that one is aware of the minimally deviant behaviors to ensure a proper diagnosis. Through prioritizing thorough clinical evaluations, care specialists are capable of launching pre-emptive intervention for potentially problematic disorders and ultimately bettering patient outcomes and quality of life. In addition to guiding immediate clinical consideration, effective evaluations carry important long-term consequences for care management in pediatric cardiology. Guidelines set for clinical assessment provide a benchmark upon which to track the progression of congenital or acquired cardiac illness and have a key influence on the progression of management in these patients. The structured approach allows practitioners to create obvious milestones for assessing treatment effectiveness and refining treatment approaches. For instance, routine clinical assessment can determine that medication should be altered or surgery should be started. Research has determined that the adherence to long-term prescribed testing regimes shows up in better health results, highlighting the very significant role of diligent assessment within ongoing patient treatment (Eldridge et al., 2016) (Figure 3.1).

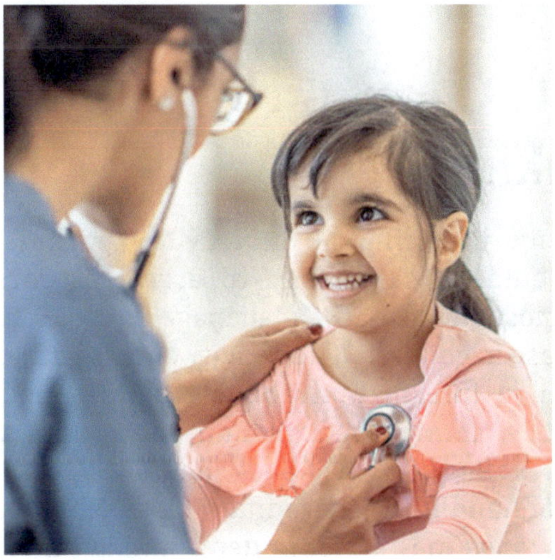

Figure 3.1. Pediatric clinical assessment.

Source: https://external-content.duckduckgo.com/iu/?u=https%3A%2F%2Fwww.lifebridgehealth.org%2Fsites%2Fdefault%2Ffiles%2Fstyles%2Ftext_and_image_535x535_%2Fpublic%2FPublic%2Fmain%2Fpediatrics%2Fcardiology%2Fpediatriccardiology.jpg%3Fitok%3DVozkw1aZ&f=1&nofb=1&ipt=8728b30da3cce84025a635323525ca6a68acab5c6d9c78b23673b389e8ef8acc.

Besides, the subjective findings by the clinician from the assessment also ensure cooperation between families and health professionals, a collaboration critical in pediatrics, as it allows parents to get involved in the decision-making process, which enables them to actively participate in their child's care. Not only does cooperation alleviate stress among parents but also enhances treatment plan compliance and follow-up visits. As parents become more actively engaged in their child's medical care, they will be more likely to value the requirement for lifestyle adjustment or ongoing monitoring, which may be necessary for individuals with chronic cardiovascular illnesses. In such cases, the role of clinical evaluation is not limited to diagnosis but is a critical component of comprehensive pediatric management.

3.1. Clinical History Taking

Taking the clinical history is paramount in pediatric cardiology to arrive at correct diagnoses and successful management of cardiac disease in children. The activity entails gathering detailed information about a child's medical history, family background, developmental history, and relevant past illness. Specifically, understanding the hereditary history of cardiac conditions may assist in determining inherited susceptibility that can influence the child's heart health. Furthermore, taking clinical history must be thorough, often with information on the child's lifestyle, activity level, and any concomitant symptoms of fatigue, chest pain, or palpitations. The skill of the clinician in eliciting such information coupled with the patient's and family's history gives a holistic view of the child's state of health and guides future diagnostic tests and treatment programs. Moreover, effective taking of clinical history enhances the clinician's ability to develop rapport and confidence with child patients as well as their caregivers. This is even more important in pediatrics since children may be reluctant to express their experiences or symptoms. Appropriateness in language and techniques of different ages can enable greater openness in communication, thus making it easier for a child to discuss his or her worries. It is equally significant to involve caregivers since they can better understand changes in behavior, adherence to treatment as directed, and potential environmental insults on the child's cardiac status. This history-taking aspect is most critical, as it creates a collaborative setting that empowers the patient and family. Through developing such communication, healthcare providers are more capable of tailoring their care to the unique situation of each pediatric patient. In pediatrics, the impact of thorough history taking goes beyond the individual clinical visit, having implications for long-term health. Not only do appropriate diagnoses help when a history is taken correctly, but it is also essential to follow-up known illness and for anticipating future complications. For instance, children who have experienced congenital heart defects may require more intense follow-up due to secondary complications in the future. Also, the implementation of evidence-based guidelines, for instance, those offered within updated frameworks, assists clinicians in making good history-taking decisions. This custom aligns with broader public health initiatives for improved cardiovascular health outcomes among children, with relevant spotlighting of efficient clinical history taking where it overlaps with prevention and treatment initiatives in pediatric cardiology (Laxmi et al., 2018; Marc et al., 2019).

3.1.1. Importance of Family Medical History

Family medical history is critical to pediatric cardiology clinical assessments, specifically in the identification of congenitally at-risk children for heart deformities and other cardiovascular illnesses. Family medical history is a valuable asset that pediatric cardiologists rely on, providing essential information that may clarify inherited patterns of heart ailment and guide prevention. This data is crucial because certain cardiac conditions, including hypertrophic cardiomyopathy and long QT syndrome, exhibit hereditary patterns. If physicians gather complete family histories, they can better assess risk and facilitate early screening interventions along genetic susceptibility lines, thereby developing improved outcomes for vulnerable children. In addition, a full family history can be helpful in interpreting some of the health conditions that exist and may complicate the child's cardiovascular disease. For instance, children with a family history of hyperlipidemia or diabetes may require an aggressive strategy for their management of risks for developing heart disease. Pediatric cardiologists can order interventions by capitalizing on such information, including changes in lifestyle and early medical interventions that can reduce the congenital heart defects' complications (Figure 3.2).

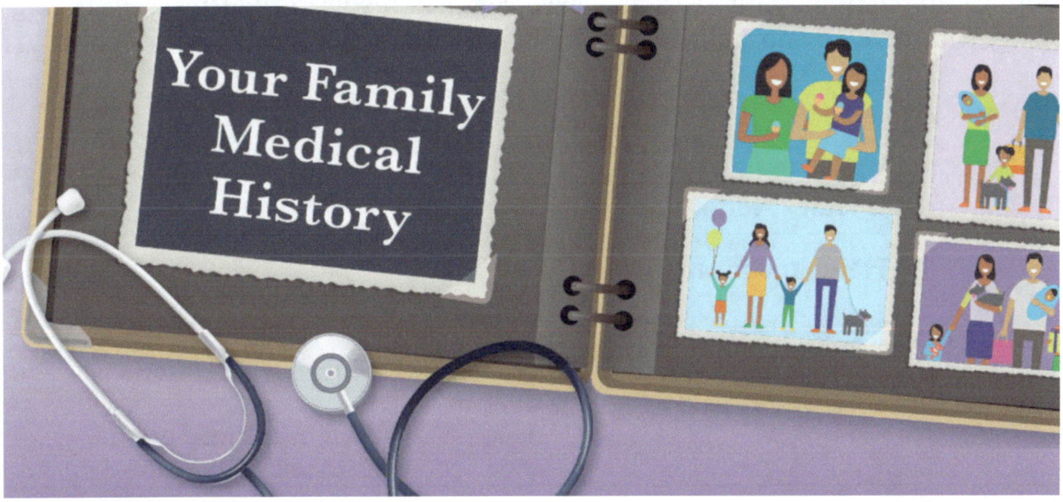

Figure 3.2. Family health history.

Source: https://www.nm.org/-/media/northwestern/healthbeat/images/health%20library/nm-family-history-tnail.jpg.

The collaboration between healthcare providers and families in establishing a comprehensive medical history makes the foundation for efficient long-term treatment planning with pediatric patients. In addition to risk assessment and treatment, family medical history is also crucial in matters of ethical concern in the pediatric cardiology treatment. In describing potential diagnoses, treatments, and results, healthcare providers must inform families appropriately about the implications of inherited traits. Family health discussions can be ice-breaking; therefore, the providers must introduce such discussions in a delicate way while ensuring that families comprehend the complexity of the genetic influence on heart health. Families with children who present signs of inherited cardiac conditions can also access genetic counseling services. Management of these variables enables the execution of a conjoining care plan that respects family patterns while promoting anticipatory care of pediatric cardiac well-being, thereby balancing clinical practice with the best outcomes for children with hereditary heart diseases.

3.1.2. Key Symptoms to Assess in Pediatric Patients

In pediatric cardiology, it is essential to recognize the primary symptoms in order to diagnose them appropriately and intervene on time. The clinical presentation of a child differs from that of adults and demands additional attention to age-specific symptoms. For instance, signs such as cyanosis—a bluish coloration of the skin, particularly around the mouth and fingertips—may suggest severe heart illnesses like congenital heart defects. In addition, the detection of a heart murmur can be a sign of pre-existing structural abnormalities or functional deficits in cardiac physiology, prompting the requirement for additional testing through echocardiography. Integration of effective evaluation techniques, such as observation of the child's growth patterns and activity tolerance, helps clinicians to determine baseline health and locate deviations that may reflect cardiac dysfunction. This proactive strategy increases the proportion of symptomatic children evaluated and treated effectively, minimizing morbidity due to delayed diagnosis. The second critical area of evaluation during pediatric patient clinical examination is evaluation of respiratory symptoms. Children with cardiopulmonary diseases may have complex respiratory distress, including dyspnea and wheezing, with cardiac and pulmonary etiologies (Figure 3.3).

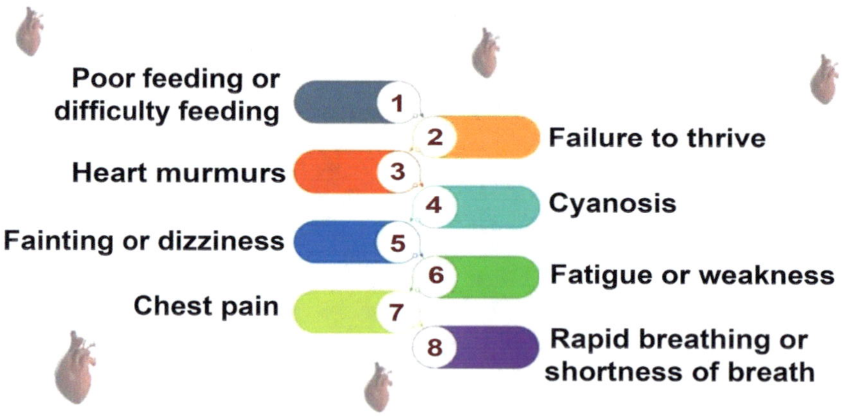

Figure 3.3. Signs of heart problems in children.

Source: https://muhilheartcentre.b-cdn.net/wp-content/uploads/2023/06/Muhil-Heart-Centre-7-1024x671.webp.

One needs to recognize the interplay between cardiac function and respiratory distress since congestive heart failure will have feeding or exertional shortness of breath in infants and toddlers. Chronic cough with dyspnea on exertion may also be a sign of cardiologically based respiratory impairment, and thus needs multidisciplinary evaluation including cardiology and pulmonary specialists. Determination of these signs in the early stages can lead to expedited diagnostic imaging and treatment interventions that are critical in mitigating the complications related to a pediatric cardiovascular patient's respiratory compromise. Lastly, the assessment of pediatric patients should, alongside pain measurement, involve determination of any noted decreased perfusion and its relevance to cardiac status. These signs like pallor, coldness of extremities, and prolonged capillary refill time can be signs of underlying circulatory issues that need to be acted on urgently. Inability of a child to meet expected milestones regarding physical activity or interactive behavior can also be indicative of impaired cardiac function. It is crucial that medical practitioners initiate a careful history-taking exercise to inquire about any history of congenital heart disease or sudden cardiac death in their families, as these are well-known to raise the suspicion of a cardiac condition. Proper evaluation of these significant findings allows for specialized treatment and monitoring with the help of newer imaging techniques, according to appropriate guidelines. Care coordination among multidisciplinary teams is most important in the effective management of children and optimal realization of health outcomes.

3.1.3. Developmental Milestones and Their Relevance

Developmental milestones are significant markers in the assessment of the development and general well-being of children, particularly in pediatric cardiology. Developmental milestones consist of a series of physical, intellectual, and emotional skills which need to be developed by children at a given age. Monitoring these developmental milestones is crucial in identifying possible delays or deviations that may reflect concealed health issues. Some of the milestones in pediatrics of cardiology have been linked to cardiovascular health, as diseases such as congenital heart defects may affect whether or not a child will be able to master these developmental tasks. Detection of delays early on through continued assessments allows clinicians to intervene optimally tailored to the individual, fostering maximal growth and developmental achievement while concurrently treating any involved cardiac conditions. The implications of developmental milestones extend beyond individual development, influencing broad clinical interventions and recommendations in pediatric cardiology. To illustrate, the American Heart Association emphasizes the significance of developmental delay identification as part of a comprehensive approach to cardiovascular disease in children. It is reported that child stroke (a burgeoning area of concern) often coincides with developmental complications. Here, emphasis on timely clinical assessments can offer important information regarding the way cardiovascular events may influence developmental trajectories in children. As has been outlined in pediatric stroke scientific statements, identification of the implications of neurological and cardiovascular interactions will contribute to improved management strategies, which ultimately translate to patients' quality of life. Furthermore, the integration of developmental assessment into regular pediatric cardiac evaluation highlights the interconnected nature between cardiovascular well-being and overall developmental development. Health care practitioners are thus encouraged to familiarize themselves with constantly changing developmental milestones criteria because it may play a role in the clinical decision-making process. Utilizing annual assessments not only makes it easier to identify developmental disorders but also facilitates an anticipatory approach in the management of children with associated cardiovascular disease. The intersection of developmental data with clinical assessment techniques underscores the need for continuous practice and research advancements in pediatric cardiology, ultimately toward improving both developmental and cardiac outcomes for child patients. Care providers are then empowered from this intersection to address the multifaceted needs of children with cardiac conditions, enhancing their overall health trajectories and quality of life.

3.2. Physical Examination Techniques

The value of physical examination skills in pediatric cardiology is underscored by their need for accurate diagnosis and effective treatment of a wide range of conditions. History-taking in detail is the backbone that allows clinicians to put physical findings into perspective in the child's global clinical status. By taking a systematic approach to examination, health professionals are more likely to identify signs of congenital heart disease or acquired heart disease. This is specifically required in children, whose symptoms are insidious or uncommon compared to adults.

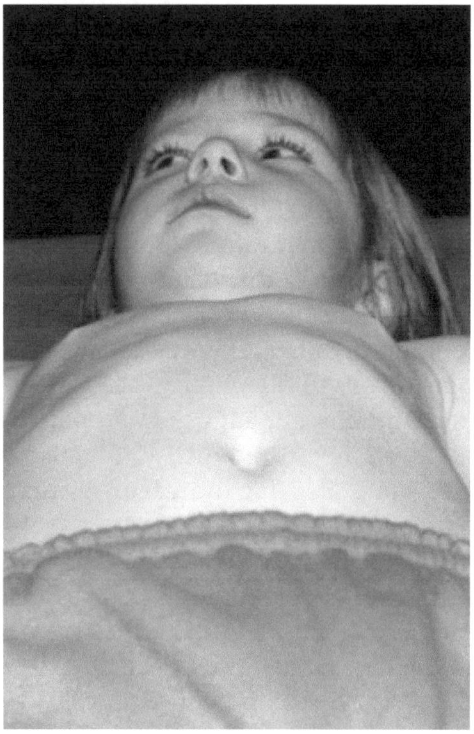

Figure 3.4. Prominence of the left side of the chest in a 3-year-old with a ventricular septal defect and a moderate left-to-right shunt that is causing enlargement of both the left and right ventricles.

Source: https://clinicalgate.com/cardiovascular-assessment-of-infants-and-children/.

A good relationship and communication with the child and his or her parents or guardians can also aid in extensive evaluation, rapport establishment, and making the patient cooperative, minimizing anxiety, and obtaining more accurate results (Brenda, 2020). The process of clinical examination typically involves a number of methods like inspection, palpation, auscultation, and percussion. All these methods yield valuable information (e.g., auscultation may identify abnormal heart sounds typical of valvular disease or other cardiac defects).

Notably, the vulnerability of children necessitates adjustment in examination method to accommodate their small body size and varied stages of development. Further, close attention to such key signs as heart rate, blood pressure, and respiration rates during examination reveals significant information regarding the cardiovascular health of the child. Recognizing that readings can vary greatly in children, clinicians must use appropriate reference ranges in order to properly diagnose issues (Brenda, 2020) (Figure 3.4).

Finally, integration of advanced technology has supplemented standard physical examination techniques in pediatric cardiology. Portable echocardiograms and point-of-care electrocardiograms are becoming more common in contemporary practice, allowing rapid and precise assessments in various clinical settings. These technologies not only improve the quality of diagnosis but also provide dynamic real-time data that informs treatment. For instance, an echocardiogram assessment may identify structural defects that cannot be clinically diagnosed through physical examination. In spite of these technological advances, it is essential that clinicians stay proficient in essential physical examination skills because they remain the mainstay of clinical assessment in pediatric cardiology. Through the integration of old practices with new technology, clinicians can optimize patient outcomes and deliver holistic care (Larry et al., 2015) (Figure 3.5).

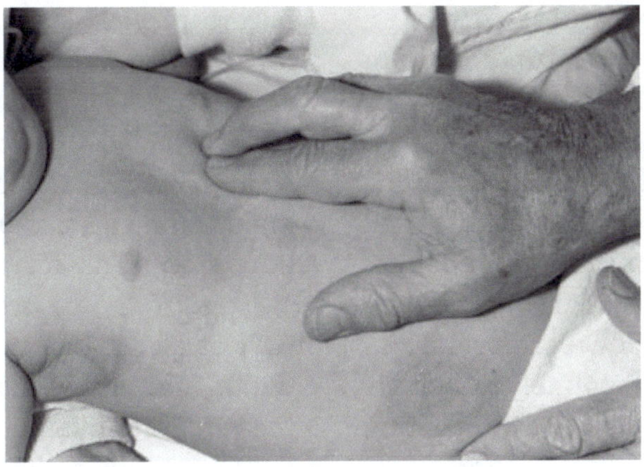

Figure 3.5. Press on the precordium to the left of the xiphoid process with the first and second digits of your right hand to detect enlargement of the right ventricle.

Source: https://clinicalgate.com/cardiovascular-assessment-of-infants-and-children/.

3.2.1. Vital Signs and Their Significance

Vital signs are critical indicators of a child's physiological status, and they constitute the first evaluation in pediatrics – including within pediatric cardiology. Measurement of heart rate, respiratory rate, blood pressure, and temperature allows the clinician to monitor vital functions that reflect the body's potential for homeostasis. In children, whose normal physiology differs significantly from adults, proper interpretation of vital signs becomes critical.

Vital Signs	Normal Values	Interpretation
Heart Rate	60-100 beats/min	Bradycardia = <60 beats/min Tachycardia = >100 beats/min
Respiratory Rate	12-20 breaths/min	Bradypnea = <12 breaths/min Tachypnea = >20 breaths/min
Blood Pressure	120/80 mmHg	Hypotension = Low Blood Pressure Hypertension = High Blood Pressure
Body Temperature	98.6°F (37°C)	Hypothermia = <95°F (35°C) Hyperthermia = >104°F (40°C)
Oxygen Saturation	> 93%	Hypoxemia = <90%

Figure 3.6. Vital signs are a set of measurements that reflect the essential functions of the body and provide a snapshot of a person's overall health status.

Source: https://www.respiratorytherapyzone.com/vital-signs/.

For instance, tachycardia, often a manifestation of the underlying cardiac distress, must be put into the normal heart rate patterns of the pediatric population. Baseline vital sign values are important for determining variations that may be manifestations of pathological processes. Also, as conditions such as congenital heart disease are prevalent in pediatric patients, understanding the variation between normal and abnormal vital signs promotes timely diagnosis and proper intervention, subsequently impacting prognosis and ultimate outcome of care. Thorough examination of vital signs is especially crucial in the diagnosis and management of pediatric cardiac illnesses. Deviation from normal can be critical, and immediate medical intervention may be warranted (Figure 3.6).

For example, in dehydration or cardiac failure, blood pressure and heart rate changes provide important information about a child's hemodynamic status. Clinicians should be able to recognize such changes in the overall clinical context. In addition, technical progress with monitoring devices has enhanced the capability to continuously monitor vital signs, leading to improved results. Repeated observation can detect subtle changes, which allow for preemptive treatment before the child's condition worsens, illustrating the important roles that vital signs play in both acute and chronic cardiac therapy. Incorporation of normal vital sign monitoring into pediatric cardiology ensures strong and sound patient treatment strategies. Vital signs also play significant roles as valuable tools for determining the efficacy of therapeutic plans in children with cardiac diseases. Response to treatment, whether pharmacologic or surgical, can be monitored through observation of changes in vital signs. For instance, a decrease in heart rate coupled with normalization of blood pressure can signal effective management of heart failure symptoms in a young patient. The dynamic nature of vital signs also makes them helpful for ongoing monitoring, enabling clinicians to adjust treatment plans in an adaptive manner. As clinical best practices evolve, especially in treating complex diseases like Fabry disease, maintaining a state-of-the-art understanding of how vital signs correlate with disease process and response to treatment becomes critical (Ort et al., 2018). In addition, organizing care within multidisciplinary guidelines that consider the integrated value of vital signs can optimize outcomes for pediatric patients who have to navigate the complexities of congenital heart disease (Berto et al., 2017).

3.2.2. Auscultation of Heart Sounds

Auscultation of heart sounds is a key component of pediatric cardiology clinical assessment, enabling clinicians to derive useful diagnostic information through a non-invasive technique. As a consequence of the technological advancements in data acquisition tools, such as the creation of large pediatric heart sound databases, clinicians have become more accepting of systematic auscultation protocols. These data sets, comprising hundreds of recordings from diverse patient populations, serve to continue educating practitioners on normal and abnormal heart sounds. Empirical evidence supports the fact that proficient auscultation not only facilitates diagnosis but also guides subsequent management decisions. As a result, the addition of technology into the auscultation process promises improved heart sound interpretation, ultimately providing a more accurate and informed approach to pediatric cardiac care (Oliveira et al., 2021). Furthermore, clinical significance of integrating machine learning algorithms in auscultation cannot be overstated. Progress made in recent years has led to the development of machines that are capable of interpreting heart sounds with high precision, thereby aiding clinicians in the detection of murmurs and arrhythmias.

Utilizing large, annotated databases, these algorithms can be trained on a rich variety of heart sounds and detect subtle variations that even experienced clinicians can overlook. In clinical trials, the use of such systems could have the capability to revolutionize the diagnosis of pediatric cardiovascular diseases, with enhanced screening capacity and inviting preventive treatment. Eventually, these technologies will be poised to improve practitioners' diagnostic capabilities, with healthier outcomes for patients and reduced need for more intrusive treatment (Oliveira et al., 2021) (Figure 3.7).

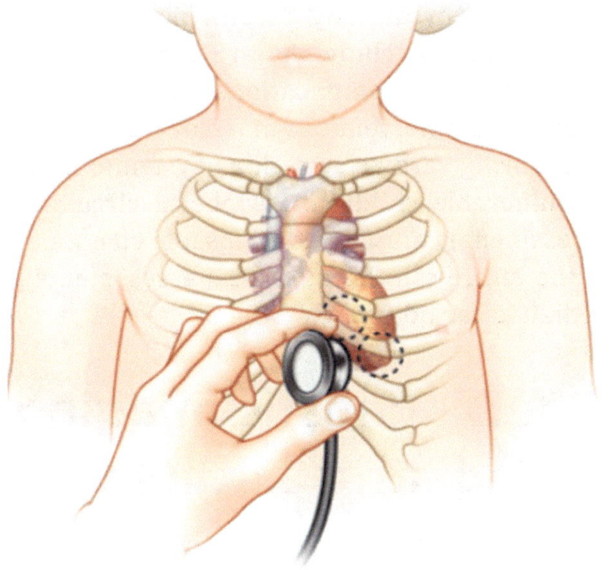

Figure 3.7. Pediatric heart sounds.

Source: https://media.springernature.com/lw685/springer-static/image/chp%3A10.1007%2F978-1-4471-6738-9_23/MediaObjects/310603_1_En_23_Fig1_HTML.gif.

In the past few years, there has been yet another technological advance in pediatric cardiology with the introduction of handheld ultrasound devices (HHUSD). Small, handheld machines have revolutionized the way exams are performed, making it possible for physicians to perform focused echocardiography at the bedside with ease never before seen. Miniaturization of the ultrasound machines, which now resemble a tablet or smartphone, allows for instant feedback and decision-making at the bedside. This positions HHUSD as not only a valuable resource for experienced clinicians but also as an educational tool for medical residents and students, with the added advantage of enhanced knowledge of cardiac anatomy and function. Besides, an article by the European Federation of Societies in Ultrasound and Medicine emphasizes the future directions of HHUSD applications in pediatric imaging for better integration of auscultation techniques with high-end imaging modalities in combined cardiac assessments (Figure 3.8).

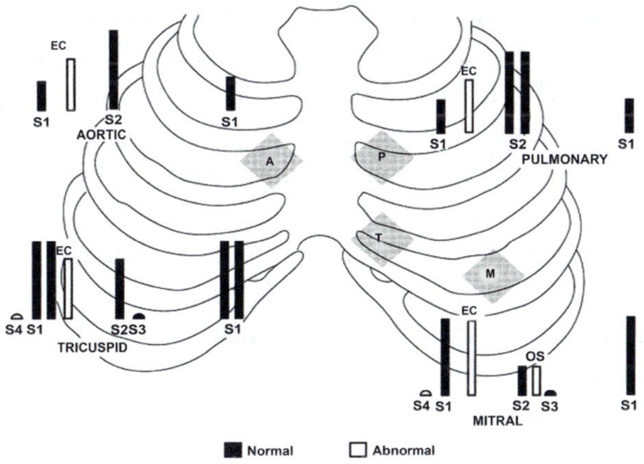

Figure 3.8. Normal and abnormal sounds in the four conventional auscultation areas. [A: aortic; P: pulmonary; T: tricuspid; M: mitral; EC: ejection click; and OS: opening snap].

Source: https://clinicalgate.com/cardiovascular-assessment-of-infants-and-children/.

3.2.3. Assessment of Peripheral Circulation

In pediatric cardiology, peripheral circulation is quite crucial in the diagnosis of cardiovascular disease, as it provides data of systemic perfusion and hemodynamics. It demands a thorough assessment with various modalities, such as echocardiographic evaluation with physical examination, Doppler ultrasound, and pulse oximetry. It begins with peripheral extremity physical examination for swelling, warmth, and color. Palpation of the pulse, using the radial, femoral, and dorsalis pedis, is quite informative regarding circulation and will be employed to identify potential circulatory compromise. Capillary refill time being abnormal also can be a sign of poor perfusion, leading the clinicians to investigate further into ensuing cardiovascular abnormalities such as congenital defects or heart failure, which is of specific interest for pediatric patients.

Hence, a systematic assessment of these parameters allows for early identification of complications that may otherwise go undetected until they are critical. Secondly, technological advancement in imaging techniques has significantly enhanced the assessment of peripheral circulation in children. Ultrasonography (i.e., Doppler imaging), has emerged as an innocuous method to assess patterns of blood flow and see vascular anatomy. This apparatus is especially beneficial in pediatric patients, who may be more sensitive to invasive studies.

Doppler ultrasound use can be utilized to identify structural anomalies in arteries and veins and conditions like arterial occlusion or thrombosis. Of particular note, the importance of peripheral circulation testing extends beyond acute diagnosis, and it is knowledge of the vascular status that can become critical in the development of treatment planning, specifically for high-risk individuals for stroke or other thromboembolic events in pediatric stroke literature (Donna et al., 2019). Thus, integrating advanced imaging techniques into routine clinical practice can facilitate improved long-term results in children. Lastly, the value of maintaining careful watch over peripheral circulation cannot be overstated, particularly in the case of newly emerging viral diseases like COVID-19. Such infections can present peripheral circulation changes through interaction of the direct virus action and the induced immune response among pediatric patients. Previous work has determined that pediatric patients with COVID-19 may experience cardiovascular complications like myocarditis, which affects peripheral blood perfusion (Siripanthong et al., 2020). This is the reason why pediatric cardiologists not only have to investigate peripheral circulation on a regular basis but also be more cautious during pandemics or infectious disease outbreaks. By careful monitoring of these changes, clinicians are amply capable of anticipating complications, making timely appropriate interventions that play a crucial role in ensuring cardiac as well as systemic health in vulnerable children. Peripheral circulation assessment is thus an indispensable component in the entire scheme of clinical assessments of pediatric cardiology.

3.3. Diagnostic Imaging in Pediatric Cardiology

Ideal diagnostic imaging is a cornerstone of pediatric cardiology practice, enabling clinicians to visualize and assess the intricate anatomy and physiology of the child's heart. Multiple imaging modalities, including echocardiography, CT, and MRI, are employed to that end. Echocardiography, often the first imaging study performed, provides real-time views of the chamber, valve, and associated vessel of the hearts. It is invasive, without radiation, and particularly suitable for neonates and children, who are more resistant to radiation injury. These characteristics make echocardiography extremely valuable not only for the detection of congenital cardiac anomalies but also for follow-up in preoperative and postoperative patients. Proper evaluation of cardiac anatomy and function has direct implications for patient management plans and determines surgical treatment, placing a high priority on total imaging protocols in pediatric cardiac assessment. In the more complex cases where echocardiography is insufficient for full evaluation, CT and MRI are superb adjuncts. While CT is particularly useful in the diagnosis of coronary artery anomalies and aortopathies, it has the disadvantage of radiation exposure—an element that deserves careful consideration, especially in children. MRI, meanwhile, offers painstaking anatomical and functional detail with no ionizing radiation and thus is superb to employ for the evaluation of cardiomyopathies and congenital heart disease.

In addition, technological advances in MRI methods, including functional imaging and tissue characterization, have greatly improved diagnostic potential. In the case of long-term disorders like cardiomyopathy, follow-up using these imaging technologies enables clinicians to monitor disease progression and modify treatment strategies accordingly. Thus, the use of a personalized strategy in imaging can provide invaluable information that has a major impact on clinical outcomes in pediatric cardiology. Integration of these imaging modalities into clinical assessment protocols not only improves diagnostic accuracy but also improves the interdisciplinary cooperation required in pediatric cardiology care. According to the American Heart Association, multidisciplinary collaborative efforts by pediatric cardiologists, surgeons, radiologists, and subspecialist nurses are essential for comprehensive patient care. This integration improves improved communication of imaging information and its implications for clinical management as well as optimizes the development of best treatment options. Additionally, the awareness of advances in imaging technology is also vital, as advances continue to increase the ability to diagnose and enhance patient safety. As pediatric cardiology continues to evolve, the growth and evolution of imaging practices will undoubtedly provide enhanced results for pediatric cardiac patients as evidence of the unique role of diagnostic imaging in this specialty niche (Alan et al., 2012; Larry et al., 2015).

3.3.1. Role of Echocardiography

Echocardiography is a crucial diagnostic imaging tool in pediatric cardiology that enables visualization and assessment of cardiac anatomy and function in infants and children across all ages. Early detection of congenital heart defects, one of the most common birth abnormalities, is made possible by echocardiography. Through a variety of techniques such as transthoracic echocardiography (TTE), doctors can achieve an immediate view of the anatomy of the heart, which can facilitate accurate evaluation of chamber volume, valve function, and occurrence of shunt or anomaly. The utility of echocardiography lies in the ability to provide hemodynamic status immediate feedback, making it most useful in monitoring patients pre- and post-operatively. Specifically, Lorusso et al. (2021) highlights the significance of echocardiography in serious assessments of children, with a focus on its usefulness not only for diagnosis but for therapeutic management and intervention as well. Echocardiography is not only limited to diagnostic imaging but functional evaluation as well that is critical in treatment planning in pediatric cardiology. For instance, it facilitates evaluation of left and right ventricular function, providing information on myocardial performance and cardiac chamber pressure measurements. These evaluations become of critical significance in children demonstrating evidence of compensation for long-term hemodynamic stresses of heart disease (Figure 3.9).

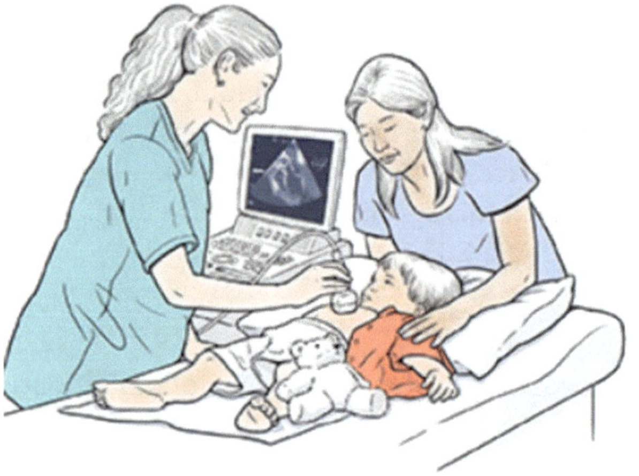

Figure 3.9. Echocardiography for children.

Source: https://www.stanfordchildrens.org/content-public/topic/images/55/434255.jpeg.

The application of advanced echocardiographic techniques, such as Doppler imaging, enhances further the ability to assess blood flow dynamics and cardiac output, supporting assistance for catheterization or surgical correction. Refinement in diagnostics highlights the applicability of echocardiography as detailed in guidelines published by organizations such as the American Society of Echocardiography based on best practice use in the pediatric clinical setting (Lorusso et al., 2021).

Further, it also plays a greater role in the management of child patients who have more complex heart surgery or require closer monitoring around the time of operation. When evaluating and guiding therapy for illnesses like congenital cardiac disease or cardiomyopathy, echocardiography is employed in diagnostic and prognostic evaluations essential to better outcomes. It not only enables preoperative planning but also for continuous monitoring of cardiac function in critically ill infants, which helps in early recognition of complications that can arise. The need for thorough echocardiographic assessment, especially in high-risk surgeries, is stressed in recent literature (Barker et al., 2020). Thus, the extent of echocardiography's function lies both in instantaneous patient care as well as long-term plans of management, and hence it is an indispensable tool in pediatric cardiology.

3.3.2. Use of Chest X-Rays

Use of chest X-rays in pediatric cardiology is an important diagnostic tool that assists doctors in assessing the cardiac conditions of children. In the case of children, anatomical disparities and developmental considerations are taken into place, chest X-rays provide useful information on the size, shape, and placement of the heart. These imaging studies not only allow for the visualization of the great vessels and the heart itself but also enable the detection of associated conditions within the lungs. The potential to detect cardiomegaly or signs of heart failure, for instance, can facilitate early interventions, making chest X-rays critically important in the initial screening for numerous congenital and acquired heart diseases.

This method, while helpful, needs to be read with caution because of the nature of pediatric patients and often requires complementation with higher modalities such as echocardiography. One other significant use of chest X-ray in pediatric cardiology is for the follow-up of chronic cardiac illnesses. Serial X-rays can reflect changes that could precipitate changes in management in children with known heart diseases or who are on therapy. In the instance of conditions such as congenital heart disease, where surgical procedures may be necessary, X-rays can be very helpful in monitoring post-operative complications. Some such conditions could be evaluation for effusion, pneumothorax, or other pulmonary complications that present post-operatively. Furthermore, incorporating chest X-rays into a multimodal protocol—performed by cardiologists, radiologists, and primary physicians—offers complete care and enhances decision-making concerning the patient status and follow-up testing necessary (Figure 3.10).

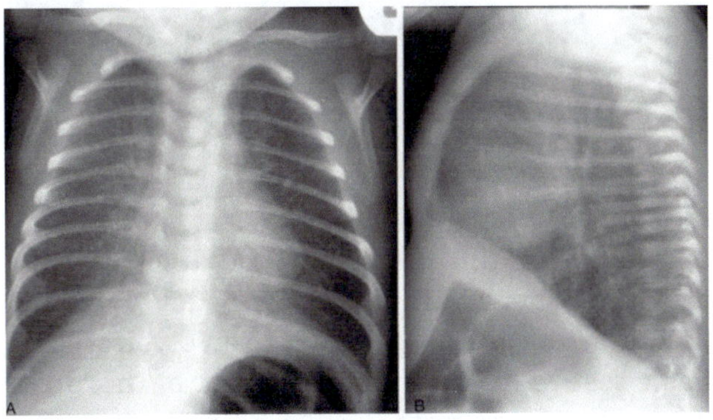

Figure 3.10. Chest radiography in pediatric cardiovascular.

Source: https://radiologykey.com/wp-content/uploads/2015/12/B9780323081764000653_f065-004ab-9780323081764.jpg.

The progression of technology and imaging techniques continuously augments the utility of chest X-rays in pediatrics. Through breakthroughs in precision medicine, machine learning algorithms have been designed that can scan large sets of chest X-ray images for abnormalities more efficiently than traditional processes.

These technologies can, in theory, bridge diagnostic gaps, integrating data from multiple sources to create good classifiers for heart diseases. Integration of these technologies can significantly speed up and improve the accuracy of diagnostics with a potential on treatment streams. Although such advancements promise a lot, regulations must be put in place for the management and interpretation of the effect of machine learning findings to bring them within achieved clinical parameters in pediatric cardiology as implemented by authorities (Bryan et al., 2021; Warnat et al., 2021).

3.3.3. Advanced Imaging Techniques: MRI and CT

Sophisticated imaging techniques such as Magnetic Resonance Imaging (MRI) and Computed Tomography (CT) are now the mainstay of clinical assessment in pediatric cardiology. These imaging techniques are particularly useful since they provide detailed anatomical visualization of the heart and surrounding structures necessary in the diagnosis of congenital and acquired heart disease in children. MRI, for instance, possesses the unique capability to assess cardiac function without the requirement of ionizing radiation and is thereby especially adapted to the child patient. The benefit of both high spatial resolution and improved soft tissue contrast enhances the clinician's capability to recognize mild abnormalities and thereby permit early intervention. As detailed in new guidelines, clinical decision-making processes with advanced imaging can play an important role in management strategies for patients with complicated cardiovascular disease (Eric et al., 2022). CT imaging, with the utilization of ionizing radiation notwithstanding, has also become an obligatory tool in pediatric cardiology, especially in vascular structure evaluation and the detection of acute thoracic ailments. The rapidity of image acquisition and ability to generate three-dimensional reconstructions make CT particularly valuable for preoperative evaluation and assessment of postoperative complications. Furthermore, technological advances such as reduced radiation doses utilizing such techniques as iterative reconstruction also enhance its safety profile in children. As more evidence indicates that precise anatomical detail obtained from CT will provide greater benefits to patients, its use for clinical assessment continues to expand. These imaging methods support risk stratification, enabling the clinician to individualize interventions in a more accurate and effective way (Jarosław et al., 2022) (Figure 3.11).

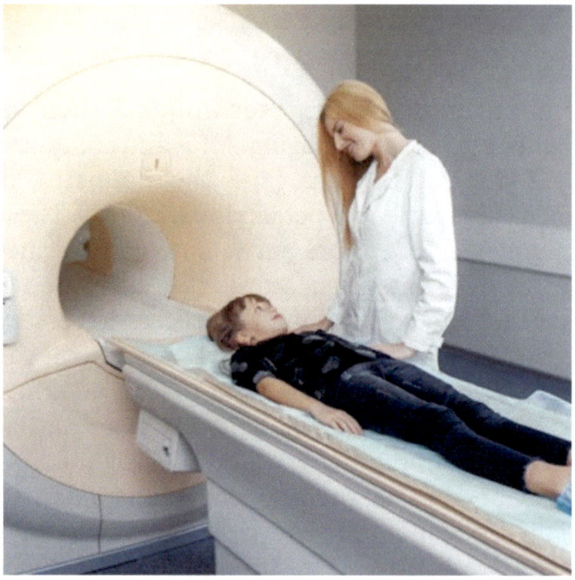

Figure 3.11. Cardiac MRI protocols differ for children.

Source: https://img.auntminnie.com/files/base/smg/all/image/2020/08/am.2020_08_06_23_16_2529_mri_scanner_kid_400.png?auto=format%2Ccompress&q=70&w=400.

The integration of MRI and CT into the practice of pediatric cardiology is not limited to diagnostics; both techniques have significant roles to be played in pre-procedure planning and educating the patient. By utilizing advanced imaging, cardiologists are able to create comprehensive maps of a child's cardiac anatomy that allow them to explain to families what may be feasible procedures. The visual aids make understanding simpler and could potentially reduce anxiety regarding intricate procedures. Secondly, advances in imaging technology open avenues for advances in treatment modalities, such as application of 3D-printed models to simulate surgeries. These models hold immense potential for maximally optimizing surgical approaches, thereby boosting procedural success rates. As pediatric cardiology continues to advance, dependency on advanced imaging techniques will continue to be important to revolutionize clinical assessment and outcomes in children (Eric et al., 2022).

3.4. Electrocardiography (ECG) in Children

Application of electrocardiography (ECG) in pediatric cardiology is a vital instrument employed in the diagnosis and follow-up of children's heart ailments. With development in pediatric cardiology, ECG has evolved from a basic test to being an integral part of thorough clinical assessment. ECG helps clinicians detect arrhythmias, conduction blocks, and other intrinsic cardiac abnormalities that are not immediately apparent on initial physical examination. Due to the unique anatomical and physiological properties of pediatric subjects, accurate interpretation of pediatric ECG requires a great deal of expertise and experience. Such intricacy emphasizes the need to utilize pediatric-trained cardiologists to interpret results with confidence, thereby offering optimal management of any detected cardiovascular ailments. In the recent years, greater appreciation of the cardiac implications of several systemic illnesses has contributed further to the relevance of ECG in children. The recent COVID-19 pandemic, for instance, has introduced concerns of cardiac involvement with the virus, even in symptom-free individuals, and therefore necessitated a conservative approach in children and adolescents actively engaged in sports. The American College of Cardiology has published guidelines advocating for extensive cardiac evaluations, including ECG screening, in young athletes who have previously had COVID-19. These measures assist in stratifying risk and identifying any potential myocardial damage that might lead to significant complications during exercise (Figure 3.12).

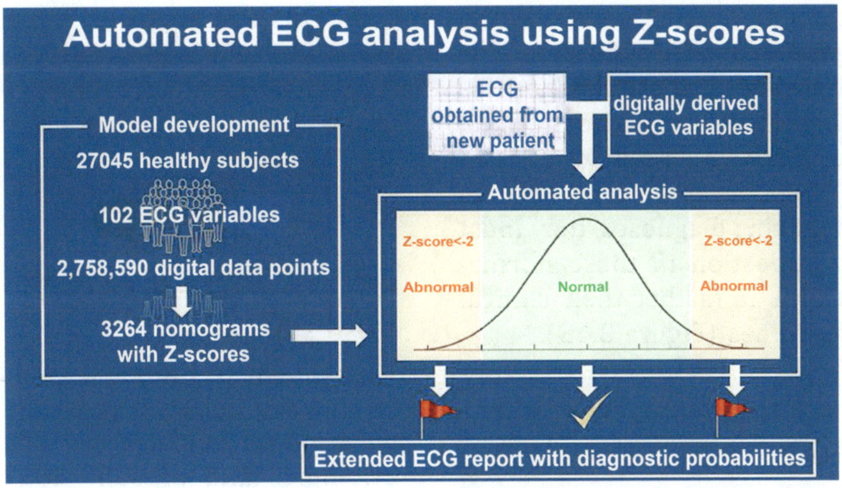

Figure 3.12. Electrocardiogram standards for children and young adults using Z-scores.

Source: https://www.ahajournals.org/doi/10.1161/CIRCEP.119.008253.

This overlap of cardiac well-being and COVID-19 marks the importance of anticipatory cardiovascular risk assessment in childhood populations, particularly high-risk groups such as athletes. Aside from acute conditions such as viral illness, congenital heart conditions also underscore the usefulness of ECG in child cardiac evaluation. Conditions like Costello syndrome with its typical craniofacial features and other systemic manifestations, including cardiac abnormalities, require vigilant surveillance through ECG tests. Patients with such rare conditions could have typical ECG patterns requiring personalized clinical approaches. The heterogeneous phenotypic presentation of RASopathies highlights the need for thorough interdisciplinary management by pediatric cardiologists and other specialists. With the use of ECG in children with complex medical illness, clinicians can make early diagnoses and implement improved management plans. Hence, ECG is not merely a diagnostic tool but a part of routine pediatric cardiac care, ensuring total health care throughout the child's life.

3.4.1. Normal ECG Patterns in Pediatric Patients

The electrocardiogram (ECG) is a valuable diagnostic tool in pediatric cardiology that provides unique information about the electrical activity of the heart. Familiarity with normal pediatric ECG patterns serves as the basis for recognizing deviations that may signal underlying cardiac disease. In children, the ECG also differs from that of adults as regards more prominent S wave in lead V1, change in QRS morphology, and age-related changes in heart rate. In addition, the conduction intervals, i.e., PR, QRS, and QT intervals, also have age-related differences that have to be taken into account during examination. These factors illustrate the importance of interpreting ECG results with age-specific standards to achieve accurate findings, which allow early identification of arrhythmias or structural heart disease that may not be apparent in the absence of age-specific evaluation. The presence of sinus arrhythmia, a common and generally benign variation with respiration variation in heart rate, is a remarkable aspect of ECG interpretation in children. This rhythm pattern may be misleading unless the clinicians know it to be a benign variant. In addition to sinus arrhythmia recognition, one should recognize other ECG features that may signify neonatal or pediatric-specific disease, such as Wolf-Parkinson-White syndrome or congenital long QT syndrome. The differential diagnosis between these conditions is important, especially since some, like congenital long QT syndrome, carry a high risk for sudden death in children. As pediatric clinicians become more proficient in making diagnoses, they must focus on ongoing education in these normal and abnormal patterns to further their clinical evaluations and outcomes (Figure 3.13).

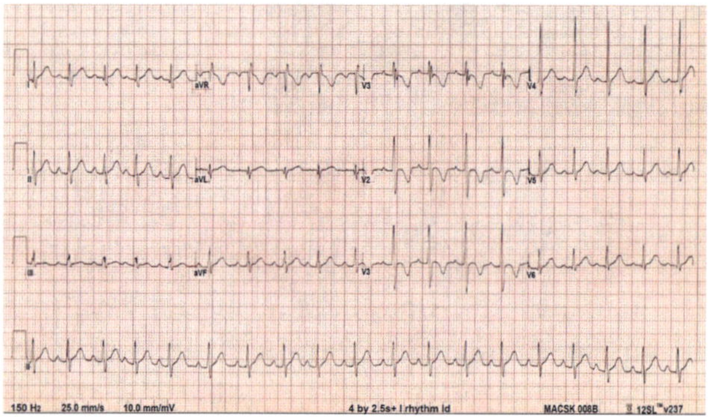

Figure 3.13. Normal pediatric ECG.

Source: https://litfl.com/wp-content/uploads/2018/08/ECG-Incomplete-RBBB-Normal-Pediatric-2-year-old.jpg.

Furthermore, the normal ECG patterns of pediatric subjects must be put in pediatric cardiology procedures literature. Studies have reported that differences in the ECG readings are caused by a multitude of factors, including genetic predisposition and the effect of growth on cardiovascular physiology.

For instance, hypertrophic cardiomyopathy (HCM) manifests in the child and adult populations with occasional distinctive ECG findings like left ventricular hypertrophy. Accurate early diagnosis through appropriate ECG interpretation can potentially trigger interventions that radically alter the disease process in these involved children, further underscoring the importance of expert ECG assessment in the setting of primary care. Lastly, the training of healthcare providers in the familiarity with normal ECG patterns allows early diagnosis and timely intervention in pediatric cardiology, confirming the indispensable role of this diagnostic test in clinical assessment (Ali et al., 2017; Brenda, 2020).

3.4.2. Common Arrhythmias in Children

Assessment of the most common arrhythmias in children is particularly difficult in pediatric cardiology because of the variability in etiologies and presentations that are taken by the diseases in children. Arrhythmias can be seen in children with a diverse range of types and the most frequently encountered are supraventricular tachycardia (SVT) and atrial fibrillation. SVT bears an inappropriately fast rate of heartbeat, leading to hemodynamic instability and symptoms of palpitations and lightheadedness. Additionally, Wolff-Parkinson-White syndrome, a genetic predisposition that affects electrical conduction in the heart, further demonstrates the complex synergy between congenital etiology and arrhythmogenic risk.

Accurate diagnosis and prompt treatment are therefore critical in preventing potential complications from such rhythm disorders. The pediatric cardiologist must exercise delicacy in identifying signs and using appropriate interventions to obtain maximum benefits in children suffering from such conditions. A meticulous clinical assessment is important in arrhythmia detection because the clinical presentation can be very age- and comorbid condition-dependent in a child. The diagnostic assessment often begins with a general history and physical examination, pinpointing symptoms like syncope, palpitations, or respiratory distress that may be related to arrhythmias (Figure 3.14).

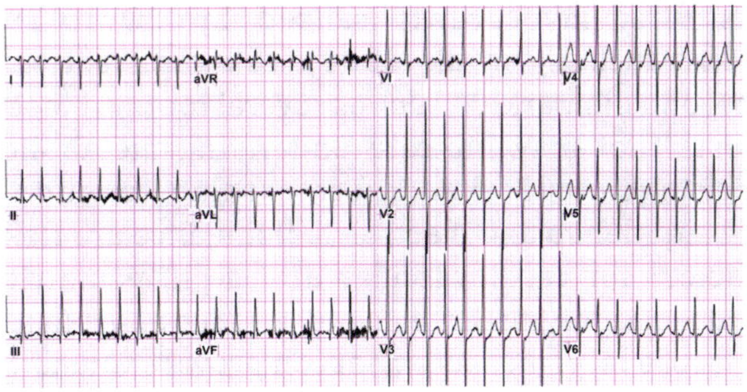

Figure 3.14. Pediatric SVT.

Source: https://emsimcases.com/wp-content/uploads/2018/05/neonatal-svt.png.

Electrocardiogram (ECG) remains the 'gold standard' for arrhythmia diagnosis, providing valuable information about the heart's electrical activity. In those cases where ECG findings are non-diagnostic, further investigations such as echocardiography and Holter monitoring can be employed to evaluate structural heart disease and detect transient arrhythmias that would otherwise go undetected on a routine ECG. Generally, the subtle clinical evaluation is important in differentiating between benign and potentially fatal arrhythmias since any undue delay in diagnosis will result in significant morbidity. Despite advances in pediatric cardiology, knowledge gaps remain regarding the long-term impact of various arrhythmias on the cardiovascular health of children. As highlighted by recent experience with pediatric stroke and its association with arrhythmias, the dynamic of the interaction between the two conditions is of extreme significance to the development of effective prevention and treatment plans (Donna et al., 2019). Further, the dynamic changing dynamics of infective endocarditis and its increasing prevalence among certain patient groups warrants the incorporation of preventive and therapeutic measures into practice (Larry et al., 2015). Physicians should provide a multidisciplinary treatment pathway in the care of children with arrhythmia so that the experts can share information and ideas for an interdisciplinary cure. In making individuals aware of the complexities of pediatric arrhythmias and driving research in this direction, the medical community can enhance cure rates and better the health of such children.

3.4.3. Interpretation Challenges in Pediatric ECGs

Interpretation of the pediatric electrocardiogram (ECG) is faced with definite challenges and needs of understand the physiology of children and the distinct nuances of electrocardiography. Compared with adults, children exhibit significant heterogeneity in heart rate, axis, and waveforms due to their age, maturity, and other congenital abnormalities. With increasing age and development of children, electrophysiological characteristics of the heart change and, therefore, the normal ECG patterns are altered. Therefore, mischaracterization of these developmental changes will lead to incorrect diagnosis. Pediatric professionals must possess expertise in the detection and putting of such differences into perspective to avoid unwarranted interventions or improper management, an element particularly evident within the acute care setting where early diagnosis is crucial. Furthermore, the existing data bank of educational resources for pediatric ECG interpretation is less advanced than that of adults, which contributes to clinician challenges. Although some interventions in education aim at common adult ECG interpretations, variation in pediatric ECG training means that a large number of healthcare workers are unable to interpret pediatric rhythms with certainty. New curricula, such as those introduced by Schrepel et al. (2021), reinforce under-pressure task-switching proficiency in ECG interpretation, as interruptions are a common feature of emergency medical settings. This educational approach is essential as it captures the reality of real-world clinical situations where pediatric patients are treated and hence better equips healthcare providers. Finally, the prevalence of conditions like hypertrophic cardiomyopathy (HCM) among children vindicates the necessity of accurate ECG interpretation. HCM, including left ventricular hypertrophy and diverse genetic mutations, may cause subtle but pathologic findings on an ECG that might be interpreted as normal physiologic variation or other benign abnormalities (Ali et al., 2017). Young patients, particularly athletes, are at risk for sudden cardiac death due to HCM, and proper and timely interpretation of ECGs is thus important in this group. The incorporation of advanced learning strategies to improve understanding by practitioners is a testament to the commitment towards ensuring patient safety through proper clinical determinations. Addressing these issues of interpretation is crucial for efficient diagnosis, treatment, and prevention of bad outcomes in pediatric cardiology.

3.5. Laboratory Tests and Biomarkers

Pediatric cardiology clinical assessment relies increasingly on laboratory tests and biomarkers to enhance diagnostic accuracy and management. They are essential for identification and treatment of cardiovascular congenital and acquired defects in children, including congenital heart disease and acquired heart disease. Biomarkers such as troponins and B-type natriuretic peptides (BNP) are diagnostic of myocardial injury and heart failure status. Higher levels of these biomarkers may also be a sign of cardiac stress, and this will result in further investigation through imaging or more invasive methods. More recent advances have highlighted the role of high-sensitivity assays for cardiac troponins, where lower levels of troponin can be detected, thereby enhancing the diagnostic yield for the detection of myocarditis or cardiac injury following infections such as viral myocarditis caused by COVID-19 (Siripanthong et al., 2020). Lab tests extend beyond biomarkers, such as several routine blood tests that may indicate underlying metabolic derangements that affect cardiac function. Dyslipidemia and electrolyte imbalance are risk factors for cardiovascular disease in pediatric patients, for instance. Lipid testing and blood glucose level measurement can provide valuable insights into the child's overall cardiovascular well-being. In this context, studies have established the necessity of early laboratory testing, especially among symptomatic or with familial histories of cardiovascular disease. In addition, routine genetic testing will be able to identify inherited disorders that susceptibility children to cardiomyopathy or arrhythmias and therefore contribute to early treatment and individualized management regimens (Chen et al., 2020). In addition, the creation of advanced imaging modalities and laboratory research has revolutionized pediatric cardiovascular assessment. Non-invasive imaging tests, such as echocardiography and cardiac MRI, supplement laboratory biomarkers to create an entire picture of a child's cardiac health. For instance, echocardiographic results can be related with elevated BNP levels, validating heart failure diagnosis. Furthermore, the potential of COVID-19-associated myocarditis reiterates the role of laboratory research in handling acute viral infection and its significance in heart health. Against the backdrop of current research on the pathophysiology of COVID-19-associated myocarditis, the need for the inclusion of biomarkers in clinical practice is exemplified; not only do biomarkers play a role in diagnosis but also response to treatment as well as long-term prognosis (Siripanthong et al., 2020).

3.5.1. Importance of Blood Tests in Cardiac Assessment

In pediatric cardiology, laboratory studies in the form of blood tests are valuable diagnostic tools in cardiovascular assessment and decision-making. They enable clinicians to quantify various cardiac biomarkers that yield evidence of underlying disease, e.g., myocarditis or cardiomyopathy. Such as troponin elevations, which trigger concern for cardiac muscle damage and require further investigation and treatment modalities specific to the child's situation. Additionally, electrolyte level measurement (i.e., potassium and sodium), is essential since changes will result in arrhythmias, and this is particularly a special concern in children. With repeated use of blood studies, the cardiac status of pediatric patients can be accurately followed by healthcare providers such that effective interventions at the earliest possible moment are made that can avoid long-term complications and thereby enhance overall results in such fragile patients. Blood test is also crucial in identifying underlying or chronic conditions which might not be directly identifiable in physical examination. For instance, pediatric patients presenting with signs indicative of hypertension can be assisted through specific assays that assess renal function and electrolyte balance based on the recent hypertension studies. As highlighted by the findings of recent research, heightened scrutiny in monitoring blood pressure and vascular well-being among children is necessary, particularly with the rising prevalence of hypertension among youth. Incorporating blood tests into routine examinations can identify these issues early enough, allowing for earlier lifestyle and treatment modifications, which are crucial in preventing the risk of future cardiovascular disease as children become adults (Lurbe et al., 2016) (Figure 3.15).

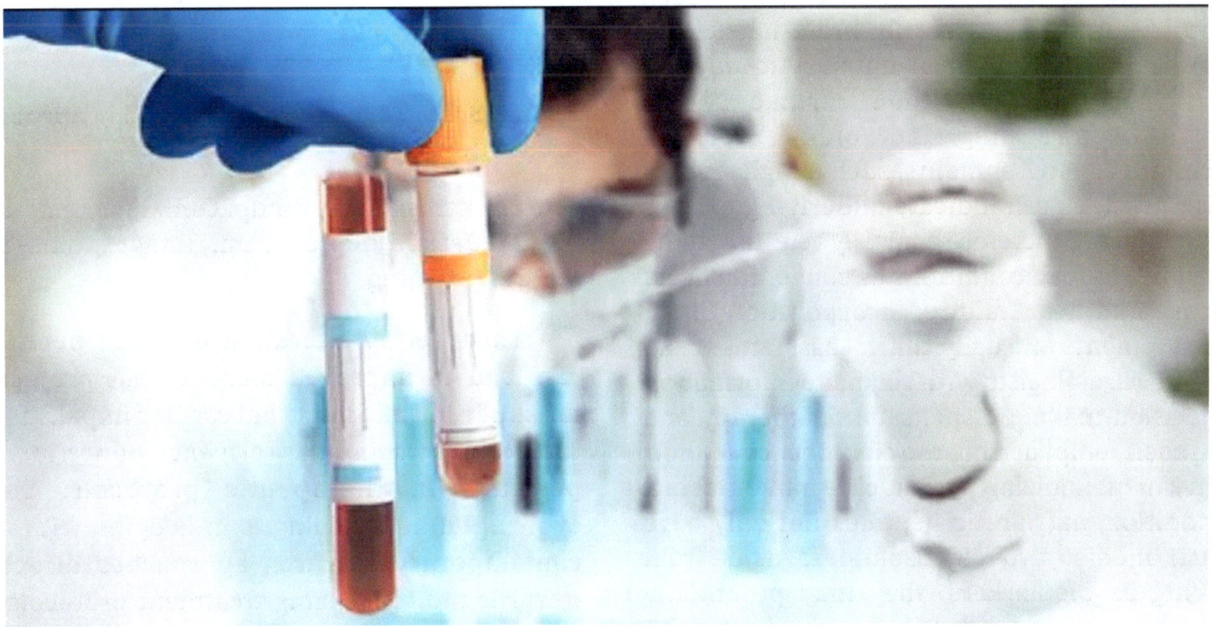

Figure 3.15. Blood test for child.

Source: https://www.manipalhospitals.com/uploads/blog/blood-test-for-kids.webp.

Where infective endocarditis is suspected, laboratory tests (particularly blood tests), have an even more pivotal role to play in confirming diagnoses and guiding therapeutic interventions. Blood cultures are pivotal in determining causative pathogens, which may significantly vary between children, hence impacting treatment strategies. Due to the complex nature of infective endocarditis, it necessitates interagency coordination from a multidisciplinary care team, as noted in current clinical guidelines favoring integrated assessment approaches with inclusion of laboratory assessments. The emergent pathogen pattern, including staphylococcal infections, demands a firm approach in pediatric patients where appropriate antimicrobial therapy is initiated early (Larry et al., 2015). Lastly, blood testing greatly enhances the ability of the clinician to make the correct choice in treatment, with greater management of pediatric cardiology cases and improved patient outcomes.

3.5.2. Role of Natriuretic Peptides

The role of natriuretic peptides (NPs) in pediatric cardiology has also gained significant interest because it is probable that they will prove to be valuable as biomarkers in the clinical assessment of heart disease in children. Such peptide hormones, primarily brain natriuretic peptide (BNP) and atrial natriuretic peptide (ANP), are released upon cardiac stress, ventricular stretching, and volume overload. In children's environments, such a high level of these peptides can indicate underlying cardiac failure and are therefore clinically relevant in the diagnosis of such conditions as congenital heart disease and heart failure. Incorporation of NP measurements into daily clinical assessment can provide cardiologists with requisite information in decision-making, dispensation of therapy, and prognosis, emphasizing the significance of their utility in maximizing patient care and outcome. In addition, natriuretic peptides not only have a dual but also two-way usefulness: aside from serving as biomarkers, they may potentially yield therapeutic benefit. In children with evidence of heart failure or volume overload, the administration of exogenous NPs can induce diuresis and peripheral vasodilation, which result in symptomatic benefit. As researchers learn more about NPs and find new applications for them, their function as endogenous regulators of fluid and electrolyte balance assumes greater significance (Figure 3.16).

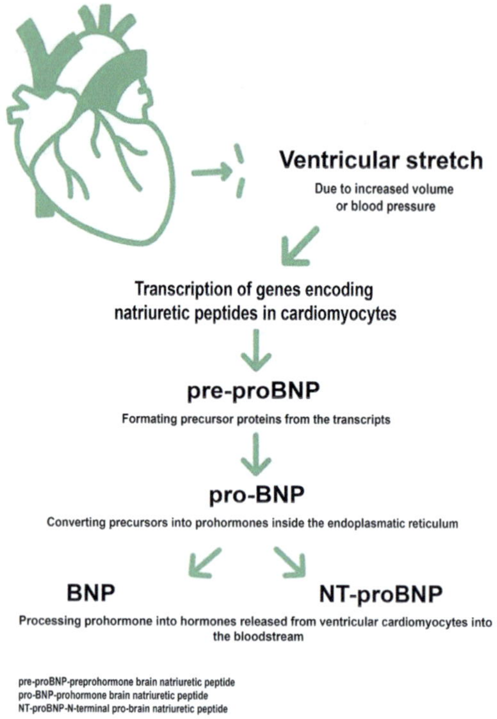

Figure 3.16. Physiology of BNP and NT-proBNP production.

Source: https://www.mdpi.com/ijms/ijms-25-08781/article_deploy/html/images/ijms-25-08781-g001.png.

Therapeutic alteration of these peptides can lead to improved management protocols for children suffering from cardiac impairment, thereby increasing the relevance of natriuretic peptides in therapeutic protocols. Such evolving understanding is in keeping with the contemporary research approaches directed towards individualizing treatment protocols to meet the unique needs of pediatric patients. Apart from their diagnostic and therapeutic purposes, recent research into the pathophysiological actions of natriuretic peptides also highlighted their involvement in broader inflammatory and cardiovascular processes. In fact, studies have begun to explore the interaction between NPs and other inflammatory biomarkers, particularly in acute settings like Multisystem Inflammatory

Syndrome in Children (MIS-C) caused by SARS-CoV-2. The appreciation of the multifaceted functions of NPs facilitates comprehensive perspectives on cardiac health, encompassing not just structural abnormalities but inflammatory processes as well. With advancing clinical practice, the incorporation of data related to natriuretic peptides functions in diagnosis and treatment of pediatric cardiovascular disease will be crucial in optimizing care and improving long-term patient outcomes, as coordinated with rigorous research activities (Lauren et al., 2020; Lorriana et al., 2021).

3.5.3. Genetic Testing for Congenital Heart Disease

Genetic testing has revolutionized the clinical assessment and treatment of congenital heart disease (CHD) in infants and children with impressive advances. Genetic testing detects chromosomal defects and gene mutations in various heart malformations, allowing early diagnosis and tailored management plans. Therapies may be initiated earlier, which allows for proactive interventions that increase outcome.

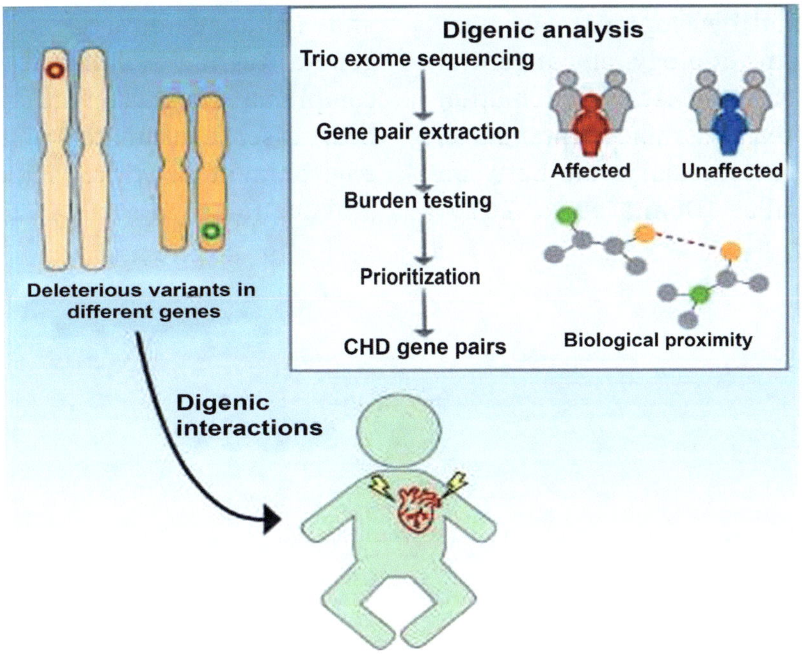

Figure 3.17. Hidden genetic causes of congenital heart disease identified.

Source: https://medicalxpress.com/news/2025-02-hidden-genetic-congenital-heart-disease.html.

Understanding of the genetic etiology of CHD not only aids in defining the prognosis but also aids in defining other comorbid conditions that might be present concomitantly, such as those associated with syndromic presentation. Moreover, inclusion of genetic information enlarges risk assessment in at-risk families for CHD and thereby generates useful information for reproductive counseling and prenatal screening decision-making in at-risk families, based on findings brought out in the context of advances in genetic counseling in pediatric cardiology (Marilyn et al., 2022). The pediatric cardiologist's role has evolved into one that not only encompasses the management of CHD but also the management of genetic information related to general patient care. Families seen with a child who has CHD will often request the potential genetic etiology for the heart defect, which can influence both medical therapy and family planning. Where genetic testing is warranted, the pediatric cardiologist will be required to negotiate discussions of the meaning of identified genetic variations or syndromes skillfully. For example, disorders like Down syndrome, which present with congenital heart anomalies as a comorbid condition, call for a longitudinal approach to follow-up that encompasses several aspects of the child's health and development. As more knowledge of genetic etiology of congenital disease is gained, cardiologists' participation in multidisciplinary teams assumes center stage, underscoring their intermediary role between geneticists and families (Donna et al., 2019) (Figure 3.17).

Furthermore, congenital heart disease gene testing has the ability to redefine existing models of diagnosis and treatment plans. With certain genetic markers for abnormalities identified, one can develop specific therapies and potential preventive interventions. This approach would shift the focus away from symptom-directed care towards prevention strategies based on leveraging genetic information. Moreover, an understanding of the genetic patterns of CHD can provide valuable epidemiological data, resulting in a deeper understanding of the pathogenesis and risks of congenital defects. In pursuing further research, the development and enhancement of methods utilized in genetic testing promise to offer increasingly comprehensive data on the etiology of congenital heart disease, ultimately enhancing the clinical environment in which pediatric cardiologists practice (Marilyn et al., 2022).

SUMMARY

In considering the intricacies of pediatric cardiology clinical assessment, it is important to note the central role that this process fills in the overall care of congenital heart disease (CHD) patients. Due to the multitude of factors that interact with one another to impact both cardiac and neurodevelopmental outcomes, assessment needs to look beyond simple anatomical evaluation. For pediatric cardiologists, embracing the role of a multidisciplinary practice that allows for the integration of the expertise of neurologists, geneticists, and psychologists can contribute to the scope of care provided. Interspecialty contact is significant, particularly with regard to the evolving evidence that implicates CHD in neurodevelopmental delay, as detailed in recent literature, which calls for an expansion of knowledge regarding the interactions between heart function and brain status (Judy et al., 2016). Optimization of clinical evaluation must include an ongoing process of applying new information to practice in order to address the needs of this susceptible group. Secondly, family-centered care in pediatric cardiology is of highest importance. The ability of the healthcare provider to share complex information regarding diagnoses, treatment plans, and potential long-term outcomes has a tremendous effect on families' emotional well-being in enduring such traumatic experiences. As shown by guideline development projects, including those published for the ICU environment, the importance of involving the family in the decision-making process cannot be overemphasized (Judy et al., 2016). Involving the family ensures that patients feel supported and also allows for an environment where healthcare professionals can take their time to examine the complex needs of the patient. With advancements in pediatric cardiology, it will be crucial to focus on family involvement in clinical assessment to improve health outcomes as well as help with better management strategies that include family values and beliefs. Finally, the future of clinical assessment in pediatric cardiology is the integration of the latest diagnostic tools and sustaining research to pinpoint the long-term implications of CHD. New imaging modalities, coupled with thorough developmental assessments, offer unprecedented insight into the complexity of heart defects and complications. For instance, as research unveils the association between CHD and neurodevelopmental disorders, it is crucial for pediatric cardiologists to create efficient diagnostic protocols for early identification and intervention (Paladini et al., 2016). With the use of most current research and technology in combination with interdisciplinary teamwork and family participation, pediatric cardiology can optimize its clinical assessment models. This multi-faceted model will eventually promote optimal health outcomes for children with CHD and families and ensure them the overall support they deserve from their healthcare providers along the care continuum.

In pediatric cardiology clinical evaluation, the initial evaluation of the child is very important in forming a complete picture of cardiovascular wellness. This often involves widespread history-taking and physical examination. Physicians should pay special attention to family history as hereditary susceptibility can go a long way in counseling diagnoses. Symptoms that occur (e.g., fatigue or cyanosis) must not be ignored as they could be evidence of occult congenital or acquired cardiac disease. Good communication with caregivers throughout this process helps to reduce anxiety and establish trust, which is important for the pediatric patient. Furthermore, the use of age-specific strategies for child engagement may improve the validity of history-taking and facilitate a cooperative atmosphere for effective evaluation. Careful evaluations are the foundation upon which specific treatment plans are developed to accommodate the unique needs of child patients. Diagnostic testing is an integral part of clinical evaluation in pediatric cardiology as it provides valuable information supplementary to clinical evaluation. Non-invasive imaging techniques, such as echocardiography, have become increasingly relevant due to the ability to visualize cardiac anatomy and function without the risk of exposing young patients to radiation. Electrocardiograms (ECG) and chest X-rays are utilized consistently to reveal electrical activity and cardiac morphology, respectively. The integration of these investigative modalities allows for an informed clinical decision-making process and allows for the guidance of subsequent management strategies. With advancing technology, practitioners can now utilize the latest tests, including cardiac MRI and genetic testing, to further assess advanced cardiovascular disease. These diagnoses not only apply to immediate management but also for the prognosis of long-term impact on the pediatric patient's health. Multidisciplinary teams collaborating with each other enhance the clinical assessment process in pediatric cardiology significantly. Healthcare professionals like pediatric cardiologists, nurses, and social workers offer diverse input that makes the quality of patient care better. Having a family-centered approach encourages treatment to include the child's overall context, such as emotional and psychosocial factors, which are not typically covered. For instance, incorporating family input can offer pertinent contextual information that is useful in enhancing diagnosis and management, and also in planning follow-up care in the future. Professional organizations offer resources and clinical guidelines for practice for the purpose of standardizing the practice of care in various institutions to allow conformity in the outcome of treatment. The emphasis on interdisciplinary collaboration ultimately aims to maximize the evaluation process, facilitating an environment conducive to integrated and compassionate care. According to N/A (2019) and Judy et al. (2016), this type of collaboration is essential to achieving optimal clinical outcomes in pediatric cardiology.

CLOSER LOOK

PEDIATRIC CARDIAC AUSCULTATION AND INTERPRETATION

Pediatric cardiac auscultation is a fundamental clinical skill involving the use of a stethoscope to listen to the heart sounds of children and infants in an effort to assess cardiovascular function and identify possible abnormalities. Due to the dynamic changing nature of the pediatric cardiovascular system, auscultation requires comprehensive understanding of developmental physiology, normal variants, and pathological findings to derive correct interpretations.

In children, the heart is situated more horizontally and tends to be more anterior in the chest when compared with adults. The anatomical difference demands a special positioning and technique when auscultation is applied. The standard locations to auscultate are the aortic area (second right intercostal space), pulmonic area (second left intercostal space), tricuspid area (lower left sternal border), and mitral area (apex of the heart, typically at the fifth intercostal space at the midclavicular line). In infants and young children, auscultation has to be conducted in a quiet room, ideally when the child is sleeping or quiet, since movement or crying can hide weak heart sounds (Figure 3.18).

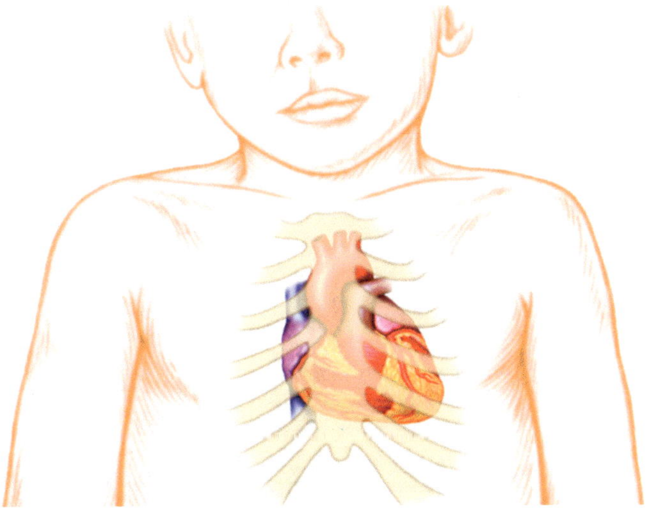

Figure 3.18. Medical illustration showing the anatomical location of the heart within a child's thoracic cavity, emphasizing its position relative to the rib cage and sternum.

Source: https://www.myamericannurse.com/wp-content/uploads/2014/07/Child-w-heart-no-dots-300B.jpg.

Usual heart sounds in children are the first heart sound (S1) and second heart sound (S2). S1 corresponds to the closure of mitral and tricuspid valves, and S2 is associated with the closure of aortic and pulmonary valves. Physiologic splitting of S2 during inspiration in children is normal and is due to delayed closure of pulmonary valve with increased venous return. This splitting is normalized by expiration; stiff or wide splitting may be a marker for an atrial septal defect or other disease processes.

Other cardiac sounds such as S3 and S4 may also be auscultated. An S3 is a physiological phenomenon in children due to their more compliant ventricles and rapid diastolic filling, but an S4 is almost always pathologic and suggests decreased ventricular compliance as in hypertrophic cardiomyopathy.

Murmurs are a frequent finding in pediatric auscultation and can be categorized as innocent (functional) or pathological. Innocent murmurs are physiological in children and are usually systolic, soft, short, and position or activity dependent. Examples include Still's murmur, which is vibratory and best heard over the left lower sternal border, and pulmonary flow murmur. Alternatively, pathological murmurs will be more intense, of harsh or blowing quality, are often pansystolic or continuous, and may be associated with other clinical signs such as cyanosis, growth failure, or respiratory distress.

The clinical significance of cardiac auscultation findings should always be set against the entire clinical presentation and, where appropriate, verified by investigations such as electrocardiography (ECG), chest X-ray, and echocardiography. Successful detection of congenital heart disease or acquired conditions such as rheumatic heart disease by auscultation can lead to early referral and treatment, crucial for optimal outcome.

References

1. Baddour, L. M., Wilson, W. R., Bayer, A. S., Fowler, V. G., Tleyjeh, I. M., Rybak, M. J., Baršić, B., et al. (2015). Infective endocarditis in adults: Diagnosis, antimicrobial therapy, and management of complications. *Circulation, 132*, 1435–1486. https://doi.org/10.1161/cir.0000000000000296 (accessed on 15th July 2025).
2. Barker, P., Lewin, M., Donofrio, M. T., Altman, C. A., Ensing, G. J., Arya, B., & Swaminathan, M. (2020). Specific considerations for pediatric, fetal, and congenital heart disease patients and echocardiography service providers during the 2019 novel coronavirus outbreak: Council on Pediatric and Congenital Heart Disease supplement to the statement of the American Society of Echocardiography. *Journal of the American Society of Echocardiography, 33*, 658–665. https://doi.org/10.1016/j.echo.2020.04.005 (accessed on 15th July 2025).
3. Bouma, B. J., & Mulder, B. J. M. (2017). Changing landscape of congenital heart disease. *Circulation Research, 120*, 908–922. https://doi.org/10.1161/circresaha.116.309302 (accessed on 15th July 2025).
4. Bull, M. J., Trotter, T. L., Santoro, S. L., Christensen, C. K., & Grout, R. W. (2022). Health supervision for children and adolescents with Down syndrome. *Pediatrics, 149*. https://doi.org/10.1542/peds.2022-057010 (accessed on 15th July 2025).
5. Chen, C., Gao, G., Xu, Y., Pu, L., Wang, Q., Wang, L., Wang, W., et al. (2020). SARS-CoV-2–positive sputum and feces after conversion of pharyngeal samples in patients with COVID-19. *Annals of Internal Medicine, 172*, 832–834. https://doi.org/10.7326/m20-0991 (accessed on 15th July 2025).
6. Davidson, J. E., Aslakson, R. A., Long, A. C., Puntillo, K., Kross, E. K., Hart, J. L., Cox, C. E., et al. (2016). Guidelines for family-centered care in the neonatal, pediatric, and adult ICU. *Critical Care Medicine, 45*, 103–128. https://doi.org/10.1097/ccm.0000000000002169 (accessed on 15th July 2025).
7. Eldridge, S., Chan, C., Campbell, M. J., Bond, C., Hopewell, S., Thabane, L., & Lancaster, G. (2016). CONSORT 2010 statement: Extension to randomized pilot and feasibility trials. *BMJ*. https://doi.org/10.1136/bmj.i5239 (accessed on 15th July 2025).
8. ElSayed, N. A., Aleppo, G., Aroda, V. R., Bannuru, R. R., Brown, F. M., Bruemmer, D., Collins, B. S., et al. (2022). Facilitating positive health behaviors and well-being to improve health outcomes: *Standards of Care in Diabetes—2023. Diabetes Care, 46*, S68–S96. https://doi.org/10.2337/dc23-s005 (accessed on 15th July 2025).
9. Ferriero, D. M., Fullerton, H. J., Bernard, T. J., Billinghurst, L., Daniels, S. R., DeBaun, M. R., deVeber, G., et al. (2019). Management of stroke in neonates and children: A scientific statement from the American Heart Association/American Stroke Association. *Stroke, 50*. https://doi.org/10.1161/str.0000000000000183 (accessed on 15th July 2025).
10. Ghany, M. G., & Morgan, T. R. (2019). Hepatitis C guidance 2019 update: American Association for the Study of Liver Diseases–Infectious Diseases Society of America recommendations for testing, managing, and treating hepatitis C virus infection. *Hepatology, 71*, 686–721. https://doi.org/10.1002/hep.31060 (accessed on 15th July 2025).
11. Gripp, K. W., Morse, L. A., Axelrad, M. E., Chatfield, K. C., Chidekel, A., Dobyns, W. B., Doyle, D., et al. (2019). Costello syndrome: Clinical phenotype, genotype, and management guidelines.

American Journal of Medical Genetics Part A, 179, 1725–1744. https://doi.org/10.1002/ajmg.a.61270 (accessed on 15th July 2025).

12. Henderson, L. A., Canna, S., Friedman, K. G., Gorelik, M., Lapidus, S., Bassiri, H., Behrens, E. M., et al. (2020). American College of Rheumatology clinical guidance for multisystem inflammatory syndrome in children associated with SARS-CoV-2 and hyperinflammation in pediatric COVID-19: Version 2. *Arthritis & Rheumatology, 73*. https://doi.org/10.1002/art.41616 (accessed on 15th July 2025).
13. Isselbacher, E. M., Preventza, O., Black, J. H., Augoustides, J., Beck, A. W., Bolen, M. A., Braverman, A. C., et al. (2022). 2022 ACC/AHA guideline for the diagnosis and management of aortic disease: A report of the American Heart Association/American College of Cardiology Joint Committee on Clinical Practice Guidelines. *Circulation, 146*. https://doi.org/10.1161/cir.0000000000001106 (accessed on 15th July 2025).
14. Kim, J. H., Levine, B. D., Phelan, D., Emery, M. S., Martinez, M. W., Chung, E. H., Thompson, P. M., et al. (2020). Coronavirus disease 2019 and the athletic heart. *JAMA Cardiology, 6*, 219–219. https://doi.org/10.1001/jamacardio.2020.5890 (accessed on 15th July 2025).
15. Kirkpatrick, J. N., Mitchell, C., Taub, C., Kort, S., Hung, J., & Swaminathan, M. (2020). ASE statement on protection of patients and echocardiography service providers during the 2019 novel coronavirus outbreak: Endorsed by the American College of Cardiology. *Journal of the American Society of Echocardiography, 33*, 648–653. https://doi.org/10.1016/j.echo.2020.04.001 (accessed on 15th July 2025).
16. Leard, L. E., Holm, A. M., Valapour, M., Glanville, A. R., Attawar, S., Aversa, M., Vidal Campos, S., et al. (2021). Consensus document for the selection of lung transplant candidates: An update from the International Society for Heart and Lung Transplantation. *The Journal of Heart and Lung Transplantation, 40*, 1349–1379. https://doi.org/10.1016/j.healun.2021.07.005 (accessed on 15th July 2025).
17. Leichtner, A. M., Gillis, L. A., Gupta, S. K., Heubi, J. E., Kay, M., Narkewicz, M. R., Rider, E. A., et al. (2012). NASPGHAN guidelines for training in pediatric gastroenterology. *Journal of Pediatric Gastroenterology and Nutrition, 56*. https://doi.org/10.1097/mpg.0b013e31827a78d6 (accessed on 15th July 2025).
18. Loren, A. W., Mangu, P. B., Beck, L. N., Brennan, L. V., Magdalinski, A. J., Partridge, A. H., Quinn, G. P., et al. (2013). Fertility preservation for patients with cancer: American Society of Clinical Oncology Clinical Practice Guideline Update. *Journal of Clinical Oncology, 31*, 2500–2510. https://doi.org/10.1200/jco.2013.49.2678 (accessed on 15th July 2025).
19. Lorusso, R., Shekar, K., MacLaren, G., Schmidt, M., Pellegrino, V., Meyns, B., Haft, J. W., et al. (2021). ELSO interim guidelines for Veno arterial extracorporeal membrane oxygenation in adult cardiac patients. *ASAIO Journal, 67*, 827–844. https://doi.org/10.1097/mat.0000000000001510 (accessed on 15th July 2025).
20. Lurbe, E., Agabiti-Rosei, E., Cruickshank, J., Dominiczak, A. F., Erdine, S., Hirth, A., Invitti, C., et al. (2016). 2016 European Society of Hypertension guidelines for the management of high blood pressure in children and adolescents. *Journal of Hypertension, 34*, 1887–1920. https://doi.org/10.1097/hjh.0000000000001039 (accessed on 15th July 2025).
21. Marian, A. J., & Braunwald, E. (2017). Hypertrophic cardiomyopathy. *Circulation Research, 121*, 749–770. https://doi.org/10.1161/circresaha.117.311059 (accessed on 15th July 2025).

22. Mehta, L. S., Watson, K. E., Barac, A., Beckie, T. M., Bittner, V., Cruz-Flores, S., Dent, S., et al. (2018). Cardiovascular disease and breast cancer: Where these entities intersect: A scientific statement from the American Heart Association. *Circulation, 137.* https://doi.org/10.1161/cir.0000000000000556 (accessed on 15th July 2025).

23. Meyer-Szary, J., Luis, M. S., Mikulski, S., Patel, A., Schulz, F., Tretiakow, D., Fercho, J., et al. (2022). The role of 3D printing in planning complex medical procedures and training of medical professionals—Cross-sectional multispecialty review. *International Journal of Environmental Research and Public Health, 19*, 3331–3331. https://doi.org/10.3390/ijerph19063331 (accessed on 15th July 2025).

24. Nielsen, M. B., Cantisani, V., Sidhu, P. S., Badea, R., Batko, T., Carlsen, J. F., Claudon, M., et al. (2018). The use of handheld ultrasound devices–An EFSUMB position paper. *Ultra Schall in der Medizing–European Journal of Ultrasound, 40*, 30–39. https://doi.org/10.1055/a-0783-2303 (accessed on 15th July 2025).

25. Oliveira, J., Renna, F., Costa, P. D., Nogueira, D. M., Oliveira, C., Ferreira, C. A., Jorge, A., et al. (2021). The CirCor DigiScope dataset: From murmur detection to murmur classification. *IEEE Journal of Biomedical and Health Informatics, 26*, 2524–2535. https://doi.org/10.1109/jbhi.2021.3137048 (accessed on 15th July 2025).

26. Ortíz, A., Germain, D. P., Desnick, R. J., Politei, J., Mauer, M., Burlina, A. P., Eng, C. M., et al. (2018). Fabry disease revisited: Management and treatment recommendations for adult patients. *Molecular Genetics and Metabolism, 123*, 416–427. https://doi.org/10.1016/j.ymgme.2018.02.014 (accessed on 15th July 2025).

27. Paladini, D., Alfirević, Z., Carvalho, J. S., Khalil, A., Malinger, G., Martínez, J., Rychik, J., et al. (2016). Prenatal counseling for neurodevelopmental delay in congenital heart disease: Results of a worldwide survey of experts' attitudes advise caution. *Ultrasound in Obstetrics and Gynecology, 47*, 667–671. https://doi.org/10.1002/uog.15852 (accessed on 15th July 2025).

28. Schneider, B. J., Naidoo, J., Santomasso, B., Lacchetti, C., Adkins, S., Anadkat, M. J., Atkins, M. B., et al. (2021). Management of immune-related adverse events in patients treated with immune checkpoint inhibitor therapy: ASCO guideline update. *Journal of Clinical Oncology, 39*, 4073–4126. https://doi.org/10.1200/jco.21.01440 (accessed on 15th July 2025).

29. Schrepel, C., Amick, A. E., Sayed, M., & Chipman, A. K. (2021). Ischemic ECG pattern recognition to facilitate interpretation while task switching: A parallel curriculum. *MedEdPORTAL.* https://doi.org/10.15766/mep_2374-8265.11182 (accessed on 15th July 2025).

30. Siripanthong, B., Nazarian, S., Muser, D., Deo, R., Santangeli, P., Khanji, M. Y., Cooper, L. T., et al. (2020). Recognizing COVID-19–related myocarditis: The possible pathophysiology and proposed guideline for diagnosis and management. *Heart Rhythm, 17*, 1463–1471. https://doi.org/10.1016/j.hrthm.2020.05.001 (accessed on 15th July 2025).

31. Warnat-Herresthal, S., Schultze, H., Shastry, K. L., Manamohan, S., Mukherjee, S., Garg, V., Sarveswara, R., et al. (2021). Swarm learning for decentralized and confidential clinical machine learning. *Nature, 594*, 265–270. https://doi.org/10.1038/s41586-021-03583-3 (accessed on 15th July 2025).

32. Wiederhold, B. K. (2020). Connecting through technology during the coronavirus disease 2019 pandemic: Avoiding "Zoom fatigue". *Cyberpsychology, Behavior, and Social Networking, 23*, 437–438. https://doi.org/10.1089/cyber.2020.29188.bkw (accessed on 15th July 2025).

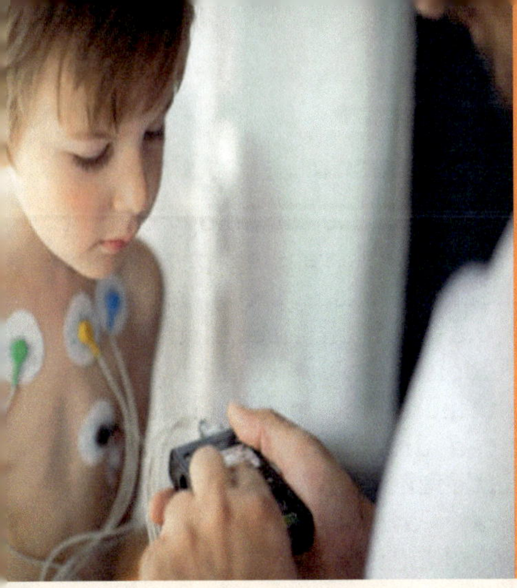

Chapter 4

DIAGNOSTIC TECHNIQUES IN PEDIATRIC CARDIOLOGY

Contents

Introduction

The specialty of pediatric cardiology has experienced phenomenal advancements during recent years primarily in the realm of diagnosis. With the unique anatomical and physiological characteristics of the pediatric patient, one must employ condition-specific diagnostic techniques that accurately assess cardiovascular disease in children. Proper diagnosis is important to offer timely and suitable intervention that potentially has the ability to substantially augment patient care. The intersection of novel imaging modalities and biomarker evaluation has entirely revamped the ability to determine causative factors for cardiovascular disease in this vulnerable population. More relevantly, understanding the complexities of such conditions as congenital heart disease and acquired heart disease necessitates a strategy for diagnosis that goes beyond established methodologies into the new. This presentation also highlights the central importance of diagnostic approaches as a foundation element of pediatric cardiology, leading on to a further discussion of the specific modalities currently in existence. With advances within pediatric cardiology, an accompanying clinical challenge appears with a corresponding need for a deeper understanding of diagnostic approaches. Detection of pediatric cardiovascular disease is frequently different from adult practice due to the differing presentation and etiologies of the child. For instance, myocarditis can have very heterogeneous clinical presentation and can be caused by infectious etiologies, such as in the recent COVID-19 pandemic (Siripanthong et al., 2020). The application of a robust armamentarium of diagnostic tools, including echocardiography, electrocardiography, and advanced imaging modalities, has been key in providing accurate diagnoses in these conditions. Moreover, utilizing knowledge obtained from previous studies and clinical experience allows practitioners to apply current knowledge to make subsequent diagnoses. This dynamic nature of the field requires intensive scrutiny of the current diagnostic techniques along with their treatment and management aspects of pediatric cardiovascular diseases. Novel diagnostic techniques in pediatric cardiology are needed not just to detect conditions at an early stage but also to tailor appropriate management plans for each individual. For example, as pediatric stroke knowledge has enhanced, it has become clear that stroke has significant effects on kids, and it calls for more sensitivity on the part of medical professionals (Donna et al., 2019). With differential rates of occurrence and diverse pathophysiologic mechanisms in such patients, early diagnosis by effective imaging and biomarker assessment remains crucial. In addition, the application of multi-disciplinary techniques of diagnostic assessment can help deconstruct the complexity of pediatric cardiology and lead to improved results. As the field expands, application of the latest technologies, such as cardiac magnetic resonance imaging and telemedicine, will further shape the future of pediatric cardiology's diagnostic procedures. This analysis will ultimately enhance the ability to provide optimal treatment for young patients with cardiovascular disease.

Importance of Pediatric Cardiology

The significance of pediatric cardiology cannot be overstated with the increasing prevalence of congenital heart disease (CHD), found in approximately 0.8% of all live births. The pediatric cardiologist plays a central part in diagnosing and managing such afflictions, utilizing advanced diagnostic equipment to evaluate the heart's function and anatomy. With higher survival rates owing to improvement in surgical and medical management, the incidence of children and adolescents with CHD is rising, creating a unique challenge for healthcare. The importance of early treatment and diagnosis is highlighted by the requirement for advanced care to effectively address complications of such congenital anomalies so that patients achieve optimal health status as they transition to adulthood (Aboulhosn et al., 2020). This highlights the critical role of pediatric cardiology in establishing screening protocols and targeted therapies based on the specific needs of young patients. In addition to congenital heart disease, pediatric cardiology also encompasses acquired diseases of the heart which may present during childhood. These consist of inflammatory diseases such as myocarditis or rheumatic fever, which, if not promptly diagnosed and treated, may lead to major morbidity. Diagnostic techniques such as echocardiography, electrocardiography, and advanced imaging such as cardiac MRI enable pediatric cardiologists to assess heart structure, function, and electrical activity with accuracy. The application of such diagnostic tools is essential in discriminating between various cardiac conditions, guiding treatment protocols, and determining suitability for surgical interventions. The evolving pediatric cardiology also emphasizes the importance of multidisciplinary collaboration, where pediatric cardiologists work together with other healthcare professionals to deliver specialized care tailored to the sophisticated needs of children (Dixon et al., 2017). This collaborative approach is essential to improving outcomes and addressing children's long-term health needs involving cardiac conditions. Beyond providing immediate clinical intervention, pediatric cardiology plays a role in education and advocacy that seeks to improve awareness on children's heart health. Through engaging with families and communities, pediatric cardiologists de-mystify cardiac complexities while sharing essential preventive information and information on early detection. This educational component is vital because the majority of children are not symptomatic even with severe cardiovascular conditions. By creating awareness on risk factors and symptoms of pediatric cardiac conditions, cardiologists empower families to seek medical attention in time. Additionally, follow-up care later in life is also vital as the patients develop, particularly for those with congenital heart disorders who may struggle with adult-onset health issues as a result of their conditions. This commitment to continuous observation and treatment sustains the role of pediatric cardiology as an essential pillar of childhood health and well-being (Aboulhosn et al., 2020).

Overview of Diagnostic Techniques

For pediatric cardiology, there needs to be a wide variety of diagnostic techniques available to adequately diagnose and manage congenital and acquired heart disease. Non-invasive diagnostic imaging technologies such as echocardiography are the most common diagnostic tools. The technique employs sound waves to produce real-time images of the anatomy and function of the heart, allowing practitioners to assess morphology, valve function, and hemodynamic properties without sedation or ionizing radiation. Application of echocardiography extends beyond diagnosis to guide treatment planning and observation over time of ongoing patient management. Its portability and ease of use make it a first-line diagnostic imaging modality of choice in children who may occasionally be unable to tolerate more invasive testing. As technology improves, advanced echocardiographic techniques, like three-dimensional imaging, promise to even further refine diagnostic accuracy and guide therapeutic intervention. Outside echocardiography, cardiac magnetic resonance (MRI) and computed tomography (CT) have also become highly regarded in the diagnostic toolbox of pediatric cardiology. Cardiac MRI provides accurate anatomical and functional details of the heart without radiation exposure, thus making it particularly well suited for the pediatric population. The modality is optimally used for assessment of complex congenital heart disease and the characterization of myocardial tissue properties. In contrast, cardiac CT offers quick high-resolution image acquisition, which is significant in the assessment of coronary anatomy and detection of congenital anomalies. MRI and CT both play a critical role in treatment planning and surgical planning, particularly with delimiting complex anatomy. Incorporation of these advanced imaging modalities in the clinical environment enhances diagnostic strengths and ultimately translates into improved patient outcomes in pediatric cardiology. Moreover, electrophysiological studies are an advancement that offers a basis for the diagnosis of arrhythmias and other heart conduction disorders among children. Electrophysiological testing involves placing catheters in the heart with the capability to assess electrical activity and conduction. Electrophysiological testing can identify the mechanisms behind an arrhythmia and guide ablative therapy as needed. As more importance is attached to pediatric stroke as an issue, particularly in relation to congenital heart disease, it is more critical than ever to achieve timely and accurate diagnosis through continuous monitoring methods. Notably, the employment of continuous electrocardiogram monitoring (ECM) has been established to be pivotal in the identification of arrhythmias that predispose children to stroke, as revealed in the latest scientific statements on pediatric stroke and cardiovascular health (Aboulhosn et al., 2020; Donna et al., 2019). This multidisciplinary initiative underscores the paramount need for ongoing innovation and integration of diagnostic techniques to ensure better patient care in pediatric cardiology.

4.1. Clinical Assessment

Pediatric cardiology clinical evaluation is a significant process that involves proper examination of a child's cardiovascular status. The detailed examination begins with a careful medical history that takes in data on family cardiovascular diseases, conditions diagnosed in the past, and the symptoms child is exhibiting. Shortness of breath, fatigue, or developmental delay symptoms typically point to related cardiac conditions for further diagnostic imaging.

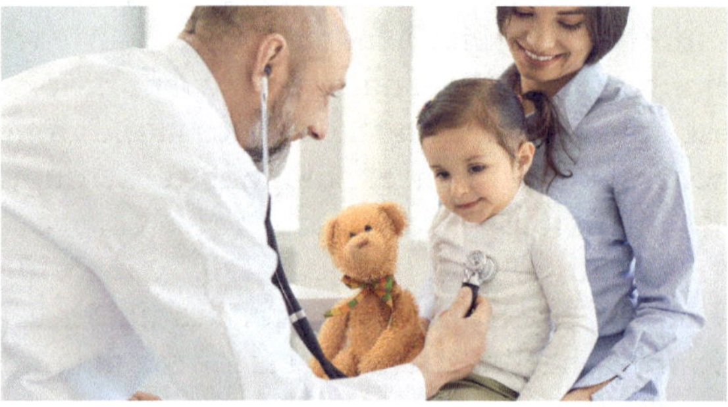

Figure 4.1. Pediatric cardiovascular assessment.

Source: https://www.springerpub.com/media/.renditions/wysiwyg/blog/Dr_.png.

With the unique anatomical and physiological patterns of children patients, physicians must apply age-adjusted assessment strategies that allow for variation in heart function and structure. Employing considerable clinical history-taking and physical examination data, healthcare providers are in a position to create an integrative picture of the child's cardiac status, forming the basis for effective diagnostic techniques. Following the initial evaluation, the clinical evaluation proceeds with a thorough physical examination that is essential in identifying signs of cardiovascular disease. The pediatric cardiologists are adept at assessing important vital signs such as heart rate and blood pressure and carefully observing cardiovascular-specific signs such as murmurs or abnormal heart sounds. The examination can also include peripheral perfusion, clubbing, or cyanosis observation, all of which could be indicative of severe cardiac anomalies (Figure 4.1).

In addition to this assessment, non-invasive modalities like echocardiography are highly valuable. Imaging modalities like these allow for dynamic imaging of cardiac performance and anatomy, enabling superior perception of congenital defects or acquired illness that is not easily discerned by physical examination. Lastly, interaction between meticulous physical examination and advanced imaging is highly amenable to precise diagnosis and appropriate treatment planning. Finally, clinical assessment involves advanced diagnostic tools and tests that further limit a child's heart condition. Electrocardiograms (ECGs) play an integral part in the assessment of defects in electrical conduction, while chest radiographs can reveal structural defects or cardiac enlargement. With the advent of technology advancements, the precision of such tests is higher, allowing for comprehensive assessments that were previously not possible. Further, detailed clinical assessments have a tendency of involving collaboration in multidisciplinary teams to consider all facets of pediatric cardiology. Interdisciplinary collaboration is crucial, particularly in managing complex cases that necessitate input from numerous specialists like geneticists, endocrinologists, as well as nutritionists. Appropriate clinical assessment thus demands interdisciplinary consideration to take into account all the factors that have an effect on a child's cardiovascular health, hence guaranteeing best results.

4.1.1. Patient History and Family Background

In pediatric cardiology, a strong understanding of patient history and family history is a critical aspect of precise diagnosis and effective treatment planning. History taking in detail (e.g., prenatal and perinatal history, symptoms in early infancy, and subsequent development milestones) can be particularly informative for understanding the patient's condition. Congenital heart defects also have individual familial patterns that must be explored; thus, understanding family medical histories can assist with the identification of genetic predispositions. For instance, the presence of rheumatic fever within a family should create close monitoring for cardiovascular sequelae and warrant the utilization of advanced diagnostic technologies such as echocardiography. If used together with careful patient history, these modalities can play an important role in increasing the diagnostic yield in the identification of underlying cardiac diseases so that timely and appropriate intervention can be done (Michael et al., 2015). Family background is also necessary to know the epidemiological factors influencing pediatric cardiology. Socioeconomic status, accessibility to healthcare, and environmental risk exposure may mold an environment with a great impact on a child's cardiovascular health. For example, children born to parents with a background of obesity have a high susceptibility to the development of cardiac defects, which necessitates an interdisciplinary strategy in assessment and diagnosis (Figure 4.2).

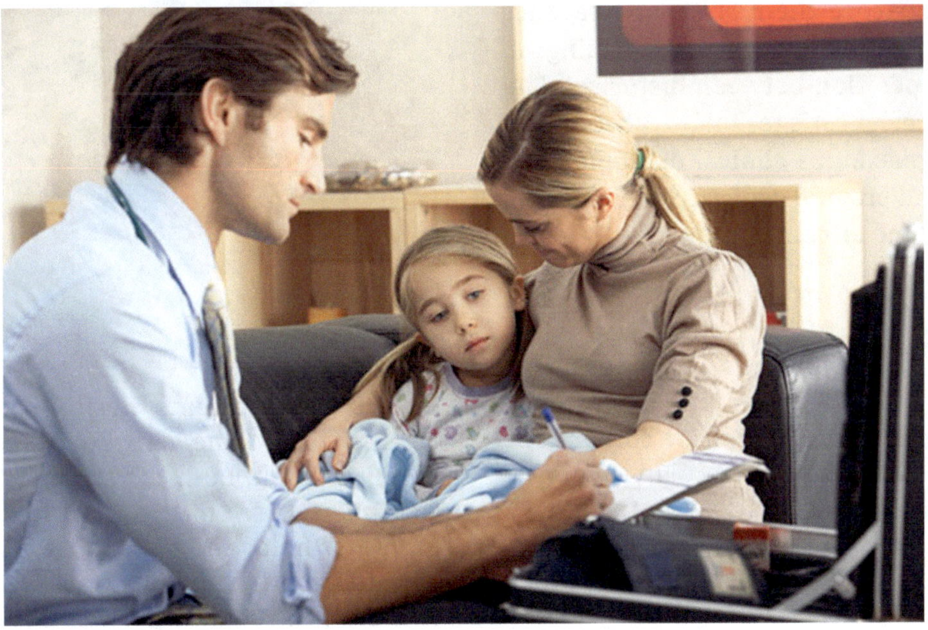

Figure 4.2. History taking in pediatrics.

Source: https://cached.imagescaler.hbpl.co.uk/resize/scaleWidth/815/cached.offlinehbpl.hbpl.co.uk/news/PGH/Epilepsy-20160921073448677.jpg.

In addition, the history of family health can be used by clinicians to prescribe individually tailored prevention. It has been shown in recent studies that there are strong associations between pediatric cardiac outcomes and social determinants of health. Therefore, utilization of a holistic approach that encompasses family and social histories can enable healthcare providers to tailor diagnostic techniques to the children's individual needs in an effective and relevant way (N/A,

2012). In addition, diagnostic technology is becoming more advanced and allowing for even simpler incorporation of patient history and family history into clinical practice. For instance, the use of Doppler echocardiography has revolutionized the identification of cardiac abnormalities even in asymptomatic individuals, particularly when complemented by extensive family histories of preconditions to particular conditions. These technological advances make possible an increased sensitivity in pediatric cardiovascular health, so disorders that would otherwise have gone undetected are more readily found. In addition, as the American Heart Association revises its guidelines to incorporate these developments, the emphasis on comprehensive histories of patients and families serves to underscore their ongoing relevance in clinical practice. Through emphasizing an integrated cooperation between historical data and innovative diagnostic techniques, healthcare providers can maximize clinical outcomes to a large degree and provide pediatric patients with more targeted and effective treatment (Michael et al., 2015).

4.1.2. Physical Examination Techniques

A complete physical examination is a cornerstone of pediatric cardiology diagnosis, allowing physicians to gather critical information regarding a child's cardiovascular status. The exam consists of inspection, palpation, percussion, and auscultation, each yielding unique information regarding the child's health. Inspection, for instance, will illustrate respiratory distress, cyanosis, or congenital abnormalities that can predate intrinsic cardiac pathology. Palpation allows doctors to assess pulses and peripheral circulation, thus identifying abnormalities of blood flow that could suggest heart disease. Percussion also provides information related to cardiac size and position, while auscultation is vital in the identification of abnormal cardiac sounds or murmurs that would require further study. The integration of these modalities is imperative in arriving at an accurate diagnosis and determining the need for further diagnostic tests or intervention. Interpretation of pediatric cardiology physical exam results can be very impactful on the patient's outcome.

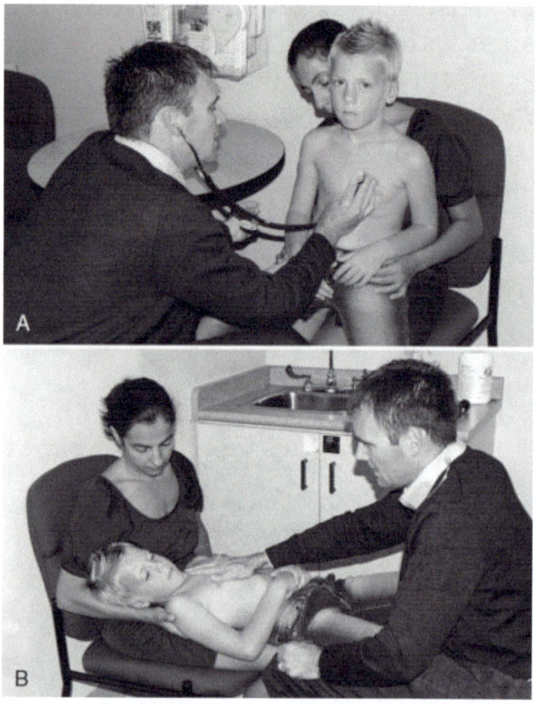

Figure 4.3. Patients hesitant to lie on the examination table can be examined on the parent's lap, in both the sitting (A) and supine (B) positions. In the supine position, the examiner holds the patient's legs against his or her sides both to help support the patient and to avoid what could otherwise be an unfortunate kick from a worried preschooler.

Source: https://nyulangone.org/files/congenital-heart-defects-in-children-doctor-examines-pediatric-patient.jpg.

Physical exam maneuvers can be supplemented with additional informative layers through diagnostic tools such as echocardiograms and electrocardiograms, but only after a skilled practitioner recognizes evidence during the physical exam that will guide the ordering of these advanced tests. For example, an auscultation result of a heart murmur may prompt an echocardiogram for assessment of structural abnormalities. Furthermore, clinical guidelines of practice emphasize the necessity of proper history and physical examination prior to invasive procedures, with the goal of minimizing potential risks (Larry et al., 2015) (Figure 4.3).

This multidisciplinary strategy not only enhances diagnostic accuracy but also fosters an interdisciplinary environment among cardiologists and pediatricians, thereby overall improving the care of cardiovascular disease in children. Clinical competence in physical examination techniques is particularly crucial in pediatric cardiology, given the unique physiological and developmental problems of infants and children. Children as patients require not only a deep understanding of cardiology but also effective communication with patients and families. Adopting child-friendly methods of examination can improve cooperation and reduce anxiety, facilitating a more effective evaluation. Of additional interest is that new guidelines emphasize ongoing education and training of healthcare staff in these essential examination skills in the face of advancing technology and diagnostic services (Alan et al., 2012). By maintaining a high degree of physical exam skill, doctors can expand their potential for diagnosis, ultimately resulting in early treatment and enhanced health for children with cardiac issues.

4.1.3. Identification of Symptoms and Signs

In pediatric cardiology, accurate identification of signs and symptoms is key to diagnosing cardiovascular disease in an efficient manner. Children have nonspecific signs and symptoms that camouflage underlying cardiac disease. Fatigue, palpitations, and breathlessness, for instance, can result from common childhood complaints or could be signs of serious illness such as cardiomyopathy or congenital heart disease. Clinical evaluation begins with a thorough history and physical examination, in which clinicians seek out external evidence of cyanosis, clubbing of the fingers, or inappropriately elevated blood pressure. Such presentations, if caught early, may initiate further workup, including diagnostic studies. Being sensitive to the subtleties in the presentation of a child and the possibility of the change in symptomatology with age and degree of development is important to arriving at a proper diagnosis and intervening appropriately. The role of rigorous clinical examinations cannot be overestimated since these provide the context against which other diagnostic techniques are employed in pediatric cardiology. Cardinal signs like chest pain (which tend to be less common in children than in adults) must increase suspicion of underlying cardiac involvement (Figure 4.4).

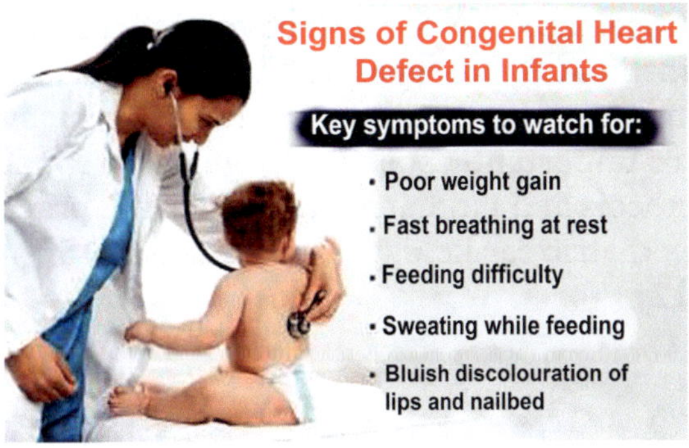

Figure 4.4. Signs of congenital heart defect in infants.

Source: https://www.facebook.com/100069816352433/posts/987070200296849/?_rdr.

Additionally, other symptoms such as failure to thrive, poor weight gain, or irritability may indicate chronic heart ailments needing prompt treatment. Due to the complexity and diversity of symptoms found in cardiovascular disease in children, medical practitioners need to be on guard to differentiate between benign and serious signs. Higher-level imaging and diagnostic technologies, including echocardiography and cardiac MRI, often follow initial assessments to provide insight into the resulting cardiac disorder, reinforcing the significance of accurate symptom identification. Symptom identification not only entails recognition but also the scope of the affiliated knowledge regarding symbiotic relationship among clinical symptoms and resulting pathophysiology. For instance, diagnosing infective endocarditis is a matter of serious consideration of risk factors such as recent intervention or underlying heart disease, since they can be likely to expose children to infection typically manifesting in unfamiliar forms. It demands a multidisciplinary model, which pools the various healthcare specialists' expertise for the purpose of improving diagnosis. For instance, recommendations by the American Heart Association emphasize the necessity of personalized management of such conditions, with diagnostic techniques to match symptomatology for effective interventions. Identification of symptoms and signs thus influences early clinical choices but even more importantly specifically guides treatment protocols and ultimately delineates the practice of pediatric cardiology (Larry et al., 2015; N/A, 2012).

4.2. Electrocardiography (ECG)

Electrocardiography (ECG) is a critical diagnostic tool in pediatric cardiology, enabling the assessment of cardiac function in the pediatric population. As a non-invasive technique, ECG records the electrical activity of the heart, acquiring vital information regarding arrhythmias, congenital heart disease, and other cardiovascular conditions prevalent in pediatric cases. The ability to detect slight changes in cardiac rhythm and form is particularly valuable since children's hearts are anatomically and physiologically different from those of adults. With clinical diagnosis using ECG, pediatric cardiologists can make accurate diagnoses, which guide the subsequent course of treatment options and interventions. The inclusion of ECG in routine cardiac evaluations ensures that potential issues are identified in the initial stages, therefore enhancing patient outcomes. Moreover, technological innovation has further increased the use of ECG in pediatric practice. With the advent of digital electrocardiography and wireless monitoring, real-time analysis is becoming even more accessible. These advances allow for an enhanced overall evaluation of a child's cardiovascular condition such that healthcare workers are able to rapidly examine ECG reports and provide timely interventions. Pediatric-specific reference values growth is another important development since it enables more precise interpretation of results that are patient age and size specific. This development shows the revolutionary impact of novel diagnostic modalities, like AI solutions in electrocardiography used to enhance predictive analytics and assist personalized care plan approaches (Karalis, 2024). In pediatric cardiology, the difficulty in performing an electrocardiogram needs to be met, particularly in relation to interpreting the results. The pediatric patients will present with exceedingly unique variations in ECG patterns that may lead to misdiagnosis if not adequately understood. Therefore, ongoing training and education for healthcare workers are of utmost importance so that correct interpretation is ensured. Additionally, ethical issues related to data privacy and security gain special importance as technology becomes more ingrained in healthcare applications. The advent of electrocardiographic monitoring systems must be held to high standards of ethics so that patient information is protected without forsaking the benefits achieved by AI-based advancements in clinical practice. As pediatric cardiology advances as a specialty, a balance has to be struck between the advantages of advanced diagnostic machinery and the ethical issues that accompany it (Stafie et al., 2023).

4.2.1. Basics of ECG in Pediatric Patients

In understanding the basics of electrocardiography (ECG) in children, it is extremely vital to understand the unique physiological and anatomical differences influencing cardiac performance in children. Pediatric ECG interpretation is very different from adult interpretation on the basis of parameters such as heart size, shape, and conductive pathways that change over age. Children possess a higher heart rate than adults, and this can result in amplitude and duration changes of the ECG waveforms. Second, axis deviation that is typical in children must be clearly known so that misinterpretation does not contribute to unjustified interventions. Thus, child clinicians must be able to recognize normal variations in a child's ECG for distinguishing between benign and pathological results. The process of acquiring an ECG in pediatric patients also requires special care in order to provide comfort as well as accuracy. Maintaining correct electrode positioning is the most critical to minimize artifacts and derive an accurate representation of cardiac function. As children are often anxious or difficult to cooperate with testing, the application of techniques that provide a soothing environment can assist in yielding a quality higher-level ECG result. Also, employing age-appropriate ECG devices more appropriate for less sturdy body structures can yield more precise data. Incorporating child-centered approaches into this process is not only helpful in obtaining clear records but also fosters a positive interaction between a child and the health assessment process in future visits, thus emphasizing the value of patient experience in pediatric cardiology (Figure 4.5).

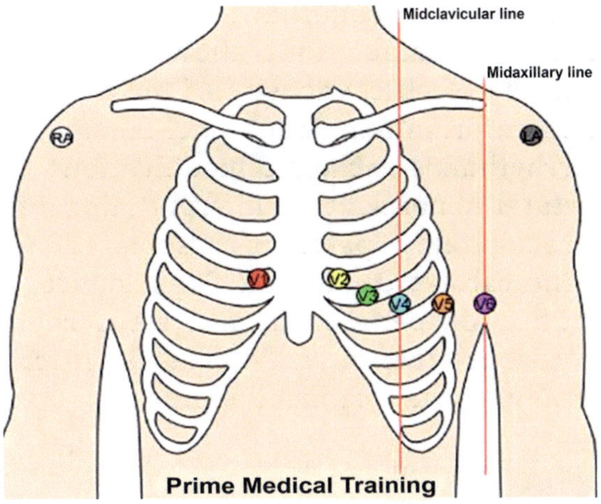

Figure 4.5. Pediatric ECG lead placement.

Source: https://www.urmc.rochester.edu/pediatrics/cardiology-fellowship/ecg-placement.

Also needed is an understanding of arrhythmias and conduction disturbances that occur specifically in this age group. Children will present with a broad spectrum of rhythm disturbances, including congenital heart block or sinus arrhythmias, which are much different from those experienced by adults. Practitioners must be able to identify life-threatening conditions versus nonsignificant variations typical of children. Other than diagnosis, management consideration for these rhythm disorders can vary from conservative observation to more intense intervention strategies, depending on the immediate diagnosis and its broader implications for the overall health of the child. In proper diagnosis and treatment advice, recognition of the complexity of pediatric ECG tracings is essential, solidifying the place of ECG as a basic diagnostic tool in pediatric cardiology (N/A, 2023).

4.2.2. Interpretation of ECG Findings

Electrocardiogram interpretation is a crucial component in pediatric cardiology to diagnose various cardiac conditions. The ECG is an outward technique that allows doctors to assess the electrical activity of the heart and obtain information about phenomena such as arrhythmias, ischemic modifications, and structural abnormalities. Interpretation relies on recognizing patterns associated with specific cardiac conditions. For instance, the identification between normal sinus rhythm and various types of arrhythmias is critical in determining the treatment approach.

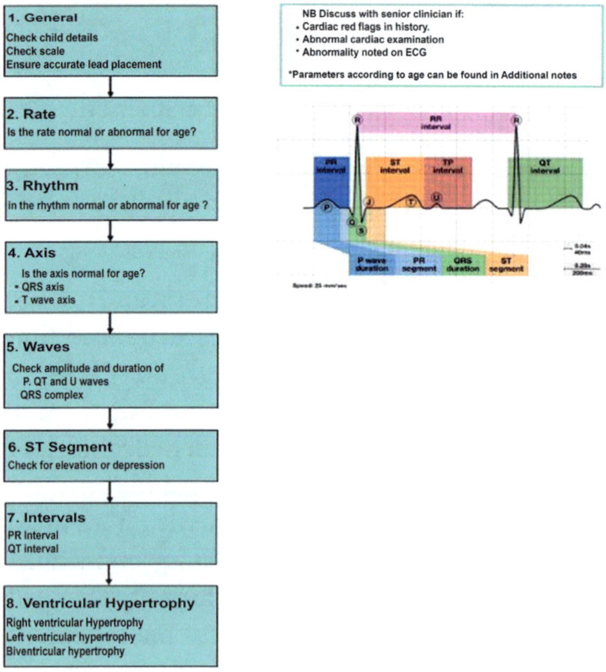

Figure 4.6. A stepwise approach to basic interpretation of a pediatric ECG.

Source: https://www.rch.org.au/uploadedImages/Main/Content/clinicalguide/guideline_index/ecg-image1.png.

As pediatric patients often present with varied symptoms, a comprehensive understanding of the nuances in ECG presentation becomes crucial to facilitate correct evaluation and management. Instructors of pediatric cardiology must prepare learners to confront the complexities in ECG interpretation, particularly in conditions that mimic real-life clinical practice environments. Modern curricula have emphasized enhancing the trainees' task-switching competency because they are frequently interrupted which can undermine their ability to read ECGs correctly. Studies have revealed that the guided education interventions that include task-switching training can improve residents accuracy and confidence during ECG interpretation when timed (Schrepel et al., 2021) (Figure 4.6).

This type of practice not only assists in building confidence but also represents the dynamic nature of emergency medicine wherein decision-making quickly makes an impact on patient outcome. Further, the application of newer imaging modalities and enhanced criteria of diagnosis still further enhances the identification of cardiac illnesses in children. For example, myocarditis (a muscular heart disease caused by inflammation) can be quite difficult to distinguish from other forms of cardiomyopathy in ECG. Guidelines now state that cardiac magnetic resonance imaging is important in accurate diagnosis, appreciating the role of various pathogens in causing inflammation (Ammirati et al., 2020). Combining traditional ECG findings with advancing imaging modalities allows pediatric cardiologists to render more comprehensive diagnoses and ultimately result in better treatment protocols. This multi-pronged approach appreciates the need for continuous education and adaptability in pediatric cardiology.

4.2.3. Common Abnormalities Detected

Among pediatric cardiology, early detection of common abnormalities has a significant effect on patient outcome. Congenital heart defects (CHDs) are among the most frequent abnormalities and represent a large group of structural defects of the chambers, valves, and blood vessels of the heart. They are typically presented by cyanosis, heart murmurs, and feeding disturbances in children. Technological innovations in the form of echocardiography and cardiac MRI enable pediatric cardiologists to visualize these structural defects in real time, enhancing accuracy in diagnosis. Early detection of CHDs not only makes timely intervention possible but also directly influences long-term management planning in the affected individuals and the establishment of a system for multidisciplinary care and follow-up. Arrhythmias also present among the common abnormalities in children, and their implications vary with the type and severity of the rhythm abnormality. Electrical conduction abnormalities can occur as tachycardia or bradycardia and manifest with symptom-related presentations like palpitations, syncope, or sudden cardiac death. Diagnostic techniques such as Holter monitoring and electrophysiological studies are critical in determining the reason and nature of these arrhythmias. By such sophisticated assessment, clinicians can distinguish between benign and problematic conditions that require immediate intervention. The versatility of equipment used for diagnostics reflects an aggregate understanding of pediatric arrhythmias, indicating the continued need for specialized interventions aimed at achieving optimal health outcomes for young patients faced with these cardiac complications. Lastly, infective endocarditis is another life-threatening condition in the practice of pediatric cardiology, likely requiring accurate monitoring and management since it's so complicated and potentially catastrophic. Its infection of the lining of the heart is usually associated with preexistent structural heart disease, making its detection important among high-risk groups. Current standards emphasize not only the diagnostic role of echocardiography but also its role in assessing the extent of valve damage and allowing for therapeutic management. As infective endocarditis becomes more complex, a team with an assortment of health care professionals is needed. Such inter-disciplinary management is critical given the disease's severity and the subtle presentation that can vary considerably among pediatric patients, which underlines the importance of intensive surveillance and intervention measures in this field (Larry et al., 2015; N/A, 2012).

4.3. Echocardiography

Echocardiography is one of pediatric cardiology's cornerstones in its diagnostic arsenal, providing real-time visual assessment of cardiac structure and function without the need for invasive methods. Echocardiography uses high-frequency sound waves to create accurate images of the heart, enabling physicians to examine congenital cardiac abnormalities, analyze cardiac function, and monitor hemodynamic status. The fact that echocardiography is noninvasive makes it especially appropriate for children, who often must undergo repeated studies. This technique not only helps in the direct identification of cardiac pathology but also helps in the decision making of continuous management, effectively directing treatment algorithms in the clinical setting. With the ongoing developments in echogenic devices, for instance, 3D echocardiography, the depth of information obtained from these studies has risen significantly, enhancing the clinician's capacity to create accurate diagnosis and treatment plans specific to the individual patient needs. Outside of initial diagnostic capabilities, echocardiography also plays an important role in the long-term management of children with congenital heart defects and acquired heart disease. Serial follow-up examinations allow ongoing observation for alterations in cardiac size and function over time in children with either congenital defects or acquired heart disease. These tests enable clinicians to measure the effectiveness of therapy interventions and, as necessary, alter treatment regimens based upon the constantly changing condition of each patient. For instance, advancements in Doppler imaging make it possible to evaluate blood flow and pressure gradients across the valves of the heart and thus gain insight into how severe valvular stenosis or regurgitation may be. Additionally, echocardiographic tests would also identify complications such as myocarditis, still a clinical challenge in pediatrics, to highlight further the need for constant monitoring with this critical diagnostic tool (Yuk et al., 2021). The integration of artificial intelligence (AI) in echocardiography can further enhance diagnostic accuracy and efficiency in pediatric cardiology. As soon as AI algorithms begin processing echocardiographic data, they can assist clinicians by identifying patterns that are difficult to spot manually. For example, AI-driven tools can reduce image interpretation time by a significant amount, allowing clinicians to focus on the immediate care and decision-making of patients. Such a technological push goes hand-in-hand with improvements in imaging modalities, with the aim of improving patient outcomes through improved accuracy of diagnosis, particularly in complex cases of congenital heart diseases. As mentioned in the recent literature, the integration of AI with echocardiographic processes is an attractive area in pediatric cardiology with developments that promise to revolutionize clinical practice as well as pose reflective consideration of ethical and privacy concerns in terms of data security as well as informed consent (Karalis, 2024).

4.3.1. Types of Echocardiography Used

The use of echocardiography in pediatric cardiology is diverse, encompassing various types of echocardiography that are appropriate for different diagnostic needs and clinical situations. Transthoracic echocardiography (TTE) remains the most common procedure and has particular worth in non-invasive assessment of child heart anatomy and function. The procedure employs transducers applied to the body surface to observe the chambers, valves, and blood flow in the heart without sedation or invasive techniques. The utility of TTE is also supplemented by the fact that it is able to generate real-time imaging, allowing clinicians to visualize dynamic cardiac function changes, especially useful in children. Moreover, advancements in technology have witnessed increases in resolution of images and Doppler capability, and therefore, TTE has emerged as a pivotal instrument for the diagnosis of congenital heart disease and other cardiac defects among children.

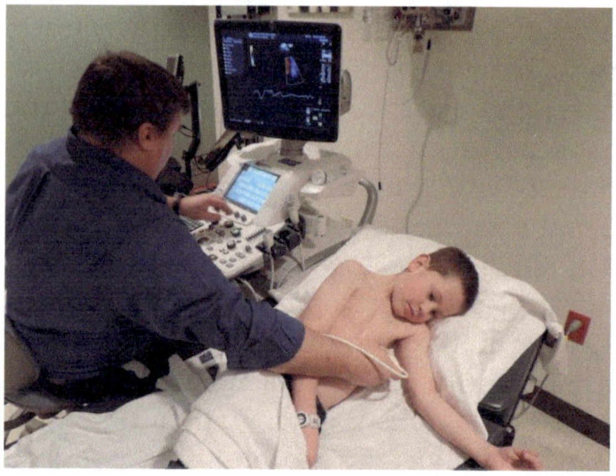

Figure 4.7. Transthoracic echocardiography (TTE).

Source: https://www.ashleyregional.com/sites/ashley/assets/pages/peds_echo.jpg.

In contrast, transesophageal echocardiography (TEE) is typically reserved for more severe cases where high-definition heart images are required. The procedure is accomplished by inserting an esophageal probe into the esophagus in order to obtain good images of the heart, obtaining very valuable information regarding structures that are difficult to image well using TTE. TEE is of most benefit with certain diagnostic workups and in the perioperative setting, where precise imaging of cardiac anatomy is critical. The procedure offers closer approximation to the heart, such that it allows for easy identification of issues such as thrombi or vegetation in infective endocarditis. Its ability to accommodate to varying clinical situations underscores the value of TEE as an adjunct procedure, especially when standard echocardiographic methods are inadequate, thus enhancing diagnostic accuracy in pediatric cardiology (Figure 4.7).

Technological developments in echocardiography have introduced new techniques such as three-dimensional (3D) echocardiography and speckle tracking imaging, which are becoming crucial tools of contemporary pediatric cardiology. Three-dimensional echocardiography possesses the unique benefit in the assessment of anatomical characteristics of congenital heart disease by yielding a spatial orientation of cardiac structures. This is superior for surgical planning and accurately evaluating ventricular function. Furthermore, speckle tracking imaging is a significant advancement by enabling measurement of deformation of the myocardium, giving evidence regarding global and regional cardiac function that might otherwise be beyond what standard techniques can readily provide. These new technologies promise not only to enhance the potential for diagnosis but also to be able to provide more individualized management strategies, especially in diseases like left ventricular non-compaction cardiomyopathy where standard imaging could be complemented by other techniques (Berceanu et al., 2017). Therefore, the evolution of echocardiographic modalities has proceeded to revolutionize the landscape of pediatric cardiology and has ensured improved patient outcomes.

4.3.2. Advantages of Echocardiography in Children

Echocardiography has become a very valuable resource in pediatric cardiology due to the fact that it is not invasive and provides a wealth of information. Compared to other modalities, echocardiography visualizes the heart's structure and function with the use of sound waves, which is safe even for neonates. This technique allows for dynamic assessment of cardiac anatomy, such as chamber size, wall motion, and valve configuration, which are crucial in the diagnosis of congenital cardiac disease and other cardiovascular diseases. Echocardiography also may be performed at the bedside, which in acute setting is extremely valuable given the necessity for rapid diagnosis. The ability to obtain real-time images significantly supports prompt interventions, which ultimately contribute to improved patient outcomes among this high-risk population, as highlighted in recent guidelines on the management of cardiovascular disease in children (Eric et al., 2022). Echocardiography also supports surveillance of patients with diagnosed heart disease, providing ongoing feedback regarding regression or progression of disease. This imaging technique allows the physician to evaluate the efficacy of treatment modalities and make adjustments in a timely fashion tailored to a specific child's anatomy. With the dynamics of their growth influencing cardiac morphology in children, echocardiographic evaluation on a regular basis is essential in following the changes. The utility of such continuous monitoring is brought to the fore in specialist reports emphasizing the necessity of continuous monitoring of children at risk of cardiovascular events, such as children with previous stroke or congenital heart disease (Donna et al., 2019). Such dynamic adaptability of echocardiography makes possible the capacity of medical caregivers to deliver the best possible care during periods of peak development. Furthermore, echocardiography is a critical teaching tool in pediatrics that teaches prospective healthcare professionals significant diagnostic skills, and enhances their knowledge of cardiac pathophysiology. From live echocardiographic examinations witnessed by residents and students, they are given exposure to clinical applications of cardiac assessments, reinforcing the theoretical bases.

This experiential education fosters an appreciation of the relationship between heart structure and function and ultimately impacts how they will be able to engage with pediatric patients. Such learning experiences are crucial in molding a new generation of clinicians skilled in the application of state-of-the-art diagnostic techniques. The integration of real clinical experience and live learning is aligned with current educational objectives in pediatric cardiology, thereby deepening the underlying foundation of cardiovascular disease in children and improving subsequent clinical outcomes.

4.3.3. Limitations and Challenges in Interpretation

The use of diagnostic techniques in pediatric cardiology is beset by limitations that can burden clinical decision-making considerably. Different anatomical and physiological characteristics inherent in the child make the diagnostic process more difficult, as imaging techniques may not have a one-size-fits-all solution. Echocardiography, for instance, while predominant technique, is sensitive to the operator's experience and patient cooperation. Diagnostic difficulties in achieving clear images in younger patients or in patients with tachypnea, among other conditions, may contribute to misinterpretation or lack of diagnosis.

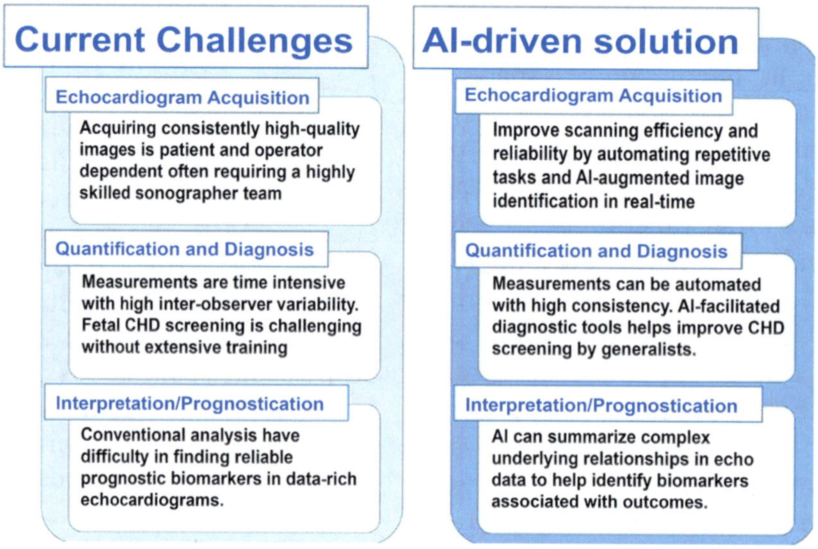

Figure 4.8. Overview of tasks in the pediatric echocardiography laboratory that could be assisted with artificial intelligence workflows.

Source: https://www.frontiersin.org/files/Articles/881777/fradi-02-881777-HTML/image_m/fradi-02-881777-g001.jpg.

Anatomical variations are also more significant in patients with congenital heart disease, making both the detection of pathologies and application of therapeutic measures more complicated. These variations demand a higher degree of experience and watchfulness in translating results because normative data collected for adults could be irrelevant to pediatric individuals, and that could lead to ill-guided management strategies (Adam et al., 2018). The incorporation of advanced diagnostic techniques, such as cardiac MRI and CT, has its own multitude of challenges. These imaging modalities are better in detail and accuracy but can be confounded by interpretation requirements for specialist training and expertise. For example, risk of overdiagnosis in structural anomaly detection could result, which in turn leads the practitioners into unnecessary treatment pathways. In children, the physiological and genetic heterogeneity complicates diagnosis, such that conditions such as hypertrophic cardiomyopathy (HCM) could present variably. The reliance on genetic testing, as valuable as it is, also presents interpretative challenges; since in roughly 40% of HCM patients, the causative genes remain unidentified, it brings into question disease prognosis and choice of treatment (Ali et al., 2017) (Figure 4.8).

This phenotypic heterogeneity serves to remind us to exercise caution in interpretation when comparing across modalities. Lastly, the temporal and developmental aspects of the interpretation of child cardiac disease cannot be overlooked. Children dramatically change as they grow, and their cardiovascular systems are no different, so that any single snapshot taken from any diagnostic imaging can be potentially limited in its application to diagnosis. Thus, longitudinal assessment may be needed, and it will become challenging to have a treatment and diagnosis timeline. Also, the psychosocial context in which care is delivered should not be overlooked; issues pertaining to diagnostic outcomes may further confound clinical interpretation. Involving the family in the process of diagnosis is necessary but can also mean variability in perception and conveying outcomes. Therefore, pediatric cardiologists must recognize these limitations and continually seek education and advancement in diagnostic skills for optimal patient outcomes, in spite of the inherent challenges that exist within interpretation (Adam et al., 2018).

4.4. Chest X-Ray

The chest X-ray is a simple investigative modality that is applied in pediatric cardiology, providing vital visual information regarding the thoracic cavity in children. It is an imaging technique that effectively identifies structural abnormalities, congenital defects, as well as other cardiovascular disorders that are not identifiable through clinical examination. It entails minimal or no radiation exposure, and thus it is extremely suitable for children, who happen to be more radiation-sensitive than adults. Moreover, chest X-rays enable clinicians to assess the size, form, and position of the heart, as well as vascular structures surrounding it, and assist in early diagnosis and treatment. By enabling rapid detection of life-threatening conditions such as cardiomegaly or pulmonary edema, chest X-rays play a central role in ensuring prompt care of pediatric cardiac patients. Though the method has its advantages, interpretation of chest X-rays in pediatric cardiology requires experience and expertise due to variations in normal cardiac morphology of younger individuals. There should be the ability to distinguish between physiological differences and pathological conditions for correct diagnosis to be established. Further, children presenting in pediatric cardiology typically have signature presentations, and so, there has to be an enlightened appreciation of age-related norms in radiologic imaging. As technology advances, incorporating machine learning techniques into radiology has the potential to improve diagnostic precision and speed. One instance is Swarm Learning, which showed promising results in handling big data sets, such as chest X-ray images, with the result that distributed data-trained classifiers are better than site-trained classifiers (Warnat et al., 2021) (Figure 4.9).

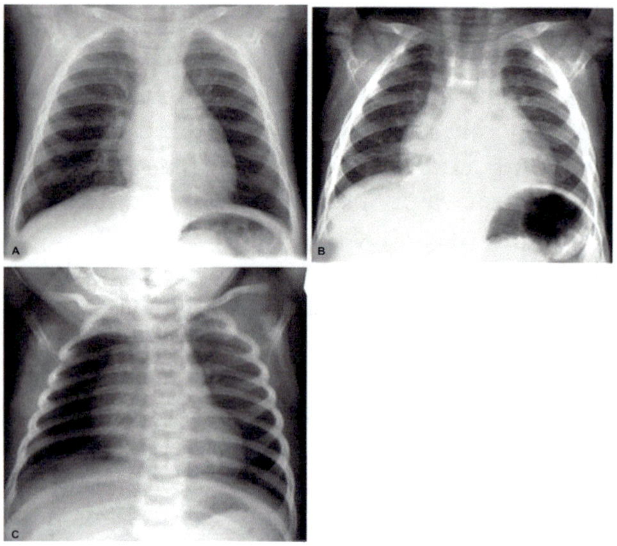

Figure 4.9. A normal chest examination in an infant. Frontal radiographs in inspiration (A) and expiration (B) show the profound impact of an expiratory film on the appearance of the heart and lungs. In another example (C), a lucent right lung reflects patient rotation to the right rather than asymmetrical pulmonary blood flow.

Source: https://radiologykey.com/chest-radiography-in-pediatric-cardiovascular-disease/.

These innovations offer promising avenues to the pediatric cardiology imaging future. Further, chest X-rays have roles beyond initial diagnosis; they are important in follow-up management and monitoring of pediatric cardiac disease. Follow-up radiographs are employed by physicians to determine long-term modifications in heart size or pulmonary blood flow in an effort to ensure that therapeutic interventions are effectively controlling the condition. This longitudinal approach is significant in the management of congenital heart disease as it offers a chance for early adjustment of care plans particular to a patient's evolving needs. Additionally, advancement of radiographic techniques, including digital imaging and low-radiation protocols, is enhancing the benefit and safety of chest X-rays. With continuous enhancement of these techniques, health practitioners are in a position to achieve a high quality of care while minimizing risks from imaging. In this sense, chest X-rays serve not only a diagnostic function but also as a core component of whole-pediatric-cardiology-care (Figure 4.10) (Bryan et al., 2021).

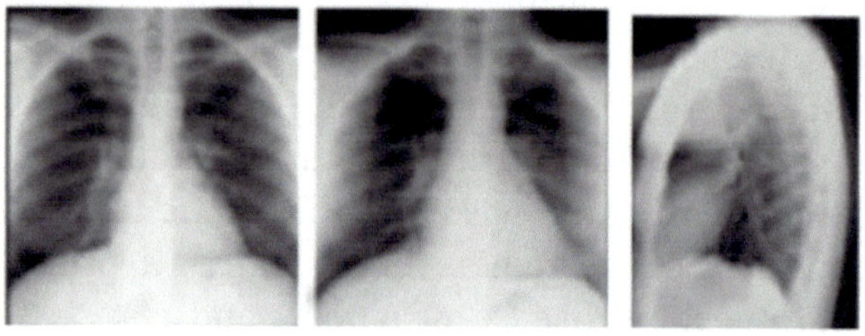

Figure 4.10. The images provided are the lateral view, AP view, and PA view, respectively.

Source: https://image.prepladder.com/prepladder/2024/04/09111015/lateral-view-AP-view-and-PA-view.webp.

4.4.1. Role of Chest X-Ray in Diagnosis

The role of chest X-ray in the diagnosis of pediatric cardiology is crucial, especially in directing clinical management and assessing the underlying anatomy. Chest X-ray is the initial imaging procedure to give an estimate of cardiac defects, enabling early treatment. Radiographs are able to identify useful information like cardiac size and form, pulmonary congestion, and its related lung findings among children. A properly read chest X-ray can indicate a large number of congenital heart conditions, among them cardiomegaly for underlying heart volume overload or hypertrophy, and abnormalities in pulmonary vascularity. Visible evidence derived from X-rays is allowed to make immediate evaluations, which in the case of pediatric patients is more important as early treatment is the main factor in significantly lowering morbidity and mortality. Secondly, understanding the inherent limitation of chest

X-ray in distinguishing some cardiovascular anomalies will encourage further investigation through other diagnostic methods. Incorporation of advanced screening technologies like chest X-ray in pediatric routine assessment has the potential to improve diagnostic validity in cardiology. The widespread availability and affordability of chest X-ray render it an accessible first-line imaging agent for clinicians. But even while it is employed as a useful tool for initial evaluation, more definitive imaging studies, e.g., echocardiogram or MRI, remain needed to define the full extent of cardiac abnormalities. Furthermore, advances in artificial intelligence and machine learning, as embodied by the Swarm Learning approach, could revolutionize the accuracy of chest X-ray interpretation. By combining distributed data and enabling classifier development with enhanced performance without violating privacy rules, such technologies could improve diagnostic accuracy, particularly by identifying subtle pathologies that may be overlooked in standard examinations (Warnat et al., 2021) (Figure 4.11).

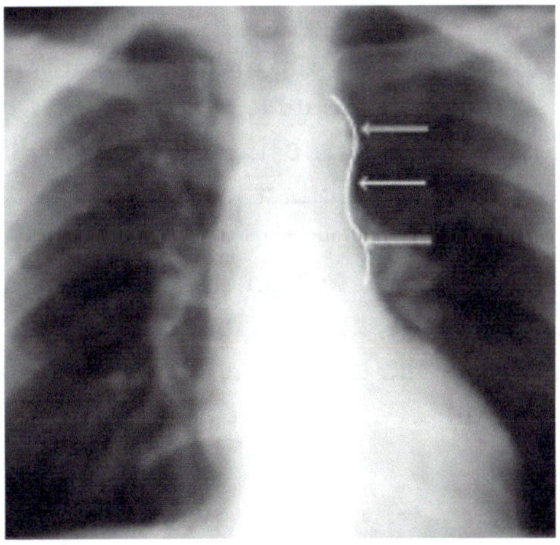

Figure 4.11. A convexity will form on the right side of the heart if the aortic arch is dilatation.

Source: https://image.prepladder.com/prepladder/2024/04/09112746/Aortic-Dilatation.webp.

Building on such advances may enhance the role of chest X-ray in an integrated diagnostic strategy for pediatric cardiology. Despite its advantages, the use of chest X-ray is also fraught with disadvantages that demand wise restraint from clinicians. X-ray interpretation has a steep learning curve due to the inherent intricacy of anatomy in children and variability of presentation in children. In addition, it is impossible to dismiss the risk of radiation exposure, especially since pediatric patients are more susceptible to such risk than adults. Practitioners must therefore balance the immediate benefit of chest X-ray with a proper understanding of its limitations and long-term consequences. This would presumably result in a more prudent use of this imaging modality in the delivery of patient-specific care, without compromising the achievement of significant diagnostic information. In conclusion, further studies and interdisciplinary cooperation will enable us to better understand the role of chest X-ray in pediatric cardiology diagnosis, ultimately resulting in patients' improved outcomes.

4.4.2. Key Indicators of Cardiac Issues

Identification of the most significant signs of cardiac disease in children should be done to ensure early and precise diagnosis and treatment. A patient who presents with cyanosis, tachycardia, and unexplained exhaustion during exertion can be a point of red flag consideration. Cyanosis as depicted by blue coloration of skin or mucous membranes is usually indicative of inadequate oxygenation and can be an indicator of underlying congenital heart disease. Tachycardia, or increased heart rate, might also suggest multiple cardiac abnormalities, including arrhythmias or cardiac failure. Additionally, symptom-free fatigue, especially post-exercise in young children, needs to be further investigated since it can signal inefficiencies of cardiac output or peripheral perfusion. Appropriate identification of these signs gives the background for subsequent diagnostic investigations, building appropriate intervention that has a great impact on the management of pediatric cardiology. Other diagnostic techniques, such as echocardiography, are crucial in determining the presence of cardiac abnormalities suggested by these clinical features.

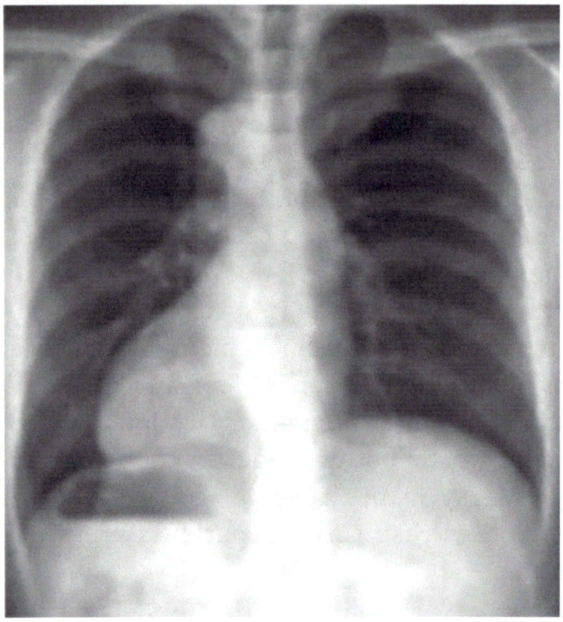

Figure 4.12. The two diaphragm domes in a normal person are not at the same level; the cardiac shadow occupies one-third of the right side and two-thirds of the left side of the thoracic cavity.

Source: https://image.prepladder.com/prepladder/2024/04/09122932/dextocardia.webp.

One of the most useful machinery, echocardiography provides accurate images of the structure and function of hearts, allowing the detection of abnormalities such as septal defects or valvular abnormality. A non-invasive but effective technique, this is particularly useful in children, where conventional invasive techniques are more dangerous. Moreover, the dynamic nature of echocardiographic assessments contributes to their value in monitoring the pattern of disease and therapeutic response, hence guiding real-time clinical decisions. Utilization of a diagnostic scheme with the incorporation of echocardiography, particularly in the context of presence of key indicators, contributes to comprehensive diagnostic accuracy in the field of pediatric cardiology and provides evidence-based focused interventions. In addition to traditional symptoms and echocardiographic assessment, the genetic and family history may yield information concerning potential cardiac issues (Figure 4.12).

A child's genetic risk is invaluable to know, especially in familial cardiomyopathy or hereditary arrhythmias as identified by nuances in family medical history. Employing a standard approach of genetic testing can allow one to identify at-risk individuals in an early state where one can have early surveillance and intervention strategies in place. Genomics and precision medicine can even offer evidence-based guidelines for treatment depending on one's genetic makeup, making interventions more efficient. These developments put greater emphasis on both the integration of clinical markers and genetic factors into the pediatric cardiology diagnostic process, both improving early detection and outcomes for children at risk for heart disease, as described in guidelines for the diagnosis and treatment of related disorders (Bryan et al., 2021; Eric et al., 2022).

4.4.3. Comparison with Other Imaging Techniques

In pediatric cardiology, the selection of imaging modalities is crucial for effective treatment and diagnosis. Echocardiography remains the cornerstone of cardiac imaging due to its non-invasive nature, lack of ionizing radiation, and potential to provide real-time data regarding cardiac function, which makes it more desirable in children. Its application extends from assessment of cardiac anatomy to hemodynamics and valvular function and therefore serves as a first-line diagnostic tool. In some of the more complex cases, however, additional imaging modalities will be needed. For example, magnetic resonance imaging (MRI) is of greater spatial resolution and tissue characterization and more capable of investigating congenital heart lesions and myocardial diseases in more detail that cannot always be resolved by echocardiography alone. While MRI enhances diagnostic capability, its longer acquisition time and need for sedation in children could limit use on a daily clinical basis. Despite the advantages of echocardiography and MRI, computed tomography (CT) has emerged as a valuable imaging modality, particularly to delineate anatomical structures and assess coronary artery disease. CT angiography provides three-dimensional images of the cardiac vasculature and potentially could be extremely valuable in preoperative planning with the presence of congenital heart disease. However, inclusion of ionizing radiation and contrast-induced nephropathy risk in pediatric patients necessitates careful consideration of its application. Additionally, technological advancements in 3D echocardiography and novel imaging modalities have been recognized to serve as adjuncts to routine echocardiography. These modalities allow for thorough assessments that can be equivalent to CT in some cases. Therefore, while each imaging modality has its own set of functions, the choice must be adapted to the individual patient need, balancing against potential risks. The role of hybrid imaging modalities, such as PET-CT, in pediatric cardiology must be mentioned. Hybrid imaging combines functional and anatomical information, which may enhance diagnostic accuracy, particularly in assessing processes like myocarditis or cardiomyopathies. However, limited data are available for long-term safety and effectiveness of these modalities in children, which has led to questions about the routine use. Furthermore, while MRI and CT more accurately define structural abnormalities, echocardiography has no substitute for immediate bedside assessment that is often most important in acute situations. When comparing these modalities, the reality that clinical context, patient age, and specific diagnostic requirements need to be accounted for becomes critical. In the long term, an integrated strategy that benefits from the strengths of various imaging modalities will lead to improved diagnosis and best clinical results for pediatric cardiology patients with opportunities for individualized patient management based on full imaging data.

4.5. Cardiac MRI

Cardiac magnetic resonance imaging (MRI) is now a focal diagnostic tool in pediatric cardiology, which yields high-resolution images that more clearly delineate cardiac structures and functions. It is a non-invasive technique that is extremely appropriate for pediatric patients since it avoids ionizing radiation used in other imaging techniques such as computed tomography (CT). Cardiac MRI excels at evaluating congenital heart anomalies, cardiomyopathies, and myocardial inflammation. Its ability to visualize the heart's anatomy and physiology in fine detail requires more accurate diagnoses and comprehensive planning of treatment. Furthermore, the development of MRI technology in the form of incorporating echo-MRI techniques has resulted in the improved visualization of dynamic heart events in real-time and paved the way for tailored therapeutic approaches to individual pathologies in children. In the diagnostic arena of myocarditis, cardiac MRI has changed clinical practice from traditional diagnostic techniques to newer imaging modalities. Since myocarditis may mimic nonspecific chest pain or heart failure in children, accurate diagnosis is necessary for appropriate treatment. Cardiac

MRI as a diagnostic standard has enabled clinicians to identify inflammatory myocardial changes noninvasively, thus preserving the risk to young people. Cardiac MRI defines hyperemic and edematous regions of fibrosis with good precision and also determines the extent of damage to the myocardium accurately, which aids in therapy determination. The accord that is brought about regarding the use of cardiac MRI in pediatric myocarditis signifies its role in delineating various etiologies of cardiac inflammation, ultimately contributing to short-term and long-term treatment, particularly for diseases that may evolve into chronic inflammatory cardiomyopathy (Ammirati et al., 2020) (Figure 4.13).

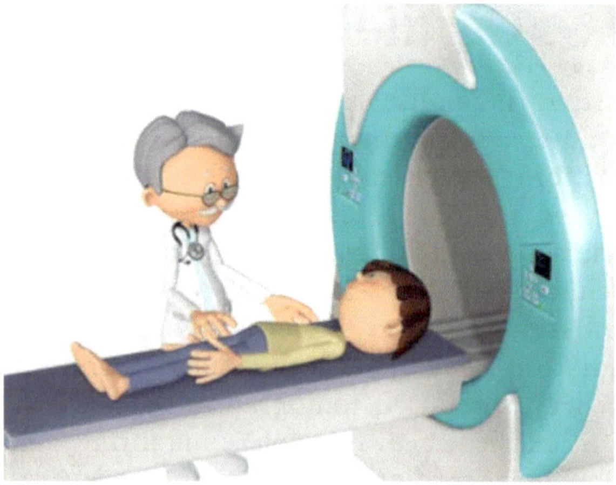

Figure 4.13. Cardiac MRI.

Source: https://i0.wp.com/www.pccoforegon.com/wp-content/uploads/2016/03/images_pediatric-cardiac-MRI.jpg?resize=400%2C300.

Despite the major advantages of cardiac MRI, its use in pediatric cardiology continues to be hindered by a number of challenges. Requirement for sedation by pediatric patients can befuddle image acquisition that is clinically useful, and this leads to variability in diagnostic results (Eric et al., 2022). Interpretation of cardiac MRI results is not only entirely reliant on specialty but also distinguishing normal developmental variants from abnormal alterations. Newer protocols designed to shorten scan times and improve image acquisition under free-breathing conditions have the capability to resolve these problems to a considerable extent. With advancements in the field, the use of cardiac MRI as part of routine clinical practice has the potential to enhance outcomes in children with heart ailments. Continuous research and communication between multispecialty teams will play an important role in optimizing this important diagnostic tool's performance and its application in pediatric cardiology, ultimately enhancing the quality of care for children.

4.5.1. Indications for Cardiac MRI in Pediatrics

The use of cardiac magnetic resonance imaging (MRI) in the pediatric setting has emerged as an essential diagnostic procedure in the evaluation of numerous congenital and acquired heart diseases. The imaging modality is non-invasive and allows for true estimation of cardiac anatomy, myocardial function, and hemodynamics without exposing children to ionizing radiation. MRI is particularly beneficial when echocardiographic data are indefinite or when better visualization is needed. For instance, cardiac MRI is critical in the assessment of complex congenital heart disease, cardiomyopathies, and ischemic heart disease in children. Moreover, the precision offered by cardiac MRI enables clinicians to define intricate anatomical relationships and assess vascular integrity, which becomes crucial for successful planning of surgical intervention. Thus, awareness of indications of cardiac MRI is crucial in order to enhance diagnostic confidence and optimize management in pediatric cardiology. In addition to anatomical imaging, the functional assessment capability of cardiac MRI confers additional advantages on pediatric cardiology. The modality allows cardiac function testing by measuring parameters like ejection fraction, stroke volume, and myocardial strain. These measurements are important in the diagnosis of progressive conditions like dilated cardiomyopathy, in which early treatment can significantly alter the prognosis. Additionally, cardiac MRI can be utilized to assess the treatment response patterns of treatment regimens, such as chemotherapy in pediatric cancer patients, who can develop treatment-related cardiac complications (Figure 4.14).

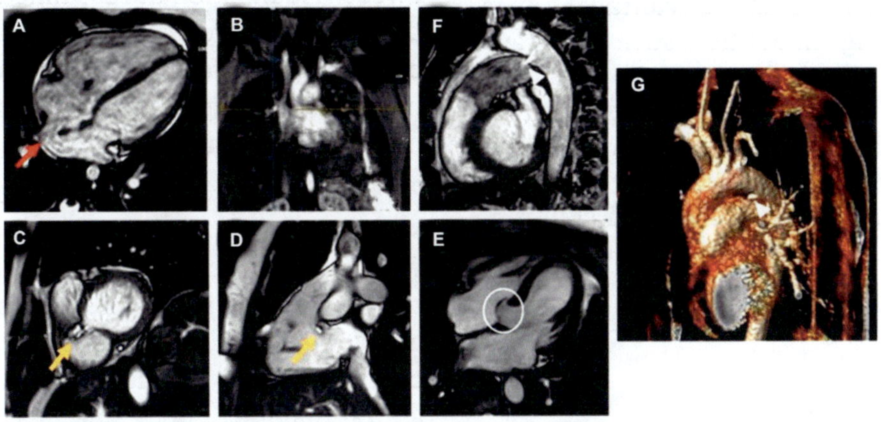

Figure 4.14. (A) 4-chamber cine SSFP image showing sinus venosus ASD (red arrow); (B) angiographic reconstruction showing the right upper pulmonary artery draining into the superior vena cava (blue and yellow cross); (C) basal short-axis cine SSFP image; (D) sagittal RV three-chamber view showing perimembranous VSD (yellow arrow); (E) 4-chamber cine SSFP image showing aneurysmal formation of the basal septum involving the adjacent septal leaflet of the tricuspid valve (white circle); (F) sagittal cine SSFP image; and (G) MRA showing PDA (arrowheads). [SSFP: Steady-state free precession; ASD: atrial septal defect; RV: right ventricle; VSD: ventricular septal defect; and PDA: patent ductus arteriosus].

Source: https://www.mdpi.com/children/children-11-00878/article_deploy/html/images/children-11-00878-g001.png.

Overall, cardiac MRI not only provides the initial diagnosis but also plays a central role in the long-term management plans, highlighting its important position on the pediatric cardiologist imaging modality arsenal. Furthermore, advances in cardiac MRI technology, such as higher field strength magnets and faster imaging sequences, have also extended the scope of its indications. These technologies allow for earlier and more accurate diagnosis of complex diseases, such as arrhythmias because of congenital heart disease or post-procedure complications of other cardiac surgeries. The most recent consensus statements stress the use of cardiac MRI in specific situations so that children are given personalized care based on their unique cardiovascular profiles (Maully et al., 2021). Despite such developments, it is still necessary for clinicians to wed clinical impression with imaging findings, particularly in the context of atypical conditions or atypical presentation. Thus, although cardiac MRI is a precious diagnostic tool in pediatric cardiology, its potency is best realized in unison with comprehensive clinical evaluations and multidisciplinary consensus. Through such an approach, clinicians are able to provide the optimal possible care to their children patient population, ultimately resulting in optimal clinical outcomes.

4.5.2. Benefits of MRI Over Traditional Imaging

Magnetic Resonance Imaging (MRI) has emerged as an important diagnostic tool in pediatric cardiology, offering some advantages over traditional imaging modalities, such as X-rays and echocardiograms. An important advantage of MRI is that it can produce high-resolution, three-dimensional images of heart anatomy without exposing pediatric patients to ionizing radiation. This aspect is particularly valuable in children, who are more susceptible to the deleterious effects of radiation exposure, especially since it has the potential to increase their lifetime risk of cancer.

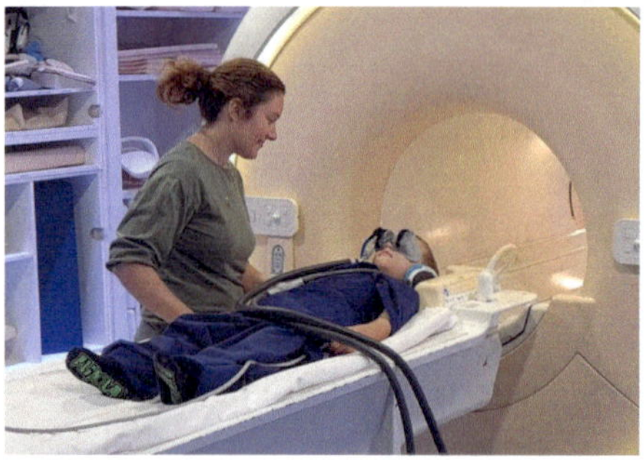

Figure 4.15. Benefits of MRI.

Source: https://cdn.wchn.sa.gov.au/assets/resized/images/WCH/children/medical-imaging/34169/mri-1_W1600_H1600_Mfit_fallback.jpg.

Moreover, MRI provides unambiguous information regarding cardiac morphology and function, enabling clinicians to evaluate complex congenital heart malformations efficiently, which are otherwise difficult to visualize using traditional imaging methods. With these advanced imaging capabilities, MRI enhances diagnostic accuracy, allowing for more informed treatment decisions, particularly in complicated situations requiring a subtle understanding of cardiac anatomy. MRI also is preferable for assessing dynamic blood flow within the heart and large arterial and venous trunks. In contrast to traditional methods that may rely on operator measurements or limited views of cardiac function, MRI uses advanced techniques such as cardiac cine MR imaging. This allows for direct visualization of real-time cardiac motion during the entire heart cycle and thus provides comprehensive functional information as well as informative insights into myocardial perfusion and wall motion abnormalities (Figure 4.15).

Furthermore, MRI can measure parameters such as cardiac volumes and ejection fraction with high precision non-invasively, making them indispensable measures for treating most pediatric cardiac disorders. By this comprehensive functional assessment, MRI is a vital diagnostic tool and means of observing heart disease development in children, and it has a direct influence on treatment and intervention strategies. Moreover, the versatility of MRI extends beyond structure and function assessment; it is also immensely beneficial in tissue characterization by way of advanced imaging techniques. Through modalities such as T2-weighted imaging and late gadolinium enhancement, MRI is capable of discriminating normal and diseased myocardial tissue, highlighting conditions like myocarditis or fibrosis that conventional imaging may not be able to pick up. This capability is particularly worthwhile in a pediatric group, in which these conditions are diagnosed early enough to create a significant impact on management and outcomes. Additionally, the use of MRI in pediatric cardiology conforms to guidelines for treating complicated aortic disease and illustrates the worth of accurate imaging assessment in individualizing treatment regimens in pediatric patients. In brief, the benefit of MRI compared to traditional imaging in pediatric cardiology is not only its capacity to provide full structural and functional evaluation but also its promise of enhancing safety and enhancing care to a vulnerable population.

4.5.3. Safety Considerations and Contraindications

Safety considerations are given top priority in pediatric cardiology when employing diagnostic processes. Processes involving echocardiography, electrocardiograms, and cardiac MRI should be comprehensively examined so that they are properly in line and beneficial for patients who are children. For instance, although echocardiography is regarded as safe, it should be comprehensively examined in newborn babies with specific birth flaws or where sedation is required. The sedation risk, particularly in preterm or low-birth-weight infants, could complicate medical decisions for practitioners. Thus, meticulous assessment of medical history and any complications arising based on aortic disease or other cardiac abnormalities is needed to prevent risks and honor patient safety (Eric et al., 2022). Contraindications to some diagnostic techniques also need to be addressed to prevent unintended effects. For instance, stress testing, potentially capable of providing substantial data regarding cardiac function, may be contraindicated in a child with known structural heart disease or refractory arrhythmias. In addition, the administration of contrast medium with cardiac MRI, which is generally harmless, poses possible risks to children with renal insufficiency or anaphylactic responses. Awareness of such contraindications allows clinicians to work on refining diagnostic approaches and assess alternatives, ensuring benefits outweigh potential risks. A well-balanced approach involves interdisciplinary teams in order to weigh the risks and ensure adequate safety protocols are in place, particularly in high-risk patient populations (Bryan et al., 2021). Finally, emphasis on safety issues and contraindications in pediatric cardiology relies on a continuum of monitoring and vigilance during the diagnostic process. Providers must remain up to date with the latest guidelines and technological developments to safeguard young patients. For example, an understanding of the ways in which chronic illness or immunotherapy can affect diagnostic decision-making is important in determining the most favorable course of action for any given patient. Guidelines also encompass the pediatric practitioner's suggestions for assessing a child's unique medical history when balancing potential advantages of diagnostic procedures with harms (Figure 4.16). By establishing an environment of safety and awareness, medical professionals can maximize the diagnostic process without causing redundant harm to vulnerable groups (Bryan et al., 2021; Eric et al., 2022).

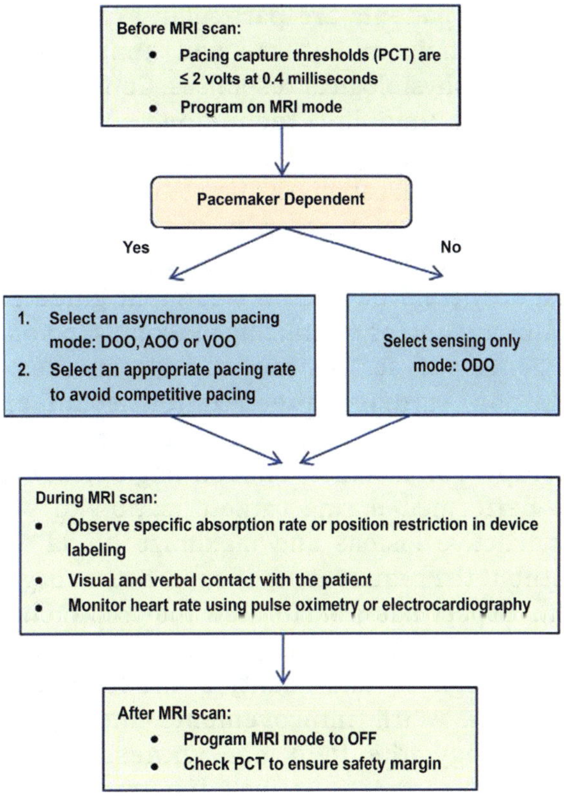

Figure 4.16. Safety considerations for MRI in patients with an MRI-conditional pacing system.

Source: https://www.researchgate.net/figure/Safety-Considerations-for-MRI-in-Patients-With-an-MRI-Conditional-Pacing-System_fig1_319694791.

4.6. Cardiac Catheterization

Cardiac catheterization is one of the most important diagnostic techniques in pediatric cardiology that enables precise evaluation of congenital and acquired cardiac and great vessel disease in patients of all ages. Cardiac catheterization is a minimally invasive form of diagnosis wherein a tiny catheter is threaded over the bloodstream to the heart, with direct measurement of cardiac chamber pressures and evaluation of the dynamics of blood flow. Pediatric patients are particularly challenging due to their miniature-sized anatomy and variable physiological responses. Consequently, advanced imaging technologies, such as echocardiography and fluoroscopy, are often combined with catheterization to obtain optimal visualization and accuracy with procedures. Overall, cardiac catheterization is not only a diagnostic aid but also a treatment guide and planning tool for optimizing outcomes in young patients with serious cardiac abnormalities. In addition, cardiac catheterization is not only used for diagnosis but is a necessary part of therapy. For instance, balloon angioplasty can be performed during catheterization to open obstructive lesions and maximize blood flow without the requirement of open-heart surgery. This aspect has transformed the treatment of congenital heart disease, enhancing the long-term prognosis and quality of life for affected children. With improvements in catheter technology, the field has witnessed novel forms of interventions, including transcatheter valve replacement and device closure. They also reduce the need for invasive procedures, which are particularly intimidating to pediatric patients and their families. To this end, the role of senior practitioners and a multidisciplinary team cannot be overstated, as they ensure each procedure is tailored to meet the particular needs of the child. As the challenges of congenital heart disease persist, so does the demand for ongoing research and optimization of cardiac catheterization procedures in children. Technological innovations in imaging, such as 3D reconstructions and improved catheter guidance systems, are continually improving procedural success and safety profiles. However, it is still challenging to minimize complications such as infective endocarditis, which is extremely serious in the case of young patients who receive such interventions (Larry et al., 2015). A strong understanding of potential risks, coupled with developments in preventive strategies, such as prophylactic antibiotics, is required to improve patient care. The evolution of cardiac catheterization as a cornerstone within pediatric cardiology is testament to its central role not only in diagnosis but also in revolutionizing treatment modalities for the diseased child's heart (Berto et al., 2017) (Figure 4.17).

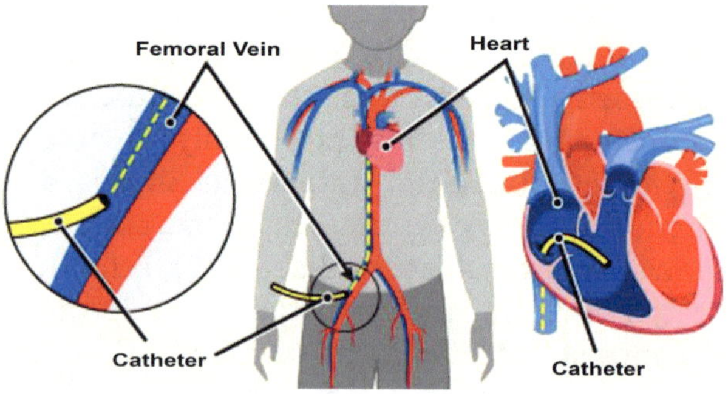

Figure 4.17. Cardiac catheterization.

Source: https://external-content.duckduckgo.com/iu/?u=https%3A%2F%2Fwww.kidshealth.org%2Fcontent%2Fdam%2Fpatientinstructions%2Fen%2Fimages%2FcardiacCath-415x233-rd5-enIL.png&f=1&nofb=1&ipt=3f56353f696fc26c7e6d649fd1eb03c06a2ad03c94350744cbc13e5e9c6294d4.

4.6.1. Purpose and Procedure of Cardiac Catheterization

Cardiac catheterization is a key role in the field of pediatric cardiology, offering a comprehensive evaluation of congenital heart disease (CHD) and other cardiac conditions. Cardiac catheterization is a minimally invasive procedure that involves introducing a thin, flexible tube, or catheter, through blood vessels into the heart. The use of cardiac catheterization extends beyond diagnosis; rather – direct visualization of the chambers of the heart and blood vessels, measurement of pressures, and measurement of oxygen saturation are all available. In addition, catheterization makes interventional treatments, such as balloon angioplasty or stent placement, available, which can alleviate obstructions or repair anatomical abnormalities of the heart. As technology and methods continue to evolve, cardiac catheterization is now an indispensable tool in managing pediatric patients with cardiovascular diseases (Aboulhosn et al., 2020). During the procedure, the patients are commonly sedated or anesthetized to ensure comfort, and the procedure is commonly carried out in a special catheterization laboratory. The clinicians utilize imaging modalities, such as fluoroscopy and echocardiography, to guide the movement of the catheter and visualize the cardiac structures in real time. Contrast agents may be employed after catheter placement to enhance the quality of images and provide exquisite anatomical information. This approach is particularly important in structural problem diagnosis, such as septal defects or valve disease, so that therapeutic decisions can be made. Successful performance of cardiac catheterization in children requires a multidisciplinary team consisting of cardiologists, anesthesiologists, and intensive care nursing staff. All team members play a critical part in ensuring procedural safety and efficacy, thereby reinforcing team-based care in pediatric cardiology (Larry et al., 2015). While its benefits are numerous, there are risks involved with cardiac catheterization, including potential complications such as bleeding, infection, or trauma to the vessels. Therefore, meticulous pre-procedural assessments play a critical part in identifying candidates for whom the benefits outweigh these risks. Post-procedure follow-up is also crucial since the patients have to be observed for any side effect or complication that might develop. Care plans typically entail initial care and follow-up in the long term; whereby ongoing observation of the patient's cardiac health will be required for proper management of congenital heart disease. With the increased number of patients with adult congenital heart disease, driven by advances in pediatric care, the role of cardiac catheterization will continue to be essential not just for diagnosis but also for planning appropriate interventions throughout the patient's life. This reason accounts for the significance of the procedure in pediatric cardiology and for the significance of constant advancements and collaborative practices in the specialty (Aboulhosn et al., 2020).

4.6.2. Diagnostic versus Interventional Uses

In pediatric cardiology, the distinction between diagnostic and interventional use of imaging modalities should be made in order to provide the best quality care to the patient. Diagnostic imaging modalities such as echocardiography and magnetic resonance imaging (MRI) are more interested in studying the structure and function of the heart without involving an implication of direct therapy.

These technologies provide very important information regarding congenital heart defects, valvular diseases, and hemodynamic abnormalities, which are essential for accurate diagnosis. For example, echocardiography enables clinicians to visualize cardiac abnormalities, quantify shunt flows, and assess ventricular function, thus influencing subsequent management. Interventional modalities, on the other hand, such as catheter-based interventions, use these diagnostic findings to facilitate treatment, having a direct impact on the outcome of patients. By non-invasive or minimally invasive intervention, interventional therapy attempts to correct structural heart defects or address arrhythmias, in effect improving the quality of life of pediatric patients. The experience with three-dimensional rotational angiography (3DRA) is an ideal example of the evolution of imaging modalities blurring the line between diagnostic and interventional application in pediatric cardiology. Although traditionally viewed as a diagnostic modality, recent reports have highlighted its role in making interventional procedures easier, especially in complicated congenital disease. For instance, data indicate that 3DRA enabled precise visualization in 67.1% of intervention cases and diagnostic utility graded higher than traditional angiography in 94% of reported cases (Stefanie et al., 2020). Such dual application not only optimizes pre-procedure planning but also minimizes radiation exposure and contrast, consistent with trends for personalized and safe patient care. With pediatric cardiology making greater use of advanced imaging technology, clinicians are challenged to reconcile maximal diagnostic accuracy with anticipation of interventional need, developing an integrated treatment model. Further, the differentiation between interventional and diagnostic uses highlights the evolving educational needs of pediatric cardiologists. Training programs are now more geared towards developing skills that span both realms, such that practitioners not only analyze diagnostic images effectively but also understand the subtleties of performing interventional procedures. The American College of Cardiology is emphasizing the requirement of robust training, as per COCATS guidelines, to sharpen the clinical skill set of cardiologists entering practice. It entails exposure to more than one imaging modality and procedural technique, fostering a balanced approach to patient evaluation and treatment (Susan et al., 2019). Ultimately, bridging the divide between diagnostic and interventional use in pediatric cardiology not only maximizes clinical outcome but also prepares future practitioners to deliver outstanding, evidence-based care to children with complex congenital heart disease.

4.6.3. Risks and Complications Associated

In pediatric cardiology, diagnostic procedures are accompanied by a set of risks and complications deserving of careful consideration. Among methods of diagnostic imaging, echocardiography, specifically transthoracic and transesophageal echocardiography, is frequently employed to assess cardiac structure and function. Procedures can provoke significant risks, however, particularly in the context of infectious disease outbreak, as with the COVID-19 pandemic. The pediatric patient, although typically less likely to develop severe illness, can also be an asymptomatic carrier of such pathogens as SARS-CoV-2, making the management and safety measures required during echocardiographic assessment more challenging. This calls for increased caution and adjusted practices to minimize viral spread and shield healthcare workers and patients alike. Because of the complexities, experts must be well-informed of the risk of echocardiography in order to optimize outcomes for patients with minimal risks in a safe clinical environment (Barker et al., 2020). Complications can also ensue from the introduction of invasive procedures, such as catheterizations, which are increasingly utilized in the pediatric cardiology field to diagnose and treat congenital heart defects. All of these operations carry intrinsic risks, including potential damage to the blood vessels and heart, as well as sedation and anesthetic risks. The rate of complication of conditions like infective endocarditis is a matter of concern when devices or prosthetics are employed, particularly with regards to long-term complications post-intervention. Surprisingly, new guidelines call for the deployment of an endocarditis team to maximize management plans in such individuals. As device-associated infective endocarditis becomes more complicated, there is a need to enhance awareness of such complications. Clinicians must emphasize prompt treatment and broad follow-up care to avoid such complications but guarantee that the right and effective treatment is given to patients (Dixon et al., 2017). Imaging techniques in response to therapy assessment and diagnosis of cardiac disease complications also pose distinctive challenges. Evolution of protocols and guidelines over time, particularly for prophylactic procedures for infective endocarditis, points towards the need for continuous watchfulness in evaluation and management processes. Pediatric cardiologists must be kept informed of shifting patterns of investigative imaging modalities and their implications. Infections like infective endocarditis can quickly deteriorate and therefore early detection and intervention are required to prevent severe morbidity. Optimization of communication among multi-disciplinary teams becomes imperative so that best management plans are put in place in a timely fashion in reaction to such diagnostic risks and complications. Finally, overcoming such pitfalls effectively is based on scrupulous adherence to evolving guidelines and an ironclad dedication towards patient safety (Dixon et al., 2017).

SUMMARY

The advancements in diagnostic technologies in pediatric cardiology foretell a new era in the management of congenital cardiac disease. The research into novel technologies, such as three-dimensional (3D) printing, has expanded the scope for personalized medical simulation and training. By using imaging technologies, such as CT and MRI, trainers can create anatomically accurate models that enhance simulation as well as hands-on practice training. This is particularly crucial given the unique challenge posed by the anatomical heterogeneity in the pediatric cohort. Of particular interest here is the possibility of modifying patient-specific models to mimic an array of cardiac pathologies and thereby facilitate personalized training opportunities, hence propelling the expertise of medical specialists in diagnosing and treating intricate cardiovascular illnesses among children (Hopfner et al., 2021). Furthermore, as new clinical problems keep emerging, such as COVID-19-associated myocarditis, pediatric cardiology practice must remain nimble and adaptable. Thorough diagnostic approaches that account for both conventional and contemporary techniques are of paramount relevance. As a case in point, when cardiac MRI is not possible, other imaging modalities such as cardiac computed tomographic angiography can be helpful in the diagnosis of patterns of inflammation and exclusion of significant coronary artery disease. Such diagnostic flexibility is imperative in a pediatric patient population that may potentially have a range of clinical presentations, highlighting the necessity for a thorough understanding of diverse diagnostic outcomes (Siripanthong et al., 2020). Ultimately, continuous development of pediatric cardiology diagnostics improves patient outcomes while also paving the way for future research and design. The convergence of cutting-edge imaging technologies and patient models is a reminder of the need for interdisciplinary cooperation, closing gaps between technology, education, and practice. As we move forward, it is imperative to keep an eye on improving diagnostic accuracy, driving educational progress, and new health challenges through research and clinical application. This team effort will be instrumental in ensuring the best possible care for pediatric patients as it pertains to cardiovascular care (Hopfner et al., 2021).

Summary of Diagnostic Techniques

Pediatric cardiology diagnostic techniques serve a crucial role in the early detection and treatment of congenital and acquired heart disease. Of the various modalities available, echocardiography is the primary non-invasive cardiac imaging modality. The technique consists of utilizing ultrasound waves to generate accurate images of heart structure and function so that clinicians are able to assess cardiac anatomy and hemodynamics without exposing children to radiation. Technological advancements in echocardiography, including three-dimensional and Doppler modalities, provide increased visualization of cardiac chambers and valves and the dynamics of blood flow. The versatility of echocardiography renders it appropriate for not only routine evaluation but also in acute presentation, which adds to its value in the pediatric cardiologist's armory. Regular training and collaboration between clinicians also enhance effective utilization of this precious diagnostic tool in the clinical environment, resulting in accurate diagnosis and proper treatment in pediatric patients with various cardiac abnormalities. Apart from echocardiography, electrocardiography (ECG) is equally a significant diagnostic tool for the diagnosis of cardiac disease among children. This process measures the electrical activity of the hearts, providing vital information regarding rhythm abnormalities, conduction abnormalities, and other cardiac dysfunctions. ECG interpretation in children is complicated since certain patterns are radically different from what they look like in adults. Pediatric cardiologists must consider age, development, and some congenital heart diseases when interpreting ECG findings. Furthermore, advances in technology of Holter monitoring and event recorders have heightened the potential for detecting intermittent or occult arrhythmias in children, potentially avoiding severe complications through early intervention. As pediatric cardiology continues to advance its knowledge, incorporating ECG data into comprehensive assessments of cardiac status illustrates the utility of this diagnostic tool in improving patient outcomes through earlier identification and tailored therapies. Additionally, cardiac MRI and CT are now mandatory imaging modalities for evaluation of late congenital heart disease, particularly when echocardiographic images are poor. Both imaging modalities provide high-quality images to allow distinct visualization and assessment of cardiac morphology and function, vascular structures, and associated abnormalities. Cardiac MRI has the added benefit of quantifying blood flow and myocardial perfusion without ionizing radiation, so it is a suitable option for serial follow-up in children. Improvement in imaging technology has also greatly improved the diagnostic usefulness of cardiac CT, which can be utilized especially in surgical planning. However, use of these imaging techniques requires careful planning for sedation protocols and patient safety, especially among vulnerable child populations. Integration of cardiac MRI and CT into practice exemplifies a multidisciplinary approach towards diagnosis and management of challenging cardiac disorders in children, stimulating interprofessional communication between pediatric cardiologists and radiologists while enhancing patient care outcomes in pediatric cardiology (Aboulhosn et al., 2020; Dixon et al., 2017).

CLOSER LOOK

PEDIATRIC ECG INTERPRETATION

Pediatric electrocardiogram (ECG) interpretation is a valuable aid to assess the electrical activity and rhythm of a child's heart. Pediatric ECG interpretation differs significantly from adult ECG interpretation due to age-related anatomical and physiological variations in heart rate, cardiac dimensions, and development of the conduction system. Analysis requires familiarity with normal pediatric ECG patterns at various ages and recognition of deviations that may signal underlying cardiac disease. One of the key aspects regarding pediatric interpretation of ECG is familiarization with normal age-specific values. Neonates and infants, for example, have a much faster heart rate than older children and adults. The normal rate in newborns ranges from 100–160 beats per minute, decreasing gradually with age to approximately 60–100 beats per minute in adolescents. Similarly, QRS axis, P morphology, and T orientation change with increasing age as the right ventricle decreases in size and the left ventricle becomes more prominent. Right axis QRS in neonatal life is normal due to in-utero physiological right ventricular dominance. In older age, left ventricular dominance is acquired and there is increasing leftward shift of the QRS axis. Hence, seemingly right axis deviation in an adult may be normal in a neonate or infant. Likewise, T waves in the right precordial leads (V1 through V3) are typically upright in the neonate but become inverted after the first week of life and can remain inverted throughout early childhood—a situation that would be abnormal in an adult but is considered normal in children (Figure 4.18).

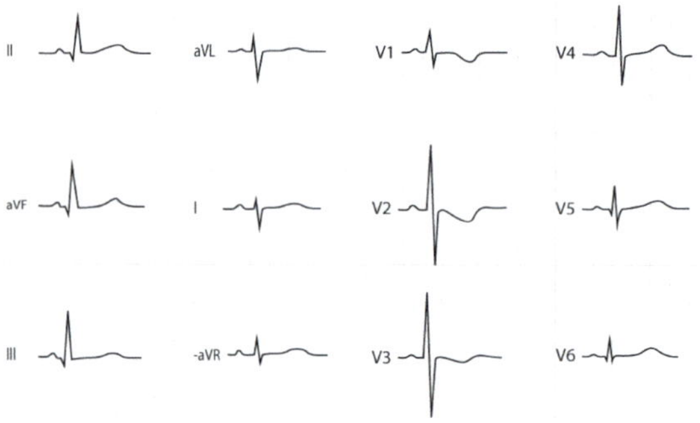

Figure 4.18. Pediatric ECG showing normal T-wave inversions in the precordial leads (V1–V3), which is a common and normal finding in children. This pattern reflects the normal physiological repolarization differences in the pediatric heart.

Source: https://ecgwaves.com/wp-content/uploads/2019/11/pediatric-ecg-t-waves-negative-inverted.jpg.

PR interval, QRS duration, and QT interval all vary with age and heart rate. Intervals are shorter in children due to increased rates and smaller heart sizes. Clinicians must use age- and heart rate-adjusted reference ranges so they do not misinterpret normal as pathologic. QT interval prolongation, for example, must be quantified in terms of corrected QT (QTc) values, and abnormality could signal risk for arrhythmias like torsades de pointes or congenital long QT syndrome.

Common pediatric ECG abnormalities include arrhythmias like sinus tachycardia, sinus bradycardia, SVT, and ventricular pre-excitation patterns in Wolff-Parkinson-White syndrome. Structural heart diseases like atrial septal defects, ventricular hypertrophy, or cardiomyopathies will also induce characteristic ECG changes like axis deviation, voltage change, or abnormal wave forms. For instance, left ventricular hypertrophy can manifest as tall R waves in left-sided leads and deep S waves in right-sided leads.

Pediatric interpretation of ECG is particularly useful in the evaluation of syncope, chest pain, palpitations, or suspected congenital heart disease. ECG may also be useful for monitoring cardiac drug effects, electrolyte imbalance, and systemic disease such as Kawasaki disease or myocarditis. However, an ECG must always be interpreted in relation to clinical history, physical examination, and other investigations like echocardiography.

References

1. Aboulhosn, J., Hijazi, Z. M., Kavinsky, C. J., McElhinney, D. B., Asgar, A., Benson, L., Daniels, C. J., et al. (2020). *SCAI* position statement on adult congenital cardiac interventional training, competencies and organizational recommendations. *Catheterization and Cardiovascular Interventions, 96*, 643–650. https://doi.org/10.1002/ccd.28885 (accessed on 15th July 2025).

2. Ammirati, E., Frigerio, M., Adler, E., Basso, C., Birnie, D. H., Brambatti, M., Friedrich, M. G., et al. (2020). Management of acute myocarditis and chronic inflammatory cardiomyopathy. *Circulation: Heart Failure, 13.* https://doi.org/10.1161/circheartfailure.120.007405 (accessed on 15th July 2025).

3. Baddour, L. M., Wilson, W. R., Bayer, A. S., Fowler, V. G., Tleyjeh, I. M., Rybak, M. J., Baršić, B., et al. (2015). Infective endocarditis in adults: Diagnosis, antimicrobial therapy, and management of complications. *Circulation, 132*, 1435–1486. https://doi.org/10.1161/cir.0000000000000296 (accessed on 15th July 2025).

4. Barker, P., Lewin, M., Donofrio, M. T., Altman, C. A., Ensing, G. J., Arya, B., & Swaminathan, M. (2020). Specific considerations for pediatric, fetal, and congenital heart disease patients and echocardiography service providers during the 2019 novel coronavirus outbreak: Council on Pediatric and Congenital Heart Disease supplement to the statement of the American Society of Echocardiography. *Journal of the American Society of Echocardiography, 33*, 658–665. https://doi.org/10.1016/j.echo.2020.04.005 (accessed on 15th July 2025).

5. Berceanu, M., Constantin, A., Donoiu, I., et al. (2017). Non-compaction cardiomyopathy–brief review. https://core.ac.uk/download/144553871.pdf (accessed on 15th July 2025).

6. Bouma, B. J., & Mulder, B. J. M. (2017). Changing landscape of congenital heart disease. *Circulation Research, 120*, 908–922. https://doi.org/10.1161/circresaha.116.309302 (accessed on 15th July 2025).

7. Dixon, G., & Christov, G. (2017). Infective endocarditis in children: An update. *Current Opinion in Infectious Diseases, 30*, 257–267. https://doi.org/10.1097/qco.0000000000000370 (accessed on 15th July 2025).

8. Ferriero, D. M., Fullerton, H. J., Bernard, T. J., Billinghurst, L., Daniels, S. R., DeBaun, M. R., deVeber, G., et al. (2019). Management of stroke in neonates and children: A scientific statement from the American Heart Association/American Stroke Association. *Stroke, 50.* https://doi.org/10.1161/str.0000000000000183 (accessed on 15th July 2025).

9. Frankel, H. L., Kirkpatrick, A. W., Elbarbary, M., Blaivas, M., Desai, H., Evans, D. P., Summerfield, D. T., et al. (2015). Guidelines for the appropriate use of bedside general and cardiac ultrasonography in the evaluation of critically ill patients—Part I. *Critical Care Medicine, 43*, 2479–2502. https://doi.org/10.1097/ccm.0000000000001216 (accessed on 15th July 2025).

10. Gewitz, M. H., Baltimore, R. S., Tani, L. Y., Sable, C. A., Shulman, S. T., Carapetis, J. R., Reményi, B., et al. (2015). Revision of the Jones criteria for the diagnosis of acute rheumatic fever in the era of Doppler echocardiography. *Circulation, 131*, 1806–1818. https://doi.org/10.1161/cir.0000000000000205 (accessed on 15th July 2025).

11. Hopfner, C., Jakob, A., Tengler, A., Grab, M., Thierfelder, N., Brunner, B., Thierij, A., et al. (2021). Design and 3D printing of variant pediatric heart models for training based on a single patient scan. *3D Printing in Medicine, 7.* https://doi.org/10.1186/s41205-021-00116-6 (accessed on 15th July 2025).

12. Isselbacher, E. M., Preventza, O., Black, J. H., Augoustides, J., Beck, A. W., Bolen, M. A., Braverman, A. C., et al. (2022). 2022 ACC/AHA guideline for the diagnosis and management of aortic disease: A report of the American Heart Association/American College of Cardiology Joint Committee on Clinical Practice Guidelines. *Circulation, 146*. https://doi.org/10.1161/cir.0000000000001106 (accessed on 15th July 2025).

13. Karalis, V. (2024). The integration of artificial intelligence into clinical practice. *Applied Biosciences, 3*, 14–44. https://doi.org/10.3390/applbiosci3010002 (accessed on 15th July 2025).

14. Law, Y. M., Lal, A. K., Chen, S., Čiháková, D., Cooper, L. T., Deshpande, S. R., Godown, J., et al. (2021). Diagnosis and management of myocarditis in children. *Circulation, 144*. https://doi.org/10.1161/cir.0000000000001001 (accessed on 15th July 2025).

15. Leichtner, A. M., Gillis, L. A., Gupta, S. K., Heubi, J. E., Kay, M., Narkewicz, M. R., Rider, E. A., et al. (2012). NASPGHAN guidelines for training in pediatric gastroenterology. *Journal of Pediatric Gastroenterology and Nutrition, 56*. https://doi.org/10.1097/mpg.0b013e31827a78d6 (accessed on 15th July 2025).

16. Levitov, A., Frankel, H. L., Blaivas, M., Kirkpatrick, A. W., Su, E., Evans, D. P., Summerfield, D. T., et al. (2016). Guidelines for the appropriate use of bedside general and cardiac ultrasonography in the evaluation of critically ill patients—Part II: Cardiac ultrasonography. *Critical Care Medicine, 44*, 1206–1227. https://doi.org/10.1097/ccm.0000000000001847 (accessed on 15th July 2025).

17. Marian, A. J., & Braunwald, E. (2017). Hypertrophic cardiomyopathy. *Circulation Research, 121*, 749–770. https://doi.org/10.1161/circresaha.117.311059 (accessed on 15th July 2025).

18. Meijboom, E. J., Oudijk, M. A., & Visser, G. H. A. (2004). Fetal tachyarrhythmia–Part I: Diagnosis. https://core.ac.uk/download/pdf/86258.pdf (accessed on 15th July 2025).

19. Plana, J. C., Galderisi, M., Barac, A., Ewer, M. S., Ky, B., Scherrer-Crosbie, M., Gáname, J., et al. (2014). Expert consensus for multimodality imaging evaluation of adult patients during and after cancer therapy: A report from the American Society of Echocardiography and the European Association of Cardiovascular Imaging. *European Heart Journal–Cardiovascular Imaging, 15*, 1063–1093. https://doi.org/10.1093/ehjci/jeu192 (accessed on 15th July 2025).

20. Schneider, B. J., Naidoo, J., Santomasso, B., Lacchetti, C., Adkins, S., Anadkat, M. J., Atkins, M. B., et al. (2021). Management of immune-related adverse events in patients treated with immune checkpoint inhibitor therapy: ASCO guideline update. *Journal of Clinical Oncology, 39*, 4073–4126. https://doi.org/10.1200/jco.21.01440 (accessed on 15th July 2025).

21. Schrepel, C., Amick, A. E., Sayed, M., & Chipman, A. K. (2021). Ischemic ECG pattern recognition to facilitate interpretation while task switching: A parallel curriculum. *MedEdPORTAL*. https://doi.org/10.15766/mep_2374-8265.11182 (accessed on 15th July 2025).

22. Shah, M. J., Silka, M. J., Avari Silva, J. N., Balaji, S., Beach, C. M., Benjamin, M. N., Berul, C. I., et al. (2021). 2021 PACES expert consensus statement on the indications and management of cardiovascular implantable electronic devices in pediatric patients. *Cardiology in the Young, 31*, 1738–1769. https://doi.org/10.1017/s1047951121003413 (accessed on 15th July 2025).

23. Shapiro, A. J., Davis, S. D., Polineni, D., Manion, M., Rosenfeld, M., Dell, S., Chilvers, M., et al. (2018). Diagnosis of primary ciliary dyskinesia. An official American Thoracic Society clinical

practice guideline. *American Journal of Respiratory and Critical Care Medicine, 197*, e24–e39. https://doi.org/10.1164/rccm.201805-0819st (accessed on 15th July 2025).

24. Siripanthong, B., Nazarian, S., Muser, D., Deo, R., Santangeli, P., Khanji, M. Y., Cooper, L. T., et al. (2020). Recognizing COVID-19–related myocarditis: The possible pathophysiology and proposed guideline for diagnosis and management. *Heart Rhythm, 17*, 1463–1471. https://doi.org/10.1016/j.hrthm.2020.05.001 (accessed on 15th July 2025).

25. Söder, S., Wällisch, W., Dittrich, S., Cesnjevar, R., Pfammatter, J.-P., & Glöckler, M. (2020). Three-dimensional rotational angiography during catheterization of congenital heart disease–A ten years' experience at a single center. *Scientific Reports, 10*. https://doi.org/10.1038/s41598-020-63903-x (accessed on 15th July 2025).

26. Stafie, C. S., Şufaru, I. G., Ghiciuc, C. M., Stafie, I. I., Sufaru, E. C., Solomon, S. M., & Hăncianu, M. (2023). Exploring the intersection of artificial intelligence and clinical healthcare: A multidisciplinary review. *Diagnostics, 13*, 1995–1995. https://doi.org/10.3390/diagnostics13121995 (accessed on 15th July 2025).

27. Warnat-Herresthal, S., Schultze, H., Shastry, K. L., Manamohan, S., Mukherjee, S., Garg, V., Sarveswara, R., et al. (2021). Swarm learning for decentralized and confidential clinical machine learning. *Nature, 594*, 265–270. https://doi.org/10.1038/s41586-021-03583-3 (accessed on 15th July 2025).

28. Wiegers, S. E., Ryan, T., Arrighi, J. A., Brown, S. M., Canaday, B., Damp, J. B., Díaz-Gómez, J. L., et al. (2019). 2019 ACC/AHA/ASE advanced training statement on echocardiography (revision of the 2003 ACC/AHA clinical competence statement on echocardiography). *Catheterization and Cardiovascular Interventions, 94*, 481–505. https://doi.org/10.1002/ccd.28313 (accessed on 15th July 2025).

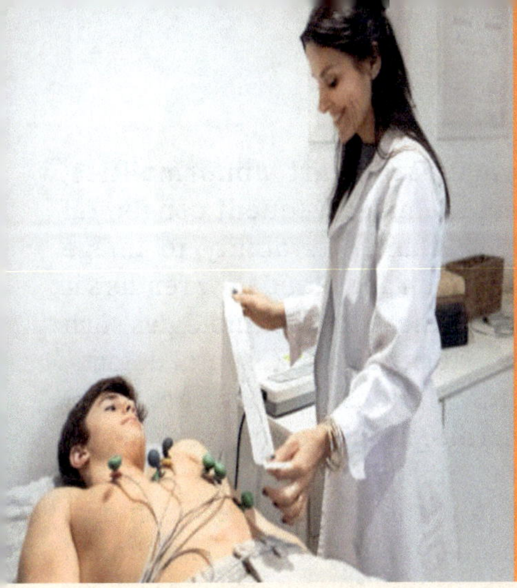

Chapter 5
ECHOCARDIOGRAPHY IN PEDIATRICS

Contents

Introduction

Echocardiography has emerged as the core pediatric diagnostic modality, particularly for assessing congenital heart disease (CHD) and other cardiac diseases in children. As cardiovascular diseases continue to rise in children, accurate and early diagnosis becomes more imperative day by day. Echocardiography offers a non-invasive technique with real-time imaging that is crucial to understanding the complex anatomical and functional characteristics of a child's heart. This imaging modality allows physicians to visualize cardiac structure and function, thereby guiding treatment and monitoring for disease progression. With advancing echocardiographic technology, improved imaging resolution and doppler capability, pediatric cardiologists now have more sophisticated tools with which to manage routine and unusual cardiac disease. The use of echocardiography in pediatrics is also unparalleled in breadth of educational and training responsibilities. There is currently a shortage of mid-level providers well-trained in performing and interpreting echocardiograms, noted by existing research on the cardiology workforce shortage. This shortage naturally limits the capacity to provide an increase in the demand for echocardiographic exams. To address this deficit, formal education programs are under consideration, aimed at mid-level providers such as Physician Assistants (PAs), who can also stretch echocardiographic services. By implementing a standardized echocardiography curriculum, medical facilities can educate practitioners to proficiency levels adequate to perform such key assessments competently. This proposed pilot curriculum should assist in mastering echocardiographic skills and interpretation to the extent that some of the pressures caused by this workforce deficiency are mitigated (Moon et al., 2017). Also, the evolution of imaging modalities such as cardiovascular magnetic resonance (CMR) compliments and enhances the role of echocardiography in pediatric cardiology. CMR provides detailed 3D imaging of cardiac anatomy and physiological data, which is particularly valuable in the treatment of congenital heart disease. The heterogeneity and potentially dynamic characteristics of CHD mandate the utilization of combinations of imaging modalities in an effort to provide comprehensive evaluations for children. With pediatric cardiologists having a better understanding and deploying these technologies into clinical practice, the synergy between echocardiography and CMR facilitates improved management plans and improved patient outcomes. Thus, the recognition of the strengths and limitations of different imaging modalities remains paramount for effective clinical decision-making in pediatric cardiology (Hughes et al., 2011).

Definition of Echocardiography

Echocardiography is a noninvasive imaging technique with high-frequency sound waves to provide dynamic images of the function and structure of the heart. Pediatric cardiology is highly dependent on this technique as a method for examining cardiac anatomy, valvular function, and hemodynamics without ionizing radiation. Echocardiography is primarily a diagnostic method for congenital heart abnormalities, which are among the most frequent congenital illness present in infants. Its ability to image dynamic cardiac motion and blood flow renders it priceless in the identification of pathologies such as patent ductus arteriosus, atrial septal defects, and other structural lesions. Furthermore, more advanced echocardiographic techniques such as Doppler imaging enhance blood flow patterns and pressures within the heart as well as inform clinical decision-making in children. The clinical uses of echocardiography extend beyond surface examination to involve extensive evaluation essential to the treatment of pediatric patients. For instance, in BPD patients, echocardiography is able to detect early pulmonary vascular disease (PVD), a disease that, if left untreated, is responsible for serious morbidity. Studies indicate that echocardiography is highly sensitive to diagnose PVD, particularly as a screening method for infants with elevated pulmonary vascular resistance. The modality's best application within this scenario illustrates its key role in pediatrics, allowing clinicians to monitor the progression of heart disease and assess the success of treatment. The diagnostic and utility value of echocardiography in pediatric cardiology is evidenced by its application in both acute and chronic cardiovascular illness (Figure 5.1).

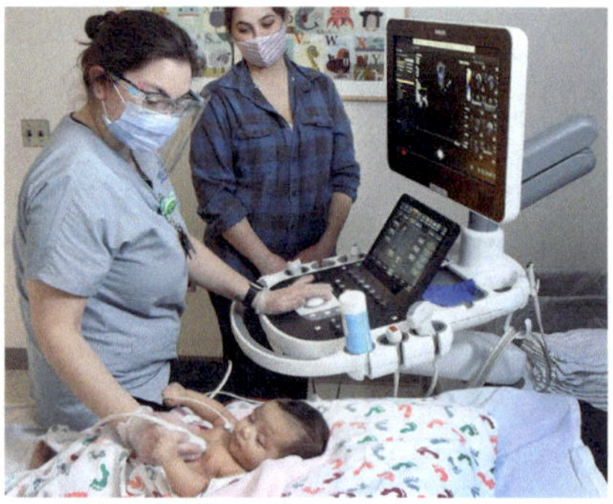

Figure 5.1. Pediatric echocardiography.

Source: https://www.hopkinsmedicine.org/-/media/heart-vascular-institute/images/mom-baby-imaging.jpg.

Technological progress in echocardiographic devices increases its application in a broad array of cardiac diseases in children. New quality measures implemented by professional organizations, such as the Adult Congenital and Pediatric Cardiology Section of the American College of Cardiology, aim at standardizing echocardiography process in a bid to ensure transparency and consistency in treatment delivery of conditions like Kawasaki disease. Through the establishment of these quality standards, the community of pediatric cardiology puts a great value on precise echocardiographic interpretation for improved outcomes. With ongoing advances in echocardiography, it remains also at the forefront of not just establishing diagnoses, but designing treatment programs and assisting long-term management plans for children with diverse cardiovascular needs. The continuous pursuit of evidence-based guidelines indicates the revolutionary capacity of echocardiography to enhance pediatric cardiac care.

Importance of Echocardiography in Pediatric Care

The use of echocardiography in pediatrics cannot be overstated, particularly considering that it is a first-line method of diagnosis for various congenital heart defects. Echocardiography allows for imaging of cardiac anatomy and hemodynamic assessment without exposing the patient to invasive testing, hence minimizing the risk inherent in diagnosis processes. With the unique anatomical and physiological characteristics of pediatric patients, echocardiography provides important information on the complexity of their cardiovascular pathophysiology. It also permits early detection of abnormalities such that timely interventions can be instituted and clinical results significantly enhanced. This diagnostic tool, therefore, plays a pivotal role in the treatment of congenital heart malformations, which is the most common birth defect, and hence forms an integral component of pediatric cardiology. Also, the non-invasive nature of echocardiography makes it particularly favorable for children, as they often require serial studies on account of the dynamic nature of growth and development. The portability of the methods facilitates bedside examination, such that even critically ill neonates can be evaluated without needing to transfer them to radiology departments, which may involve additional risk. The growing application of telemedicine and digital technology improves access to ultrasound consultation, including echocardiographic evaluation, particularly in remote areas. With the evolution of medical care in responding to challenges brought about by the COVID-19 pandemic, echocardiography remains resolute, offering effective monitoring and follow-up for children. Accordingly, the benefits of echocardiography extend beyond its immediate diagnostic capabilities, supporting continuity of pediatric cardiology care and improving patient management approaches in general. Apart from its application to diagnosis, echocardiography also holds significant implications for research into the genetic basis of congenital cardiovascular malformations (CVMs) because it aids in the development of correlations between phenotypic presentations and underlying genetic abnormalities. Recent developments in genetic testing, for example, next-generation sequencing, have uncovered novel associations between genetics and CVMs, open up new vistas for the incorporation of genetic information into clinical practice. Echocardiography enables this link by producing an accurate two-dimensional image of heart anatomy, upon which genetic counseling can be directed and recurrence likelihood predicted in families with CVM. While integration with genetic testing will introduce challenges and opportunities, it confirms the necessity for ongoing communication between genetics and cardiology to optimize therapeutic intervention and improve long-term patient outcome.

Lastly, the combination of echocardiography with genetic information adds strength to the complete treatment plan for children suffering from cardiovascular diseases, thereby becoming the cornerstone of contemporary pediatric cardiology practice (Cui et al., 2020; Landis et al., 2016).

5.1. Historical Background

The path of echocardiography in pediatrics is rooted in the early developments in ultrasound technology that started in the middle of the 20th century. The early developments were focused on the domain of adult heart care, where the use of ultrasound waves was employed to generate visual representations of heart structure and function. As research spread, it became apparent that congenital heart malformations—a significant source of morbidity and mortality among infants—needed a specialized solution for pediatric patients. Pioneers in the field of echocardiography began exploring such applications, and as a result of that, the method along with the technology applied improved such that visualizing and evaluating conditions of the heart in pediatric patients became increasingly more accurate than before. This led to the advent of specialized echocardiographic methods that were capable of satisfying the unique anatomical and physiologic characteristics of children. The integration of non-invasive techniques, such as non-invasive electrocardiography (NI-ECG), was a pivotal step in the tracking of the heart of the fetus and neonate. As noted in recent reviews, NI-ECG has been vastly helpful in establishing the health of the fetus and neonate using its long-term tracking ability and ease of use over traditional usage using adhesive electrodes (Jaroš et al., 2024). The benefits of textile electrode use have been placed under more scrutiny, including a shift toward embracing patient-centered approaches while simultaneously addressing common complications like skin irritation. Computer-aided diagnostic technology advances further underscore the need for continuous innovation in the field since it has the potential to enhance the classification of neonatal and fetal health at critical points during development, providing clinicians with necessary information that can lead to early intervention. Historical accounts identify how institutional support has affected the development achieved in pediatric echocardiography. As evidence of such development, publications like the Jefferson Alumni Bulletin document the ongoing advancement in improving echocardiographic techniques and their application in pediatrics (N/A, 1978). The collective work of physicians, investigators, and educators has created an intuitive understanding of cardiac physiology in children that improves with technology. The historical record not only points up significant advances but also testifies to the commitment of the medical community to greater diagnostic capability and therapeutic alternatives. On reflection of these advances, it is clear that the history of echocardiography in children is one of ongoing innovation and devotion to greater health in compromised groups.

5.1.1. Development of Echocardiography Technology

Echocardiography technology has seen phenomenal evolution since its inception, greatly enhancing the diagnostic capability at the bedside of pediatric clinicians. Initially, echocardiography was done through two-dimensional imaging, which, despite being helpful, only enabled visualization of complex cardiac structures to a partial degree. The advent of three-dimensional (3D) echocardiography revolutionized the diagnosis of pediatric cardiovascular anomalies. This technical advancement facilitates high-resolution imaging of flow dynamics and anatomical relationships, which can facilitate improved evaluation of congenital heart disease in children. Thanks to this better visualization, cardiologists can make the right intervention and management decisions aimed at ultimately improving patient outcomes. Continuous evolution of echocardiography is a reflection of its position at the forefront of pediatric cardiology, emphasizing the need to work on improving technology to handle the unique challenges presented by younger patients. Furthermore, technological advancement in echocardiography has concurrently supported the development in pediatric practice. The use of Doppler imaging has enabled clinicians to more precisely assess hemodynamic states, attaining valuable information regarding the velocity profiles and pressure gradients in the heart and blood vessels. This information is particularly vital in the management of valvular disease and pulmonary hypertension, which are challenging to diagnose in pediatric patients due to the dynamic nature of their physiology. In addition, technology advancement in the guise of portable echocardiography machines has addressed issues of access, allowing one to perform echocardiograms in nearly any environment outside mainstream hospitals. Such democratization of care not only enhances early detection of cardiovascular pathology but also allows for prompt interventions that have direct bearings on better overall health outcomes among pediatric patients (Liang et al., 2025) (Figure 5.2).

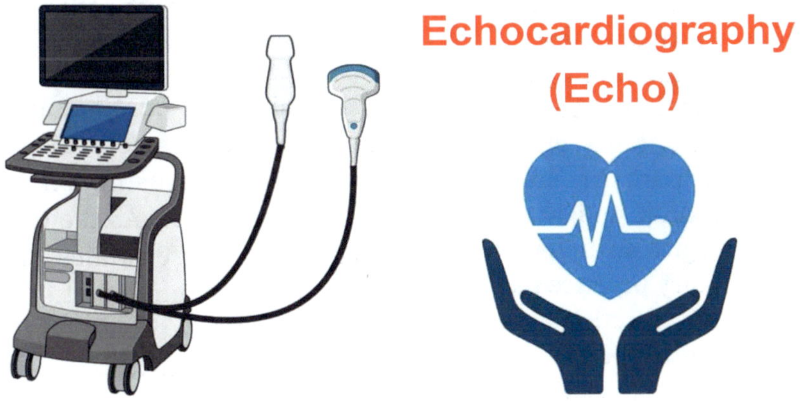

Figure 5.2. The development of echocardiography technology.

Source: https://microbenotes.com/wp-content/uploads/2023/09/Echocardiography-Echo.jpeg.

With evolving technology in echocardiography, integration of artificial intelligence (AI) with echocardiographic images holds vast potential for pediatric use. AI-guided tools are engineered to enhance accuracy and rapidity in interpreting images, reducing dependency on operator skill and perhaps eradicating inconsistency in diagnostic testing. AI-assisted systems have the capacity to examine vast data sets, allowing clinicians to identify subtle anomalies not readily detectable. By streamlining the workflow and making decisions easier, AI solutions can further enhance the pediatric cardiologist's abilities so that children are provided with ideal care in a timely fashion. However, there are challenges at hand in the widespread adoption of AI-assisted systems, particularly concerning training, cost, and ethics. Increased efforts towards standardization of medical staff education and interdisciplinary cooperation will be essential in overcoming such challenges and realizing the maximum potential of echocardiography in pediatric cardiology (Hughes et al., 2011).

5.1.2. Milestones in Pediatric Echocardiography

The past decades have seen tremendous evolution of pediatric echocardiography, and each milestone has provided increased comprehension and management of congenital and acquired cardiac defects among children. While technology was initially a limiting factor for echocardiography, the challenges posed by the small and rapidly contracting neonatal and small child hearts were also significant. In spite of this, major advancements in imaging technology, such as the development of portable echocardiography units and more effective ultrasound transducers, have made it possible to have accurate and detailed cardiac assessments. Such advancements not only maximized diagnostic function but also allowed for timely interventions, which are most critical in the improvement of outcomes in pediatric patients. As such, pediatric echocardiography has become more than an adjunct diagnostic modality but a central part of standard cardiology evaluation in children, with the ability to tailor management strategies on an individual patient basis. Interdisciplinary practice has also played a significant role in facilitating pediatric echocardiography methods. The coming together of a combination of specialties—e.g., pediatric cardiology, radiology, and genetics—has made it possible for cardiovascular disease in children to be diagnosed and treated multi-disciplinarily. This synergy is particularly evident in the management of complex cases, such as those with syndromic diseases such as pseudoxanthoma elasticum (PXE) that may occur not only in cardiovascular complications but also in dermatological and ophthalmological scenarios (Azi et al., 2024). Identification of such multisystem involvement has been essential in bringing to light the importance of multidisciplinary teams in the enhancement of the efficacy of interventions and patient care. In addition, this partnership ensures the development of educational programs that equip healthcare professionals, such as physician assistants (PAs) and nurse practitioners (NPs), with the skills required to perform echocardiography efficiently, for addressing prevalent workforce deficits in the field (Moon et al., 2017).

Finally, pediatric echocardiography has a promising future for additional advances driven by technological advances, education, and research. Emerging technologies such as machine learning and artificial intelligence have the potential to increase diagnostic speed and accuracy and thus improve pediatric echocardiography efficiency. Furthermore, the development of standardized training curricula for healthcare professionals will enhance echocardiographic care quality, enabling uniform levels of capability in various medical settings. By closing gaps in training and putting mechanisms of continuous enhancement into effect, pediatric echocardiography will continue to develop, focusing on achieving optimal patient outcomes. As the technology continues to develop, future studies will have a significant function in finding additional applications and determining the relevance of echocardiography to general pediatrics.

5.1.3. Evolution of Techniques and Methodologies

Evolution of pediatric echocardiographic modalities has been shaped by milestones that enhance diagnostic capability and therapeutic efficacy. Two-dimensional (2D) echocardiography was the first mainstay, which allowed clinicians to visualize cardiac structures with a plane representation. With this modality, congenital heart defects could be detected but no detailed functional analysis was feasible. With time, introduction of three-dimensional (3D) echocardiography revolutionized the field by giving a closer look into cardiac morphology. This revolution was particularly productive in pediatric cardiology, where visualization of precise morphology is critical for planning treatment. The development of advanced imaging devices, such as tissue Doppler imaging and speckle tracking, has also enhanced the evaluation of cardiac function, providing data regarding myocardial motion and performance that have not been previously available. In the past few years, the advent of transportable echocardiography has provided a pivotal transformation in the accessibility of pediatric cardiac evaluations. Traditional echocardiography once required heavy machinery and specialized medical facilities, limiting its use in emergency departments or rural clinics. But with portable equipment, physicians are now able to perform echocardiograms at the bedside of the patient, greatly improving the timeliness of diagnosis and potential treatment. Additionally, they make real-time monitoring of high-risk infants and neonates possible, better and more safely addressing their special physiological needs during crucial times. Being able to conduct echocardiographic examination outside of standard facilities is particularly beneficial for premature babies, who may experience a variety of complications, including those related to cardiac output and other cardiovascular reaction to extrauterine life, as seen through recent thesis work (Miletín et al., 2021). Furthermore, the progress in echocardiography has been propelled by cross-disciplinary team efforts that have fostered creativity. For example, progress in genetic studies, including that regarding Turner syndrome, have highlighted the relevance of knowing the genetic basis of cardiac abnormalities within the pediatric population. Such information has pushed towards a more focused use of echocardiography so that clinicians can selectively tailor assessment according to hereditary disease. The Turner Resource Network is one such group that illustrates the potential of coalitions between multiple stakeholders to highlight awareness and treatment of congenital illnesses. As such techniques evolve, the integration of echocardiography with genetic data provides a more holistic platform for pediatric cardiology, paving the way for improved patient outcomes and personalized care strategies (Backeljauw et al., 2015).

5.2. Types of Echocardiography

Echocardiography is a necessary pediatric diagnostic tool that employs various modalities to assess cardiovascular status in children. The three essential types are transthoracic echocardiography (TTE), transesophageal echocardiography (TEE), and fetal echocardiography. The most common type is TTE, wherein a portable ultrasound machine is placed against the chest and uses the chest wall as a window to visualize the heart in real-time. This less invasive procedure is especially useful for pediatric patients because it requires minimal preparation and can be completed without sedation. TEE, on the other hand, employs the insertion of a probe into the esophagus to obtain close-up views of the heart structures. Though TEE is more accurate, it is typically reserved for complex cases or when TTE is inconclusive. Fetal echocardiography has greatly improved prenatal detection of congenital heart disease and its early intervention. In children, it is required to accurately diagnose congenital heart disease (CHD), and this involves echocardiography as a part of the diagnosis. Current studies show that CHD is prevalent among newborns, particularly among newborns with heart murmurs during physical examinations. Echocardiographic evaluations of these neonates find a strong association between the heart murmurs produced and congenital abnormalities, with ventricular septal defects among the most prevalent abnormalities detected. As pointed out by the findings, the association with echocardiography and clinical presentation highlights the significance of comprehensive cardiac evaluations in high-risk neonates. Specifically, research has indicated that almost 51.6% of infants diagnosed with heart murmurs possessed some form of CHD, which highlights the importance of employing echocardiographic techniques in pediatric cardiology (انتشاری مقدم et al., 1389). The differential effectiveness of echocardiographic techniques also means that there needs to be skilled professionals in the pediatric domain. Research has shown that echocardiographers who have received additional training exhibit more diagnostic skill than less experienced echocardiographers, such as housemen. This precision is especially critical in managing conditions such as atrial septal defects, commonly overlooked at diagnosis. This variation highlights the necessity of specialized echocardiographic education to enhance early detection and management of cardiovascular disparities in children. The primary role of clinical examination and subsequent echocardiographic assessment cannot be overstressed, particularly as the techniques improve and become increasingly specific. The more pediatricians are engaged with advanced echocardiographic methods, the better the potential for improved outcomes in the management of congenital cardiovascular disease will be (Bailey et al., 2004).

5.2.1. Transthoracic Echocardiography (TTE)

Transthoracic echocardiography (TTE) is now a routine modality in pediatric cardiac diagnostic studies, enabling noninvasive assessment of cardiac structure and function in a vulnerable population. TTE employs sound waves to produce dynamic images of the heart, permitting essential information about structural abnormalities and functional deficits that are not infrequent in children. The value of TTE is least apparent in the assessment of congenital heart disease, where early diagnosis and characterization can lead to prompt management. TTE is also very important in assessing acquired conditions such as infective endocarditis, by which the extent of infection can be followed and cardiac function can be properly assessed so that management approaches can lead to more favorable outcomes among pediatric patients with these severe diseases (Scalia et al., 2016). Pediatric application of TTE is also made easier by advances in imaging technology, for example, that of three-dimensional (3D) echocardiography, which can allow extensive cardiac anatomy imaging. The enhanced imaging capability offers better appreciation of anatomical relationship, crucial in planning surgical or intervention procedures. For instance, the high-precision views acquired using 3D echocardiography can lead to more rational decisions regarding the timing and type of surgery for congenital heart disease. Secondly, TTE is also a key part of current patient management, which allows for the analysis of temporal changes as well as longitudinal pediatric research studies in patients with acquired or congenital heart disease (Scalia et al., 2016) (Figure 5.3).

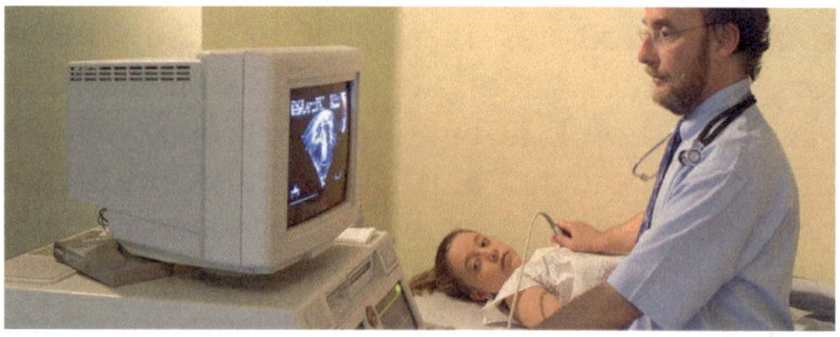

Figure 5.3. Transthoracic echocardiography (TTE).

Source: https://drkshitijsheth.com/assets/img/service/inner/1.jpg.

In isolated conditions such as Hutchinson-Gilford progeria syndrome (HGPS), TTE is a useful tool in the follow-up of cardiovascular abnormalities that significantly affect morbidity and mortality among the patients with this disease. HGPS children have variable cardiac presentations of arrhythmias and fibrosis, and these can be detected by echocardiographic studies. The comprehensive cardiac evaluation provided by TTE is vital to comprehending the impact of defective prelamin A processing on cardiac performance and therefore patient management. With each advance of knowledge from current research to sort out the complexity of cardiac involvement in genetic disease, TTE will remain an important part of diagnostic and follow-up management for all pediatric populations with the unique cardiac adversity.

5.2.2. Transesophageal Echocardiography (TEE)

Transesophageal echocardiography (TEE) is an essential modality in pediatric cardiology, enhancing diagnostic accuracy and management of various cardiovascular ailments.

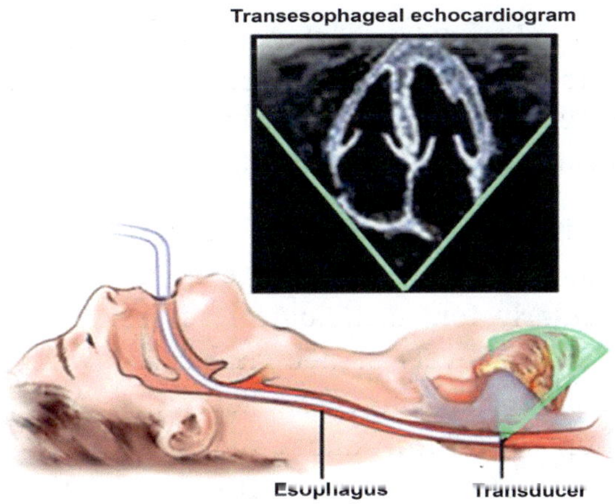

Figure 5.4. Transesophageal echocardiography (TEE).

Source: https://lh4.googleusercontent.com/proxy/9Z_Pmg1UjQFxBR0zvCVHw0jL0_il592q760CMLeH3d_9UKgq8RyMJQRao2nwZjugkEbPx7H-KwNVnA.

Compared to transthoracic echocardiography, TEE provides superior imaging, particularly in obese or lung-disease subjects with a younger age, where transthoracic imaging may be impaired. TEE allows for direct visualization of cardiac structures, whereby clinicians can assess congenital heart disease, valvular disease, and other complex anatomical malformations easily. This degree of precision is absolutely critical in children, in whom minute abnormalities can have profound clinical implications. Because of the necessity for early and precise diagnosis, TEE has emerged as a crucial operation within pediatric cardiac assessment, helping with preoperative diagnosis and postoperative monitoring (Figure 5.4).

The management and diagnostic function of TEE in diseases such as infective endocarditis (IE) is particularly intriguing. Echocardiography is pivotal to managing infective endocarditis across all stages of illness, from important areas such as diagnosis and surgical planning to management. Because of its greater imaging resolution, TEE can diagnose vegetations as well as other IE-related complications before conventional imaging can. In addition, the application of newer techniques such as real-time three-dimensional echocardiography provides added value to intracardiac infection imaging, allowing for comprehensive assessment of the disease extent. Such enhanced diagnostic power is particularly important in the pediatric group, where timely intervention might be mandatory to avoid potentially life-altering effects (Scalia et al., 2016). With continued progress in the field of echocardiography, the integration of emerging imaging modalities into TEE will revolutionize pediatric cardiology. Advances such as tissue Doppler imaging and optimization of three-dimensional echocardiographic modes provide improved understanding of congenital heart disease. These advances not only facilitate enhanced anatomical and functional assessment of cardiac structures but also allow for safer and more efficient interventions. The ongoing evolution of standard training and accreditation pathways for pediatric echocardiography only further supports the necessity for expert-level expertise in TEE performance in order to best care for children. Thus, TEE acts as a witness to the rapid evolution of pediatric cardiac imaging, which the reader can translate to better clinical results and enhanced patient safety (Ades et al., 2008).

5.2.3. Fetal Echocardiography

The employment of fetal echocardiography is a significant advancement in prenatal medical care that may lead to early identification of congenital heart diseases that may affect a growing fetus. The fetal echocardiography can be done as early as 18 to 20 weeks of gestation through various imaging modalities. Cross-sectional echocardiography is the primary method, which can be complemented with M-mode echocardiography and pulsed Doppler ultrasonography. These techniques combined enable accurate imaging of cardiac anatomy, which is as good as postnatal echocardiographic studies. Ten cardiac structural anomalies were described in a study involving 168 pregnancies, showing the possibility of in utero diagnosis. Since with antenatal diagnosis of congenital heart disease, health care providers can provide genetic counseling, tailor labor and delivery planning, and decide on postnatal management and potential pregnancy termination, thereby transforming the therapy for congenital diseases in children (Golbus et al., 1985). Fetal echocardiography is not just a diagnostic process but also a core part of multidisciplinary care planning and family support. Accurate prenatal diagnosis of congenital heart defects allows coordinated team effort of pediatric cardiologists, obstetricians, and neonatologists. Care teams can be ready to intervene immediately after birth, which could include surgical interventions or observation in specialty facilities. Further, such planning alerts parents with important information so that they could make informed decisions concerning their child's future well-being. The significance of these early diagnoses cannot be overstated, as they enhance the worldwide outcome in concerned infants and allow for proper provision of healthcare resources. As advances are made in medical knowledge, implications for pediatric cardiology are profound and revolutionary (Golbus et al., 1985) (Figure 5.5).

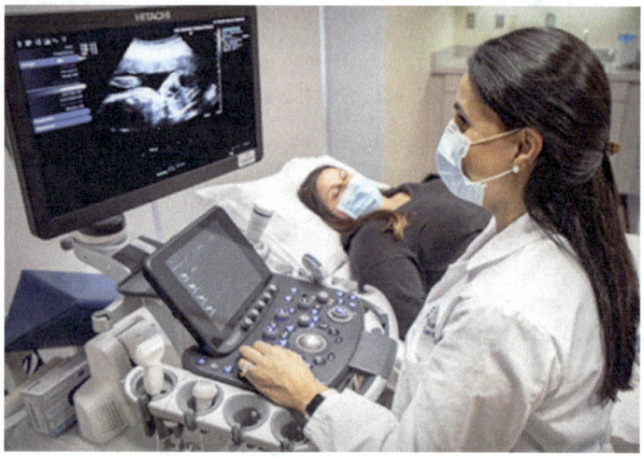

Figure 5.5. Fetal echocardiography.

Source: https://health.ucdavis.edu/media-resources/children/images/Page-Content/services/pediatric-heart-center/fetal-echocardiogram-dr-sunderji.jpg.

The implementation of point-of-care ultrasound (POCUS) practice in neonatology, particularly for cardiological assessment, can elevate the levels of neonatal care of infants with potential congenital heart disease even further. POCUS introduces a level of diagnostic capacity during the neonatal period that is possible through rapid assessments essential for timely interventions. Nonetheless, although POCUS has progressed in a range of neonatal care fields—from assessing cardiac function to ensuring device placement—it is employed differently in usual practice. The development of fetal echocardiography as an antenatal screening technique can encourage increased utilization of POCUS by neonatologists, hence optimizing proper management of severe cardiac conditions following birth. Nevertheless, this movement calls for extensive training of medical professionals to be competent at using these techniques safely and effectively, hence enhancing the overall environment of pediatric care.

5.3. Indications for Echocardiography in Pediatrics

Echocardiography is a valuable tool for pediatric medicine, particularly in the early detection of congenital heart disease (CHD). Importantly, early fetal echocardiography (EFEC) has revolutionized the detection of CHD in utero, and this can be done as early as the 12th to 16th week gestation. This advancement is conducive to timely intervention that can significantly affect the neonate's outcome. During this window of time, application of the aneuploidy sonographic markers enables physicians to identify risky pregnancies and the necessity for additional assessment. Studies have shown the efficiency of EFEC, proven to possess a very high diagnostic accuracy as compared to the regular screening at other gestational weeks, thereby justifying the requirement for early echocardiographic assessment in cases of familial histories of CHD or other genetic disorders, ultimately influencing pediatric cardiology clinical management guidelines (Abed et al., 2016). The echocardiography referrals extend beyond prenatal screening; it also plays a significant role in the diagnosis of cardiovascular diseases in infants and children. Pediatric practitioners will have a tendency to use echocardiographic assessment when patients present with certain symptoms and signs, such as heart murmurs, cyanosis, or failure to thrive. These are manifestations of underlying cardiac defects that need to be assessed further. In addition, echocardiography is an important management tool in children with known cardiac disease, providing useful information regarding the success of intervention and disease progression. Given its innocuity and ability to produce real-time images of cardiac structure, echocardiography is now a foundation stone of pediatric cardiology, facilitating early diagnosis and management of life-threatening conditions in this vulnerable population (Chintala et al., 2005). Kawasaki Disease, as a significant cause of acquired heart disease in children, is representative of the application of echocardiography in pediatrics. Inflammatory Kawasaki Disease can lead to coronary artery aneurysms that are a risk to future cardiovascular morbidity, such that early detection is important to successful management. In a case reported in a 19-month-old child with Kawasaki Disease, echocardiography allowed for early assessment of coronary artery dimensions and identification of bilateral giant aneurysms. These findings bring to the foreground the importance of continued echocardiographic evaluation in pediatric patients presenting with symptoms of Kawasaki Disease. Early echocardiographic examination enables the clinicians to initiate necessary treatments, such as intravenous immunoglobulin therapy, to prevent cardiac complications and promote better health outcomes among the children. Overall, echocardiography has an important role in the diagnosis, treatment, and management of childhood cardiac illness, maintaining its position in the promotion of child health (Chintala et al., 2005).

5.3.1. Congenital Heart Defects

Congenital cardiac defects (CHDs) are a heterogeneous group of structural defects of the heart, which occur during fetal life. They are the most frequent form of congenital anomaly, affecting an estimated 1 in every 100 live births. Early detection and diagnosis are crucial as these defects have the potential to lead to severe morbidity and mortality if left untreated. The evolution of echocardiography has revolutionized CHD management by providing non-invasive, real-time imaging that is crucial for diagnosis and follow-up. Clinicians are able to visualize structures of the heart, assess blood flow, and evaluate chamber size with high precision using echocardiograms, which allows for the initiation of appropriate intervention strategies. Furthermore, the pervasiveness of echocardiography has made it a valuable resource not only in complicated presentations but also as a routine pediatric examination, thereby enabling its earlier detection of congenital abnormalities which may otherwise go undetected until adult life.

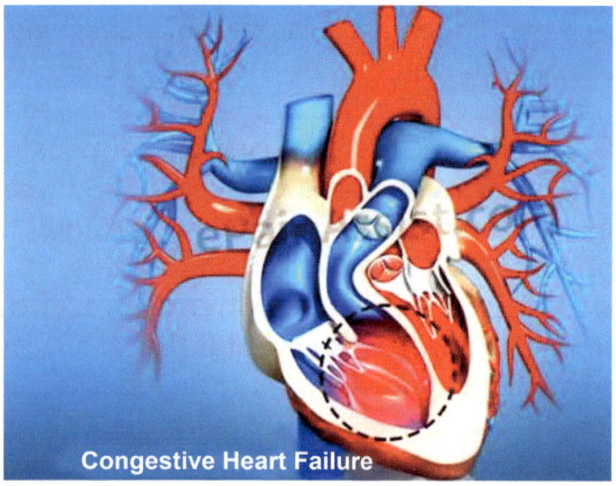

Figure 5.6. Critical congenital heart disease.

Source: https://external-content.duckduckgo.com/iu/?u=https%3A%2F%2Fwww.healingheartdiseasenaturally.com%2Fwp-content%2Fuploads%2F2017%2F12%2Fcongenital-heart-disease.jpg&f=1&nofb=1&ipt=7a80c0876b76a180f0079b1dbdcd20b435b9cadf8f534bb41c8346906b3145d8.

Another significant advantage of echocardiography is that it can adapt to the variable nature of children. As the child grows and cardiovascular demands change, so does the presentation of underlying congenital defects. Certain conditions, such as left ventricular outflow tract obstruction, may be cryptic until a child with this lesion develops heart failure or developmental delay. Employing advanced echocardiographic techniques, including three-dimensional imaging and Doppler flow imaging, can yield data about dynamic changes in the heart as patients mature. This adaptability underscores the necessity of repeated echocardiographic evaluations to re-assess previously diagnosed cardiac defects and to screen for new complications that arise with the passage of time. By doing this, physicians can institute early therapeutic interventions, thus achieving better long-term results in CHD patients (Figure 5.6).

The management of isolated congenital abnormalities shows its pivotal role in determining care. For example, when surgical intervention is warranted, precise echocardiographic imaging outlines anatomy problems key to procedural planning and conduct. Such cases as closure of a right coronary artery fistula are evidence of this function, in which echocardiography assists in preliminary diagnosis and follow-up afterwards. Complications like infective endocarditis occurring following heart surgery further demonstrate the need for routine echocardiographic follow-ups for detection of initial changes in cardiac function or complications. All such forward thinking, as in clinical examples, concurs with present guidelines emphasizing the role of extensive patient education in combination with surveillance in effective management of such multifactorial congenital diseases in order to contain the associated morbidity and mortality (Montalto et al., 2012).

5.3.2. Acquired Heart Conditions

Acquired cardiovascular disorders in children are a significant clinical challenge because they can develop due to various reasons, including infections, metabolic disorders, and other systemic illnesses. One of the best examples of this is how human immunodeficiency virus (HIV) infection influences the heart. Westerhof-

Grueters et al. have demonstrated that children and young adults with HIV infection can experience subclinical myocardial dysfunction when there is preserved left ventricular (LV) ejection fraction. The use of emerging echocardiographic techniques, such as three-dimensional speckle tracking echocardiography, has been helpful in the assessment of such individuals. Evidence attests that LV global longitudinal strain (GLS) is significantly reduced in HIV individuals compared to healthy controls, thereby establishing the significance of echocardiography in identifying early cardiac complications that go unnoticed in clinical assessment (Ajassa et al., 2019).

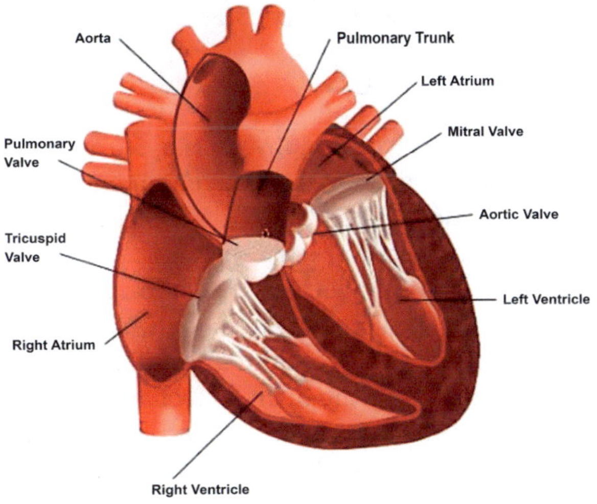

Figure 5.7. Acquired heart disease causes.

Source: https://lh4.googleusercontent.com/proxy/zPLsJpEgVGF8BuyCC_JV71CULzIS8tZAn3pjB-pU_23sjS9_vFqR8Brs60atbuZDL4InGpQfWVhZLtERVUPge7y7AU4lhvvY7KRTWc14Vzaubx4B8rFLr_pj6WTQwEqgH-t2k3fpeN8koWZWs9bU82_uUnqVpf_iyGUJVfgnBPU.

Another important domain of acquired heart conditions in children is the evaluation of patients with chronic kidney disease (CKD). The cumulative effects of CKD can lead to severe cardiovascular alterations, such as left ventricular dysfunction and pathological ventricular remodeling. The advancements in cardiac imaging technologies, particularly cardiac magnetic resonance (CMR) imaging, have facilitated a better understanding of these changes in a more superior manner. The literature emphasizes that CKD patients have elevated native T1 relaxation times, which are markers of myocardial fibrosis and, therefore, reflect the cardiac manifestation of the disease process. These imaging technologies along with echocardiographic assessment enable the clinicians to detect and monitor potential cardiac complications in children with CKD, thus imparting better management strategies and outcomes in this at-risk population (Mangion et al., 2018) (Figure 5.7).

Finally, an integrated therapy of acquired heart disease in pediatric patients must involve the application of several diagnostic modalities, including echocardiography and other imaging methods. The dynamic nature of echocardiographic approaches allows for more accurate determination of cardiac function, which is vital for effective timing of intervention and treatment.

In addition, the relationship between acquired cardiac conditions and systemic disease emphasizes the importance of collaborative multidisciplinary practices between pediatric cardiologists, nephrologists, and infectious disease specialists. As greater appreciation is realized of the subtleties of these conditions, it becomes increasingly evident that echocardiography not only plays a pivotal role in diagnosing acquired cardiac conditions but also in coordinating global care that maps cardiac as well as systemic health issues in children. Understandings of the intricacies of these relationships will ultimately enhance quality of life and patient outcomes.

5.3.3. Preoperative and Postoperative Assessments

The preoperative assessment is highly valuable in the pediatric patient, particularly in those patients who are undergoing echocardiography to screen for cardiac illness. A full preoperative assessment includes an adequate history, physical examination, and pertinent imaging tests that direct surgical strategy. This assessment enables caregivers to identify any potential risk factors for the patient's cardiovascular status, such as congenital abnormalities or previous cardiac interventions. In addition, preoperative echocardiography can elucidate the complexity of cardiac anatomy and consequently explain the pathophysiologic mechanisms in the child. These assessments ultimately contribute to optimizing surgical outcomes by ensuring that surgical teams are adequately informed and prepared for any complications that may arise during surgery. Postoperative assessments are just as vital in the life cycle of pediatric cardiac care, as they quantify the short-term and long-term outcomes following surgery. Identification of several postoperative morbidities, particularly in pediatric cardiac surgery, is required to protect the patient's safety and ensure quality assurance. Morbidities may include a host of complications such as neurological events (e.g., seizures), unplanned re-operations, and major adverse cardiac events, as summarized in contemporary literature (Brimmell et al., 2017). Careful monitoring of these outcomes allows healthcare providers to develop targeted interventions aimed at optimizing recovery and minimizing complications. Additionally, postoperative echocardiography not only serves to assess the function of the repair heart but also to identify any late-onset complications that require additional therapy. Furthermore, serial monitoring by echocardiography is crucial in assessing long-term viability in pediatric recipients of heart transplantation, where preoperative and postoperative assessment forms the basis of patient care. Infant heart transplantation requires meticulous pre-transplant evaluation for ascertaining the viability of the donor heart and overall health of the recipient. The process of healing requires scrupulous surveillance of rejection or other untoward effects, which may appear within months post-surgery (Billingham et al., 2011). Last question, a sound foundation in preoperative and postoperative assessment is at the heart of improving survival and long-term quality of life of pediatric patients that has undergone cardiac intervention that allows for timely intervention and enhanced clinical outcomes.

5.4. Techniques and Procedures

Pediatric echocardiography employs a range of methods and procedures significant in diagnosing and assessing congenital and acquired cardiac disease in children. Some of the significant methods include the use of transthoracic echocardiography (TTE), which involves placing an ultrasound transducer against the child's chest to capture real-time images of the heart and chambers. This effective and safe non-invasive method is favored by clinicians for its ability to examine cardiac anatomy, chamber size, and patterns of blood flow without sedation or invasive testing. Another advantage of echocardiography is its portability since equipment is utilized across a variety of settings from outpatient clinics to emergency rooms, making it a valuable asset for pediatric cardiology. In complicated cases, and particularly in situations where anatomy cannot be visualized by the conventional technique, transesophageal echocardiography (TEE) can be employed. This involves advancing an esophageal ultrasound probe through the esophagus to provide improved images of posteriorly located heart structures. TEE is very useful in suspected cardiology disease, such as atrial septal defect or to evaluate coronary circulation. According to pediatric cardiology observation studies, for example, described in recent developments from leading journals, utilization of TEE may add substantially to the precision of diagnoses, influencing intervention strategies and management plans appropriately (Bernasconi et al., 2019). Finally, the clinical scenario will determine whether to utilize TTE or TEE, both with their particular advantages adding value to comprehensive pediatric cardiac assessments. Addition of Doppler techniques to echocardiography has greatly enhanced the possibility of hemodynamic assessment in children. Color Doppler and pulsed-wave techniques prove extremely useful in ascertaining the direction and velocity of blood flow within cardiac structures, thus helping to identify valvular heart disease or congenital abnormalities leading to disparate hemodynamic effects. Such rigorous scrutiny not only facilitates diagnosis but is also central to monitoring the sufficiency of therapeutic intervention post-procedure, as in the case of infective endocarditis where proper complication detection in a timely manner is paramount (Montalto et al., 2012). With increasing sophistication in pediatric echocardiography, ongoing advance in imaging technology and technique will increasingly yield more accurate diagnosis, thus improve patient outcomes and reduce morbidity due to cardiac disease in this vulnerable group.

5.4.1. Patient Preparation and Positioning

Ideal patient preparation and positioning are the key factors in the successful execution of echocardiography, particularly in pediatric patients. Keeping patients relaxed and adequately prepared prior to the procedure aids in the obtainment of high-quality images. This can typically involve engaging the child to explain the process in a soothing and familiar context. The children are uneasy when given medical procedures, and this makes them move and hence taint the quality of the echocardiographic images. Having caregivers involved during the preparatory procedures can thus act to decrease anxiety, resulting in a more cooperative setting. By creating a setting of security and trust, the healthcare providers can make the success of optimal imaging probable. Placing the child correctly for an echocardiographic examination is also essential. Different views will require specific placements, and it is necessary that the child be positioned comfortably in a way that these views can be taken without any distress. One example is placing the child supine with the left lateral decubitus that is useful in visualizing the anatomy of the hearts. Also, factors related to age must be taken into consideration; for example, babies may need additional support or stabilization in order to attain the desired posture. Pillows or specially designed stabilizers can prove useful in attaining the desired positioning, especially in children who cannot sustain stable positions on their own. Adequate positioning does not only enhance the quality of diagnostic images but also adds to an overall patient and healthcare team experience. Patient positioning and preparation also have implications for procedural outcomes in echocardiography. It has been demonstrated in studies that technical issues might arise when the patient is poorly prepared or positioned and lead to inconclusive results or the need to repeat testing. Particularly, children may show different levels of cooperation, which are products of psychological needs as well as bodily comfort. For instance, studies have shown that a relaxed child is more likely to give accurate measurements, giving medical professionals a greater sense of assurance in their diagnosis. This adaptability to the child's specific needs is proven by the echocardiography guidelines in favor of age-based approaches. As a result, optimizing pre-procedure regimens can substantially enhance echocardiographic testing effectiveness in children, since the literature discusses variability of imaging modalities and their application in clinical settings (Achenbach et al., 2015; Aumann et al., 2008).

5.4.2. Image Acquisition and Interpretation

In pediatric echocardiography, image acquisition is as crucial to make sure of safe and informative scans. This begins with the choice of appropriate transducer frequencies in a precise manner to provide maximum resolution based on the size and clinical condition of the patient. This calls for a fine appreciation of how different imaging modalities influence cardiac structure visualization, particularly in very-low-birth-weight infants (VLBWIs) whose vulnerable anatomy poses special challenges in the majority of situations. For instance, the techniques employed during the modal acquisition phase must be well optimized to achieve accurate measurements of parameters like tricuspid annular plane systolic excursion (TAPSE) that are critical in determining myocardial function in these vulnerable patients. Effectiveness of the imaging technique has a direct effect on the diagnostic potential, emphasizing the involvement of trained personnel in the production of good-quality images required for subsequent interpretation (Fern et al., 2020) (Figure 5.8).

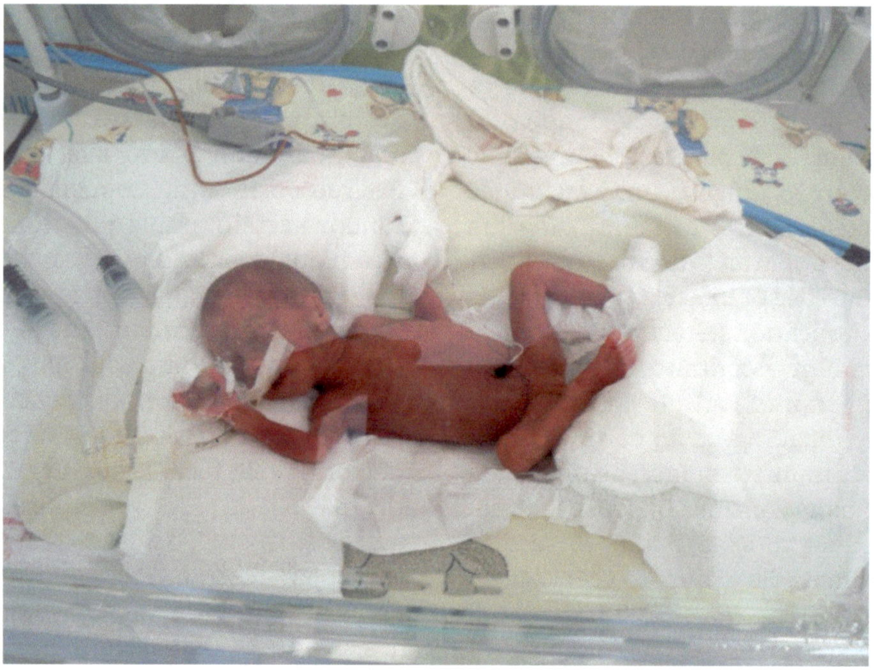

Figure 5.8. Very low birth weight infants (VLBWIs).

Source: https://upload.wikimedia.org/wikipedia/commons/6/6a/Nina_wcze%C5%9Bniak.jpg.

Once the images are acquired, interpretive phase is prominent and calls for careful assessment of echocardiographic information achieved. Interpretation is difficult in children since the cardiac physiology is dynamic and parameters such as gestational age and postnatal age have variable influences on echocardiographic findings. Utilization of advanced techniques such as two-dimensional speckle-tracking echocardiography (2DSTE) allows clinicians to derive valuable insights into left ventricle function that are significant in the management of conditions such as bronchopulmonary dysplasia (BPD). A research study on VLBWIs is discussed to demonstrate how echocardiographic measurements evolve over time and how they could be associated with increased NTproBNP levels and thus aid risk stratification and management among these patients. Hence, echocardiographic data interpretation not only directs clinical decisions but also broadens pathophysiological mechanisms understanding (Fern et al., 2020). Rendering reference values for varying echocardiographic parameters is critical in the delivery of true image interpretation and has been emphasized in recent studies among children. Metanalyses results that have been obtained have provided a wide view of left ventricular strain parameters, including global longitudinal strain (GLS), that is crucial when evaluating myocardial health in children. With mean GLS values defined close to –20.2%, these thresholds create invaluable comparative data that can be useful in clinical practice. These normal reference ranges bridge the gap between images obtained and their clinical value, further validating the requirement for systematic image acquisition and interpretation to enable effective pediatric practice. Furthermore, the presence of a normal apex-to-base longitudinal strain gradient demonstrates the dynamic nature of cardiac performance as children grow up, providing essential information in the assessment of pediatric patients' cardiovascular health (Figure 5.9).

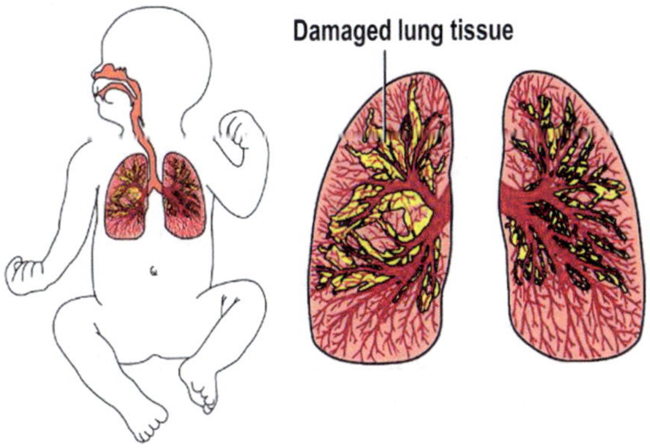

Figure 5.9. Bronchopulmonary dysplasia (BPD) lung damage.

Source: https://www.nhlbi.nih.gov/health/bronchopulmonary-dysplasia.

5.4.3. Use of Doppler Ultrasound in Echocardiography

The use of Doppler ultrasound in echocardiography has revolutionized the diagnosis and management of pediatric patients, particularly those with congenital heart disease. The device enables doctors to measure blood flow velocities and direction in the Great vessels and heart, providing valuable information on hemodynamics. Through the application of color Doppler imaging, physicians can visualize and quantify the flow of blood in real-time and thus assess the diastolic and systolic performance of the heart structures very accurately. The non-invasive nature of Doppler ultrasound is especially advantageous in pediatric wards, as children are more susceptible to exposure to radiation, and so the diagnostic procedure becomes safer for them. The ability to view flow dynamics over time also assists the clinician in making pragmatic decisions for the need of operative procedures or ongoing observation by optimizing patient outcomes. Doppler ultrasound has proven to be extremely helpful in advanced cases to understand subtle flow mechanics in infants and neonates. Evolution of new techniques, such as two-dimensional speckle tracking, can capture nuances in patterns of blood flow that more traditional Doppler methods may not detect. Evidence indicates that despite possible remaining artifacts for these newer imaging tools, these can greatly enhance the validity of hemodynamic assessment when used appropriately. The studies on diastolic inflow jets, for instance, identify the potential barriers, such as artifacts and phase variations with respect to cardiac phases, which necessitate a careful interpretation of ultrasound results in children. Such advances pave the way for more accurate diagnosis and personalized treatment protocols, thereby improving the overall treatment of congenital heart disorders in children (Fadnes et al., 2016) (Figure 5.10).

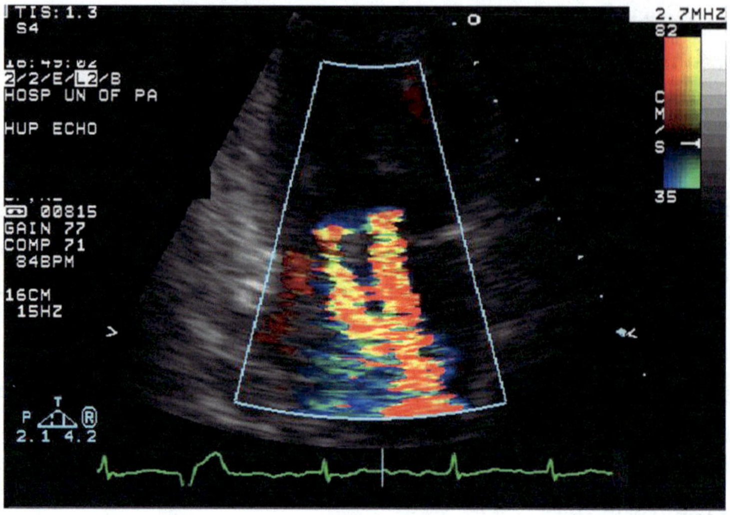

Figure 5.10. Doppler ultrasound in echocardiography.

Source: https://pedecho.org/media/images/image21.png.

Moreover, increasing demand for echocardiography, driven by the increasing incidence of pediatric cardiovascular conditions, adds momentum towards adopting a systematic approach for the training of professionals in this delicate area. With reported shortages in trained cardiovascular professionals being felt, there is a need to develop optimal education programs for medical caregivers, including physician assistants (PAs) and nurse practitioners (NPs), who may not have had extensive experience with echocardiography. Pilot program proposals with the intention to equip PAs with theoretical education and procedural skills in echocardiography are vital to this workforce issue-solving. By adopting templates such as Entrustable Professional Activities (EPAs), these programs would help ensure that future practitioners achieve proficiency in Doppler ultrasound skills and, consequently, enhance pediatric echocardiography access across various healthcare environments (Moon et al., 2017).

5.5. Challenges in Pediatric Echocardiography

Pediatric echocardiography has a myriad of challenges unique to those presented in adult cardiology. One major issue is the anatomical and physiological variation of pediatric patients. Neonates and infants have lower cardiac sizes and elevated heart rates, making it imperative for techniques and equipment specialized to image these accurately. Such variations in development are to be known by pediatric cardiologists as inaccurate interpretations can yield misdiagnosis or delayed treatment. The pediatric patient also typically has complicated congenital heart disease that involves experience in dealing with deranged hemodynamics and structural abnormalities. This complexity underscores the value of ongoing training and education for healthcare professionals who practice in this discipline, as the consequences are especially severe in the case of pediatric care where interventions must be prompt in order to impact long-term outcomes. Anatomical difficulty is accompanied by the variation in cooperation and behavior among children, making echocardiographic assessments challenging. As opposed to adults, children may be less able to remain still or comply with instructions during the course of the test, affecting image quality and diagnosis. These issues are avoided in pediatric echocardiography by needing to resort to creative solutions at times, like using childlike distractions or even sedation in some cases, to present the optimum imaging conditions. These approaches add layers to the procedure and are time-consuming, with a negative impact on the efficiency of cardiac examinations in clinical practice. In addition, the presence of the parents during the duration of the echocardiogram is crucial because their reassurance will prevent anxiety among the children, with the overall impact being enhanced results. Thus, the use of an effective communication strategy with both parents and the young patients is included in the echocardiography procedure. In addition, the implementation of new technologies presents opportunities and challenges alike to pediatric echocardiography. With advances such as three-dimensional imaging and contrast echocardiography comes more precise diagnostic accuracy at the cost of greater training and adaptation required from clinicians. The constantly evolving nature of the imaging modalities necessitates that clinicians stay up to date with the latest guidelines and the latest literature to deliver optimal care. For instance, recent studies delineated the importance of quality metrics in monitoring and improving pediatric cardiac care, particularly in conditions such as Kawasaki disease, in which an early intervention significantly alters disease outcomes (Cotts et al., 2020). In addition, as demonstrated in studies giving an overview of the challenges of cardiac imaging among patients with chronic ailments like kidney disease, the data obtained through advanced cardiac imaging techniques can enhance pediatric cardiology knowledge across various patient groups (Mangion et al., 2018). As the field advances, becoming more a prototype of lifelong learning is imperative to combat these challenges effectively and provide optimal patient care (Figure 5.11).

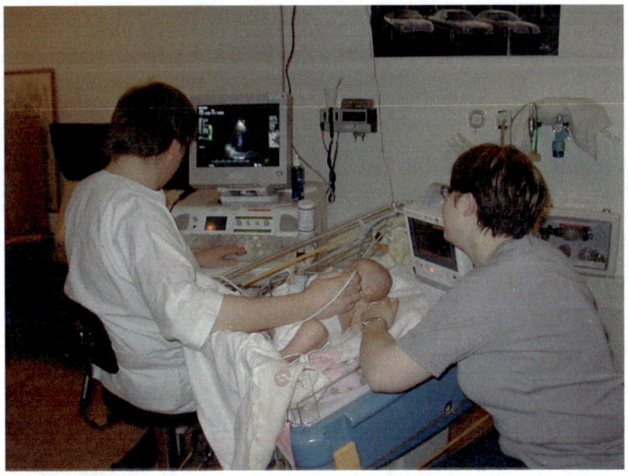

Figure 5.11. Challenges in pediatric echocardiography.

Source: https://www.hopkinsmedicine.org/-/media/heart-vascular-institute/images/mom-baby-imaging.jpg.

5.5.1. Anatomical Differences in Children

Anatomical differences between the child and adult populations significantly influence pediatric echocardiography practice. Children's hearts exhibit certain structural differences, such as reduced chamber size, differences in wall thickness, and variations in vascular association. These differences necessitate certain echocardiographic techniques to deliver appropriate assessment and diagnosis. In addition, pediatric cardiac physiology is distinct (e.g., relatively faster heart rate), and this impacts the timing and interpretation of echocardiographic images. Clinicians need to be aware of these differences in anatomy because misinterpretation may result in incorrect management or missed diagnosis. Thus, pediatric cardiologists must be mindful of such differences so that they use age-based protocols in echocardiography to treat their child patients successfully. In addition, growth and development of a child's cardiovascular system further complicate echocardiographic evaluation. As children mature, their cardiovascular anatomy completely transforms (e.g., from fetal to postnatal circulation). These modifications influence echocardiographic measurements, with certain normal values having wide variability based on the child's age and size. Practitioners must therefore be highly trained in recognizing age-dependent normative data, particularly in chamber and vessel dimensions. These are required to recognize pathologies such as congenital heart disease, which can occur in a child differently from an adult. Clinicians are asked to synthesize this broad knowledge base of anatomical and physiological growth patterns as they interpret echocardiographic results in order to ensure timely and accurate interventions. In addition, advances in imaging technologies have supplemented the pediatric echocardiography landscape, improving the visualization of these anatomical variations. Techniques like three-dimensional echocardiography and Doppler imaging bring high-resolution insights into cardiac structure and function that were not possible before. These advances are particularly well-suited to identify subtle congenital abnormalities that would otherwise be missed by standard two-dimensional imaging. As Bernasconi et al. (2019) asserts, the continuous progress of pediatric cardiology supports the incorporation of new diagnostic techniques, which can enhance the outcome of patients to a considerable extent. Besides, as Drivas et al. (2015) have explained in detail, there are important differences in scanning methods between adults and children that must be respected to ensure adequate assessment and management of congenital heart disease. Thus, staying current on technological advancement while appreciating anatomical differences remains important for optimal pediatric cardiac practice.

5.5.2. Patient Cooperation and Sedation Issues

Pediatric patients' echocardiography often encounters severe challenges related to cooperation and sedation. Cooperation is a requirement due to the fact that children may not have the ability to remain immobile for a prolonged time, which is critical to ensure optimal visualization throughout the echocardiogram procedure. Children and young children are likely to be nervous or scared when they are presented with medical environments and procedures. This emotional response can result in movement and failure to cooperate with instructions, finally compromising the quality of echocardiographic results. It is thus essential to formulate successful methods of ensuring patient cooperation, which may incorporate the involvement of parents, adequate information on preparation, and creating a reassuring environment that minimizes anxiety. Sedation is then an issue of major concern when dealing with overcoming patient cooperation obstacles during pediatric echocardiography. While most of these are managed by non-invasive imaging in an awake, relaxed child, those requiring a thorough examination, especially in ill children, may require sedation. Sedation method is not standardized, and while most pediatric offices get by on minimal sedation to ensure the comfort of the child, deeper levels of sedation may be required if the resultant echocardiographic examination is particularly complex or long. This need for sedation also generates further consideration, such as safety and observation of the patient throughout procedure. It is important that healthcare staff are under strict guidelines to ensure that the sedation employed is within the child's clinical requirement and different responses, both maximizing the accuracy of echocardiogram and the child's overall experience with procedure. Secondarily, anesthetic modality selection and administration can often be the determining factor for the success of the echocardiographic examination. The heterogeneous application of sedative drugs and techniques must be most wisely planned, since their appropriateness varies widely from child to child on the basis of age, health status, and personality. Some research indicates that minimal anxiolysis or sedation with topical anesthetic is commonly used; yet more complicated cases may necessitate deeper levels of sedation with a broader range of pharmacological interventions to maintain the comfort and safety of the child (Sacit et al., 2011). These findings highlight the need for ongoing investigation and refinement of sedation regimens in pediatric echocardiography to enable individual children to receive the imaging necessary for accurate diagnosis without undue distress or diminished cooperation (Bhatt-Mehta et al., 1998).

5.5.3. Limitations of Echocardiographic Technology

Echocardiography, while a pillar in pediatric cardiology due to its lack of invasiveness, has several inbuilt limitations. One of the primary issues is the interpretation of Doppler readings, which can be operator-sensitive as well as patient-sensitive based on age and body type. For pediatric patients, variations in anatomy and small size can affect the angle and orientation of the ultrasound beam, leading to suboptimal images. Besides, flow measurement reliability also relies on the precise placement of the transducer, which can be complicated in pediatric patients. This makes it dependent on a high level of skill from the sonographer, which can be difficult to achieve at all times in less skilled centers and may have an impact on the validity of conclusions reached through echocardiographic examination (Alverson et al., 1985). Apart from technical issues, echocardiographic technology is also limited by its ability to assess certain pathophysiological conditions with accuracy. Structural abnormalities and conditions like congenital heart disease may appear in a manner that their imaging presents interpretive challenges. For instance, conditions such as atrial septal defects cannot always be well visualized if defect size and location do not fall into the best available windows of an echocardiogram. Further, Doppler techniques, while revolutionary, are only useful in the presence of proper flow; states of diminished flow can offer false reassurance with resultant inappropriate or delayed clinical responses (Smart et al., 2014). Thus, the intrinsic limitations in visualization and quantification must be understood as fundamental regulators of pediatric echocardiography diagnostic outcomes. While the diagnostic accuracy and procedural effectiveness have been enhanced by the evolving echocardiographic methods, the technology is still limited by its dependence on technological factors and operator expertise. Incorporation of advanced imaging modalities, such as three-dimensional echocardiography, mitigates some limitations but imposes new ones. Such advanced techniques may not be in widespread usage or even feasible in all health centers, particularly in those of lower capacity. Therefore, differences in access to such types of equipment bring about disparities in health care services, preventing their incorporation into standard practice. Lastly, while echocardiography is a core pediatric diagnostic imaging modality, it is imperative to appreciate its limitations for effective clinical decision-making and whole patient care (Alverson et al., 1985; Smart et al., 2014).

5.6. Advances in Echocardiography

Recent advances in echocardiography have significantly improved our understanding of cardiovascular function in children, especially in infants and neonates. These advances include high-resolution imaging techniques and 3D echocardiography, which allow for accurate imaging of the heart structures. Thus, doctors can now evaluate better congenital heart defects and other cardiovascular conditions in infants where conventional two-dimensional echocardiography is insufficient. The incorporation of Doppler imaging also bettered our ability to evaluate blood flow dynamics, thus improving diagnostic accuracy. Furthermore, these new echocardiographic developments help proactively monitor, enabling intervention earlier, which can lead to improved long-term outcomes in children. The coupling of advanced echocardiographic techniques with novel biomarkers has opened new paradigms for personalized pediatric management. Continuous blood flow monitoring under the guidance of real-time echocardiographic imaging has contributed to the improvement of hemodynamic conditions in malformed hearts. In contemporary clinical practice increasingly focused on precision medicine, echocardiography improvements promote the individualized treatment of patients according to their own unique anatomical and physiological profile. Exactly, Mathur et al. (2017) identifies the need to form stable hemodynamic boundaries in order to counteract cerebral injuries in preterm infants, thereby a convergence between high-tech echocardiography and neuroprotective measures. The convergence highlights the capability of echocardiography to not only diagnose but also direct therapy in pediatrics. Besides, echocardiographic technology development can offer a significant contribution to the care of neonates through a more reliable monitoring of circulatory health and cardiac output among critically ill newborns. Upcoming research points out the importance of such advancements in facilitating bedside evaluation-guided timely interventions. As an example, Bernasconi et al. (2019) points out the manner in which advances in various pediatric specialties like cardiology and neonatology have significantly increased our knowledge of the treatment and epidemiology of acquired and congenital heart disease. As practitioners rely more and more on these advances, echocardiography is an important driver for improving patient outcomes and further developing knowledge about pediatric cardiovascular disease, making it an essential tool in contemporary medicine.

5.6.1. 3D Echocardiography

The advancement of echocardiographic technology has significantly enhanced the diagnosis and treatment of congenital heart disease in children. Among these advancements is 3D echocardiography due to its ability to provide high-quality anatomical images of the heart, particularly in children. 2D echocardiography is limited in its ability to accurately represent complex congenital cardiac defects, but with 3D echocardiography, more detailed understanding of the three-dimensional structures and interrelations within the heart is possible. This is important for pediatric cardiologists since exact imaging of heart anatomy can guide both diagnosis and therapeutic interventions. Furthermore, advances in software and imaging technology have decreased the technical sophistication of 3D echocardiographic data acquisition and interpretation, which erased most of the technical challenges previously which made this modality less desirable for use in routine clinical settings among children. In echocardiography among children, 3D imaging has revolutionized the diagnosis and treatment of congenital heart disease. Through providing real-time, dynamic images of cardiac anatomy, 3D echocardiography enhances procedural guidance of interventional therapy, such as device positioning and surgical repairs. Visualization of intricate anatomy and spatial relationships between structures can also significantly assist in surgical planning and teamwork communication. The ability to produce reproducible and precise models of the heart from 3D datasets also facilitates preoperative simulation, wherein surgical teams can anticipate issues and adapt their strategies. These innovations lead ultimately to improved surgical outcomes and postoperative care in children with congenital heart disease, further establishing the robustness of advanced imaging techniques in pediatric cardiology (Figure 5.12).

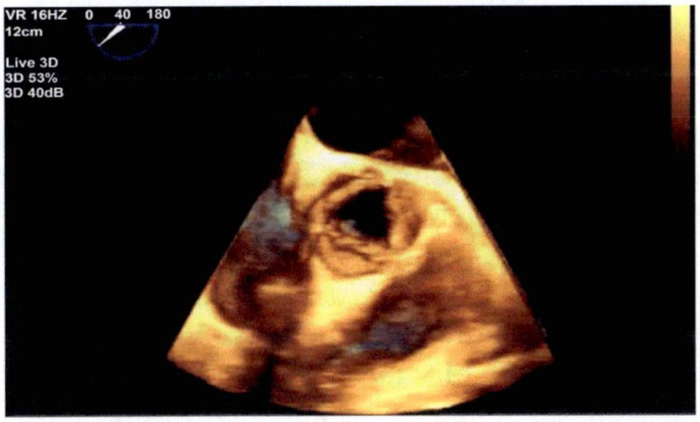

Figure 5.12. 3D echocardiography.

Source: https://www.thinking3d.ac.uk/assets/images/echocardiography/fig3-cardiovascular-image-3.png.

While future uses for 3D echocardiography are hopeful, there remain limitations, particularly in constructing normative data in children. In accordance with current research, it is critical to establish standard nomograms that reflect sensitivity to variance in age, body dimensions, and pathophysiology in an effort to effectively interpret 3D echocardiographic data in children.

Studies have shown that while currently available nomograms provide adequate coverage for left ventricular parameters, there is a critical deficiency of information for the right ventricle and atria, which are no less important in the overall assessment of the function of the heart (Assanta et al., 2025). Secondly, the continuous developments in 3D echocardiographic devices necessitate ongoing updating of training and accreditation processes in pediatric echocardiography (Ades et al., 2008). Therefore, an effort to consolidate the strengths of practitioners and researchers must be made to optimize the utility of 3D echocardiography and make it a workable tool in the pediatric sector, ultimately leading to better patient care and clinical outcomes.

5.6.2. Contrast Echocardiography

In pediatric cardiology, contrast echocardiography has been a useful imaging modality, with improved visualization of cardiac anatomy and greater accuracy in the diagnosis of congenital heart disease. Conventional echocardiography is limited, particularly with the newborn and infants where anatomical detail is obscured by poor acoustic windows and small body sizes. By adding contrast agents—such as microbubble technology—doctors can greatly improve the quality of echocardiographic images. These agents provide improved delineation of cardiac chambers and coronary vessels and enable the detection of complex congenital abnormalities that would otherwise not be detectable. This is particularly significant because early diagnosis and treatment of cardiac abnormalities are essential in maximizing outcomes among children. Thus, the inclusion of contrast agents in echocardiography not only augments diagnostic capability but also may alter treatment plans that are patient-specific. Also, the value of contrast echocardiography is not only improved imaging but is utilized in guiding clinical management of congenital heart disease. The technique enables detailed assessment of hemodynamic parameters, such as shunting and vascular flow patterns, essential in planning interventional therapy or surgical intervention. As mortality rates for congenital heart disease have come down significantly with the help of technology like contrast echocardiography, precise imaging technology becomes ever more vital. Clinicians must apply the detailed information obtained from the contrast studies to formulate personalized treatment plans that may involve surgical repair or catheter-based strategies, thus tailoring the strategy to a patient's unique anatomical and physiological deficits. This increased ability to visualize and assess the anatomy of hearts collectively contributes to improved care pathways within this vulnerable group. Pediatric imaging technology continues at the leading edge of innovation, and future developments with contrast echocardiography will continue to enhance diagnosis and treatment planning. New technologies such as three-dimensional imaging and real-time imaging capabilities will transform clinicians' interpretation of echocardiographic data. Enhanced contrast agents may provide even greater visualization of cardiac anatomy, enabling more informed decision-making and less danger from procedure complications. Besides, with the pediatric cardiovascular disease medical community facing the challenge of congenital heart disease, the role of contrast echocardiography will be increased, encouraging training program innovations for healthcare workers. The value of effective imaging methods has a significant role in creating detailed educational schemes, enhancing communication among multidisciplinary teams, and ultimately enhancing the quality of care delivered to pediatric patients. With these advances, the future of echocardiography is extremely bright in the management of congenital heart disease in children and highlights its pivotal role in pediatric cardiology in the current era (Anwar et al., 2018; Drivas et al., 2015).

5.6.3. Integration with Other Imaging Modalities

In pediatric practice, the combination of echocardiography with other imaging modalities significantly enhances therapeutic care and diagnostic precision. More sophisticated imaging modalities such as magnetic resonance imaging (MRI) and computed tomography (CT) augment echocardiography by providing precise anatomical detail that can be extremely useful in the assessment of complex congenital heart disease. While echocardiography is optimally suited to evaluating functional elements of cardiac form, MRI offers superior visualization of tissue characteristics, facilitating more precise characterization of myocardial disease. The combination of these techniques not only provides integrated evaluation of the cardiovascular system but also underlies evidence-based clinical decision-making for interventional strategies. Lastly, integration of echocardiography with molecular imaging technologies introduces new dimensions to pediatric cardiovascular assessment. The emergence of biomarkers, particularly from the genetic school, is a demonstration of the need to pair echocardiographic discoveries with molecular and functional imaging. For example, the next-generation sequencing-derived characterizations are increasingly identified to possess the ability to identify genetic variants associated with cardiovascular malformations and thus guide echocardiographic evaluation. The explanation of these integrative approaches ends up in improved individualized care for patients, with multidisciplinary teams combining genetic data with echocardiographic data to better predict cardiovascular outcomes and in turn modify treatment approaches (Landis et al., 2016). In the end, interspecialty utilization of echocardiography along with other imaging modalities not only dispels diagnostic ambiguity but also aids disease monitoring. New technologies, as documented in the recent advances in biomarkers of diseases like cardiac disease, offer additional pathways to enhance the merging of imaging techniques. The biomarkers allow for cardiac involvement to be ascertained through non-invasive methods; whereby imaging typical changes are an indication of underlying biochemical and physiological changes within the heart. This multi-dimensional approach eventually supports an improved understanding of pediatric cardiology, providing the foundation for further research focused on creating new biomarkers and refining imaging protocols for better patient care (Blair et al., 2019).

SUMMARY

The application of echocardiography in pediatrics has greatly enhanced diagnostic capability in the diagnosis and treatment of congenital and acquired heart diseases in children. As outlined in recent studies, echocardiography is not only a non-invasive but highly valuable examination in the evaluation of cardiac function and morphology, thus enabling timely intervention. Precision of echocardiographic parameters can play a key role in determining the outcome of the patient, particularly in conditions like pulmonary hypertension, where early detection is crucial. Interestingly, in children with cystic fibrosis, specific echocardiographic parameters, such as pulmonary artery diameter, were found to be independent predictors of pulmonary hypertension, hence underlining the modality important role in pediatric cardiology (Aghahosseini et al., 2018). This underlines the significance of regular echocardiographic evaluation in children in an attempt to monitor heart health and make informed clinical decisions. In addition, telemedicine with echocardiography has provided doors of new opportunities for greater accessibility and control of pediatric cardiac diseases. Research has shown that teleconsultation has the same efficacy as traditional face-to-face consultation but is cost-neutral (Dowie et al., 2008). This change not only addresses the growing demand for pediatric cardiology services but also assures that children, especially those in underserved populations, receive timely cardiac assessments. The integration of telecardiology as an ancillary to conventional methods can optimize resources and enhance patient management protocols, thereby decreasing healthcare system burden. The novel method complementing the classical use of echocardiography is in support of the fact that advanced imaging modalities are imperative to counter the complexity of pediatric cardiovascular disease. In conclusion, the advancement of echocardiography in pediatrics is a critical milestone in the field of pediatric cardiology. Its ability to enable early detection and continuous monitoring of cardiovascular conditions cannot be overstated. Embracing both traditional echocardiography and telemedical approaches, medical practitioners can ensure an integrated approach that is responsive to the varied needs of child patients. All subsequent studies must focus on maximizing diagnostic criteria in addition to exploring the integration of new technologies in echocardiography aimed at improving the quality of care for children with cardiac diseases. As the global industry develops further, maintaining a priority on accessibility, accuracy, and innovation will be needed in helping to propagate healthier outcomes for youth patients nationwide.

Echocardiography is of relevance in the management and assessment of children with various cardiac conditions. Of note in this imaging method is its capability to evaluate heart structure and function in HIV-infected children. Findings have indicated that three-dimensional speckle tracking echocardiography (3DSTE) can detect subclinical myocardial dysfunction in HIV-infected children and young adults even with a normal left ventricular ejection fraction. Detection of lesser global longitudinal strain (GLS) in such patients compared to control subjects mainly highlights the need for routine echocardiographic evaluation in such a patient group so that they can be detected early with potential cardiac complications and appropriate measures can be taken for diminishing cardiovascular risk as well as outcomes (Ajassa et al., 2019). Kawasaki disease also presents peculiar challenges in the prediction of the risk of coronary artery aneurysms (CAAs) in another crucial area of pediatric echocardiography. One recent study developed a risk model that utilizes both echocardiographic and demographic parameters to stratify patients based on their risk of CAAs early during the course of fever. The model demonstrated excellent discriminative performance, with high c-statistics in the development and validation groups. This stratification into low, moderate, and high-risk groups facilitates clinicians to tailor monitoring and treatment strategies according to individual patient risk, thus maximizing long-term patient management for Kawasaki disease and overall care (Baker et al., 2019). In addition, incorporation of advanced echocardiographic techniques has expanded the scope of diagnostic capability and therapeutic surveillance in pediatric cardiology. For instance, 3DSTE not only provides improved visualization of complex cardiac structures but also helps with motion analysis of cardiac walls, which is crucial to ascertain deformation and strain patterns. This technology comes in handy for the early detection of potential left ventricular and right ventricular dysfunctions that might be overlooked using standard echocardiographic methods. On-going revisions in echocardiographic protocols and ongoing upgradation of clinical personnel in sophisticated imaging modalities are needed to provide optimal patient care and accurate diagnosis in children, highlighting the evolving echocardiography scenario (Ajassa et al., 2019; Baker et al., 2019).

CLOSER LOOK

THREE-DIMENSIONAL (3D) ECHOCARDIOGRAPHY IN PEDIATRIC USE

Three-dimensional (3D) echocardiography has revolutionized cardiac imaging with better visualization of cardiac anatomy and function compared to conventional two-dimensional (2D) methods. In pediatric cardiology, 3D echocardiography plays a critical role in the evaluation of congenital heart diseases (CHDs), intervention planning, and improving diagnostic accuracy with fewer geometric assumptions. It provides real-time, three-dimensional imaging of the heart, allowing clinicians to quantify intricate structural relationships and spatial orientations, particularly valuable in the small, dynamic hearts of infants and children.

One of the key advantages of 3D echocardiography in children is its ability to provide en face views of septal defects and valves. This is highly beneficial in the assessment of semilunar valves and atrioventricular valves and also in the evaluation of atrial and ventricular septal defects. With 3D imaging, septal defects may be better visualized with regard to position, size, and shape, and thus accurate diagnosis and planning for catheter-based or surgical repair can be established. Similarly, valve morphology, motion, and leaflet coaptation can be examined in greater detail, which is important in preoperative planning and postoperative evaluation in repair or replacement of valves.

In patients with complex congenital heart disease, such as double outlet right ventricle (DORV), transposition of the great arteries (TGA), or single ventricle physiology, 3D echocardiography offers accurate spatial relationships that are difficult to grasp on the basis of 2D imaging. The 3D models allow better understanding of anatomical complexity, particularly beneficial for surgical planning and parental counseling. In addition, progress in 3D echocardiographic software allowed for virtual dissections, cropping, and rotation views to facilitate complete cardiac evaluation.

Real-time 3D echocardiography, or 4D echocardiography, also enhances intraoperative and catheterization lab procedures. For example, for atrial septal defect closure or valve repair, 3D echocardiography provides real-time imaging, reducing procedural time and complications. Transesophageal echocardiography (TEE) in 3D also increases procedural accuracy by offering high-definition visualization of intracardiac structures during interventions.

Measurement of cardiac function, including left and right ventricular volumes and ejection fraction, is another significant application. 3D echocardiography is more accurate and reproducible than 2D echocardiography, as 2D echocardiography relies on geometric assumptions that are invalid in abnormally shaped ventricles. In children with heart failure and cardiomyopathies, this means more accurate longitudinal follow-up and therapeutic treatment.

However, pediatric imaging is limited by reduced acoustic windows, elevated heart rates, and patient movement. Improvements in technology still increase image resolution, frame rate, and ease of use. Utilization of pediatric-specific probes and sedation regimens may enhance image quality in infants and noncompliant children.

References

1. Abed, M. M., Caiaro, A., Ceccacci, I., et al. (2016). Reliability of early fetal echocardiography for congenital heart disease detection: A preliminary experience and outcome analysis of 102 fetuses to demonstrate the value of a clinical flow-chart designed for at-risk pregnancy management. https://core.ac.uk/download/54531071.pdf (accessed on 15th July 2025).
2. Achenbach, S., Al-Mohaissen, M., Alberti, K., Armbrust, R., Asferg, C., Bland, J., Buchanan, M., et al. (2015). Quantitative planar and volumetric cardiac measurements using 64 MDCT and 3T MRI vs. standard 2D and M-mode echocardiography: Does anesthetic protocol matter? https://core.ac.uk/download/36778517.pdf (accessed on 15th July 2025).
3. Ades, A., Bosch van den, A. E., Dubin, A. M., et al. (2008). What is new in pediatric cardiac imaging? https://core.ac.uk/download/pdf/8277958.pdf (accessed on 15th July 2025).
4. Aghahosseini, F., Bakhshayeshkaram, M., Hassanzad, M., Jamaati, H., et al. (2018). CT-measured pulmonary artery diameter as an independent predictor of pulmonary hypertension in cystic fibrosis. https://core.ac.uk/download/161841179.pdf (accessed on 15th July 2025).
5. Ajassa, C., Capotosto, L., Cavallari, E. N., D'Ettorre, G., et al. (2019). Assessment of biventricular function by three-dimensional speckle tracking echocardiography in adolescents and young adults with human immunodeficiency virus infection: A pilot study. https://core.ac.uk/download/231747596.pdf (accessed on 15th July 2025).
6. Alverson, D. C., & Berman, W. (1985). Assessment of hemodynamic function with pulsed Doppler ultrasound. https://core.ac.uk/download/pdf/82549222.pdf (accessed on 15th July 2025).
7. Anwar, S., Barach, P., Bhatla, P., Biglino, G., et al. (2018). 3D printing is a transformative technology in congenital heart disease. https://core.ac.uk/download/212858839.pdf (accessed on 15th July 2025).
8. Assanta, N., Cantinotti, M., Capponi, G., Franchi, E., Giordano, R., Gowda, K., Kutty, S., et al. (2025). Normal values for speckle-tracking echocardiography in children: A review, update, and guide for clinical use of speckle-tracking echocardiography in pediatric patients. https://core.ac.uk/download/657094534.pdf (accessed on 15th July 2025).
9. Attard Montalto, S., Bailey, M., DeGiovanni, J. V., Galea, G., et al. (2012). Mitral valve infective endocarditis following device occlusion of a coronary artery fistula. https://core.ac.uk/download/46602339.pdf (accessed on 15th July 2025).
10. Aumann, R., Hinterseer, M., Kozlik-Feldmann, R., Lang, D., et al. (2008). Creation of ventricular septal defects on the beating heart in a new pig model. https://core.ac.uk/download/16432659.pdf (accessed on 15th July 2025).
11. Azi, C. I., Carsrud, N. D. V., DelGiodice, M. J., Egli, D., et al. (2024). The multisystem impact of *Pseudoxanthoma elasticum* (PXE): Systemic manifestations, multidisciplinary management, and diagnostic and therapeutic advances. https://core.ac.uk/download/621451766.pdf (accessed on 15th July 2025).
12. Backeljauw, P. F., Bondy, C., Cernich, J. T., Chernausek, S. D., et al. (2015). Proceedings from the Turner Resource Network symposium: The crossroads of health care research and health care delivery. https://core.ac.uk/download/83230247.pdf (accessed on 15th July 2025).

13. Bailey, M., Grech, V. E., Mercieca, V., Spiteri, A., et al. (2004). A comparison of clinical pediatric murmur assessment with echocardiography. https://core.ac.uk/download/46601893.pdf (accessed on 15th July 2025).

14. Baker, A. L., Burns, J. C., de Ferranti, S., Dedeoglu, F. G., et al. (2019). Risk model development and validation for prediction of coronary artery aneurysms in Kawasaki disease in a North American population. https://core.ac.uk/download/323067004.pdf (accessed on 15th July 2025).

15. Benavente Fernández, I., Lubián López, S. P., Méndez Abad, P., Zafra Rodríguez, P., et al. (2020). Myocardial function maturation in very-low-birth-weight infants and development of bronchopulmonary dysplasia. https://core.ac.uk/download/288159239.pdf (accessed on 15th July 2025).

16. Benítez Iglesias, R., Caballero, R., Cabello, N., Calvo, E., et al. (2016). Cardiac electrical defects in progeroid mice and Hutchinson-Gilford progeria syndrome patients with nuclear lamina alterations. https://core.ac.uk/download/81578585.pdf (accessed on 15th July 2025).

17. Berceanu, M., Constantin, A., Donoiu, I., Istrătoaie, O., et al. (2017). Non-compaction cardiomyopathy – brief review. https://core.ac.uk/download/144553871.pdf (accessed on 15th July 2025).

18. Bernasconi, S., Borrelli, M., Caffarelli, C., Corsello, G., Di Pinto, R., Gaeta, V., Iovane, B., et al. (2019). Report on advances for pediatricians in 2018: Allergy, cardiology, critical care, endocrinology, hereditary metabolic diseases, gastroenterology, infectious diseases, neonatology, nutrition, respiratory tract disorders and surgery. https://core.ac.uk/download/286528671.pdf (accessed on 15th July 2025).

19. Bhatt-Mehta, V., & Rosen, D. A. (1998). Sedation in children: Current concepts. https://deepblue.lib.umich.edu/bitstream/2027.42/90049/1/j.1875-9114.1998.tb03900.x.pdf (accessed on 15th July 2025).

20. Billingham, M., Boucek, M., Boucek, D., Cho, S., Choo, D. M. S., Griffiths, G., et al. (2011). Heart transplantation in pediatric patients: Twelve-year experience of the Asan Medical Center. https://core.ac.uk/download/pdf/8556395.pdf (accessed on 15th July 2025).

21. Blair, I. A., Farmer, J., Hersch, S., Larkindale, J., et al. (2019). The current state of biomarker research for Friedreich's ataxia: A report from the 2018 FARA biomarker meeting. https://core.ac.uk/download/228066295.pdf (accessed on 15th July 2025).

22. Brimmell, R., Brown, K. L., Bull, K., Chigaru, S., et al. (2017). Definition of important early morbidities related to pediatric cardiac surgery. https://core.ac.uk/download/79526687.pdf (accessed on 15th July 2025).

23. Chintala, K., Forbes, T. J., & Reddy, S. V. (2005). Cardiovascular involvement in Kawaski disease. https://core.ac.uk/download/46602916.pdf (accessed on 15th July 2025).

24. Cotts, T., Dahdah, N., Davidson, A., Harahsheh, A. S., et al. (2020). Development and utility of quality metrics for ambulatory pediatric cardiology in Kawasaki disease. https://core.ac.uk/download/286361330.pdf (accessed on 15th July 2025).

25. Cui, M. D., Huang, M. D., Jia, Y., et al. (2020). Chinese expert consensus on critical care ultrasound applications at COVID-19 pandemic. https://core.ac.uk/download/322850186.pdf (accessed on 15th July 2025).

26. Dowie, R., Franklin, R. C., Mistry, H., Rigby, M. L., et al. (2008). A pediatric telecardiology service for district hospitals in south-east England: An observational study. https://core.ac.uk/download/337059.pdf (accessed on 15th July 2025).

27. Drivas, P., Greil, G. F., Mitchell, F. M., Prasad, S., et al. (2015). Cardiovascular magnetic resonance: Diagnostic utility and specific considerations in the pediatric population. https://core.ac.uk/download/83923979.pdf (accessed on 15th July 2025).

28. Fadnes, S., Lovstakken, L., Rodriguez-Morales, A., Segers, P., et al. (2016). Assessing the performance of ultrafast vector flow imaging in the neonatal heart via Multiphysics modeling and *in vitro* experiments. https://core.ac.uk/download/74712692.pdf (accessed on 15th July 2025).

29. Fineman, J. R., Guslits, E., Keller, R. L., Nawaytou, H., et al. (2020). Clinical utility of echocardiography in former preterm infants with bronchopulmonary dysplasia. https://core.ac.uk/download/287623787.pdf (accessed on 15th July 2025).

30. Fowler, S., Hamvas, A., Hardi, A., Holland, M. R., et al. (2016). Reference ranges of left ventricular strain measures by two-dimensional speckle-tracking echocardiography in children: A systematic review and meta-analysis. https://core.ac.uk/download/84831896.pdf (accessed on 15th July 2025).

31. Golbus, M. S., & Silverman, N. H. (1985). Echocardiographic techniques for assessing normal and abnormal fetal cardiac anatomy. https://core.ac.uk/download/pdf/81145316.pdf (accessed on 15th July 2025).

32. Güleç, S., & Aydin, T. (2011). Sedation for esophagogastroduodenal endoscopy. https://core.ac.uk/download/pdf/26760290.pdf (accessed on 15th July 2025).

33. Hughes, M. L., Ntsinjana, H. N., & Taylor, A. M. (2011). The role of cardiovascular magnetic resonance in pediatric congenital heart disease. https://core.ac.uk/download/1895946.pdf (accessed on 15th July 2025).

34. Jaroš, R., Marnani, R. A., Martinek, R., Pavlíček, J., et al. (2024). Advancements and challenges in non-invasive electrocardiography for prenatal, intrapartum, and postnatal care: A comprehensive review. https://core.ac.uk/download/636657853.pdf (accessed on 15th July 2025).

35. Kim, J. H., Safarulla, A., & Shalygin, N. (2018). Current neonatal applications of point-of-care ultrasound. https://core.ac.uk/download/322438600.pdf (accessed on 15th July 2025).

36. Landis, B. J., & Ware, S. M. (2016). The current landscape of genetic testing in cardiovascular malformations: Opportunities and challenges. https://core.ac.uk/download/84831326.pdf (accessed on 15th July 2025).

37. Liang, G., Liang, J., & Ma, X. (2025). Transesophageal echocardiography: Revolutionizing perioperative cardiac care. https://core.ac.uk/download/644449667.pdf (accessed on 15th July 2025).

38. Mangion, K., Mark, P. B., McDowell, K., Rutherford, E., et al. (2018). Characterizing cardiac involvement in chronic kidney disease using CMR—a systematic review. https://core.ac.uk/download/132211551.pdf (accessed on 15th July 2025).

39. Mathur, A. M., & Vesoulis, Z. A. (2017). Cerebral autoregulation, brain injury, and the transitioning premature infant. https://core.ac.uk/download/83101016.pdf (accessed on 15th July 2025).

40. Miletín, J. (2021). Nízký srdeční výdej u extrémně nezralých novorozenců a mozkové intraventrikulární krvácení. https://core.ac.uk/download/481707159.pdf (accessed on 15th July 2025).

41. Moon, S. (2017). Echocardiography curriculum development for physician assistants using entrustable professional activities. https://core.ac.uk/download/215924737.pdf (accessed on 15th July 2025).

42. N/A. (1978). *Jefferson Alumni Bulletin–Volume XXVIII, Number 1 Fall 1978.* https://core.ac.uk/download/46965646.pdf (accessed on 15th July 2025).

43. Scalia, G. M., & Sedgwick, J. F. (2016). Advanced echocardiography for the diagnosis and management of infective endocarditis. https://core.ac.uk/download/322428045.pdf (accessed on 15th July 2025).

44. Smart, S., van Raan, A. F. J., & Waltman, L. (2014). Exploring the relationship between the engineering and physical sciences and the health and life sciences by advanced bibliometric methods. https://core.ac.uk/download/388668614.pdf (accessed on 15th July 2025).

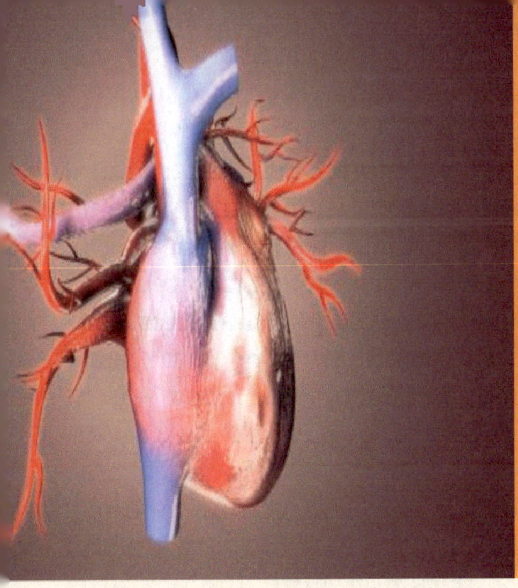

Chapter 6
CONGENITAL HEART DISEASES – ACYANOTIC

Contents

Introduction

The world of congenital heart diseases (CHD) is a very problematic and challenging one in pediatric practice. Of all the diversity of these cardiac abnormalities, acyanotic heart diseases are especially extremely prevalent. They are non-cyanotic conditions where defects in structure of the heart impair normal blood circulation in the heart. Atrial septal defects (ASD) and ventricular septal defects (VSD) are two of the most prevalent conditions that belong to this category. The prevalence of CHDs highlights the necessity for high-level research to establish the rate and extent of such defects among neonates since early diagnosis is vital for proper care. It was recently noted that in 459 suspected cases, the prevalence of congenital heart disease was 2.86%, with the prevalence of acyanotic lesions being considerably higher than their cyanotic counterparts, and this emphasizes the importance of intervention and awareness early on (Farooqui et al., 2010). Acyanotic heart defects generally have subtle presentations, which are easy to overlook, thus making diagnosis more challenging. These are less severe than cyanotic lesions but can lead to severe morbidity if untreated. Atrial septal defect, for instance, may lead to right heart volume overload to result in PAH, an increasingly severe condition, as happened in a case where an infant with an isolated ASD presented with severe PAH. This case is significant in demonstrating the necessity of close follow-up and early intervention; intervention can have a dramatic clinical impact, as demonstrated when ASD closure led to dramatic decrease in PAH and resolution of chronic recurrent respiratory infections (Andrews et al., 2012). Acyanotic congenital heart disease management is more than successful surgical correction. It involves a multidisciplinary approach with cardiovascular specialists, pediatricians, and the family support network. Early diagnosis and screening are crucial in optimizing outcomes for affected infants since these conditions can lead to complications like heart failure or growth retardation if not treated. Educational workshops targeted towards general practitioners and the public will ensure awareness of potential signs and symptoms and hence facilitate earlier intervention. The study of acyanotic congenital heart disease in this chapter aims to shed light on the importance of early diagnosis and appropriate medical treatment to improve the quality of life for children. By exploring the complexity of the conditions, the chapter aims to establish a better understanding of the knowledge of congenital heart disease and its relevance to child health.

Definition of Congenital Heart Diseases

Congenital heart diseases (CHDs) are a variety of structural and functional cardiac defects at birth. They may affect the walls, valves, and vessels of the heart and present in a wide spectrum of clinical features. Acyanotic congenital heart diseases are characterized by normal oxygen saturation of the blood, with a marked difference from cyanotic lesions when oxygen cannot be supplied properly. Abnormalities such as ventricular septal defects (VSD) and atrial septal defects (ASD) are commonly termed acyanotic, facilitating proper oxygenation despite structural impairment. The defects significantly impact heart function and ultimately the wellbeing of the respective individuals if left untreated. It is necessary to know the unique characteristics and implications of acyanotic congenital heart diseases to formulate appropriate management strategies and improve patient outcomes. The impact of acyanotic congenital cardiac defects extends far beyond the immediacy of physiological barriers and has a profound influence on a patient's nutritional status and overall health. Research has indicated a disturbing prevalence of undernutrition among children with CHD, noting that defect nature, comorbid conditions, and socio-economic status can drive its progression. In a study in Nairobi, undernutrition was prevalent among nearly 48% of children with CHD and highlighted the complicated interaction between cardiac disease and nutrition needs (Yahya et al., 2022) (Figure 6.1).

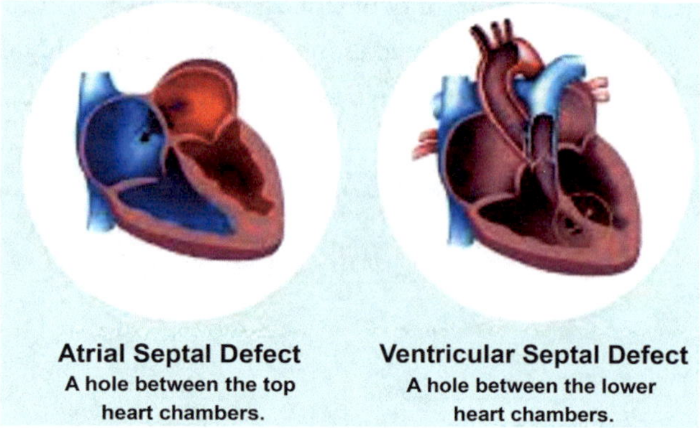

Figure 6.1. Types of congenital heart diseases (CHDs).

Source: https://encrypted-tbn0.gstatic.com/images?q=tbn:ANd9GcTccEuI1iZYMEnCSZVoOF79PbOGAdadE8EMvw&s.

Due to such complexities, utilizing a multidimensional approach in the management of acyanotic defects by means of appropriate surgical intervention at the right time and nutritional support according to the child's individual needs is vital. Accurate diagnosis is one of the key aspects in the successful management of congenital heart disease. Advanced techniques of diagnosis, including conventional radiography and cardiac catheterization, have enabled a more precise appreciation of structural and functional abnormalities associated with such conditions. Proper diagnosis is crucial, especially with the potential for surgical correction in most CHD. The technical procedures not only delineate the anatomical lesions but also permit estimation of hemodynamic effects, thus enabling individualized treatment regimens (Lester et al., 1965). Further, discrimination between acyanotic and cyanotic defects will give us information regarding urgency and type of intervention to be carried out. Due to such subtleties, an integral understanding of congenital heart diseases - particularly the acyanotic subgroup - is required in order to achieve optimal clinical outcomes and attain permanent wellness.

Overview of Acyanotic Heart Diseases

Acyanotic heart disease forms a leading category of congenital heart disease, which is characterized by the absence of cyanosis among these patients because of proper oxygenation of the blood. All the entities of atrial septal defects (ASDs), ventricular septal defects (VSDs), and patent ductus arteriosus (PDA) fall into these disorders. These disorders result from structural heart abnormalities that impede effective circulation of blood and can lead to pulmonary hypertension or heart failure if not diagnosed. While acyanotic heart diseases are less severe than their cyanotic counterparts, early diagnosis and detection are necessary. The manifestations are variable with some patients having fatigue, dyspnea, or growth retardation, but clinical alertness is essential for pediatricians to enable timely intervention and management of the conditions. Notably, the nuances involved in acyanotic defects are further highlighted in less frequent presentations, such as the congenital Gerbode defect, in which a defective connection between the left ventricle and right atrium occurs. This condition most exemplifies the diagnostic challenge inherent with revealing less frequent acyanotic defects because presenting signs may simulate those of more prevalent cardiac diseases. A systematic literature review of the Gerbode defect discusses a range of clinical presentations—from dyspnea to asymptomatology—and emphasizes the necessity of multimodal diagnostic management. Best management is based on early diagnosis of the defect and individually tailored treatment modalities, wherein surgical closure of the defect is recommended over device closure, particularly due to complexity in conditions and unpredictable manifestations (Winter et al., 2024) (Figure 6.2).

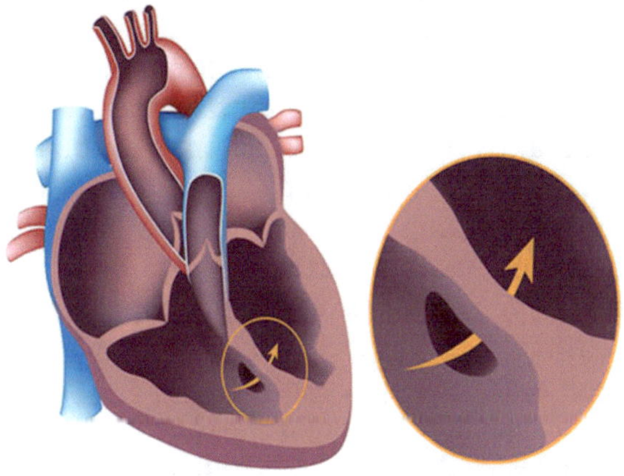

Figure 6.2. Acyanotic congenital heart disease.

Source: https://www.homeocareclinic.in/acyanotic-heart-disease-causes-symptoms-treatment/.

Furthermore, the relationship between acyanotic heart diseases and other diseases is becoming more pertinent, especially in the context of the COVID-19 pandemic's impacts on child populations. As many resources have been diverted to combat the pandemic, children who are already afflicted with such conditions as acyanotic heart defects have been subjected to higher health risks and had their usual care interrupted. The implications extend to the domain of matters of child vaccination policy, being safety, efficacy, and risk management of transmission, which these advances validate as strengthening the call for an extensive panorama of knowledge in pediatric cardiac disease within the overarching issue of public health, and they reiterate the call for prudence in the surveillance of cardiovascular consequences of the effect of extrinsic stimuli on acyanotic heart disease patients (Lababidi et al., 2024).

Importance of Understanding Acyanotic Conditions

An accurate understanding of acyanotic conditions is critical to healthcare professionals and patients with congenital heart disease. These conditions, like defects in the region of the atrial septal and ventricular septal areas, result predominantly in an increase in pulmonary blood flow without noticeable cyanosis. By understanding the pathophysiological mechanisms and related complications, healthcare professionals can apply appropriate immediate intervention. Appropriate management can prevent progression of symptoms, such as pulmonary hypertension or heart failure, which may arise from undiagnosed defects. For families, the knowledge of these diseases helps detect signs and symptoms needing treatment, thus encouraging an active care strategy in accordance with the guidelines available from healthcare authorities and medical organizations, as highlighted in the ESC Guidelines (Baumgartner et al., 2020). The psychological and emotional effects of acyanotic congenital heart diseases are just as significant to bear in mind. Children with these conditions tend to have difficulties that are associated with their health status, which may affect their development milestones. Parents and caregivers need to be informed to be able to provide support to their child's physical and emotional needs. The need for frequent monitoring and surgical or non-surgical interventions is critical to understand. Educational knowledge of community resources and support groups can also help families overcome barriers to ultimately achieving a higher quality of life. Great stress should be placed on ongoing education regarding acyanotic heart disease in order to reduce anxiety and condition families to any lifestyle adjustments (Hayes et al., 2019). The medical community has to do its part in eliminating the misconceptions regarding acyanotic congenital heart disease, especially their relative severity in comparison to cyanotic disease. Educational programs for healthcare providers and the general public can facilitate better understanding of these defects in the context of their impact on long-term health. Through specialist training, medical professionals can acquire skills in early identification of acyanotic conditions, with improved diagnosis, and modulating treatment protocols to the patient. By facilitating collaboration between the health teams, families, and patients, overall management of such conditions can be facilitated. Continuing observation of best practices and evolving therapy changes will continue to contribute to current knowledge, enabling patients with acyanotic congenital heart diseases to receive the comprehensive care required to thrive (Baumgartner et al., 2020).

6.1. Types of Acyanotic Heart Diseases

Acyanotic heart disease is among the significant classifications of congenital cardiac malformations that lack cyanosis, or blue color, indicating absence of oxygenation of blood.

These malformations are primarily related to raised pulmonary blood flow, because of left-to-right shunting of the blood. Among the common types are atrial septal defects (ASDs), ventricular septal defects (VSDs), and patent ductus arteriosus (PDA). All these malformations share certain characteristic hemodynamic consequences. For example, ASDs allow blood to flow between the atria, leading to right atrial and ventricular volume enlargement, while VSDs allow communication between the ventricles, leading to congestive heart failure if not treated. The prognosis and management in these patients vary and are solely based on the size of the defect and hemodynamic effect, which highlights the importance of early diagnosis and treatment. The consequences of acyanotic heart malformations are greater than acute clinical presentation; they can initiate long-term sequelae if not effectively managed. In conditions like PDA, for instance, the persistent shunting of blood leads to left atrial enlargement and ultimately pulmonary hypertension, thus potentially converting a formerly acyanotic condition into its more severe variants typically anticipated of cyanotic heart disease. Atrial septal and ventricular septal defects would follow the same path, adding to the load of the right half of the heart. The existing information about the conditions is based on the latest studies that have highlighted the interplay of various mechanisms in acyanotic heart diseases' pathophysiology (Luo et al., 2019). These involve the grounds for more research to be done to improve treatment procedures and results of patients. Treatment of acyanotic heart defects typically involves a multidisciplinary management plan with medical treatment and surgical intervention in certain instances. In minimal defects, close follow-up may be sufficient because certain patients can recover through spontaneous closure, especially in ASD. Larger or symptomatic defects will typically require surgical correction. Recent advancements have also augmented the importance of catheter-based interventions, with less invasive options that may reduce recovery time and associated complications (Baumgartner et al., 2020). Treatment should entail ongoing follow-ups, which should be tailored according to the type of defect and the requirements of each patient. With continued advances in technology and technique, more emphasis on the early diagnosis and intervention would yield improved long-term result in patients with acyanotic cardiac diseases (Figure 6.3).

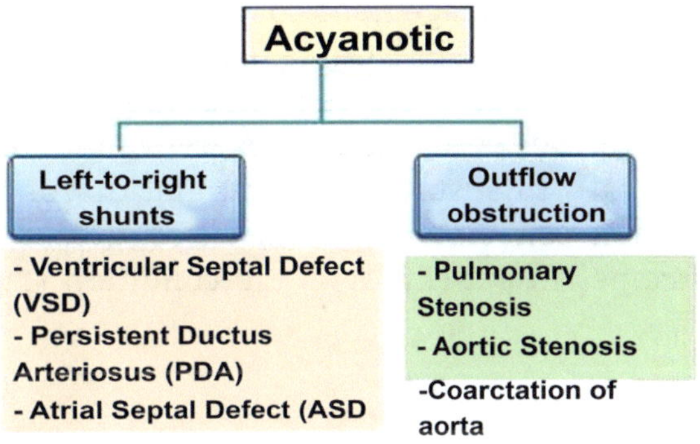

Figure 6.3. Types of acyanotic heart diseases.

Source: https://cdnintech.com/media/chapter/64469/1512345123/media/F1.png.

6.1.1. Ventricular Septal Defect (VSD)

The cardiac anatomy is important in the pathogenesis of congenital conditions like Ventricular Septal Defect (VSD). VSD is defined by a faulty opening within the ventricular septum, that is, the wall between the left ventricle and the right ventricle. This defect causes a left-to-right shunt, increasing blood volume flowing to the lungs. VSD may vary in severity from minimally defective and asymptomatic to more severe defects that, left untreated, will cause pulmonary hypertension and heart failure. The impact of VSD on hemodynamics is multifaceted as it not only affects oxygenation of blood but also causes additional stress on the ventricles and the pulmonary circulation, which contributes to the overall clinical picture of acyanotic heart diseases. Diagnosis of VSD involves both clinical evaluation and advanced imaging techniques. Auscultation typically reveals common heart murmurs, a background for further study through echocardiography, providing an express image of the defect and resultant hemodynamic consequences. Azizova et al. (2020) particularly emphasizes the recognition of concomitant anomalies adding to the clinical course of patients with VSD. These include persistent left superior vena cava, which can complicate surgical procedures or catheterization. Accurate diagnosis of VSD and potential future complications must be made in order to develop an optimal treatment plan which best addresses the individual patient's cardiac anatomy and physiology. Treatment of VSD varies on several factors, including size of defect, presence of symptoms, and concomitant cardiovascular anomalies. Small, asymptomatic, uncomplicated VSDs are often treated with observation alone, since spontaneous closure will develop in infancy. More profound defects will need surgical intervention or medical management to prevent related complications such as heart failure or pulmonary vascular disease. ESC Guidelines recommend that individualized treatment based on each patient's situation and risk factors is most important in determining the appropriate management strategy. Baumgartner et al. (2020) observes that clinical decisions are made in accordance with the latest guidelines to ensure an ethical and thorough care strategy. Thus, VSD, although one of the more common congenital heart diseases, demands thorough evaluation and management for optimal outcomes in patients with the condition (Figure 6.4).

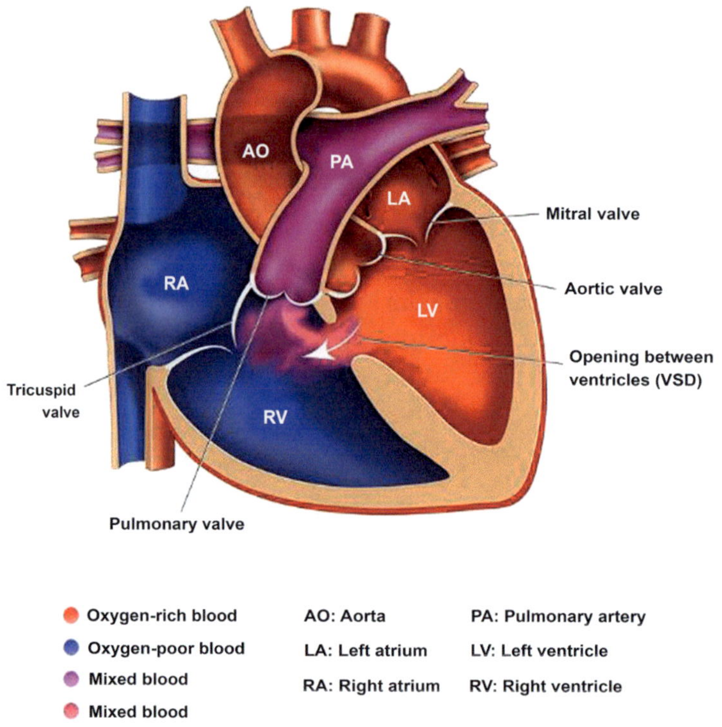

Figure 6.4. Ventricular septal defect.

Source: https://www.tomwademd.net/acyanotic-congenital-heart-lesions-part-1-from-pedscases-with-additional-resources/.

6.1.2. Atrial Septal Defect (ASD)

Atrial Septal Defect, also abbreviated as ASD, is a prevalent form of congenital heart disease that falls under the category of acyanotic defects (i.e., patients do not present with significant cyanosis in infancy). ASDs are a defect in the septum between the left and the right atria of the heart, resulting in an abnormal flow of blood from one chamber to the other. The condition allows for shunting of oxygen-rich blood from the left atrium into the right atrium, increasing blood flow to the lungs. The effects of this left-to-right shunt can lead to complications such as right heart volume overload, pulmonary hypertension, and arrhythmias unless treated. As observed by research, symptomatic presentations related to ASD, including PAH, are rare in infancy, but if and when they occur, they can result in serious complications that necessitate urgent medical intervention (Andrews et al., 2012).

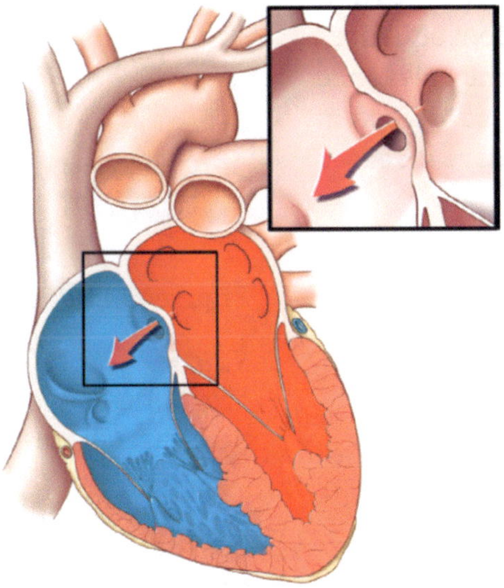

Figure 6.5. Atrial septal defect with flow from the left atrium to the right atrium, as depicted by the red arrow.

Source: https://obgynkey.com/acyanotic-congenital-heart-disease-5/

The implications of untreated ASD are significant, with some infants having severe respiratory insufficiency as a result of right atrial and ventricular overload. One case study emphasizes the need for intervention in such complications and how a child who presented with recurrent respiratory issues and failure to thrive due to severe PAH secondary to an isolated ASD (Andrews et al., 2012) showed a notable decline in pulmonary artery pressure after repair of the defect via surgery, leading to improved respiratory function and improved growth in the affected infants. This illustrates the immediate correlation between early medical treatment of ASD and having the capability to avoid the cascade of undesirable effects that may result from untreated cases. Surgical repair of ASDs is therefore indicated, particularly in symptomatic cases, to maximize quality of life and reduce severe morbidity as a sequel to the condition. Understanding the epidemiological prevalence of ASDs is similarly crucial in realizing its clinical impact. Of many types of congenital heart defects, acyanotic forms—such as ASDs—are particularly more prevalent, occurring in about

67.1% of cases of total congenital heart disease in pediatric populations (Umer et al., 2018). ASD may often be accompanied by other defects, including ventricular septal defects, and thus constitutes a significant priority area for pediatric cardiology. Detection at an early stage, usually through echocardiography, enables effective therapeutic measures that can greatly enhance patient outcomes. With treatment and awareness measures enhancing with time, it is increasingly crucial to continue research on ASD so as to maximize management approaches and identify more about the long-term consequences on the patients, thus maintaining the relevance of this acyanotic congenital cardiac defect in the larger context of congenital heart diseases (Figure 6.5).

6.1.3. Patent Ductus Arteriosus (PDA)

Patent Ductus Arteriosus (PDA) is a significant acyanotic congenital heart disease as a result of failure of the ductus arteriosus, an artery that must close in the early postnatal period. This duct in normal infants shunts blood past the fetal lungs and delivers it from the pulmonary artery to the aorta. If not closed, babies will exhibit tachypnea, feeding difficulties, and failure to thrive due to the augmented pulmonary blood flow. It may lead to complications such as left heart volume overload and pulmonary hypertension unless it is closed. Prompt diagnosis and appropriate therapy of PDA are essential to avoid the complications and enhance patient outcomes as cases that are left untreated can result in severe morbidity. The definitive treatment for PDA has evolved to emphasize the use of percutaneous closure devices as the most suitable alternative to surgery. Following guidelines, this less invasive technique has been reported to have low complication rates, enabling quicker recovery for children. However, complications can arise, including device embolization, necessitating surgical or percutaneous retrieval procedures. An example is that a new snaring technique has proved useful for retrieving embolized devices and demonstrates the adaptability of available interventional cardiology practices to address unexpected complications. The operators must remain vigilant during and post-procedure, as there may be such complications, and an individualized approach for each patient can help meet their unique anatomical and physiological status (Figure 6.6).

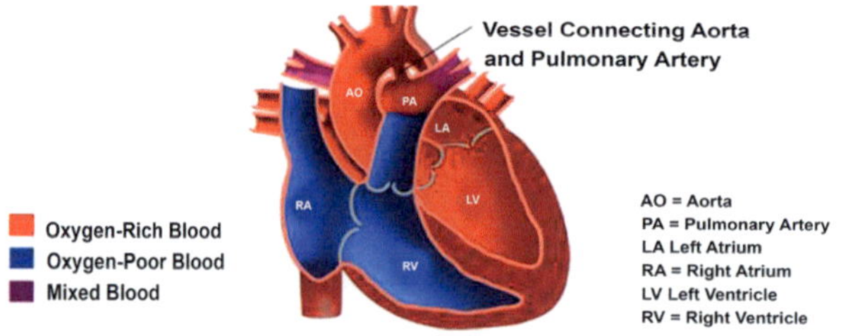

Figure 6.6. Patent ductus arteriosus.

Source: https://www.tomwademd.net/acyanotic-congenital-heart-lesions-part-1-from-pedscases-with-additional-resources/.

The example of the case of an untreated 29-year-old man with PDA illustrates the severe consequences that can occur as a result of congenital cardiac malformations, one of which is infective endocarditis. His presentation with vegetations in the pulmonary artery illustrates a rare and complex interplay between PDA and secondary infection and needs surgery. Following vigorous treatment, including vegetation excision and PDA ligation, massive reverse remodeling took place, which highlights the potential for recovery following intervention. Such cases indicate the importance of early surgery not only for palliation but also for complete care in cases of PDA, who may be at risk of developing complications more than simple hemodynamics (Cool et al., 2025). Improvements in clinical knowledge regarding PDA have created the demand for further research and practitioner awareness, which is still essential to enhance treatment modalities and patient care approaches (Fransiska et al., 2024).

6.2. Causes and Risk Factors

Acyanotic congenital heart disease most commonly results from a host of causes that may broadly be categorized into genetic and environmental factors. Genetic predisposition is a significant factor to consider, with certain chromosomal anomalies such as trisomy 21 (Down syndrome) having a high prevalence of cardiac malformations. Family patterns also show that congenital factors are at play in the risk of developing congenital heart disease. Understanding these genetic predispositions is crucial to early diagnosis and intervention, particularly in individuals with a positive family history for cardiovascular defects. Teratogenic exposure in utero by the mother—certain drugs or toxic agents—has been known to predispose to cardiac defects. This intricate interplay of the environment and genetics emphasizes the importance of proper prenatal care and parental counseling in averting risk associated with acyanotic congenital heart disease. In addition to environmental and genetic causation, maternal health conditions and lifestyle also greatly contribute to the risk for congenital heart disease. Obesity and diabetes have been indicated to enhance the risk of heart defects in newborns. Maternal diabetes, for instance, may be a factor of fetal development that results in structural heart defects through altered metabolic conditions. Pregnancy smoking has also been associated with a myriad of adverse effects, including increased risk of congenital heart defects. All of these lifestyle factors underscore the importance of public health programs to encourage maternal health during pregnancy and prior to it. Most optimally effective education and provision can enable pregnant women to make informed health choices to reduce the risks of acyanotic congenital heart disease, ultimately resulting in improved outcomes for the mother and the child. Finally, maternal age has been identified as a critical risk factor in the development of acyanotic congenital heart diseases. Research has indicated that women of older maternal age, typically 35 years and older, are at higher risk of having offspring with congenital heart malformations. The increased risk is possible due to age-linked genetic mutation, as well as an increased likelihood of developing chronic illnesses that complicate pregnancy. With population trends showing a rise in the age of first pregnancies, awareness of this population trend is crucial among healthcare providers. In order to manage the implications of mature maternal age, they must take patients through proper screening and counseling services to reduce potential risks associated with congenital heart disease. By incorporating such information into prenatal practice, health care providers are able to provide enhanced maternal-fetal health results and reduced prevalence of acyanotic congenital heart defects, as advised through standards emphasized in the practice (Baumgartner et al., 2020; Stout et al., 2018) (Figure 6.7).

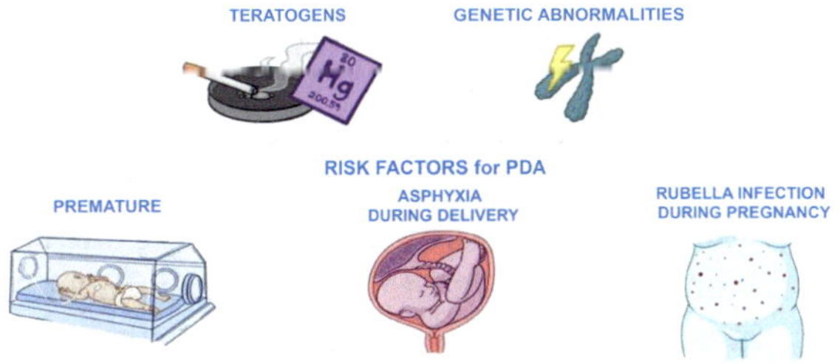

Figure 6.7. Common causes and risk factors of acyanotic congenital heart disease.

Source: https://www.osmosis.org/_next/image?url=https%3A%2F%2Fd16qt3wv6xm098.cloudfront.net%2F1VCWd7y2TkK3yYg-xe5i_l1ISJCdGxrs%2F_.jpg&w=3840&q=75.

6.2.1. Genetic Factors

The etiology of congenital heart diseases (CHDs), particularly acyanotic CHDs, involves complex, multifactorial genetics. According to published studies, genetic predisposition contributes significantly to the development of structural heart malformations. Certain chromosomal defects and single-gene mutations have been implicated in specific conditions such as atrial septal defect (ASD) and ventricular septal defect (VSD), which are prevalent among acyanotic heart malformations. Such genetically determined susceptibilities tend to occur in families and point towards an inheritable factor worthy of a rigorous investigation. Moreover, karyotype analysis has established that a considerable percentage of CHD patients have identifiable genetic syndromes, thereby lending support to the hypothesis that genetic makeup is a causative factor in the occurrence of these conditions. As we delve further into the genetic causation, it seems that understanding the causes of them is necessary for early detection and potentially preventive interventions. In addition to chromosomal abnormalities, the involvement of environmental factors playing along with genetic factors cannot be underestimated. The idea of gene-environment interactions is increasingly being recognized in cardiovascular development. For instance, teratogenic exposure during key periods of development, for instance, drug or environmental toxicant exposure in pregnancy, can increase inherent genetic susceptibility to produce acyanotic cardiac malformations. Perturbation in signaling pathways during cardiogenesis has been found to be induced by such interactions, skewing normal myocardial development. This interactive dynamic suggests that while genetics form the basis of potential heart malformations, environmental stimuli can trigger or dampen the development of such defects. Integrated strategies directed at genetic counseling and environmental study therefore become necessary in an effort to maximize outcomes among affected individuals and their families. The genetic influences have implications beyond the extent of identifying the presence of congenital heart defect; they also extend to the long-term health implications of the diagnosed person. As it is clear from studies, people suffering from congenital heart disease, particularly those who underwent operation, may suffer from neurodevelopmental impairments caused by genetic influences. For instance, data prove that adolescents with complicated congenital heart disease experience severe cerebral volume loss, which is related to cognitive and executive dysfunction impairment, especially those with more complex cyanotic types compared to acyanotic types. That informs us that some genetic factors may not only influence structural heart malformations but also underlying neurodevelopmental pathways (cognitive outcomes, $P < 0.05$). These findings emphasize the imperative of long-term cardiac and neurodevelopmental follow-up of acyanotic congenital heart disease patients, working interventions to mitigate long-term consequences as the etiology of genetic influences still continues to be illuminated (Buchmann et al., 2017; Golalipour et al., 2011).

6.2.2. Environmental Influences

The cause of congenital heart diseases (CHD), including acyanotic conditions, is decided by outside influences in critical times of pregnancy. Some teratogenic exposures, for instance, some medications, alcohol, and infectious agents, have been seen to impair fetal cardiac development. For instance, maternal obesity and diabetes may create a metabolic environment that predisposes the offspring to CHD. Besides, poor prenatal care can exacerbate these risks through limiting essential screenings and interventions, especially for high-risk populations. As repeating the European Society of Cardiology recommendation, healthcare professionals should consider these environmental elements when assessing patients' risks for the onset of acyanotic heart diseases (Baumgartner et al.,

2020). By addressing issues of maternal health and environmental protection, interventions can be explicitly designed to limit these risks and improve outcomes for children as well as mothers. Geographic patterns in congenital heart disease (CHD) also indicate environmental disparities impacting rates of prevalence. Current research conducted in numerous regions of China illustrates that birth prevalence varies substantially by geographic and socioeconomic factors, highlighting a high correlation between these and incidence of CHD. Increased prevalence rates were observed in the economically developed countries where medical care is more readily available and early screening is prevalent (Zhao et al., 2020) (Figure 6.8).

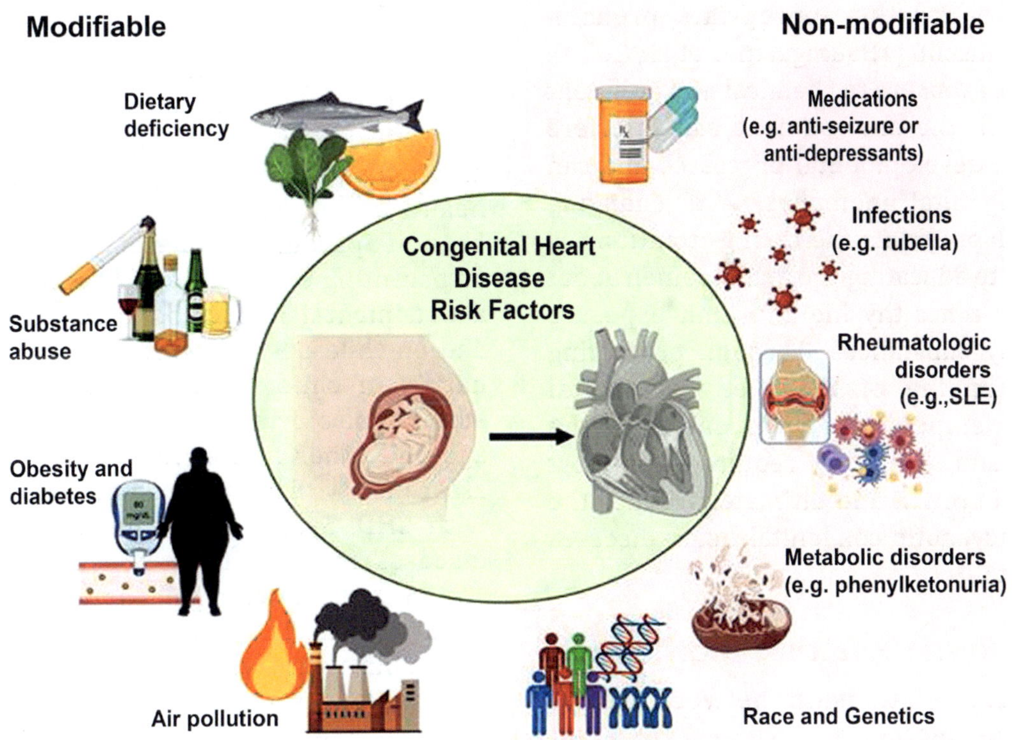

Figure 6.8. Risk factors of congenital heart disease. Modifiable risk factors associated with congenital heart disease include diet, obesity, substance abuse, and air pollution, whereas nonmodifiable risk factors include rheumatologic disorders, genetic variants, specific medications, and infection.

Source: https://www.frontiersin.org/files/Articles/635280/fcvm-08-635280-HTML/image_m/fcvm-08-635280-g001.jpg.

Conversely, under-reporting of CHD exists in lower-income and rural populations due to the lack of resources and healthcare centers. Such findings indicate that environmental factors of CHD are necessary, which indicate interventions not just against biological causes but also against the overall context of socioeconomic disparities. By comprehending the multifactorial environmental causes of CHD, public health intervention can be more effectively designed to reduce incidence and improve healthcare access. The interplay of lifestyle variables and maternal exposures is also an essential part in comprehending environmental determinants of acyanotic congenital cardiac diseases. All these factors have been proven through studies to significantly impact fetal development outcomes by influencing nutrition, exposure to stress, and environmental poisons. Nutritional deficiencies, particularly of essential vitamins such as folic acid, have also been linked to increased risks for CHD, hence reiterating the necessity for the appropriate prenatal nutrition counseling (Baumgartner et al., 2020). Additionally, exposure to chemical and pollutant substances in the environment can interfere with normal developmental processes and can lead to congenital anomalies. With changing public health programs, increasing attention has been drawn to educating pregnant women about how to lead a healthy life and limit exposure to unhealthy substances. Through promoting an understanding of these environmental influences, empowering women with the knowledge and skills they require to support healthy fetal growth and ultimately reduce the burden of acyanotic congenital heart diseases becomes vital.

6.2.3. Maternal Health Conditions

The intricate relationship between health status of the mother and congenital heart diseases, especially acyanotic ones, calls for an understanding of how directly a mother's health status affects fetal development. Maternal health status of uncontrolled diabetes, obesity, and advanced maternal age has been associated with elevated risk of congenital heart defects among newborns. For instance, gestational diabetes can result in hyperglycemia during moments when organogenesis is crucial, and this can result in structural heart malformations. Furthermore, the presence of maternal disease affects not just the baby's physical health but also maternal psychological statuses, as evidenced by increased stress and anxiety levels. These affective factors may complicate the care process, introducing difficulties that can influence the developmental trajectories of infants with CHD and thus underline the imperative interface between maternal health and congenital heart disease in the neonate. In addition to the immediate consequences for fetal development, maternal health conditions dictate long-term outcomes among children with acyanotic heart disease. Research has shown that babies born to mothers who have some medical conditions are at greater risk for developmental delay, intrauterine growth restriction, and psychosocial problems in early life. Maternal mental health is significant as well; mothers who perceive either their health or the health of their baby as having been jeopardized experience greater levels of parenting stress, which in return can have a detrimental impact on parenting practices and on child development. The interconnected nature of child health and maternal health status is also evident in findings that maternal age and other measures of health are highly associated with cognitive ability among children with CHD. Systematic treatment of maternal diseases may optimize support to mothers and children toward enhanced health-related quality of life. The shared social and economic conditions under which families operate worsen the challenges of congenital heart diseases. The majority of families with acyanotic heart defects are confronted by a complex healthcare environment that is potentially determined by socioeconomic status and health service access. It has been established through research that the lower socioeconomic-class mothers have other barriers to accessing prenatal care and ongoing support, thereby impacting their own health and their children's as well. The impact of such disparities can be astonishing in that developmental delay is more commonly reported among children who are less privileged. In addition, parenting stress is likely to increase in families that are both struggling financially and dealing with the challenges of raising a child with a chronic illness. The need for integrative healthcare interventions directed towards favoring maternal well-being and reversing the consequences of socioeconomic disadvantage is essential in improving long-term outcomes of children with acyanotic heart disease, as indicated by evidence related to effective care models in various healthcare systems (Cangas-Isacaz et al., 2025; Smith et al., 2017).

6.3. Symptoms and Diagnosis

The clinical presentation of acyanotic congenital heart disease (ACHD) is usually varied by the lesion and its hemodynamic consequences. Tachypnea, diaphoresis, and poor exercise tolerance are common symptoms that may present in infants and toddlers. These result from the augmented pulmonary blood flow of lesions like atrial septal defects or ventricular septal defects. Because these heart defects allow left-to-right shunting of the blood, the patients may come with the signs of increased cardiac workload, leading to symptoms of heart failure if left untreated. Moreover, parents also know very little about their child's condition, as noted in a study where 59% of parents accurately identified the congenital heart disease of their child but fewer than one-third were able to diagrammatically locate the heart lesion, indicating vast knowledge gaps for symptoms and outcomes (Chau et al., 2004). The diagnostic approach to acyanotic congenital heart disease most often begins with a comprehensive history and clinical examination supported by reliance on advanced imaging techniques, such as echocardiography. This nonoperative testing not only assists in visualization of the structural cardiac abnormalities but also assesses the degree of blood flow alteration within the cardiac chambers. Lastly, chest X-rays and electrocardiograms (ECGs) may provide further data regarding heart shape and size as well as the dynamics of blood flow. The identification of prototypic clinical findings, such as a murmur indicating a turbulent blood flow through an abnormality, is of valuable significance in initiating further investigation. Despite these improvements in diagnosis, the heterogeneity of symptoms can lead to delays in diagnosis, thus the necessity of increased awareness among parents and medical workers (Cullen et al., 2013). At diagnosis, acyanotic congenital heart diseases are treated multimodally to maximize benefits for the patient. This may include comprehensive family education regarding potential symptoms to be observed, such as changes in exercise tolerance or respiratory distress, and a nutritional supplement to promote growth and development among affected children. Coordination with pediatric cardiologists, nurses, and social workers is ensured so that families are provided with a comprehensive description of their child's condition and relevance to everyday life. New evidence demonstrating adult congenital heart disease patients commonly experience compromised quality of life underscores the importance of early diagnosis and treatment, which significantly impacts long-term health (Cullen et al., 2013). This collaboration aims not only to address present health issues but also to educate families to promote the care of their children in the future.

6.3.1. Common Symptoms in Infants and Children

It is important to be aware of common child and infant symptoms for early identification of congenital heart diseases (CHD), particularly for acyanotic conditions. Acyanotic CHD infants usually have a range of typical clinical presentations, including symptoms such as fast breathing and feeding. In fact, one research has revealed that rapid breathing is the most prevalent presenting symptom in neonates with CHD, occurring in around 43.4% of cases. Difficulty in feeding comes close, with around 20.77% of children being affected. Prompt recognition of such symptoms is important, as this can enable timely intervention that can go a long way in enhancing overall prognosis and handling of the afflicted children. Unless closely monitored, the undiagnosed conditions can lead to catastrophic results that deteriorate the health of the infants, thereby highlighting the need for healthcare professionals to be on the lookout for heart defects in symptomatic infants (Mir et al., 2019) (Figure 6.9).

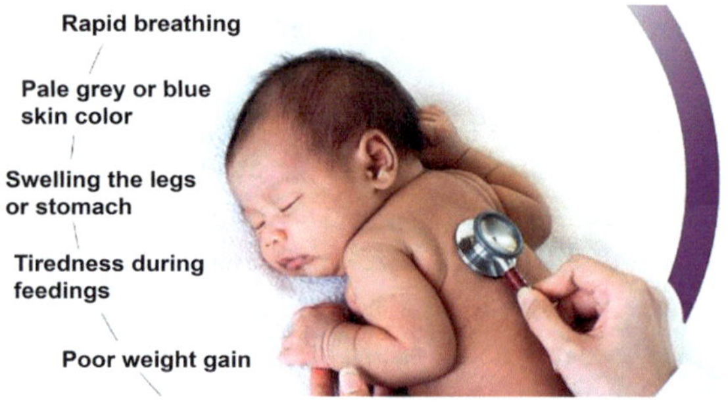

Figure 6.9. Acyanotic congenital heart diseases (ACHD) symptoms.

Source: https://external-content.duckduckgo.com/iu/?u=https%3A%2F%2Fkdahweb-static.kokilabenhospital.com%2Fkdah-2019%2Ftips%2F1644583788.jpg&f=1&nofb=1&ipt=4c008ea02e38b46bf98ea67151cb02834bc8295c7f2795bfc239bbb1c0ea704e.

Other than for respiratory distress and feeding, cyanosis can also be a critical indicator of intrinsic cardiac malformations. In neonates, cyanosis is typically manifested in the form of blue discoloration of skin or mucous membranes secondary to insufficient oxygenation. Although cyanosis is more commonly associated with cyanotic heart disease, it is also present in a group of acyanotic diseases where compromised blood flow causes diminished oxygenation of the systemic circulation. Cyanosis presents as a presenting symptom in approximately 17.2% of neonates with CHD. The presence of this symptom is important to identify as it usually portends the need for urgent medical evaluation and potential intervention. Infant variability of the presentation of the symptoms emphasizes the necessity of a comprehensive clinical assessment to distinguish cyanotic from acyanotic forms of cardiac malformations (Mir et al., 2019). Other non-specific signs, such as decreased urine production, and shock, also require evaluation in the context of congenital heart disease. These signs may be caused by the circulatory alterations due to the heart malformation. Among the population studied, approximately 8.1% of neonates had shock, as evidenced by markedly decreased urinary output, which can be an indicator of organ dysfunction. Although respiratory infections such as those caused by respiratory syncytial virus (RSV) may worsen these conditions, the combination of presentations of different illnesses makes standard diagnostic channels cumbersome. Therefore, healthcare providers must exercise a wholistic approach in the diagnosis of CHD, considering the symptomatic pattern as well as diagnostic imaging, e.g., echocardiography, to confirm CHD diagnoses. This wholistic practice is essential in achieving maximum outcomes in infants with acyanotic disease because timely diagnosis and treatment are associated with prognostic success here.

6.3.2. Diagnostic Imaging Techniques

Of all the diagnostic imaging techniques used in assessing congenital heart conditions, particularly acyanotic ones, echocardiography is the cornerstone. It is a non-invasive technique that relies on sound waves to produce images of hearts' structure and function in real time. Because of its ability to visualize anatomy of the heart, clinicians can identify abnormalities such as septal defects and valvular disease without exposure to radiation. The functional assessment provided by echocardiography is critical in determining the hemodynamic significance of noted anomalies. As described in contemporary guidelines, correct synthesis of echocardiographic results with presentation may have a significant influence on management strategies in congenitally affected individuals. The growing reliance on echocardiography underscores its worth in terms of making early and accurate diagnoses that eventually lead to improved patient outcomes in patients with these congenital defects (Azizova et al., 2020) (Figure 6.10).

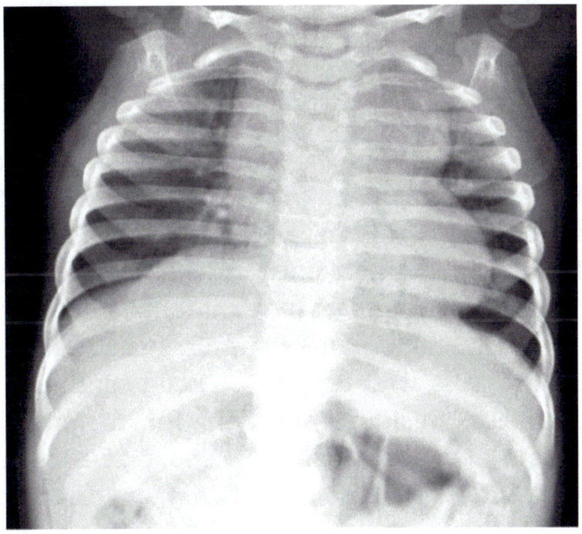

Figure 6.10. Diagnostic imaging techniques utilized for assessing congenital heart diseases.

Source: https://prod-images-static.radiopaedia.org/images/5964933/8b7c93613763fc37070b6fad2f379e_big_gallery.jpeg.

Other than echocardiography, magnetic resonance imaging (MRI) is similarly gaining increasing relevance in the evaluation of congenital heart disease. MRI proves to be particularly useful in complex anatomy evaluation and higher-resolution functional studies than echocardiography. MRI is particularly valuable in patients where accurate imaging of the pulmonary vasculature and aorta is crucial. Furthermore, MRI provides details on myocardial perfusion and tissue characterization, which are extremely valuable in the treatment of patients with concomitant conditions. On integration of the findings on MRI with those on echocardiography, doctors gain better insight into the health status of the patients, allowing them to pursue tailored therapeutic approaches. Most notable, recent research highlights the potential of MRI to aid in diagnosis of associated anomalies, such as persistent left superior vena cava — a key consideration in surgical management and intervention (Azizova et al., 2020). Computed tomography (CT) is also a significant diagnostic imaging technique for the evaluation of congenital heart diseases. While long-standing less so in pediatric patients due to issues with radiation exposure, technological advancements in CT imaging, including coronary CT angiography, have made it a valuable resource in the assessment of vascular abnormalities and complex congenital lesions. CT imaging has a distinct ability to provide high-resolution three-dimensional reconstructions of cardiac and vascular anatomy and is useful both for diagnosis and preoperative planning. Especially for those patients presenting with suspected abnormalities such as coarctation of the aorta or anomalous pulmonary veins, CT will serve to explain anatomy and potential concomitant conditions well. As the clinician progresses through the series of diagnostic modalities at hand, accurate interpretation of CT findings alongside other imaging techniques is required to direct treatment plans, to result in better case management of cases involving congenital heart disease (Baumgartner et al., 2020).

6.3.3. Role of Echocardiography

Echocardiography is a valuable tool in diagnosing and treating congenital heart diseases (CHDs) and, particularly, in the case of acyanotic lesions such as atrial septal defects (ASDs) and ventricular septal defects (VSDs). Echocardiography is an imaging modality that is free of invasiveness and allows for precise visualization of the anatomy of the heart as well as hemodynamics, making it easy for doctors to assess the anatomy and function of congenital defects. Recurrent use of transthoracic echocardiography offers real-time imaging of cardiac function and is particularly useful in routine examinations (Figure 6.11).

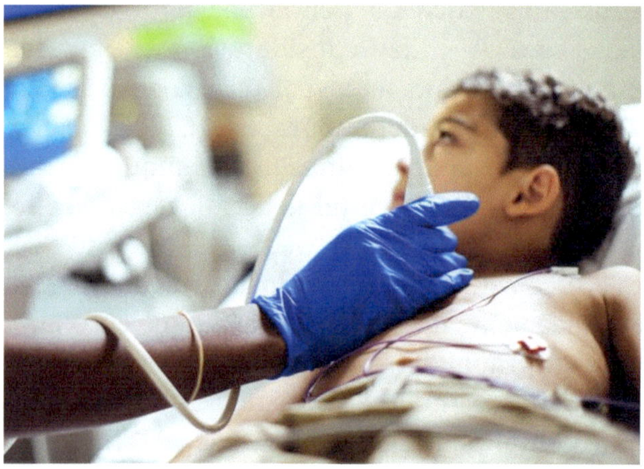

Figure 6.11. The echocardiogram is created using an ultrasound machine connected to a microphone-shaped transducer, which is placed near the part of the anatomy to be examined.

Source: https://drshreepaljain.com/wp-content/uploads/2023/12/boy-having-cardiac-imaging-700x500.jpg.

In patients with CHD, its early identification through echocardiographic assessment also significantly contributes to clinical outcomes and channels timely interventions, ultimately reducing risks of complications due to untreated defects. This initial imaging gives a clearer path for holistic treatment plans, and thus its importance in pediatric cardiology and more is asserted. Advances in technology on echocardiography have optimized its role in addressing acyanotic congenital heart disease. Transoesophageal echocardiography (TOE) is now a powerful ally to the traditional transthoracic approach, particularly in the management of complicated cases or when traditional views are limited. According to recent reviews, TOE not only offers good visualization during interventional procedures but also aids in guiding trans-catheter procedures such as ASD closure and VSD repair with precision. This capability is of specific importance in adulthood when the majority of individuals with congenital heart defect reach maturity. The integration of advanced imaging technologies has a direct bearing on the effectiveness of treatment, demonstrating that advancements in echocardiography are essential in pushing interventional cardiology forward for routine as well as rare congenital disease (Giordano et al., 2025). Furthermore, ongoing evolution of echocardiography entails its utilization in longitudinal follow-up of patients suffering from congenital heart disease throughout their lives. Medical practitioners must make note of the fact that acyanotic defects have patients who often come with underlying symptoms that change and progress with age, hence need continuous follow-up. Besides follow-up for diagnostic reasons, echocardiography also tracks post-interventional course to confirm that corrective procedures are effective and to identify any acute complications. Along with the rising incidence of CHDs to adulthood, particularly in conditions such as atrial septal defects, detailed imaging assessment has become an integral part of chronic healthcare management (Cri et al., 2024). Thus, echocardiography not only forms part of initial diagnoses but also as an ongoing resource within the management strategy of congenital heart disease.

6.4. Treatment Options

The treatment modalities for acyanotic CHD are diverse, as is the wide range of conditions that come under this category. Treatment modalities usually include both surgical and non-surgical modalities tailored to each individual patient's anatomy, age, and clinical presentation. Non-surgical management consists of medical management to manage symptoms and interventional modalities like catheter-based interventions. Surgical intervention may involve corrective surgery, where the aim is to repair structural heart anomalies, or palliative surgery intended to relieve symptoms without necessarily completely correcting the defect. Tailoring comes in here in that patient outcomes are maximized and the treatment plan is more tailored based on the condition and the severity. In recent years, collaborative models of care have been seen as a possible means of expanding access to treatment for acyanotic CHD, particularly in LMICs. One such initiative is the Rashtriya Bal Swasthya Karyakram, which initiated the "Sishu Sathi Scheme" in West Bengal, India. This public-private initiative provides monetary support to patients who require cardiac surgeries so their families can cover much-needed treatments regardless of their economic status. These initiatives not only cured thousands of patients but also benefited over 27,000 people from 2013 through 2022 (Das et al., 2024). This new funding model not only is a respite to the financial burden but also signifies the government's intervention in treatment protocols for confronting challenges involving congenital heart defects. The technology improvements in surgical interventions have further enhanced the options for treatment presented to the patient with acyanotic CHD. Among these advances, pulmonary valve replacement has grown far more prevalent, especially in the context of adult congenital heart disease (ACHD). Prosthetic choice is varied and ranges from bioprosthetic valves to newer transcatheter technologies. The process of valve selection is also complex, based on the history of the patient, the delicacy of their specific heart anomaly, and long-term prognosis anticipation (Ashfaq et al., 2024). Such developments not only improve short-term operative outcomes but patient quality of life as well, supporting ongoing development and refinement of treatment guidelines in this critical area of healthcare.

6.4.1. Medical Management

In the treatment of congenital heart diseases, particularly the acyanotic varieties, medical management plays an essential role in the provision of optimal patient outcomes. Such diseases, characterized by the existence of left-to-right shunts, encompass the likes of ventricular septal defect and atrial septal defect. Medical management encompasses numerous therapeutic interventions aimed at symptom relief, prevention of complications, and improvement in global cardiac function. It is important for healthcare professionals to be updated with the latest guidelines when they progress through treatment pathways. The ESC Guidelines emphasize the importance of implementing accessible scientific evidence in clinical setting, as well as taking into account the unique patient circumstances and healthcare policy. This method of practice guarantees that medical management remains patient-focused, eventually enhancing the quality of care delivered (Baumgartner et al., 2020). Pharmacological treatment of acyanotic congenital heart diseases typically consists of drugs which can improve complications and improve hemodynamics. Diuretics, for instance, are generally used in relieving fluid overload as well as congestive heart failure symptoms due to increased pulmonary blood flow. Further, drugs such as angiotensin-converting enzyme (ACE) inhibitors can enhance cardiac output by reducing afterload. Health care professionals also have to consider long-term repercussions of these drugs that might encompass side effects and interactions. This pharmacotherapy knowledge is informed by the guidelines, which offer recommendations regarding the selection and utilization of medicines for patient efficacy and safety (Hayes et al., 2019) (Figure 6.12).

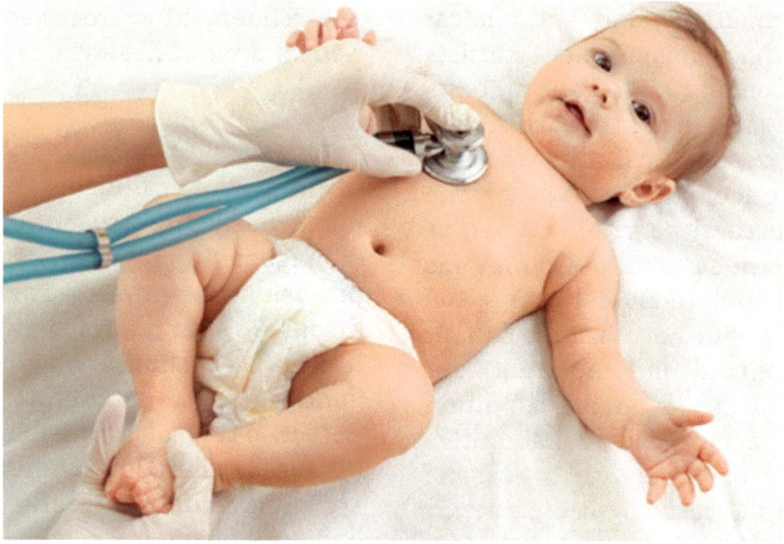

Figure 6.12. Managing congenital heart diseases.

Source: https://external-content.duckduckgo.com/iu/?u=https%3A%2F%2Fckbh.ckbirlahospitals.com%2Fstorage%2Fbmb%2Fuploadedfiles%2Fgallery%2F1674647389_Congenital-Heart-Disease-in-Child.jpg&f=1&nofb=1&ipt=cd2b8c4410bad597a7ccef176cb425f5e89b94415eb276f0be9e06c3752a3b8d.

Ongoing assessment and adjustment of medical treatment are essential components of a successful management program for patients with acyanotic congenital heart disease. Furthermore, patient and family education should not be overemphasized in patient care. Patient and family education, as well as family involvement in decision-making, engages patients in following their treatment programs and facilitates a more therapeutic physician-patient relationship. This shared model is in good agreement with the overall principles set forth in the ESC Guidelines, which include the emphasis on the value of informed patient consent and shared decision-making. By empowering families through education on their conditions, potential therapies, and lifestyle modification, clinicians can facilitate enhanced management of acyanotic congenital heart conditions. Engaging the patients in their own treatment not only increases adherence to doctor's instructions but also optimizes the effectiveness of the therapeutic treatment, hence making the road to recovery more participatory and collaborative (Baumgartner et al., 2020). Patient education is thus a core element within the overall framework of medical treatment for congenital heart diseases.

6.4.2. Surgical Interventions

Congenital heart disease (CHD) surgical interventions, particularly acyanotic defects, have evolved significantly with time, where the outcomes and survival rates of patients have improved. Advances in surgical interventions, such as open-heart surgery and catheter-based therapies, allow for structural defects to be intervened upon early. In cases like atrial septal defects or ventricular septal defects, the application of minimally invasive methods has decreased hospital stays and complications while enhancing recovery times. Significantly, these interventions are not just physical corrections but also the long-term developmental and psychosocial impact on children and their families. The hemodynamic burden of the described abnormal blood flow relieved by surgical correction significantly impacts the overall quality of life, and therefore constant monitoring and supportive management becomes imperative for optimal development and quality of life in children with CHD (Smith et al., 2017). Current practice is a multi-disciplinary method for assessment and execution of the operation with careful balancing of benefits versus risks.

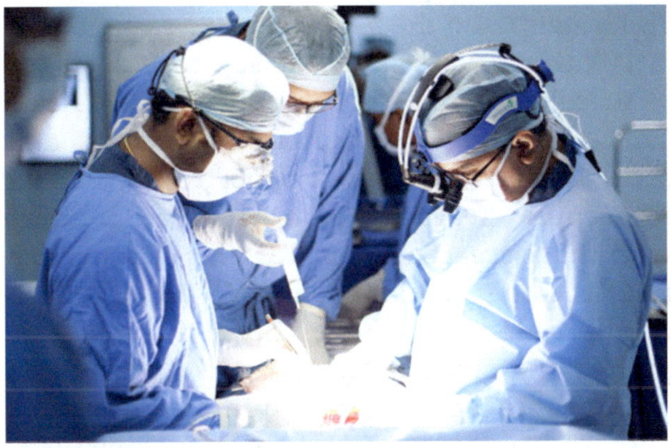

Figure 6.13. Surgical interventions for congenital heart diseases (CHDs).

Source: https://www.bcmch.org/asset/uploads/common/93228970861bc4cffa63d0.jpg.

Surgeons, cardiologists, and pediatricians collaborate to create personalized plans considering the complexity of the defect, patient's overall health, and susceptibility to comorbidities. Interestingly, newer technologies like transcatheter closure procedures reduce the need for open-heart surgery with equally beneficial outcomes. These methods make possible the correction of diseases such as patent ductus arteriosus or small atrial septal defects with less morbidity and shorter recovery times. Even more complex operations, such as the Fontan procedure, are possible for fixing single ventricle physiology with significant effects on survival. Therefore, the role of surgical interventions in the management of acyanotic congenital heart diseases cannot be overstated; not only does it alter the immediate medical situation but also the patient's general outcome in the long term (Prakoso et al., 2024) (Figure 6.13).

Despite the positive impact of surgical intervention, the post-operative issues involve prolonged follow-up treatment for children suffering from acyanotic defects. The outcomes often involve greater rates of growth retardation and developmental delay, as evidenced in studies conducted in various settings, including South Africa. These investigations indicate that even though outcomes from operations can be considered satisfactory to meet set standards, the difficulty involved in providing long-term health care for these patients cannot be overlooked. Regular surveillance for developmental milestones and educational intervention must be done to counteract the likely psychosocial consequences that accompany congenital heart disease. In addition, as the parents navigate the emotional and practical difficulties of the child's plight, supportive interventions are priceless in determining adaptations and offering holistic care. Consequently, surgery must be part of a holistic package of continuous medical and developmental treatment (Smith et al., 2017).

6.4.3. Long-Term Care and Monitoring

Long-term care and monitoring for patients with acyanotic congenital heart diseases are essential components of a comprehensive management plan. Individuals diagnosed with these conditions often require lifelong follow-up to monitor cardiac function, growth, and development. Regular check-ups can help identify any potential complications early, ensuring timely intervention. According to the European Society of Cardiology (ESC) guidelines, doctors must use prudent clinical judgment when assessing each patient's unique condition and health profile (Baumgartner et al., 2020). The rationale behind using individualized assessment is that acyanotic heart defects may lead to varying degrees of hemodynamic change as a function of time, which requires dynamic adjustments in treatment strategies to adapt to the fluctuating health status of the patient. In addition to routine clinical evaluation, long-term patient care for acyanotic congenital heart disease patients can also comprise a multidisciplinary team. The team, which includes cardiologists, pediatricians, nutritionists, and physical therapists, collaborates to address all the health issues of the patient. Routine monitoring of weight, exercise tolerance, and psychosocial status is required as it helps in the evaluation of the overall health status and quality of life of the patients. The ESC emphasizes the importance of including preventive measures, such as routine echocardiography and exercise testing, to ensure optimal health outcomes and provide adequate control of potential complications like arrhythmias or heart failure (Hayes et al., 2019). Education and counseling are also a key element of long-term management of these patients. Families must be thoroughly educated regarding their child's condition and the treatment consequences, so they can recognize warning signs that will necessitate immediate medical care. Support groups and educational materials can foster a supportive community environment as well as a vehicle for sharing experience and solutions. It would not be an exaggeration to state that the significant contribution made by caregivers is extended to supporting the patient through compliance with prescribed medical treatment and lifestyle modification required for long-term health. Based on the ESC guidelines, the responsibility of healthcare professionals is not just related to medical management but also ensuring that families are empowered and supported for the life-long journey of coping with acyanotic congenital heart disease (Baumgartner et al., 2020).

6.5. Complications Associated with Acyanotic Heart Diseases

Acyanotic heart illnesses, which are characterized by the absence of cyanosis, often present with a variety of complications that can have meaningful implications for patient outcomes. These illnesses typically arise from structural abnormalities in the heart that lead to abnormal circulation, such as atrial septal defects or ventricular septal defects. These forms of defects can result in volume overload of the heart, and secondary left ventricular hypertrophy, leading to eventual heart failure if not treated. Along with the increased pressures, the patients can also develop secondary pulmonary hypertension due to elevated blood flow through the pulmonary circulation. Chronic elevation of pressure causes vascular remodeling along with irreversible lung injury, thus making these patients difficult to manage. If not treated, not only do such complications decrease quality of life, but they are also potentially life-threatening, and therefore early diagnosis and treatment in these patients is essential. The other significant concern in patients with acyanotic heart disease is endocarditis risk, infection of the innermost lining of the heart. The risk occurs in the case of abnormal flow dynamics resulting in murky blood flow through cardiac structures, predisposing them to bacterial colonization. The issue lies in identifying at-risk individuals who should be given prophylactic antibiotics for invasive procedures. Although the current guidelines put much emphasis on such preventive practices, compliance remains non-uniform. The outcomes of endocarditis are quite devastating, typically resulting in severe morbidity and mortality unless diagnosed and treated in a timely manner. Subsequently, the medical community continuously updates guidance and advice with the focus on improving the results of disease treatment, paying attention to the irreplaceable significance of timely patient education and communication in reducing associated risks (Baumgartner et al., 2020; Stout et al., 2018). Finally, psychosocial effects of acyanotic heart diseases cannot be ruled out. Such people are belatedly developed as well as face interpersonal problems to a great extent due to the medical burden. Family relationships can be strained as caregivers are subjected to frequent medical appointments, hospitalization, and prolonged treatment, which yield stressors of a personal nature. Furthermore, delayed diagnoses create avoidable complications, which serve to exacerbate these psychosocial problems. To manage these complexities, an integrative approach to care in which attention is given not only to the physical symptoms of the disease but also to the emotional and social well-being of patients and families must be implemented. With the evolving scenario of congenital heart disease management, there can be an emphasis on efficient long-term approaches offering continuous support and care to acyanotic heart disease patients (Baumgartner et al., 2020; Stout et al., 2018).

6.5.1. Heart Failure

Heart failure is a serious one that can strike patients with congenital heart diseases, particularly in acyanotic forms. It generally arises from structural defects of the heart, such as atrial septal defects (ASD) and ventricular septal defects (VSD), which may induce volume overload of the heart. The increased amount of blood flow across the heart chambers may ultimately make the heart muscle become less efficient, resulting in decreased cardiac output. Acyanotic heart disease patients, although often presenting in an initially asymptomatic state, may go on to develop heart failure if the conditions are left uncorrected. Detection and monitoring of heart function are therefore essential components of the management plan, and underscore the necessity for early intervention to prevent complications in such patients. The metabolic ramifications involved in heart failure in acyanotic congenital heart disease patients are significant. Evidence has revealed that metabolic dysregulation plays an important role in the pathogenesis of heart failure in such patients. For instance, alterations in metabolic profiles, including differences in some metabolites, can be utilized to obtain some information on the pathophysiological processes involved. A recent work emphasized the potential of metabolic profiling in differentiating between cyanotic and acyanotic congenital heart diseases and identified some metabolites as potential biomarkers for disease severity and progression. This untargeted metabolic strategy not only accelerates the knowledge of energetics in heart failure but also creates opportunities for personalized treatment regimes based on the unique needs of the individual patients (Vimal et al., 2021) (Figure 6.14).

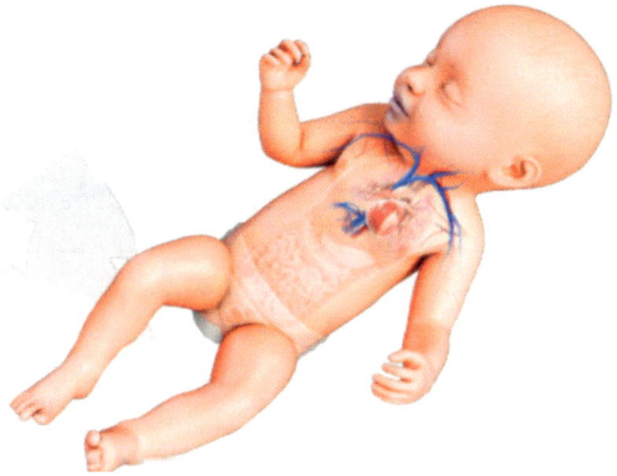

Figure 6.14. Heart failure.

Source: https://www.acepnow.com/wp-content/uploads/2018/05/ACEP_0518_pg22b.png.

The management of heart failure in acyanotic congenital heart disease involves a multi-disciplinary approach through different therapeutic strategies. Based on the European Society of Cardiology (ESC) Guidelines, clinicians need to make decisions on both pharmacological and non-pharmacological interventions to maximize patient outcomes. Diuretics and angiotensin-converting enzyme (ACE) inhibitors are frequently used to relieve symptoms and enhance hemodynamics. However, it is also important that healthcare professionals work in association with patients to extensively inform and engage them in their treatment regimen. This not only helps adhere to the treatment plan but also helps monitor and adjust therapies based on the evolving clinical course of the patient, therefore completely managing heart failure (Baumgartner et al., 2020).

6.5.2. Pulmonary Hypertension

One of the fascinating consequences of congenital heart diseases (CHDs), particularly in the acyanotic types, is pulmonary hypertension (PH). PH is a consequence of the enhanced flow of blood through the pulmonary arteries. This may occur due to structural defects of the heart such as atrial septal defects or ventricular septal defects. Besides making the clinical management of such cardiac defects more complicated, PH aggravates the overall condition of the patients. The pathophysiologic mechanism involves elevated pulmonary artery pressures causing right ventricular stress, which ultimately results in the efficacy of the heart's pumping mechanism. Therefore, patients with acyanotic CHDs begin experiencing signs of heart failure, which again decreases the quality of life and necessitates more complex treatment options that may include drugs that decrease pulmonary pressures and improve cardiac performance. The relationship of malnutrition with outcome in children with congenital heart defects has been adequately studied, particularly in the developing world where access to optimal nutrition care may be limited. Dadang et al. (2015) documents a significant association of malnourishment and increased mechanical ventilation and intensive care unit stay among patients who have had cardiac surgery in children. This finding is particularly relevant when considering the progression of pulmonary hypertension in malnourished children with acyanotic defects. Malnutrition does not only block the growth, but also prevents the body's response to surgery, which can lead to higher rates of postop complication, like that regarding PH. Therefore, nutritional deficiency needs to be treated when designing total care for children with these kinds of conditions. Furthermore, knowledge of environmental and hereditary elements that contribute to the occurrence of acyanotic congenital heart diseases is critical when it comes to preventive measures. It has been established through research that there is a direct linkage of maternal exposure to environmental contaminants and the occurrence of CHDs (Figure 6.15).

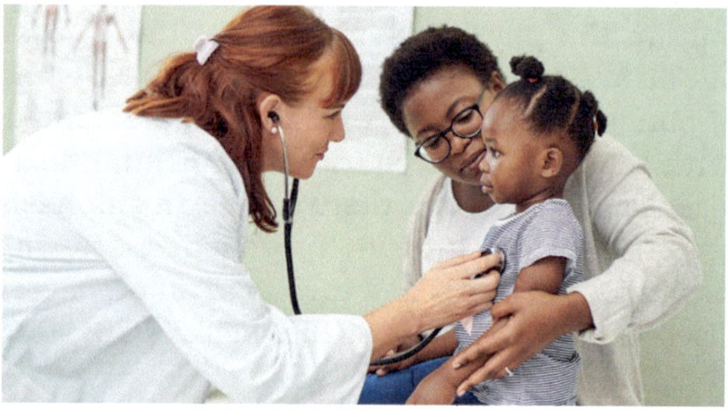

Figure 6.15. Pediatric pulmonary hypertension.

Source: https://www.hopkinsmedicine.org/-/media/images/health/1_-conditions/high-blood-pressure/pulmonary-hypertension-hero.jpg?h=500&iar=0&mh=500&mw=1300&w=1297&hash=B134577368CD813403B04222DB75EF1E.

Kumari et al. (2025) points out how air and water contamination caused by adjacent industrial processes can significantly increase the risk of congenital anomalies, along with those that lead to pulmonary hypertension too. It is this environmental risk factor that public health interventions are addressing in order to make a significant contribution to reducing the occurrence of congenital heart disease and its complications, including pulmonary hypertension. This cross-disciplinary response underscores that imperative integrated health strategies should incorporate not just short-term surgical interventions but also long-term management and prevention services intended to fortify maternal health and environmental integrity.

6.5.3. Arrhythmias

Arrhythmias, or irregular rhythms of the heart, are a significant component of the clinical course of the acyanotic congenital heart diseases. Unlike cyanotic defects leading to reduced oxygenation of the blood, acyanotic congenital heart diseases may lead to electrical abnormalities in the form of arrhythmias caused by structural abnormalities of the heart. These disruptions can be caused by defects such as atrial septal defects or ventricular septal defects, defects that alter normal electrical impulse flow required for a coordinated heartbeat. Arrhythmias are predisposed to complications such as heart failure and stroke; therefore, clinicians should have high suspicion for their development in such patients with structural abnormalities. The diagnosis and monitoring of arrhythmias in acyanotic congenital heart disease require a comprehensive strategy, merging clinical acumen with advanced diagnostic equipment. Electrocardiograms (ECGs) remain a central component in the detection of arrhythmias, enabling clinicians to analyze the rhythm, rate, and overall electrical conduction of the heart. Furthermore, continuous monitoring equipment can assist in recording transient arrhythmias, which are not always detectable during a standard ECG. The adoption of clinical guidelines by influential organizations plays an important role in the management of these conditions to the highest feasible practices; these guidelines help medical practitioners modify their approach to patient profiles so that treatment strategies may be in alignment with existing best practices (Baumgartner et al., 2020; Stout et al., 2018). Treatment for arrhythmia in the presence of acyanotic congenital heart disease typically involves a combination of lifestyle modification, medications, and, if need be, surgery. Medication usually includes antiarrhythmic drugs to restore normal rhythm and prevent further worsening. But these drugs must be administered with caution considering potential interactions and the overall health of patients. In cases where pharmacological therapy is unsuccessful, catheter ablation or pacemaker implantation is an option to re-establish normal electrical function. With such complicated cases, shared decision-making between healthcare professionals and patients is crucial, emphasizing the need for customized treatment protocols that correspond with individual patient values and preferences (Stout et al., 2018).

6.6. Prognosis and Quality of Life

The prognosis for acyanotic congenital heart disease (CHD) patients is generally healthier compared to their cyanotic counterparts, largely due to the advances in medical treatment and surgery technology. Early diagnosis, facilitated by increased prenatal screening and improved imaging techniques, allows for the conditions to be kept under control from an early stage, thus significantly enhancing the long-term success rate for the patients. Most acyanotic cardiac anomalies such as ventricular septal defects or aortic coarctation can be effectively treated with medical therapy or surgery with excellent outcomes in survival. The overall survival rate of children with acyanotic CHDs has improved substantially, according to recent studies, and this benefits an expanding population of adults with these lesions. This trend emphasizes the necessity of ongoing research and clinical follow-up regarding long-term outcomes, including comprehensive care models that address both physical well-being and psychosocial adaptation (Baumgartner et al., 2020). Quality of life (QoL) in patients with acyanotic congenital heart defects is influenced by a multifaceted set of factors including age at diagnosis, defect nature, treatment, and comorbidities. Patients also report QoL subjectively, a description of the experiences that not only include the physical limitations imposed on them by the heart defect but also emotional and social challenges. For instance, children may worry about their well-being and its impact on psychosocial growth and relationships. Furthermore, the long-term results of surgical and medical treatments will also impart complications that alter a patient's QoL, which will require holistic measures incorporating psychological assessment along with medical evaluation. Thus, healthcare professionals are compelled to adopt a holistic approach while assessing the quality of life in these patients to address physical as well as emotional health (Zhao et al., 2020) (Figure 6.16).

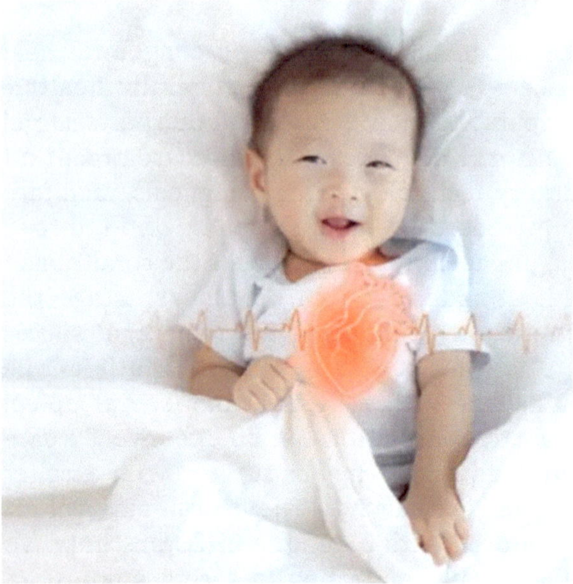

Figure 6.16. Quality of life (QoL) for individuals with acyanotic congenital heart disease.

Source: https://chblob.icloudhospital.com/thumbnails/4-81959c18-0dda-40d5-b952-b3efa1fa72e7.webp.

The prognostic profile and quality of life of patients with acyanotic congenital heart disease also highlight the importance of a multidisciplinary treatment strategy. Coordination of cardiologists, surgeons, pediatricians, and mental health specialists is essential in devising tailored treatment plans not only to treat pending health issues but with foresight to address threatening problems before they ensue. Care transition from pediatric to adult services can be a possible hindrance; thus, patient and family readiness for transfer is of utmost priority. Effective communication and proper support systems can go a long way in enhancing compliance with treatments and self-management skills in patients as they age. Studies indicate that comprehensive care models with regular follow-up and proactive psychological care vastly improve long-term outcomes and quality of life for acyanotic CHD patients, illustrating the evolving nature of congenital heart disease management (Baumgartner et al., 2020).

6.6.1. Life Expectancy for Acyanotic Patients

The mortality of acyanotic patients with CHD is far less than that of their cyanotic patients. This is owing to the advancements in medicine and technology, early detection, and well-planned treatment. Acyanotic lesions such as atrial septal defects and ventricular septal defects normally facilitate normal oxygenation of the blood, subsequently resulting in fewer life-threatening complications at an early age. Evidence indicates that with proper surgical intervention and ongoing medical care, most patients of acyanotic conditions are able to enjoy a normal life until adult age. In addition, the success of the interventions is noted through the high rate of patients diagnosed during the first year of life, and therefore early intervention is crucial in charting their prognosis of long-term health (Akcevin et al., 2023). Additionally, research has shown that intervention type and timing significantly influence the determination of life expectancy in acyanotic patients. Infancy operations are more likely to yield good outcomes than surgeries at a later age. For instance, a study in East Java concluded that noncyanotic types of CHD are prevalent among patients diagnosed at the time they were in their initial years, with successful nonsurgical treatment accounting for the majority of cases (Finariawan et al., 2018). This shows the importance of early diagnosis to facilitate early intervention and monitoring of the health of the patients. Furthermore, the availability of healthcare facilities, such as national health insurance programs in terms of funding, is also an important factor to ensure optimal patient outcomes. Offering these patients complete care can also play an important role in their quality of life, as well as in their overall lifespan. It should, however, be mentioned that while acyanotic patients typically have favorable prognoses, these types of patients also have long-term effects of their illnesses. Research indicates that after surgery, the majority of acyanotic patients can develop complications such as arrhythmias, exercise intolerance, or congestive heart failure as they age. Thus, lifelong follow-up and management are necessary to address these potential consequences to health. Additionally, the psychological and social determinants of living with a congenital heart defect also influence a patient's perception of quality of life. Therefore, while the life expectancy of acyanotic patients may be promising, they require a complete approach to care—comprising medical, psychological, and social support—to enjoy overall well-being throughout their lifespan (Akcevin et al., 2023).

6.6.2. Impact on Daily Activities

Congenital heart diseases (CHD) or the acyanotic ones, have significant impacts on day-to-day life as well as the quality of life of the patients. CHD may cause different physical disabilities because patients tend to experience trouble with endurance and muscle strength. It has been proven by research that those with congenital heart disease who are adults experience a notable decrease in functional capacity, as reflected by compromised performance on such tests as the six-minute walk test. Such impairment could impede participation in activities of daily life, which are normally taken for granted, hence impacting social interaction and overall satisfaction with life. In the young, these impairments may restrict involvement in physical activities that serve a role in socialization and development, thereby extending the effects of CHD into the realm of psychosocial health and functioning. In addition to physical impairment, cognitive functioning is also adversely affected in patients with acyanotic congenital heart disease. Studies indicate frailty, as quantified by markers such as muscle strength and overall functioning, is associated with cognitive function in these patients. Cognitive impairment also may amplify the challenge posed to daily activities of living, since executive function plays a central role in planning and executing tasks, ranging from simple cleaning and cooking to more complex social interaction. For example, they may have a harder time managing their own finances or organizing social gatherings, which subsequently makes them more reliant and can impact their mental health in a negative manner. This multifaceted impact requires an entire picture perception and primary assessment of frailty in adult congenital heart disease patients, as it directly relates to whether they can maintain day-to-day activities independently and with purpose (Topcuoglu et al., 2024). Moreover, strengthening interventions and functional capacity improvements have the promise of augmenting activities of daily living in acyanotic congenital heart disease patients. Tailored exercise programs can correct targeted impairments that occur in this population, such as peripheral muscle strength and endurance deficits, as shown in recent studies. There is evidence to suggest that focused rehabilitation can yield measurable improvements in activities of daily living, and overall gain in independence and quality of life. Addressing the combined physical and cognitive demands of these patients, health professionals can implement approaches that minimize the adverse effects of frailty. Thus, early intervention and a care system with support would significantly diminish the impact of congenital heart diseases on functioning in daily life and enhance overall satisfaction with life (Topcuoglu et al., 2024).

6.6.3. Psychological and Social Considerations

Psychosocial issues play a very crucial role in the management of individuals with congenital heart diseases (CHD), particularly acyanotic conditions. CHD patients are likely to have a unique form of psychological problems resulting from their condition that influence their mood as well as social behavior. The stress involved in repeated hospital admissions, potential surgery, and restrictions on lifestyle can lead to feelings of isolation and distress. Also, the outward appearance of a medical condition, e.g., surgical scars, can attribute body image issues and affect self-esteem in children as they become incorporated into social relationships. With addressing these psychological concerns, health workers are better able to support not just the medical needs but the total well-being of such children, enhancing resilience and self-esteem as they grow. In addition to psychological impacts, the social mechanisms engaged in children with acyanotic CHD are significant. Families can experience considerable stress to deal with the child's ongoing needs, disrupting family relations and social connections. Parents may become socially constrained by care demands or worry about their child's well-being and thus suffer from social isolation and diminished support. Siblings may also have any variety of emotional responses to the circumstances of their brother or sister, ranging from jealousy or bitterness to a strong protective response. This home environment not only affects the individual child's well-being but also the family environment in general. Family counseling and community support interventions can fortify the social infrastructure needed to provide care for not just the child with CHD but the family, allowing for healthier social interactions and coping. Up-to-date studies emphasize the necessity of organized interventions to improve physical and psychological health outcomes for children with CHD. For instance, a comprehensive program to enhance physical activity level was shown to maximize peak exercise capacity significantly and yield a positive impact on children with congenital heart disease who had active living attitudes (Callaghan et al., 2021). These interventions are useful in desensitizing the experience of chronic illness by equipping children with proper mechanisms for coping constructively with peers and their own self-image. Moreover, public health organizations' recommendations suggest that doctors should integrate psychological and social issues into the overall treatment regimen of children with CHD (Baumgartner et al., 2020). Tackling such problems enables doctors to support the whole person by enhancing emotional resilience as well as the quality of life in children with the consequences of congenital heart conditions.

SUMMARY

The prevalence of acyanotic congenital heart diseases (CHD) justifies continued study and medical treatment particularly for this population. Acyanotic lesions, such as Atrial Septal Defect and Ventricular Septal Defect, have been characterized as the most common presentations of children with CHD, according to recent studies. For instance, in a study, it was identified that 74.26% of children had acyanotic CHD and, therefore, early diagnosis and treatment of the conditions are needed to ensure optimal patient outcomes (Pasha et al., 2023). With a focus on early detection of such defects, clinicians can avoid complications and make the patient healthier in the long term. This proactive strategy is essential not only for enhancing acute care but also for educating the family in regard to management techniques. Moreover, the relationship between oral health and systemic status in children with acyanotic CHD highlights the importance of overall care. Statistics obtained from a pediatric population indicate that 50% of the patients had dental problems, mainly caries disease, which is common in this population (Pasha et al., 2023). These findings indicate that acyanotic heart defects have consequences that extend beyond the cardiovascular system, entering into general health and quality of life. By combining cardiology with dental care, practitioners can adopt a more comprehensive approach, addressing the interconnected causes of health that figure heavily in these children. Encouraging behaviors such as regular dental check-ups and oral hygiene can lead to improved health results and thus a superior multidisciplinary healthcare strategy for this high-risk population. The implication of these findings calls for a multi-directional approach in treating congenital heart diseases. It is important that further academic studies are conducted to improve knowledge about acyanotic CHD and resulting health complications. As evidenced in the existing literature, including the caries prevalence in these patients, there remains space for intervention that is innovative and can close interventional gaps between dental and cardiac care (Patrícia et al., 2024). Future studies are recommended to explore the long-term effect of the combined healthcare strategies on the quality of life and overall health status among children with acyanotic CHD. Through prioritizing this topic of research, the medical community can then progress to develop more cohesive routes of care that foster not only survival but also improved health and well-being for children who are managing these complexities.

To know congenital heart diseases (CHD) with emphasis on acyanotic types is to learn about the variety of structural heart defects not typically presenting with cyanosis. Acyanotic defects such as atrial septal defect, ventricular septal defect, and patent ductus arteriosus are characterized by left-to-right shunt of the blood. This has the effect of lowering the volume load of the heart and lung and can lead to congestive heart failure if not addressed. Unlike cyanotic defects, acyanotic lesions allow for normally acceptable oxygenation of the blood. Pulmonary hypertension or other complications as a long-term implication signify the significance of early detection and care. Awareness of these potential consequences is required for clinicians as well as families of children with CHD, so that appropriate follow-up and anticipatory management strategies are started right from infancy to childhood. Acute challenges of acyanotic congenital heart diseases go beyond physiological and also affect the overall ecosystem of general healthcare. It is, for instance, the acute economic burden of long-term management and care of CHD patients that places a strain on healthcare systems as well as families. Unpaid care also comes from relatives and plays a central role in coping with such challenges. Such caregivers also experience undue physical and mental burden as a consequence of caregiving responsibilities, which can lead to negative effects on their overall health and economics. The mutual relationship between the health outcomes for the patient and caregiver highlights the significant need for health care systems to implement caregiving support strategies. Such support can include educational resources, mental health services, and economic assistance programs that acknowledge the sacrifices made by informal caregivers, thus promoting a more sustainable model of CHD care (Kisangala et al., 2024). New innovative methods in the diagnosis and treatment of acyanotic congenital heart diseases, particularly with brain imaging techniques, have shed new light on the complexity of such conditions. It has been proposed by studies that acyanotic defects may affect the neurodevelopmental pathway in affected babies. The use of brain magnetic resonance imaging (MRI) and other methods for assessment of brain maturation can provide clinicians with a more accurate indication of potential developmental delay and the related co-morbidities. The development of scoring systems, including the paralimbic-related subcortical brain dysplasia score, enables clinicians to better predict outcomes for CHD patients. Identification of subcortical abnormalities can guide focused interventions to support neurodevelopmental health in these patients, emphasizing the importance of attending to both cardiac and neurological aspects of care in depth (Reynolds et al., 2024). As technology improves, it holds the potential to optimize early treatment and improve quality of life for children with acyanotic congenital heart disease.

CLOSER LOOK

MONITORING AND FOLLOW-UP IN PEDIATRIC AND ADULT CHD CLINICS

Congenital heart disease (CHD) is a spectrum of structural cardiac defects at birth from simple lesions such as atrial septal defects to complex states such as single ventricle physiology. Advances in medicine and surgery have significantly increased survival, and thus more and more children are reaching adulthood with CHD. Long-term health effects thus necessitate systematic follow-up and surveillance in adult and pediatric CHD centers.

Follow-up is begun early in pediatric CHD clinics after diagnosis—either prenatally, at birth, or infancy—and then at regular intervals based on defect complexity and interventions performed. Primary objectives are to assess cardiac function, follow growth and development, detect complications early, and maximize quality of life. Echocardiography forms the basis of surveillance with non-invasive assessment of heart structure and function. ECGs, Holter monitoring, MRI, CT scanning, and exercise testing can be utilized for more detailed testing or in the event of symptoms.

Pediatric cardiologists also treat associated comorbidities such as arrhythmias, pulmonary hypertension, complications of cyanosis, and delays in neurodevelopment. Nutritional counseling, exercise guidance, and psychosocial evaluation are often integrated into treatment. Interestingly, parent and caregiver education involves being able to recognize clinical deterioration and the implication of the condition, therapies, and drugs.

As CHD children develop, transition planning is of the highest importance. They experience transition from pediatric to adult-oriented care. Transition is an explicit, multidisciplinary process that includes educating the patient, teaching self-care, and choosing an appropriate adult CHD (ACHD) provider. If effective transition is not executed, patients have a risk of being lost to follow-up, leading to late complication detection and outcome. Adult CHD clinics are endowed medical facilities with cardiologists trained in both adult and congenital heart disease. Adults with CHD must be followed their entire lives, even if they were "fixed" in childhood, since most lesions are not curable but rather treated. Follow-up visits are intended to uncover advancing valvular insufficiency, ventricular impairment, arrhythmias, and complications of previous surgeries or interventions. Sophisticated imaging, electrophysiology, and cardiac catheterizations may be needed.

Adult CHD patients, particularly women, require reproductive health counseling since pregnancy is extremely hazardous based on the type and severity of the defect. Preconception counseling, risk stratification, and shared care with maternal-fetal medicine specialists are provided by ACHD clinics. Endocarditis prophylaxis, exercise safety, mental illness, and career guidance are also key concerns.

Multidisciplinary team care is the calling card of best CHD care during lifetime. Such teams can include cardiologists, cardiac surgeons, nurses, psychologists, social workers, and genetic counselors. Registries and electronic health records support continuity of care and follow-up on long-term outcomes.

References

1. Akcevin, A., Ates, M. S., Er, Z. C., Sal, E., et al. (2023). Measurement of primary hemostasis potential with platelet function analyzer to investigate the predictive effect on post-operative blood loss in cyanotic and acyanotic pediatric patients. https://core.ac.uk/download/578386981.pdf (accessed on 15th July 2025).
2. Andrews, T., Berlinger, A., Bull, K., Chan, L., Corno, A., Diab, K., Dickinson, J., et al. (2012). Bronchial compression in an infant with isolated secundum atrial septal defect associated with severe pulmonary arterial hypertension. https://core.ac.uk/download/pdf/27063040.pdf (accessed on 15th July 2025).
3. Ashfaq, A., Faateh, M., & Shahanavaz, S. (2024). Percutaneous and surgical pulmonary valve replacement options in adult congenital heart disease: A review. *Current Treatment Options in Pediatrics.* https://www.semanticscholar.org/paper/9a2c5513ecc164ebd6a019f5f952662cc6ee1242 (accessed on 15th July 2025).
4. Azizova, A., Önder, Ö., Arslan, S., Ardalı, S., & Hazırolan, T. (2020). Persistent left superior vena cava: Clinical importance and differential diagnoses. *Insights into Imaging, 11.* https://doi.org/10.1186/s13244-020-00906-2 (accessed on 15th July 2025).
5. Barr, R., Green, C., Sande, C., & Drysdale, S. B. (2019). Respiratory syncytial virus: Diagnosis, prevention and management. *Therapeutic Advances in Infectious Disease, 6.* https://doi.org/10.1177/2049936119865798 (accessed on 15th July 2025).
6. Baumgartner, H., De Backer, J., Babu-Narayan, S. V., Budts, W., Chessa, M., Diller, G. P., Lung, B., et al. (2020). 2020 ESC Guidelines for the management of adult congenital heart disease. *European Heart Journal, 42*, 563–645. https://doi.org/10.1093/eurheartj/ehaa554 (accessed on 15th July 2025).
7. Buchmann, A., Hagmann, C., Huber, R., Klaver, P., et al. (2017). Brain volumes predict neurodevelopment in adolescents after surgery for congenital heart disease. https://core.ac.uk/download/85224721.pdf (accessed on 15th July 2025).
8. Callaghan, S., Morrison, M. L., McKeown, P., Tennyson, C., Sands, A. J., McCrossan, B., Grant, B., et al. (2021). Exercise prescription improves exercise tolerance in young children with CHD: A randomized clinical trial. *Open Heart, 8*, e001599. https://doi.org/10.1136/openhrt-2021-001599 (accessed on 15th July 2025).
9. Cangas-Isacaz, A., Espín-Sambache, B., Mena-Noroña, D. A., Valdivieso-Andrade, E. J., Ortiz-Prado, E., Arias-Rodríguez, F. D., Izquierdo-Condoy, J. S., et al. (2025). Epidemiological characterization of congenital heart disease at different altitudes in Ecuador: A four-year retrospective study in a pediatric referral hospital. https://core.ac.uk/download/651327830.pdf (accessed on 15th July 2025).
10. Chau, A. K. T., Cheuk, D. K. L., Cheung, Y. F., Choi, Y., et al. (2004). Parents' understanding of their child's congenital heart disease. https://core.ac.uk/download/37881538.pdf (accessed on 15th July 2025).
11. Cool, C. J., Putra, I. C. S., Kamarullah, W., Sukmadi, N., Pramudyo, M., Dewi, T. I., & Raharjo, P. (2025). A 29-year-old man with uncorrected congenital patent ductus arteriosus presenting with heart failure and pulmonary artery vegetations removed during surgery: A case report. *The American Journal of Case Reports, 26.* https://www.semanticscholar.org/paper/

cec79b810e3a3136b2f1cd3b92aa32fec7655db7 (accessed on 15th July 2025).

12. Crișan, S., Băghină, R. M., Luca, S. A., Pătru, O., Lazăr, M., Văcărescu, C., Rus, M., et al. (2024). From ECG to imaging: Challenges in the diagnosis of adult congenital heart diseases. *Journal of Clinical Medicine, 13.* https://www.semanticscholar.org/paper/bf13fe1ce4fd24d8fb16f91604368853a69d85b4 (accessed on 15th July 2025).

13. Cullen, S., Deanfield, J., Fteropoulli, T., Newman, C., et al. (2013). Quality of life of adult congenital heart disease patients: A systematic review of the literature. https://core.ac.uk/download/9982967.pdf (accessed on 15th July 2025).

14. Das, D., Dutta, N., Das, S., Sharma, M., Chattopadhyay, A., Ghosh, S., & Nandy Das, J. (2024). Public–private partnership for treatment of congenital heart diseases: Experiences from an Indian state. *World Journal for Pediatric and Congenital Heart Surgery, 15*, 439–445. https://www.semanticscholar.org/paper/f4e37295d75b09684006c19cccc8cde55570cb34 (accessed on 15th July 2025).

15. Farooqui, R., Haroon, U. F., Niazi, A., Rehan, N., Butt, T. K., & Niazi, M. (2010). Congenital heart diseases in neonates. https://core.ac.uk/download/544153620.pdf (accessed on 15th July 2025).

16. Finariawan, F., Mahmud, S. A., & Syifa. (2018). The characteristics and distribution of congenital heart disease in outpatient clinic and inpatient ward of RSUD Dr. Soedono Madiun East Java in year 2015. https://core.ac.uk/download/295457925.pdf (accessed on 15th July 2025).

17. Giordano, M., Scognamiglio, G., Gaio, G., Marzullo, R., Palma, M., Barracano, R., Fusco, F., et al. (2025). The role of trans-esophageal echocardiography in the interventional cardiology of adult congenital heart diseases. *Journal of Clinical Medicine, 14.* https://www.semanticscholar.org/paper/6e9d06972a262e8b952265156faacd785ca0929a (accessed on 15th July 2025).

18. Golalipour, M. J., Mirfazeli, A., Nikyarspi-Sup, B., Qourbani, H., et al. (2011). Prevalence and pattern of congenital heart disease among neonates in Gorgan, Northern Iran (2007–2008). https://core.ac.uk/download/52204847.pdf (accessed on 15th July 2025).

19. Hayes, D., Wilson, K. C., Krivchenia, K., Hawkins, S. M. M., Balfour-Lynn, I. M., Gozal, D., Panitch, H. B., et al. (2019). Home oxygen therapy for children: An official American Thoracic Society clinical practice guideline. *American Journal of Respiratory and Critical Care Medicine, 199*, e5–e23. https://doi.org/10.1164/rccm.201812-2276st (accessed on 15th July 2025).

20. Kisangala, E., Mbivnjo, E. L., Webb, E. J. D., Barrett, B., Rukundo, G. Z., Namisango, E., & Heslin, M. (2024). Health and economic impact of caregiving on informal caregivers of people with chronic diseases in sub-Saharan Africa: A systematic review. *PLOS Global Public Health, 4*, e0004061. https://doi.org/10.1371/journal.pgph.0004061 (accessed on 15th July 2025).

21. Kumari, A., & Shukla, S. D. (2025). Risk factor profiling in congenital heart disease: Maternal and foetal determinants. https://core.ac.uk/download/655504575.pdf (accessed on 15th July 2025).

22. Lababidi, G., Lababidi, H., Bitar, F., & Arabi, M. (2024). COVID-19 vaccines in the pediatric population: A focus on cardiac patients. *Canadian Journal of Infectious Diseases and Medical Microbiology, 2024*, 1–12. https://doi.org/10.1155/2024/2667033 (accessed on 15th July 2025).

23. Lester, R. G. (1965). Radiologic diagnosis of congenital heart disease in children. https://core.ac.uk/download/51294242.pdf (accessed on 15th July 2025).

24. Luo, G. P., Zhao, J., Zhu, Y., Zhu, Y., Chen, B., Ma, R., Tang, F., et al. (2019). Sirt1 promotes autophagy and inhibits apoptosis to protect cardiomyocytes from hypoxic stress. *International Journal of Molecular Medicine.* https://doi.org/10.3892/ijmm.2019.4125 (accessed on 15th July 2025).

25. Mir, A. B., Jan, M., Ali, I., Ahmed, K., & Radhakrishnan, S. (2019). Congenital heart disease in neonates: Their clinical profile, diagnosis, and their immediate outcome. *Heart India, 7,* 80–80. https://doi.org/10.4103/heartindia.heartindia_3_19 (accessed on 15th July 2025).

26. Nunes, P. L. S., Lisboa, V. M., Costa, R. C. N., Ferreira, M. C., Ribeiro, M. F. R., Guedelha, L. P. S., & Costa, C. P. S. (2024). Clinical, epidemiological and dental characterization of children with congenital heart diseases. *Concilium.* https://www.semanticscholar.org/paper/ab34b69b54a4e708735e4ac29f8dfccaf1c8c208 (accessed on 15th July 2025).

27. Pasha, W., Ramchand, R., Khokhar, R., Sathio, S., Kanwal, M., & Aurangzeb, A. (2023). Congenital heart diseases pattern among children presenting to tertiary care hospital. *International Journal of Health Sciences.* https://www.semanticscholar.org/paper/1083d18a90ed4326287a2f1020f98c20e5921b80 (accessed on 15th July 2025).

28. Prakoso, R. (2024). The current strategy in managing congenital and structural heart disease: Find and treat them appropriately. https://core.ac.uk/download/618247692.pdf (accessed on 15th July 2025).

29. Reynolds, W., Votava-Smith, J. K., Gabriel, G. C., Lee, V., Rajagopalan, V., Wu, Y., Liu, X., et al. (2024). Development and validation of a paralimbic related subcortical brain dysmaturation MRI score in infants with congenital heart disease. *medRxiv (Cold Spring Harbor Laboratory).* https://doi.org/10.1101/2024.04.21.24306144 (accessed on 15th July 2025).

30. Sihotang, F. A., & Putri, V. (2024). Dealing with a nightmare: A case report of successful percutaneous treatment of an embolized occluder device complicating a minimal-fluoroscopy patent ductus arteriosus closure. *Cureus, 16.* https://www.semanticscholar.org/paper/2cf130ee501abc0756404ab44e2c15c942886616 (accessed on 15th July 2025).

31. Smith, R. (2017). Neurodevelopment, quality of life and burden of care of young children who have undergone cardiac interventions in central South Africa: Three-month and six-month post cardiac intervention outcomes. https://core.ac.uk/download/188772618.pdf (accessed on 15th July 2025).

32. Somasetia, D. H., Marwali, E. M., Portman, M. A., Haas, N. A., Darmaputri, S., & Sastroasmoro, S. (2015). Does malnutrition influence outcome in children undergoing congenital heart surgery in a developing country? https://core.ac.uk/download/192686893.pdf (accessed on 15th July 2025).

33. Stout, K., Daniels, C. J., Aboulhosn, J., Bozkurt, B., Broberg, C. S., Colman, J. M., Crumb, S. R., et al. (2018). 2018 AHA/ACC guideline for the management of adults with congenital heart disease: A report of the American College of Cardiology/American Heart Association Task Force on Clinical Practice Guidelines. *Circulation, 139.* https://doi.org/10.1161/cir.0000000000000603 (accessed on 15th July 2025).

34. Topcuoglu, C., Vardar Yagli, N., Aykan, H., Ertugrul, I., Karagoz, T., & Sağlam, M. (2024). Exploring frailty: Muscle strength, functional capacity, activities of daily living and cognition

in adult congenital heart disease. *Disability and Rehabilitation, 47*, 3137–3143. https://www.semanticscholar.org/paper/818b9b9267128f74b9666875f194799a6585c1aa (accessed on 15th July 2025).

35. Topcuoglu, C., Vardar Yagli, N., Ertugrul, I., Aykan, H., Karagoz, T., & Saglam, M. (2024). Comparison of peripheral muscle strength, functional capacity and activities of daily living in frail and non-frail adult individuals with congenital heart disease. *European Journal of Preventive Cardiology.* https://www.semanticscholar.org/paper/587e226a8e71cbbaa388b3ab1b3a3f2a20fbc491 (accessed on 15th July 2025).

36. Umer, H. M., Arshad, M. U., Mudassar, F., Slam, A. U., Junaid, S., Asghar, R. M., & Aslam, F. (2018). Pattern of congenital heart diseases in paediatric age group. https://core.ac.uk/download/553166207.pdf (accessed on 15th July 2025).

37. Vimal, S., Ranjan, R., Yadav, S., Majumdar, G., Mittal, B., Sinha, N., & Agarwal, S. K. (2021). Differences in the serum metabolic profile to identify potential biomarkers for cyanotic versus acyanotic heart disease. *Perfusion, 38*, 124–134. https://doi.org/10.1177/02676591211042559 (accessed on 15th July 2025).

38. Winter, L., Strizek, B., & Recker, F. (2024). Congenital Gerbode defect: A left ventricular to right atrial shunt—State-of-the-art review of its general data, diagnostic modalities, and treatment strategies. *Journal of Cardiovascular Development and Disease, 11*, 166. https://doi.org/10.3390/jcdd11060166 (accessed on 15th July 2025).

39. Yahya, S. (2022). Prevalence and factors associated with undernutrition among children with congenital heart disease at three tertiary hospitals in Nairobi, Kenya. https://core.ac.uk/download/597995955.pdf (accessed on 15th July 2025).

40. Zhao, L., Chen, L., Yang, T., Wang, T., Zhang, S., Chen, L., Ye, Z. W., et al. (2020). Birth prevalence of congenital heart disease in China, 1980–2019: A systematic review and meta-analysis of 617 studies. *European Journal of Epidemiology, 35*, 631–642. https://doi.org/10.1007/s10654-020-00653-0 (accessed on 15th July 2025).

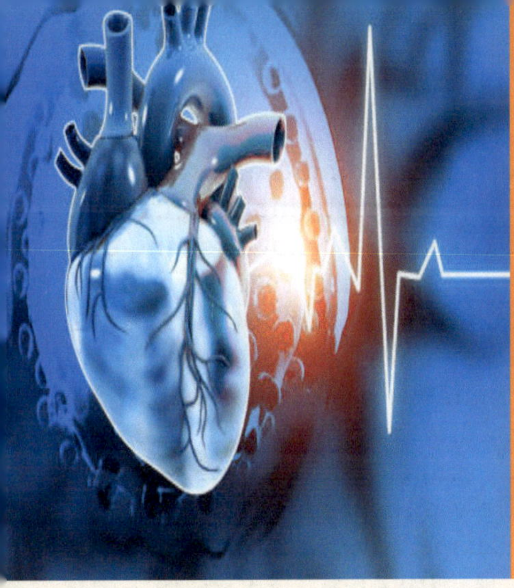

Chapter 7

CONGENITAL HEART DISEASES – CYANOTIC

Contents

Introduction

Congenital heart disease is a general class of diseases that manifest from congenital heart defects during birth, cyanotic congenital heart disease being particularly significant due to its complexity as well as the gravity of potential health impacts. The diseases, presented with right-to-left shunt, lead to a systemically deoxygenated system of circulation, the implications of which are cyanosis, fatigue, and dyspnea. The various presentations of cyanotic heart defects necessitate a complete understanding of both their clinical manifestations and pathophysiological bases. This complexity only serves to demonstrate the importance of prompt diagnosis and treatment, as early management can significantly influence life expectancy and quality of life in those affected. A good illustration in this context is Fallots pentalogy; a cyanotic congenital heart anomaly that is uncommon and characterized by the presence of five distinct anomalies of the cardiac structure, one of which is an atrial septal defect. Diagnosis is typically established after thorough clinical evaluation supported by various imaging techniques, such as echocardiograms and chest X-rays, which reveal the structural anomalies of the defect (Rom et al., 2025). A crucial aspect of the management of congenital heart diseases lies in accurate severity assessment, as prognosis widely differs depending on the specific nature of the defect and whether accompanying anomalies are present. In addition, clinical management should include a multidisciplinary team of cardiologists, surgeons, and geneticists to achieve the best outcome on treatment of the afflicted patients, asserting categorically that holistic management is necessary in the management of such complex conditions. Furthermore, interactions between congenital heart disease and other systemic illness, such as thyroid hormone resistance, can complicate clinical management. As in one case report with a patient having both a complex cyanotic heart defect and thyroid hormone resistance, preoperative preparation needed to be carefully managed in an attempt to balance the physiological differences present in both conditions (Fedorczak et al., 2025). Such occurrences are designed to highlight the intricate interplay of various organ systems and the need for personalized therapeutic interventions. The observation of such associations is not just designed to highlight the need for interdisciplinary practice in healthcare facilities but also necessitates ongoing research and education among healthcare practitioners for greater understanding and effectiveness of treatment of congenital heart diseases, with a specific focus on their cyanotic forms.

Definition of Congenital Heart Diseases

Congenital heart disease (CHD) represents a spectrum of structural cardiac abnormalities that result during fetal life. The defect may involve the walls of the heart, valves, arteries, and veins and lead to abnormal circulation through the heart and to the remainder of the body. This defect may lead to a wide variety of clinical presentations, which may vary from minimal to extensive, life-threatening conditions demanding urgent medical care. The pathogenesis of CHDs is multifactorial, most likely due to genetic susceptibility and in utero exposure. More current data, however, indicate the incidence of CHDs has remained fairly constant at around 1 case per 100 live births, and this implies the importance of exposure and appropriate prenatal assessment in the care of these illnesses. Early treatment and diagnosis are significantly enhanced, and an intimate awareness of these diseases by both providers and caregivers is imperative. Cyanotic congenital heart diseases (CCHDs) are a series of CHDs with low oxygen levels in the blood, leading to cyanosis—a bluish discoloration of the skin and mucous membranes. Tetralogy of Fallot, Transposition of the Great Arteries, and Tricuspid Atresia are a few conditions under this category, each with varied physiological derangements and requiring proper treatment strategies. Pathophysiology of CCHDs typically involves shunt channels that redirect deoxygenated blood into systemic circulation, thus compromising oxygenation of peripheral tissues. This can lead to precipitating acute and severe clinical issues like arrested growth, intolerance to exercise, and susceptibility to life-threatening arrhythmias. Thus, early and accurate diagnosis is crucial, and careful monitoring and surgery in the majority of cases to correct anatomical defects. Treatment of congenital heart diseases, particularly cyanotic forms, demands a multidisciplinary team consisting of cardiology, cardiothoracic surgery, and pediatrics. Therapy of such abnormality tends to be successful if a specially formulated approach and the typical features and needs of each patient are taken into account. Recent technological developments in interventional cardiology and surgery have revolutionized the prognosis of the majority of children with CCHDs to lead relatively healthier lives. Nevertheless, the complicating nature of the diseases necessitates ongoing follow-up in adulthood since patients will always have residual problems or complications depending on the initial diagnosis. In addition, there are procedure guidelines that have been implemented to direct healthcare providers in assessment, management, and treatment of such patients with a view to enhancing general outcomes (Baumgartner et al., 2020). Aside from this, communication between obstetricians and cardiologists has increasingly been necessary when it comes to the development of care plans, especially considering the impact of maternal conditions in pregnancy (Laxmi et al., 2020).

Overview of Cyanotic Heart Diseases

Cyanotic heart conditions are characterized by the presence of a right-to-left shunt or other malformations resulting in under-oxygenation of blood, presenting as cyanosis or blue color of the skin. Cyanotic heart conditions are typically seen in infancy and can lead to severe morbidity in a child's life if left undetected and treated early. Of the various cyanotic heart diseases, Tetralogy of Fallot (TOF) remains the most common and is found in approximately three out of every 10,000 live births (Ahamd et al., 2025). Hypoplastic left heart syndrome and complete atrioventricular septal defects with imbalance are uncommon but serious defects that can lead to severe complications if they are not dealt with early. Early diagnosis and intervention of these conditions are critical in maximizing outcomes and reducing mortality rates attributed to congenital heart disease in neonates. The value of fetal echocardiography is crucial to contribute towards the diagnosis of cyanotic heart disease during gestation and, consequently, impact the treatment protocol of affected neonates. This technology allows for the detection of major cardiac defects, allowing timely interventions that have a major impact on prognostics. One study looking back at results from fetal echocardiography proved that a high proportion of fetuses had already been diagnosed with severe cardiac malformations, and the usefulness of this diagnostic tool (Duman et al., 2024) (Figure 7.1).

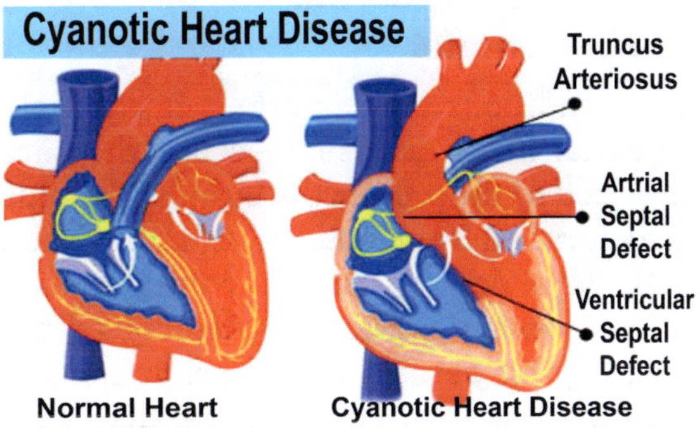

Figure 7.1. Cyanotic heart disease.

Source: https://images.medindia.net/patientinfo/950_400/cyanotic-heart-disease.jpg.

Specifically, prenatal diagnosis of ailments such as hypoplastic left heart syndrome and critical aortic stenosis can prepare parents and medical teams for postnatal treatment and surgery in anticipation. Such proactive measures indicate the benefit of early diagnosis for the proper management of congenital heart disease. The application of sophisticated imaging modalities, such as echocardiography and multidetector computed tomography angiography (MDCTA), has optimized the diagnostic performance in the detection of cyanotic heart diseases. While echocardiography is the primary modality for intracardiac anomaly evaluation, MDCTA is applicable in visualizing extracardiac appearances and complications. In one comparison study involving correlations among these imaging modalities, there were high agreements in measurements, particularly for cardiac morphology (Ahamd et al., 2025). This emphasizes the use of a combination of modalities for complete evaluations, leading to effective treatment strategies. Continual development and enhancement of such diagnostic methods are required to enhance patient management in congenital heart diseases such that clinicians can offer timely and appropriate interventions to patients suffering from such complicated ailments.

Importance of Understanding Cyanotic Conditions

Cyanotic conditions are important in the field of congenital heart diseases because they are characterized by the presence of cyanosis, or blue skin discoloration from inadequate oxygenation of blood. Physiologic reasons for cyanosis are a result of several structural defects of the heart and great vessels that disrupt normal flow and oxygenation. For instance, disorders such as Tetralogy of Fallot and transposition of the great arteries are complex cases requiring prompt diagnosis and intervention. Only with a thorough understanding of these complexities can medical professionals come up with effective treatment plans and improve patient outcomes. Additionally, recognition of cyanotic heart disease signs and symptoms opens the door to early intervention, which is important in preventing long-term sequelae such as growth retardation and developmental delay, pointing therefore to the importance of education and awareness of these potentially life-threatening conditions. Beyond direct clinical utility, knowledge of cyanotic conditions has implications for public health. Appropriate diagnosis and management of these congenital heart defects can reduce hospital re-admission rates and the cost of healthcare as a result of complications of un-treated cyanosis. Early detection and intervention can also improve the quality of life of the victims, enabling them to engage more deeply in day-to-day activities. Furthermore, practitioners must remain adept at detecting presentation differences among populations since environmental and genetic influences can significantly affect incidence and severity of cyanotic heart diseases. From the integration of such knowledge of differing factors, practitioners can further tailor methods of prevention and screening, eventually precipitating an active strategy to cardiac management in the case of congenital heart disease. In addition to clinical and public health perspectives, awareness of cyanotic conditions fosters research and innovation improvement. Increased understanding of the pathophysiology of this congenital heart diseases may lead to further research on selective therapies and surgical interventions to improve patient outcomes in the long term. Recent findings indicate the potential contribution of cellular senescence to cardiac health and disease; thus, investigation of these associations may deliver novel therapeutic strategies for the treatment of cyanotic diseases. An understanding of the genetic, environmental, and physiological determinants of cyanosis is crucial in designing protocols of broad-spectrum treatments that address not only the current health needs but also the emerging health trends of patients. As the ESC Guidelines also state, healthcare professionals have the responsibility to apply the latest scientific evidence along with patient-centered care in mind, particularly in the case of complex, multifactorial conditions like cyanotic heart disease (Baumgartner et al., 2020). Ultimately, it can lead to improved clinical outcomes, more preventative efforts, and continued evolution of treatment practice (Calcinotto et al., 2019).

7.1. Types of Cyanotic Heart Diseases

Cyanotic heart diseases are a type of congenital cardiovascular malformations that have a significant impact on systemic blood oxygenation, leading to exaggerated cyanosis, a bluish color produced by deoxygenated hemoglobin. Among all other cyanotic heart diseases, one of the most prevalent types is Tetralogy of Fallot (TOF). TOF comprises four anatomic abnormalities: ventricular septal defect, pulmonary stenosis, right ventricular hypertrophy, and overriding aorta. These malformations lead to abnormal blood circulation such that deoxygenated blood is exposed to oxygenated blood. As a result, patients with TOF are likely to be cyanotic at birth, an effect which, if not treated, may lead to severe complications. Other cyanotic defects of high severity are transposition of the great arteries and total anomalous pulmonary venous return, both of which also need to be treated immediately for improving the oxygen saturation and well-being of the child. Besides the anatomical abnormalities caused by such heart defects, the clinical course of cyanotic heart diseases usually involves complex surgical management. Surgery generally aims to repair or palliate the abnormal anatomy in a manner that re-establishes normal hemodynamics and optimizes oxygenation. Currently, patients with congenital heart disease, including those leading to cyanosis, attain variable amounts of surgery on the basis of individual anatomical variations and pre-operative conditions. Retrospective analysis of the surgical procedures for congenital heart disease recommended that diagnosis and early intervention are essential to improving patient survival and outcome, particularly in the presence of arteriovenous malformations (Abulimiti et al., 2025) (Figure 7.2).

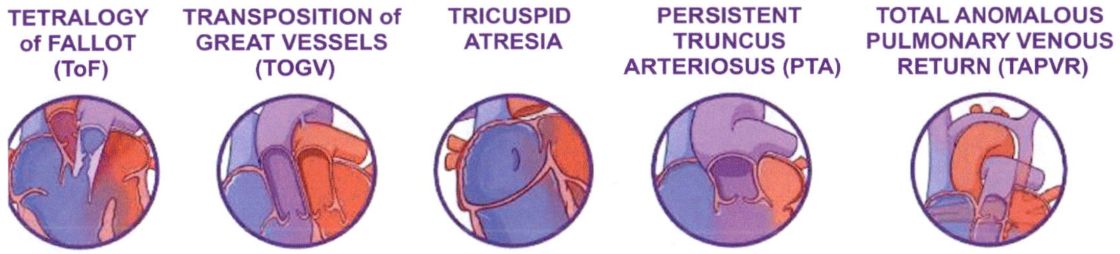

Figure 7.2. Types of cyanotic congenital heart disease.

Source: https://external-content.duckduckgo.com/iu/?u=https%3A%2F%2Fosmose-it.s3.amazonaws.com%2FSHcF4dygSH2mNU6IByyyR6lRQ1iJnjKd%2F_.jpg&f=1&nofb=1&ipt=fa97d961e3cd44299bce10e46990087276f72830b4f8ec2e426ad020af1ac410.

Such management can reduce substantially the risk of infective endocarditis, a serious complication that may develop alongside such congenital malformations. The severity and nature of cyanotic heart disease have a profound impact on both immediate management strategies as well as long-term treatment and outcome for the patient involved. For instance, studies have demonstrated that patients with more severe congenital heart disease (e.g., ones requiring severe surgical repair) may experience a greater frequency of postoperative complications and a longer recovery period (Patel et al., 2024). Care and monitoring of the patients extend beyond the operating room to prolonged follow-up, which would include routine echocardiography to assess cardiac function, in addition to pulmonary complication screening and other risk factors. Because of the heterogeneity of the population, multidisciplinary care is important in order to individualize best strategies for therapy and to deliver overall care to these patients with cyanotic heart diseases throughout their lifespan.

7.1.1. Tetralogy of Fallot (TOF)

Tetralogy of Fallot (TOF) is a type of combination cyanotic congenital heart disease, consisting of four various structural malformations of the heart. They are a ventricular septal defect (VSD), pulmonary outflow tract obstruction, right ventricular hypertrophy, and an overriding aorta straddling across both ventricles. The presence of these abnormalities can severely compromise the oxygenation of the blood perfusing the body, leading to cyanosis—a measurable bluish discoloration of the skin. This condition is best identified early in life, and symptomatic presentations range from feeding difficulty and lethargy to significant cyanosis with exertion. Because of this, timely diagnosis and intervention are mandatory to optimize the quality of life for involved patients, who typically require surgical correction to normalize hemodynamics and increase oxygen delivery to peripheral tissues. Surgical management of TOF has evolved significantly since its initial description in the latter part of the 19th century. Early surgery has significantly enhanced survival and quality of life in patients, who otherwise had high mortality associated with uncorrected defects. Despite improvements in operative strategies and postoperative care, patients with TOF—both those who undergo reparative surgery and those who do not—continue to have a wide range of complications later in life. These have implications such as right ventricular failure, arrhythmias, and need for additional procedures including pulmonary valve replacement or closure of residual defects. Understanding how chronic pulmonary regurgitation results in these is significant because it usually causes progressive right ventricular dilation and dysfunction over time and will ultimately necessitate further intervention (Khan, 2025) (Figure 7.3).

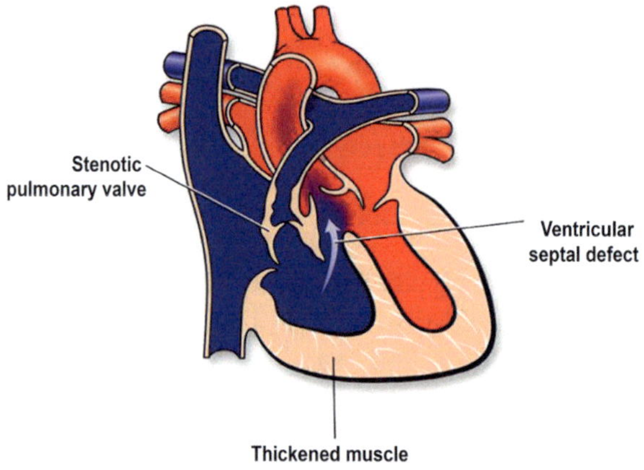

Figure 7.3. Tetralogy of Fallot.

Source: https://external-content.duckduckgo.com/iu/?u=https%3A%2F%2Fwww.heart.org%2F-%2Fmedia%2Fimages%2Fhealth-topics%2Fcongenital-heart-defects%2F50_1683_51_tof.jpg&f=1&nofb=1&ipt=c32360d92066858bc59e696e822e5f49b477739681f0e18ed98a0233c23d9f1b.

In addition, the importance of multidisciplinary management of dental and medical care for TOF patients cannot be overstated. TOF patients often have issues beyond cardiac defects that are common in congenital heart diseases, like issues that affect the teeth based on poor oral hygiene. As evident from current studies, it is essential to provide attention to these oral conditions prior to cardiac surgery to treat potential focal infections that may lead to complications such as infective endocarditis. An integrated approach involving inclusive treatment under pediatric cardiologists, dentists, and other specialists can effectively enhance the overall health status for these patients. Effective interventions underscore the need for early and multi-faceted medical management by stressing that a diverse method can not only contribute substantially towards both oral as well as cardiac health status, but also enhance the overall quality of the patient's life (Khan, 2025).

7.1.2. Transposition of the Great Arteries

Transposition of the great arteries (TGA) is one of the most critical forms of cyanotic congenital cardiac disease, characterized by a spatial malrelationship between the aorta and pulmonary artery. In the normal heart, the aorta originates from the left ventricle and supplies oxygenated blood to the systemic circuit, while the pulmonary artery originates from the right ventricle and conveys deoxygenated blood to the lungs to be oxygenated. In TGA, the major arteries reverse positions, resulting in a situation where the systemic and pulmonary circulations remain completely isolated. Therefore, although the body's tissues are supplied with deoxygenated blood, the lungs cannot receive sufficient blood flow, with the result that severe cyanosis occurs, which is clinically evident and necessitates immediate medical attention.

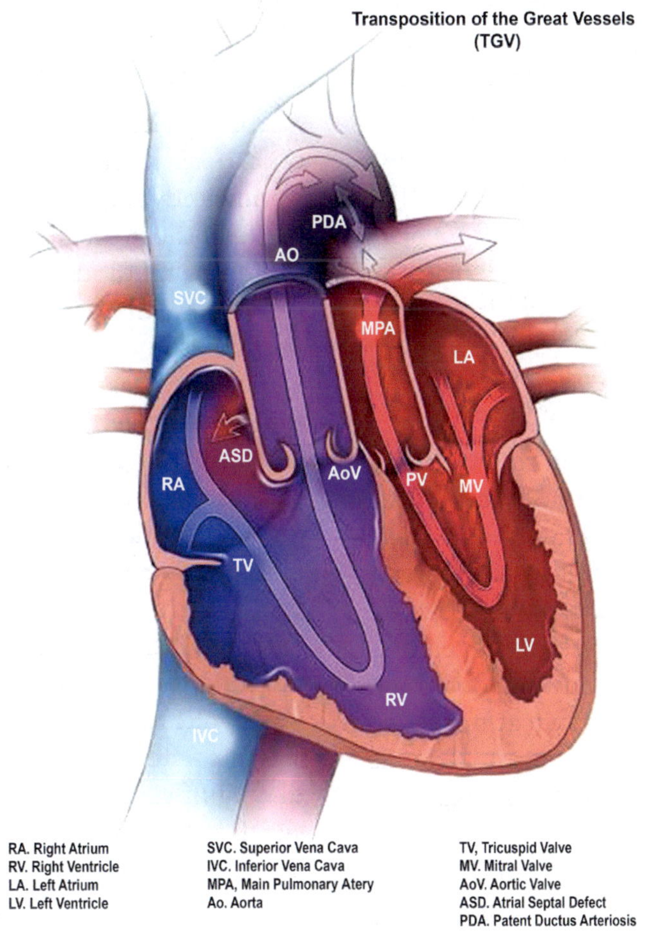

Figure 7.4. Transposition of the great arteries (TGA).

Source: https://external-content.duckduckgo.com/iu/?u=https%3A%2F%2Fhealthjade.net%2Fwp-content%2Fuploads%2F2020%2F03%2Ftransposition-of-the-great-arteries.jpg&f=1&nofb=1&ipt=62ef9e5b2010146decbaaec22669f196e911b098b6e489802f0feb4827817c6c.

The condition, if left untreated, can be fatal, thus necessitating early surgical correction to reestablish normal circulatory physiology (Eilers et al., 2021). TGA management is aimed at early diagnosis and intervention because the prognosis is better with early treatment. Stabilization in the initial stages may involve the giving of prostaglandin E1, which maintains ductal patency and guarantees some measure of oxygenated blood will gain entry into the systemic circulation through the patent ductus arteriosus (PDA). Therapy with surgery, which is typically performed during the initial weeks of life, consists of an arterial switch procedure that relocates the aorta and pulmonary artery to their normal anatomical positions. The repair not only corrects the immediate clinical presentation of cyanosis but also offers long-term cardiac function and growth. With the advancement in surgical techniques and perioperative care, mortality of this procedure has really improved, and TGA has become a condition that can be controlled (Eilers et al., 2021) (Figure 7.4).

The importance of continued research into long-term status in TGA patients cannot be overstated. With better survival rates, research is increasingly focused on the quality-of-life post-surgery in such individuals, with such research into cognitive development, activity level, and psychosocial adjustment. In addition, detection of the potential for related complications, such as arrhythmias and ventricular dysfunction, is essential for further management. As suggested by studies, patients may present with varying signs and symptoms related to cyanotic spells, which illustrate the complexity of managing congenital heart defects like TGA (Ilyas et al., 2021). Physicians aim to design comprehensive care plans that encompass not only surgical correction but also follow-up and management of any underlying illness long-term, ultimately improving life outcomes in those afflicted by this serious congenital heart defect.

7.1.3. Tricuspid Atresia

Tricuspid Atresia (TA) is a leading manifestation of cyanotic congenital heart disease without a functioning tricuspid valve, which ultimately abolishes normal passage of blood from the right atrium to the ventricle. This maldevelopment leads to a complex interplay of hemodynamic changes and inadequate oxygenation of the blood during passage in the bypass lung circulation. Clinically, infants with TA are often brought in with symptoms such as cyanosis, difficulty feeding, and failure to thrive, which will have negative impacts on their overall health and developmental courses.

Early detection of these symptoms is crucial as it provides early intervention that significantly improves the prognosis and quality of life of those affected. With enhanced prenatal screening methods, hopes of early diagnosis are growing, with hopes of better management and prognosis in infants with this condition (Yogi et al., 2025). Presentation of Tricuspid Atresia is typically a spectrum of symptoms depending on the impaired delivery of oxygen. As evident in case studies, such as a 16-month-old Nepalese girl who had typical cyanosis and acute malnutrition, the outcome of left untreated TA is death. In this case, the child was diagnosed with TA type IB, thus highlighting the variety of forms the condition comes in. After initial misdiagnosis and application of alternative treatment modes, the ultimate emergency procedure highlighted the significance of early surgical treatment for survival. Surgery recovery is typically turbulent, as in this patient, but marks a turning point in the management of cyanotic congenital heart diseases. The case portrays the role of health education and awareness for provision of timely and appropriate care (Yogi et al., 2025) (Figure 7.5).

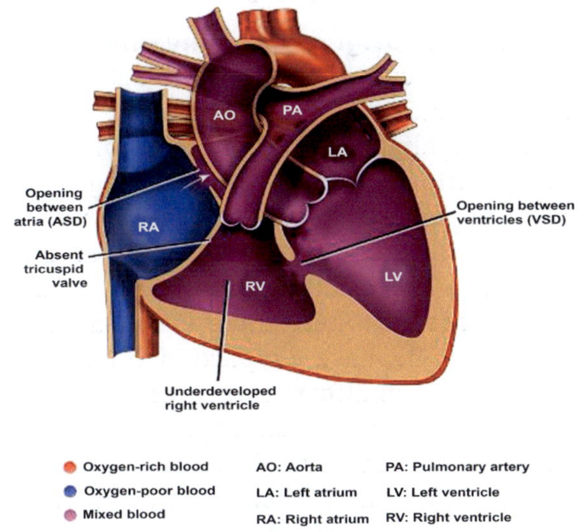

Figure 7.5. Tricuspid atresia.

Source: https://www.chop.edu/conditions-diseases/tricuspid-atresia.

Tricuspid Atresia Management is intricate measures that typically begin with surgery along with ongoing medical management. This can include a series of staged operations that target providing adequate pulmonary blood flow and maximizing the performance of the systemic perfusion.

For instance, surgical interventions such as the Fontan procedure have proved essential in long-term treatment of TA, allowing functionality of single ventricles without causing complications resulting from severe cyanosis. The case of a 10-month-old boy patient confirms the challenge of diagnosing TA, where preliminary symptoms were in the form of respiratory infections and were thus late in seeking adequate attention. Constant observation and review are essential aspects to confirm the patient's health is regularly observed and well addressed with the lapse of time. These integrated methods not only improve survival rates but also better the quality of life among individuals who have Tricuspid Atresia.

7.2. Causes and Risk Factors

Awareness of the etiology and risk factors of cyanotic congenital heart diseases (CCHDs) helps in early diagnosis and optimal therapy. Both genetic and environmental components have been known to contribute significantly to the etiology of the diseases. Chromosomal abnormalities, like Down syndrome, are usually associated with congenital cardiac malformations, like forms of Tetralogy of Fallot, which make up a significant proportion of the former. Further, fetal exposure to teratogens during gestation, including maternal infections (e.g., rubella), and other drugs has been implicated in the potential increase of CCHD development. The interaction of these environmental and gene factors further contributes to the complexity of heart development and underscores the need for comprehensive prenatal care in eliminating such risks and securing optimal outcomes for high-risk newborns with cyanotic heart disease. Apart from genetic predispositions, lifestyle and maternal health also significantly contribute to risk factors associated with CCHDs. Conditions related to pregnancy such as diabetes and hypertension may negatively affect fetal cardiovascular development. Aside from maternal predispositions, maternal lifestyle factors such as smoking, drug abuse, and inadequate diet have been shown to increase the risk of congenital heart defects. For instance, some nutritional deficiencies, namely folic acid, have been associated with a heightened frequency of heart abnormalities. Review of such risk factors is of paramount significance not only for prevention but also for increasing parental knowledge, as attested by some reports of lacunae in parental knowledge regarding the nature of their child's heart disease and associated risks. Making sure that mothers are provided with the correct information is able to empower them to make healthier lifestyle choices which would counterbalance such risks.

Greater knowledge about etiology and risk factors is particularly crucial in clinical practice, where parents' vigilance is crucially engaged in the progression of cyanotic heart diseases. Research shows that, although the majority of parents know their child's diagnosis, they lack total insight into the nature and implication of the condition (Atiq et al., 2008) (Figure 7.6).

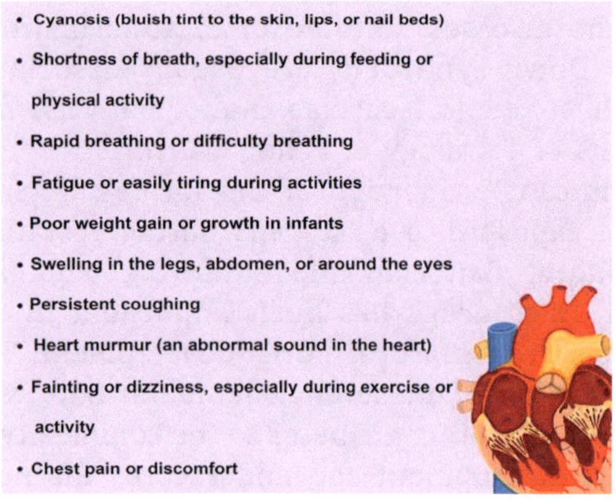

Figure 7.6. Cyanotic congenital heart diseases (CCHDs) symptoms.

Source: https://continentalhospitals.com/uploads/mceu_94219417311701511346716.jpg.

Such a lack of information can hinder effective communication between families and healthcare providers and, in turn, affect health outcomes.

Another area of serious concern is that many parents could be inadequately informed about the possible hereditary nature of such conditions, further complicating how to tackle and understand CCHDs within families. Therefore, implementing teaching programs in order to enhance parental education and effectively communicating information regarding the etiology and risk factors of cyanotic congenital heart diseases is required in order to improve the health literacy and outcomes of infected neonates (Atiq et al., 2008).

7.2.1. Genetic Factors

The genetic origins of congenital heart disease, particularly cyanotic heart disease, are multifactorial and complicated. Current research highlights the importance of genetic predisposition in the form of single-gene mutations and chromosomal abnormalities as primary factors in the etiology of these conditions. For example, disorders such as Down syndrome, where there is an additional chromosome 21, have a typical high frequency of congenital malformations of the heart, including atrioventricular septal defects and ventricular septal defects. Conversely, variations in some genes have been implicated in the maldevelopment of the heart, suggesting that precise genetic pathways could be involved to some extent in the origin and development of cyanotic congenital heart disease. Identification of such genetic contributions makes it possible to learn more about individual risk factors, paving the way for targeted interventions and prenatal screening to prevent the impact of such disorders. Moreover, the identification of genetic risk factors emphasizes the significance of environmental factors that can augment genetic vulnerabilities. Work has indicated maternal effects, notably nutrient levels during pregnancy, to have an impact on genetic expressions related to the development of the heart. For example, evidence points towards maternal 25-hydroxyvitamin D levels as possible determinants of children's risk for congenital heart diseases, though flaws in methodology among past research call for careful interpretation of such findings (Walker et al., 2025). This interaction underscores the need for an integrated perspective that considers both genetic and modifiable determinants. By making the interactions between these factors clearer, medical professionals can develop more individualized management and preventive regimens that acknowledge the complexity of congenital heart diseases, especially among high-risk populations (Figure 7.7).

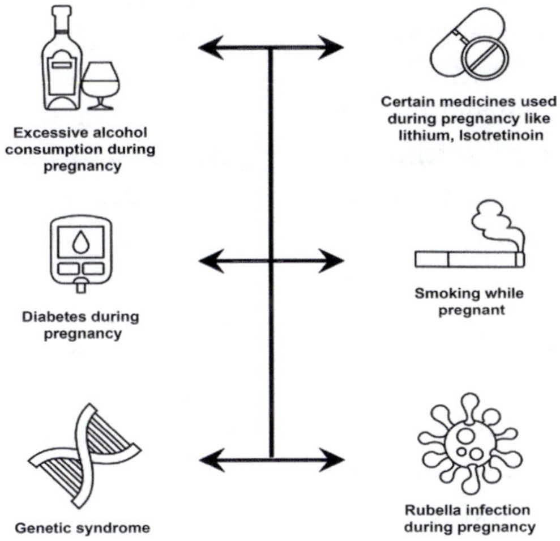

Figure 7.7. Risk factors for congenital heart diseases.

Source: https://drraghu.com/wp-content/uploads/2022/07/Cong.-heart-diseas.jpg.

Additionally, the adult congenital heart disease (ACHD) situation emphasizes long-term impacts of early genetic influences on health outcomes. As advances in medical therapy continue to spur better survival rates among children with cyanotic congenital heart diseases, knowledge of the genetic influences driving surgical and post-operative outcomes has become essential. Current data from large-scale databases show that age, the complexity of the congenital anomaly, and underlying disease are critical determinants of mortality following surgery (Osawa et al., 2024). This new information necessitates continued research on genetic markers that can potentially predict surgical risk and outcomes to enable directed care strategies to be formed. Lastly, the comprehension and integration of genetic factors into clinical practice not only enhance the management of patients but also augment the understanding base of congenital heart diseases during life.

7.2.2. Environmental Influences

Environmental determinants of congenital heart diseases (CHDs), particularly cyanotic ones, demonstrate a complex interaction between genetic vulnerabilities, maternal health, and social determinants of health. Different research studies have established that exposure to teratogens during intrauterine growth, such as some drugs, toxins, and infections, greatly increases the risk of developing CHDs. For instance, maternal smoking during pregnancy has been related to higher rates of cardiac abnormalities among neonates, particularly cyanotic anomalies. Additionally, the mother's health condition, i.e., diabetes and obesity, increases the risks further. This provides an indication of how crucial it is for the mothers to become aware of their condition and seek healthcare attention to limit the environmental risks, thereby reducing the occurrence of congenital heart defects in generations to come, as the intricate dynamics laid out in the ESC Guidelines underscore (Baumgartner et al., 2020). Moreover, socio-economic determinants have also been proven to influence the prevalence of cyanotic congenital heart diseases. Research among diverse populations has indicated great variability according to income levels and geographical locations. Based on a large-scale study involving over 76 million Chinese births, researchers established that the high-income provinces had a much higher prevalence of CHDs than the low-income provinces. This trend points towards the potential contribution of healthcare access, the quality of prenatal care, and health education in different settings to ultimately affect maternal choice and exposure to the environment during pregnancy (Zhao et al., 2020).

Therefore, the environmental determinants need to be interpreted not only from the individual behavior but also in larger socio-economic contexts, which affect this behavior and its ensuing health results. In addition, the geographic distribution of congenital heart diseases holds indications towards revealing the environmental determinants of the prevalence of these diseases. As exemplified in the previous study, regional disparity in CHD rates suggest that environmental determinants are not homogeneously distributed. A number of elements, including urbanization, industrial exposure, and contamination of the environment, differ widely between urban and rural settings. For instance, rural to urban migration may induce increased exposure to contaminants and changes in diet, impacting maternal and fetal growth. Therefore, it is crucial to study these regional variations for the development of effective targeted public health interventions and programs aimed at mitigating the rising prevalence of cyanotic heart diseases. Through targeting the environmental causes of such conditions, efforts may be made towards reducing their prevalence and improving overall reproductive and child health results.

7.2.3. Maternal Health Conditions

Maternal health status significantly influences the occurrence and severity of congenital heart diseases (CHDs), particularly cyanotic forms, which are typically underlaid with complex medical interventions. Maternal health conditions can include maternal diabetes, maternal hypertension, and maternal age that can endanger the maternal and fetal health. Maternal diabetes, for instance, is closely linked with the formation of CHDs through genetic-environmental interplay during fetal development's sensitive periods. Furthermore, advanced maternal age is associated with an increased risk of chromosomal abnormalities that make the occurrence of CHDs more likely, primarily the cyanotic varieties that lead to insufficient oxygenation of the body. Knowledge of such maternal health conditions is vital for early identification, effective prenatal care, and risk stratification with the aim of realizing improved outcomes for the affected infants and minimizing the associated emotional trauma among parents. Prenatal diagnosis has been a significant factor in the treatment of congenital heart disease, allowing for adequate preparation in anticipation of cyanotic defect situations. There are many benefits of prenatal diagnosis; it allows parents the choice of termination of pregnancy for severe CHD with a poor prognosis or prepares them better for postnatal management if they choose to continue pregnancy. Worth mentioning, the lesions such as ductus arteriosus-dependent CHD and complicated obstructive lesions inflict serious risk on the life of a newborn and need early action. If the diagnosis is made prenatally, doctors can organize the delivery logistics, typically in high-level tertiary facilities with the ability to deliver immediate care, thus reducing morbidity and mortality among affected infants. Such preventive activity not only improves clinical outcome but also regulates parents' anxiety regarding the unknowns of the health of their child. Other research also indicates the newly emerging interaction of gut microbiota with congenital heart disease and hints that maternal conditions of health influence the infant's microbiome structure and have implications for their health. For instance, congenital heart disease-affected infants also typically present with dysbiosis—a alteration of the intestinal microbial communities—which also potentially plays a part in inflammatory processes in their heart disease. Interventions, such as the administration of probiotics like *Bifidobacterium longum* ssp. *infantis*, have been studied in the clinic to see their impact on gut health and plasma cytokine levels in such infants. While results to date have shown some potential in the control of inflammation and infectious complications, more work is required to define the effectiveness of these interventions on a large scale in the realm of maternal health and its consequences for congenital heart disease treatment.

7.3. Symptoms and Diagnosis

Identification of the symptoms of cyanotic congenital heart diseases (CCHDs) is important in terms of performing early diagnosis and intervention. The patients will typically present with a distinct constellation of signs that reflect compromised oxygenation due to structural cardiac defects. The most frequent symptoms are cyanosis, which is characterized by blue coloration of the mucous membranes and skin, due to deoxygenated blood being circulated to the body. Other presentations include respiratory distress, infantile weakness of feeding, and failure to grow. These presentations range from mild to severe, with some patients having intermittent cyanosis that worsens with illness or activity. Detection of these clinical presentations is key in allowing medical practitioners to advance with the correct diagnostic examinations at the optimal time, potentially saving patient lives and preventing disastrous complications of untreated conditions with CCHDs (Baumgartner et al., 2020). Cyanotic congenital heart diseases tend to be diagnosed by a blend of clinical evaluation and advanced imaging modalities. Physicians are able to utilize echocardiography as an initial line of diagnostic tool, which carries out real-time imaging of cardiac structure and function. Non-invasive imaging enables significant assessment of the anatomy of the heart and can help in the identification of shunting lesions and other anatomical abnormalities that lead to cyanosis. Diagnostic criteria involve meticulous patient history and physical examination too, which ensure a general insight into the state of the patient. In complex cases, a cardiac MRI or CT scan may be warranted to gather more information about the structural function and integrity of the hearts. This multi-dimensional diagnostic approach is essential as it directs therapy strategies and forecasts clinical outcomes in patients with CCHDs (Stout et al., 2018). Laboratory studies supplement imaging in the diagnosis of cyanotic congenital heart diseases. Arterial blood gas examination can measure oxygen saturation levels and show hypoxemia—an important finding for defective oxygenation with heart anomalies. Furthermore, the presence of metabolic acidosis can also suggest subnormal tissue delivery of oxygen, which raises a strong suspicion of a cyanotic process. Genetic analysis is also indicated when a syndromic connection is suspected or to guide family counseling. Besides, sound management of CCHDs is targeted at collaboration within a multidisciplinary team to ensure compliance with clinical guidelines in offering effective patient care. Consistency with the latest evidence-based practice is necessary for health care practitioners when dealing with the symptoms and ensuring accurate diagnosis in patients afflicted with such complex congenital heart diseases (Baumgartner et al., 2020).

7.3.1. Common Symptoms in Infants

The manifestation of symptoms in infant patients with cyanotic congenital heart disease (CHD) is typically not clear-cut but important in early diagnosis and management. Infant patients with cyanotic CHD present cyanosis, a blue coloration of the skin, particularly over the lips, tongue, and peripheral limbs, due to insufficient oxygenation of the blood. This symptom is especially prevalent when the infants are crying or feeding since this aggravates the babies respiratory distress. The identification of such signs at an early age can lead to early medical interventions, which are mandatory due to the high mortality if left untreated cyanotic heart defects. Also, a significant proportion of these infants may also be detected to be lethargic or have poor weight gain, which combined with cyanosis, suggests potential cardiovascular compromise warranting immediate medical evaluation (Duman et al., 2024).

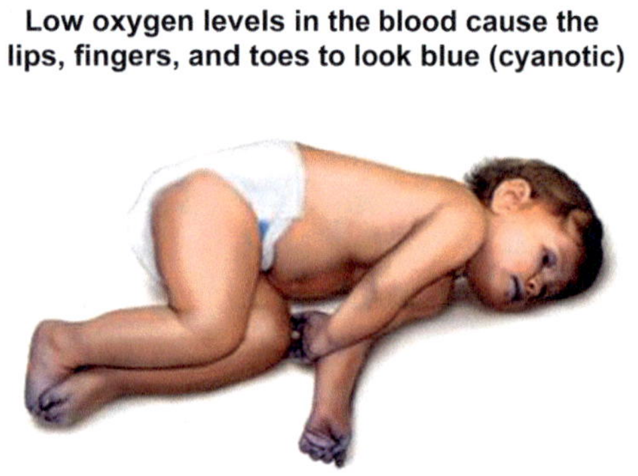

Figure 7.8. The main symptom of cyanosis is a bluish color of the lips, fingers, and toes, caused by the low oxygen content in the blood.

Source: https://medlineplus.gov/ency/article/001104.htm.

Another common symptom among cyanotic CHD infants is tachypnea or rapid breathing rate, usually caused by the body's compensation for diminished oxygenation. Infants with the condition can also exhibit irritability and distress due to compromised circulatory competence. Respiratory distress can sometimes be mistaken for a typical pediatric cold. Caretakers thus must distinguish between normal neonatal fluctuation and indicators that are of concern. Furthermore, there must be constant monitoring of an infant's respiratory and cardiovascular condition since symptoms can fluctuate while performing various activities such as feeding or position. Such a presentation of symptoms demands high alertness from parents as well as health professionals, especially in early life when such conditions are determined and can lead to life-saving interventions (Khedewy et al., 2024) (Figure 7.8).

Extensive clinical assessment and adequate parental education regarding symptoms of cyanotic CHD may have a positive bearing on the outcome for the affected babies. The parents must be alerted to the signs of respiratory distress like grunting, retractions of the chest wall, and alteration of the color in the skin. Ability to recognize such symptoms may enable caregivers to seek medical intervention early, thereby resulting in earlier diagnosis and treatment. Prenatal echocardiographic evaluations and subsequent neonatal screening can contribute significantly to the detection of such anomalies before the onset of noteworthy manifestations and reducing morbidity rates. Broadly speaking, heightened awareness of normal cyanotic CHD symptoms is important for optimal immediate and long-term care of susceptible infants (Duman et al., 2024; Khedewy et al., 2024).

7.3.2. Diagnostic Imaging Techniques

Technological improvements on diagnostic imaging modality have significantly affected the profession of congenital heart condition diagnosis, particularly cyanotic heart diseases. Among all the modalities employed, echocardiography is the backbone for cardiac imaging due to its non-invasive nature and efficiency in imaging cardiac anatomy. Transthoracic echocardiography, more so, provides real-time assessment of cardiac function, chamber size, and septal defect. This technique allows clinicians to measure hemodynamic parameters and identify the presence of shunts, an important characteristic of cyanotic heart disorders. Also, echocardiography's ability to provide color-flow Doppler images enhances the diagnosis of abnormal blood flow patterns, thereby helping in diagnosis and subsequent treatment of these complex conditions. As described in the ESC Guidelines, physicians are encouraged to incorporate more advanced imaging techniques like echocardiography in their tool chest to enhance clinical decision-making (Baumgartner et al., 2020). Echocardiography is extremely useful in the initial assessment, but advanced imaging modalities like magnetic resonance imaging (MRI) and computed tomography (CT) are increasingly utilized for additional anatomical definition and functional evaluation (Figure 7.9).

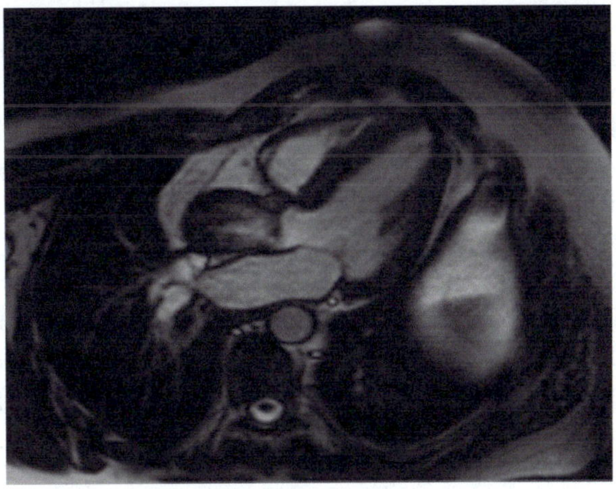

Figure 7.9. MRI in the assessment of congenital heart disease.

Source: https://cdn.agilitycms.com/applied-radiology/MediaGroupings/4000/Deshpande_figure02c.jpg.

Cardiac MRI has excellent soft tissue contrast and three-dimensional imaging, which makes it exceptionally valuable in the assessment of complex anatomical features that are a characteristic of cyanotic heart diseases. It creates panoramic images of the heart and great vessels morphology and enables surgical planning and post-operative assessment. Similarly, CT angiography can also be employed to evaluate vascular structures and anomalies that are responsible for the cyanotic presentation. Utilization of these imaging techniques facilitates advanced understanding of etiology in congenital heart disease, ultimately resulting in the optimal treatment modalities appropriate to the patient's requirements (Stout et al., 2018). Utilization of these advanced diagnostic imaging techniques within medical practice underscores the importance of a multidisciplinary team in the treatment of congenital heart diseases (Kampouris et al., 2018). Multidisciplinary treatment by cardiologists, radiologists, and surgeons enhances the precision of diagnosis and optimizes patient care. As noted by the guidelines, it is important that clinicians use clinical judgment in conjunction with these imaging modalities to create well-informed and individualized treatment decisions. Clinician-patient shared decision-making can also greatly improve treatment adherence by ensuring interventions align within patient comorbidities and preferences. Ultimately, utilizing the strengths of various diagnostic imaging techniques makes comprehensive evaluation of cyanotic congenital heart diseases possible, paving the way for improved outcomes and improved quality of life for individuals with these diseases (Baumgartner et al., 2020).

7.3.3. Role of Echocardiography

Echocardiography is an essential tool in the diagnosis and treatment of congenital heart diseases, particularly those cyanotic. The technique allows clinicians to achieve real-time visualization of heart structures, making proper diagnosis of defects possible. In cyanotic congenital heart diseases such as Tetralogy of Fallot and transposition of the great arteries, echocardiography helps determine the effectiveness of surgery and subsequent complications. The ability to quantify hemodynamic parameters, image shunts, and evaluate valve function has emphasized the importance of echocardiography in personalizing treatment approaches. By integrating clinical information into echocardiographic evaluation, clinicians are able to enhance patient care through early and informed clinical decision-making, thus supporting the preeminent position of this imaging modality in the management of congenital heart disease. Transthoracic echocardiography is particularly valuable in follow-up of patients with surgical repair of congenital heart disease. For example, after surgical repair of Tetralogy of Fallot, late effects like pulmonary regurgitation can occur, for which follow-up by regular echocardiograms is required to assess the function of the right ventricle and to identify residual lesions. Echocardiography not only helps in identifying the postoperative complications but also in assessing the hemodynamic status of patients during follow-up. These findings are critical when planning subsequent intervention, such as reoperations or catheter-based intervention. The subtle information derived from echocardiography allows medical teams to predict long-term results more accurately and treat complications in patients with a history of cyanotic congenital conditions, thus improving overall treatment and surveillance practice (Ashraf et al., 2019). Furthermore, echocardiographic use goes beyond monitoring and diagnosis since it facilitates immediate decision-making in acute clinical situations. In acute pulmonary regurgitation after correction of congenital lesions, echocardiography is quick to identify hemodynamic alterations that may call for instant intervention. Visualization of shunt, such as an unsuspected right-to-left shunt via a patent foramen ovale, provides important information to guide therapeutic modalities and interventions. As directed in powerful clinical recommendations like those of the European Society of Cardiology, echocardiography plays an imperative role in the comprehensive management of congenital heart disease, emphasizing the need that the providers make use of such bits of information in clinical decision-making (Baumgartner et al., 2020). The comprehensively integrated information rendered by echocardiography ultimately ensures that patients are given the appropriate and timely treatment specifically tailored to their evolving cardiac disorders.

7.4. Treatment Options

Management of cyanotic CHDs needs a team approach that accommodates variegation of the condition of each patient. The management typically spans between surgical interventions, pharmacologic treatment and long-term supportive therapy. Early detection and treatment are important since all these conditions have the capacity to lead to serious morbidity if left untreated. Palliative maneuvers in some cases need to be done to augment oxygenation and systemic perfusion before definitive surgical correction. The nature of these maneuvers would follow the specific anatomical and physiological deviances within the heart and hence indicate the need for personalized treatment options based on certain patient factors and general condition. Surgical procedures are still a cornerstone of treating cyanotic congenital heart disease. These may include such procedures as the creation of shunts to enhance blood flow or the complete reconstruction of the involved cardiac structures. These operations tend to be for individualized malformations, such as transposition of the great arteries or tetralogy of Fallot, and attempt to restore normal hemodynamics. These operations are usually, however, preceded by careful consideration of perioperative and long-term hazards. An important factor is the long-term follow-up of complications such as heart failure or arrhythmias, which could need further procedures after initial correction, and thus indicate a need for an overall care plan that evolves with the patient as they grow and create their own unique health profile. Surgical therapy, however, is not the sole treatment modality employed in the management of cyanotic congenital heart disease, as pharmacological therapy also plays a significant role in alleviating symptoms and risk of complications. For instance, congenitally affected infants are significantly predisposed to infection with respiratory syncytial virus (RSV), which may make their condition worse and lead to unnecessary hospitalization. Administration of monoclonal antibodies, such as palivizumab, has been shown to reduce RSV morbidity in patients, demonstrating the effectiveness of preventive interventions in their treatment regimen (Cyran et al., 2011). Furthermore, continued research into promising new therapies and future vaccines against such organisms is imperative to optimize outcomes in this population since the cost of current prophylaxis highlights the economic burden of treatment in these high-risk individuals (Diller et al., 2009). This multidisciplinary treatment strategy is not only important in terms of achieving maximum clinical outcomes, but it is also important to the quality of life of children with cyanotic congenital heart disease.

7.4.1. Surgical Interventions

Treatment of cyanotic congenital heart diseases at times needs surgical interventions that can essentially alter the prognosis and quality of life in patients suffering from such conditions. Surgical techniques have evolved significantly and enabled surgeons to operate on complex anatomical defects characteristic of such conditions. For instance, in disorders such as Tetralogy of Fallot, one of the most common forms of cyanotic heart disease, surgical correction is typically a series of operations to improve blood circulation and oxygenation. Not only do these treatments enhance physical capacities, but they extend lifespan also, as many become adults, especially where available health facilities can offer advanced surgery. In countries with limited access to these life-saving procedures, pediatric survival remains crucially low, as indicated by the fact that less than 10% of patients with congenital heart disease live for more than a decade without surgery (Amin et al., 2024). Aside from life-saving interventions, the long-term impact of surgical interventions on cognitive outcomes in children with cyanotic congenital heart disease has increasingly been studied in recent years. Studies have always revealed that cognitive impairments can still remain following surgical repair, and the care must be holistic to address this. A study comparing children with congenital cardiac malformations reported striking disparities in cognitive performance between children with cyanotic and acyanotic heart disease, highlighting the intricate relationship between surgical status and intellectual function (Kamal et al., 2024) (Figure 7.10).

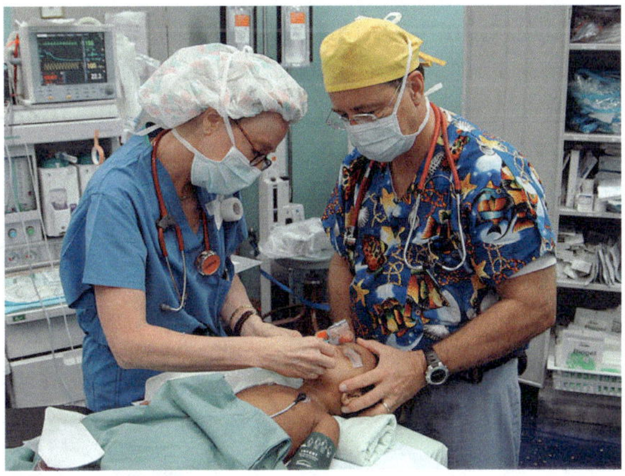

Figure 7.10. Cardiac surgery in children with congenital heart disease.

Source: https://www.childheartspecialist.com/wp-content/uploads/2016/03/children-heart-disease-non-cardiac-surgery.jpg.

Though the corrective surgeries do yield the undisputed immediate physiological benefit, continued vigilance is still warranted to ensure and regulate cognitive function in these patients. It is this multi-faceted approach that ensures practitioners not only treat the anatomy of the heart but also address the brain's development as an integral part of the comprehensive treatment plan. With the improvement in operating techniques, the landscape of cyanotic congenital heart disease care is evolving. Early treatment, choice between open heart surgery and minimal invasive therapy, and postoperative rehabilitation are of primary importance in arriving at better results. Timely surgery is of great consideration, in which early interventions can improve not only survival rates at the time of operation but also subsequent neurodevelopmental outcomes. Research has shown that children who are subjected to correctional surgery at younger ages were found to exhibit enhanced cognitive function as opposed to their peers who are treated late. Hence, enhancing surgical timing and techniques can provide astounding strides in the life quality of these children, which means that surgical intervention can be a cornerstone in the treatment and management of congenital heart disease (Kamal et al., 2024).

7.4.2. Medications and Management

Treatment of cyanotic congenital heart disease is multifactorial and involves both non-pharmacologic and pharmacologic modalities. Cyanotic patients can present with reduced oxygenation and, therefore, have numerous systemic implications. Medication plays an essential role in alleviating these issues, particularly in the treatment of secondary complications such as arrhythmias. The neonatal immature myocardium renders them extremely vulnerable to rhythm disturbances, and these can be caused by overpowering physiological stressors in the early postnatal life. With the restriction of pharmacologic interventions in this age group due to their own physiological concerns, the selection of the drug is crucial. Earlier studies show that arrhythmias can lead to long-term development problems, complicating treatment further (Anjan et al., 2024). Thus, the healthcare provider has to tread the thin line between drug therapy's short-term curative benefits and potential long-term harmful effects (Figure 7.11).

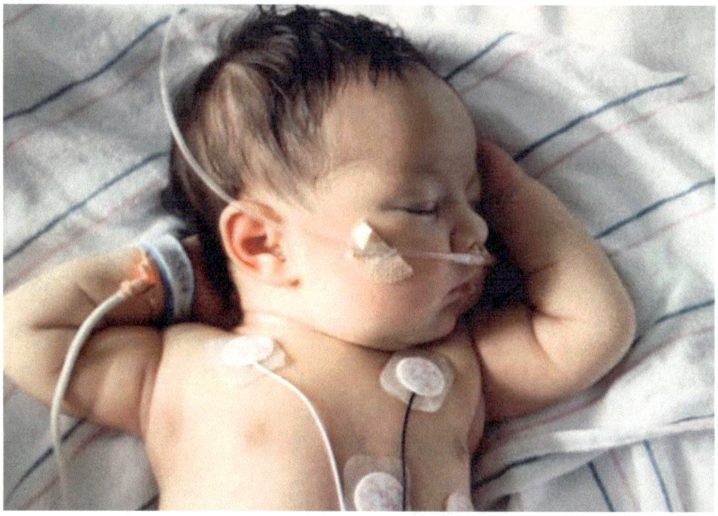

Figure 7.11. The management of congenital heart diseases.

Source: https://www.heart.org/-/media/Images/Health-Topics/Congenital-Heart-Defects/Survivor-photos/Sloan-in-hospital.jpg?h=533&w=800&sc_lang=en.

Anticoagulation therapy is another imperative part of cyanotic congenital heart disease treatment, particularly in children presenting with thrombotic complications. As CHD carries the inherent risk of bleeding and thrombosis, the children will present with an increased risk of venous thromboembolism (VTE) owing to altered hemodynamics. Standard treatment methods, such as heparin or warfarin, may not be optimal in all cases owing to the variability in dosage and monitoring needs. Recent research regarding the efficacy and safety of dabigatran, a direct thrombin inhibitor, has yielded positive outcomes. Findings reported dabigatran to have particular promise as a safer and more effective option for children with CHD, reporting increased complete resolution of thrombi compared to control treatment (Albisetti et al., 2024). This new data favors a trend towards more personalized methodologies of anticoagulation in these complex diseases tailored to the individual needs of the child. Under the background of recent developments in pharmacologic care for cyanotic congenital heart disease, there is a call for continued research. New medications and treatment protocols need to be followed by reputable research into their safety and efficacy in the specifically pediatric patient. As noted, dabigatran VTE acute management trials identify robust benefits in CHD children with the potential to further simplify treatment models (Albisetti et al., 2024). Such cases' complexity and scarcity, however, bring inherent sample size constraints, warranting cautious data interpretation. Future research will have to target large-scale, multicenter trials to establish more robust data, ultimately guiding clinical practice guidelines for pharmacologic management in this unique population. By taking a research-driven approach, the medical community can evolve therapeutic strategies that address both acute clinical challenges and promote better long-term outcomes for those with cyanotic congenital heart disease.

7.4.3. Long-Term Care and Follow-Up

Long-term follow-up and care in CCHD patients are essential components of care that play a significant role in survival as well as quality of life. Due to the multistage physiological adaptation of their body, these individuals might require round-the-clock monitoring. Regular follow-up visits need to be conducted to assess cardiac function, watch for complications, and make early interventions when necessary. Specifically, infants with tetralogy of Fallot are at risk of developing right ventricular outflow tract obstruction in later life for which surgical revisions may be necessary. Furthermore, total care involves multidisciplinary management with cardiologists, pediatricians, and allied health professionals to address not only cardiac disease but also the psychosocial determinants of care. These comprehensive management strategies result in improved functional outcomes and help families adapt to the adversity of living with CCHD (Eilers et al., 2021). Transition from pediatric care to adult care is another critical aspect of long-term follow-up for CCHD patients. Cardiac requirements change as the patients grow older, and they possess unique health issues. Effective transition protocols need to have at the patient's bedside and the provider's bedside, familiarization with the specific congenital defect as well as its implications. Transitioned care models with adult cardiologists who are conversant in CCHD enable the transition because they offer subspecialty experience in management of long-term sequelae such as arrhythmias, heart failure, and management of other comorbidities. Education is an integral part of the transition, with a focus on changes in lifestyle and self-care measures that can lead to longevity and enhance the quality of life overall. These preventive interventions coupled with regular cardiac assessments enable clinicians to recognize and address potential complications prior to the transition (Baumgartner et al., 2020). Moreover, follow-up over the long term also fosters a network of support for patients and families, a critical component of emotional and psychological well-being. The regular exposure to health care practitioners can enhance fear about illness management and provide access to mechanisms for overcoming the challenges that CCHD poses. Support groups offer patients and families a venue to exchange experiences, raise concerns, and learn from one another. Moreover, technology progression, such as telemedicine consultations, can enable patients and healthcare teams to be in contact at all times, especially for patients who are from rural communities. The development of multi-dimensional care pathways involving physical, emotional, and social support services ultimately leads to better outcomes and a better quality of life for cyanotic congenital heart disease survivors (Eilers et al., 2021).

7.5. Impact on Quality of Life

The complexities of congenital heart diseases, particularly cyanotic heart disease (CyHD), have a deep impact on the quality of life in patients with it. Children with CyHD typically face a range of challenges not merely physical in nature. Studies indicate that the psychosocial status of these patients can be greatly impacted. According to a research study, kids with isolated cardiac defects were able to attain the same HRQoL as their peers. However, children who have CyHD tend to have lower HRQoL and more distress than other children. This further means that severity and complexity of their condition are apt to result in serious emotional and social complications, thus calling for the need of holistic care measures addressing physical health as well as mental wellness within pediatric cardiac management (Liu et al., 2022). Further, even the nature of treatment pursued has an important contribution to make in deciding the quality of life among children suffering from congenital heart diseases. Invasive procedures, although often necessary for the treatment of complex heart defects, have the secondary implication of being able to result in a decline in HRQoL among patients. Research has indicated that adolescents who have undergone such procedures exhibit elevated anxiety and emotional distress. These findings underscore that medical therapies, although life-sustaining, may have unexpected psychological implications and hence emphasize the importance of incorporating mental health care into treatment protocols for CyHD patients. Healthcare professionals must take into account not only the immediate clinical outcomes of treatment but also the long-term effects on the quality of life of patients (Liu et al., 2022). Such an integrative approach optimizes the chance of congenital heart disease management including recovery and emotional stability. Finally, the implications of these discoveries extend to the broader societal circles, where awareness and knowledge of congenital heart ailments must be strengthened considerably. Families coping with the confines of CyHD are usually isolated and stressed, impacting their overall quality of life. While clinicians are putting the ESC guidelines into practice, it is important that they also apply such psychosocial factors in taking into account long-term prognosis for families and patients. Evidence indicates the need for policies that enable access to psychological resources and community support systems for CyHD-affected families to improve resilience and global HRQoL. Moreover, increased awareness through community education programs can become the doorway to reducing stigma and enhancing the support system of such families and thus leading to improved health outcomes.

7.5.1. Physical Limitations and Challenges

The synergistic interaction of the cyanotic congenital heart diseases with physical disabilities presents unsurmountable obstacles for people with such conditions. These challenges usually stem from the intrinsic physiological derangements of the cyanotic heart diseases (e.g., faulty oxygenation of blood) leading to manifestations of exertional dyspnea and fatigue. These constraints greatly affect the general quality of life since patients can end up unable to engage in appropriate activities for their age or lead an active life. According to clinical guidelines, the effectiveness of management approaches is highly dependent on individualized adjustments of interventions to patient-specific requirements, thus emphasizing the significance of shared decision-making between healthcare professionals and patients when dealing with these day-to-day challenges (Stout et al., 2018). The consequences of CyHD extend past immediate symptoms, affecting the patient's tolerance level and capacity to engage in various activities. Progressive right-sided heart failure (RHF) is a condition faced by most patients through increased workload on the heart, reducing exercise tolerance and functional capacity (Marvin et al., 2018) (Figure 7.12).

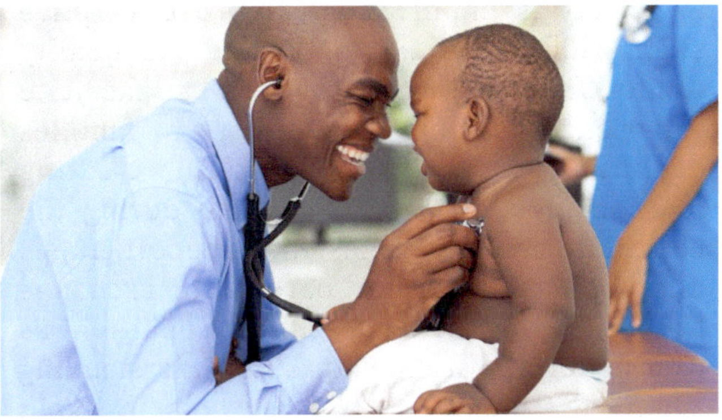

Figure 7.12. The repercussions of cyanotic heart diseases extend beyond immediate symptoms, affecting the patient's physical endurance and capacity for engagement in various activities.

Source: https://www.cdc.gov/heart-defects/media/images/checkup.jpg.

The cumulative burden of these physical limitations can also give rise to emotional and psychological struggles as individuals come to terms with the reality of their condition. Advances in treatment modalities can mitigate some of the physical struggles, but the ubiquitous nature of such limitations emphasizes the requirement of an integrated support system with both medical and psychosocial components. Such a comprehensive approach may empower patients to overcome barriers induced by their health issues. To gain an improved understanding of physical limitations of cyanotic heart diseases, it is critical to examine how current clinical guidelines are applied. The American College of Cardiology and American Heart Association call for individualized care plans that not only consider the disease's biological impact but also social determinants of patient participation (Stout et al., 2018). This practice promotes the philosophy that quality care is about adapting interventions to supplement the patient's lifestyle and life circumstances. Through the use of an integrated model of care that involves monitoring progress, placing significant importance on patient education, and promoting shared decision-making, it is possible to limit the detrimental effect of physical impairments that define cyanotic heart disease. These methods can assist in providing improved patient outcomes and quality of life so that individuals can more effectively manage their physical challenges.

7.5.2. Psychological and Emotional Effects

The psychologic effect of congenital heart diseases (CHD), particularly cyanotic forms, plays an important role in impacting the quality of life in patients. The patients commonly experience chronic disease, which can lead to anxiety and depressive disorders. Research indicates that CHD can imbue an omnipresent state of emotional distress due to frequent medical interventions and health challenges experienced throughout life. Thus, these problems are likely to hinder formation of a firm self-image since the patients will regard themselves as other or inferior to others. The long-term nature of these health complications, coupled with the unpredictability of attendant symptoms, fosters an environment of psychological anxiety that compromises their ability to adapt socially and emotionally as they grow up. Evidence also suggests that emotional effects manifest in diverse ways based on the severity of the illness. Research shows that patients with late stages of CHD have a higher chance of exhibiting psychosocial maladjustment (i.e., higher levels of anxiety and depression, particularly in females). This also points towards the necessity to consider gender differences in emotional responses; female patients had higher frequencies of disturbances in mental health, reporting more somatic symptoms and higher frequencies of withdrawal of emotions. These disparities highlight the necessity of tailored psychological treatment that deals with the specific difficulties faced by more severely affected cases of congenital heart disease, promoting enhanced coping and emotional stability in such vulnerable patients (Areias et al., 2013). Social support and psychological adaptation in cyanotic CHD patients also highlight the emotional makeup of such individuals to cope with daily life. A robust social support system can help buffer some of the adverse effects of the condition and contribute positively to mental health outcomes. It has been established through research that those with positive family and peer support have less anxiety and improved psychosocial adjustment while those without such support show social withdrawal and behavioral problems. Therefore, establishing solid relationships and interpersonal support becomes essential to foster emotional resilience among congenital heart disease patients. Future interventions must prioritize the development of supportive care environments that not only address the medical issues of the disease but also reinforce psychological and emotional strengths to foster quality of life (Cullen et al., 2013).

7.5.3. Social Integration and Support

The experience of congenital heart disease, and indeed cyanotic conditions, in children and families demonstrates the widespread impact of social integration and support upon health status. Families finding themselves coping with the challenges of dealing with such severe medical conditions have a tendency to be socially isolated due to the intensive care and repeating hospitalizations required. Such loneliness can be supplemented by the psychological loads of the diagnosis, such as anxiety and concern for the future of the child. It is then crucial that there should be social support groups that can help share such loads, since successful relationships with family, friends, and peer networks can provide emotional support and material assistance during difficult moments. It can strongly improve psychosocial outcomes and, consequently, foster resilience in families with the burden of congenital heart diseases (Baumgartner et al., 2020). Family inclusion in society is important to improve adaptive coping measures and maximize the quality of life. Organized care programs can facilitate experience sharing and support to families dealing with a similar problem, creating relationships that are invaluable during the healthcare process. For instance, support groups offer opportunities for parents to exchange tips on coping with the child's condition, as well as forging friendship and understanding among the members. The psychological gain from such contacts can outweigh feelings of loneliness, thus enhancing overall well-being. On the other hand, community resources such as counseling agencies and educational seminars can increase the family's capacity to seek assistance, when necessary, further enhancing social integration and support networks. These are particularly relevant because they can neutralize the extreme stress of the complexity of cyanotic congenital heart diseases (Kozik, 2019). Furthermore, investigations have advanced medicine technology and therapies, raising the chances of survival among children with cyanotic congenital heart diseases but with social integration as a key motivator of long-term success. Even though the medical practices of today are focusing on physical health outcomes, the necessity of attending to the emotional and social sides can easily be exaggerated. Best assisted by a holistic method that is aware of both the clinical aspects of care and the need for social integration are the families. Interventions should not only address the physical rehabilitation of the child but also the psychosocial well-being of families, such as ensuring they are provided with inclusive support systems. Fostering an acceptant and understanding society within communities can help in social integration, subsequently addressing improved quality of life for children suffering from congenital heart diseases and their respective families (Baumgartner et al., 2020).

SUMMARY

The pathophysiology of congenital heart diseases, and specifically cyanotic conditions, demonstrates that a delicate understanding of their complexities is critical to clinical management and patient outcome. Cyanotic congenital heart diseases present multi-faceted challenges that span the range from levels of physiological disturbances that can meaningfully impact the lives of neonates who are so afflicted. These conditions, Tetralogy of Fallot most notably, have been identified as the most prevalent ones in this group, as seen in the findings of Aga Khan University Hospital where the majority of the neonates diagnosed with the condition had a large proportion. Diagnosis therefore early and interventions timely are crucial, as they have a close correlation with survival rates and overall prognoses. The mutual dependency between surgical and medical management in the treatment of cyanotic congenital heart diseases complications requires an integrated strategy. Based on findings of most research studies, outcomes revealed a 63.6% survival rate among neonates who had been subjected to the appropriate treatment, which demonstrated that the only most important determinant in optimizing the prognosis of such patients is medical management (بالاخانی et al., 1387). Also, the relationship of congenital heart disease with other disorders, such as brain abscess in conditions like cyanotic heart defects, makes treatment more severe for patients (بالاخانی et al., 1387). In dealing with such an intricate situation, healthcare workers must take into account not just short-term surgical treatment but also the general management of concomitant diseases. Lastly, the treatment process of congenital cyanotic heart diseases is one that involves patient and research development commitment in the long term. Future work should be directed towards the enhancement of diagnostic approaches, therapeutic modalities reinforcement, and the establishment of good support systems for families handling such life-altering situations. The value of interdisciplinarity in teamwork cannot be stressed highly enough as this maintains a holistic strategy towards comprehending as well as managing both the immediate and the indirect complexities of such afflictions. As we strive to refine our practice as well as expand our knowledge base, emphasis on continuing research as well as patient-centered practice will be imperative in improving the quality of life for congenital heart patients in the cyanosis spectrum.

In the context of congenital heart diseases (CHDs), cyanotic states are unique in presenting problems that have a significant impact on patient prognosis and management. Cyanosis, the condition represented in blue coloration of the skin as a marker for the absence of properly oxygenated blood, is a significant indicator of underlying cardiovascular malformations. Tetralogy of Fallot, Transposition of the Great Arteries, and Total Anomalous Pulmonary Venous Return are notable cyanotic states. These conditions typically need early corrective surgery to restore structural abnormalities and improve oxygenation. Hence, an understanding of the pathophysiology and clinical correlations of such diseases is important for clinicians. Due to the complexities involved, the management of cyanotic CHD patients necessitates a multidisciplinary team that involves pediatric cardiologists, surgeons, and nursing staff to treat the whole person from the time of diagnosis until the end of life. The prognosis of a cyanotic heart patient largely depends on the nature and degree of the disease along with the nature and quality of intervention and timing. Improved technology in cardiology, particularly in well-funded centers, has revolutionized the specialty for the management of these congenital anomalies. Still, unequal access to care remains in low- and middle-income countries, where there is limited infrastructure that has the potential to amplify the mortality rate that comes with congenital heart defects (Yang et al., 2021). As the evidence suggests, children with congenital heart defects are at greater risk, with many of these being diagnosed later and where there are insufficient medical facilities, resulting in poorer outcomes. Therefore, health care facilities must make it a priority to improve and implement improved diagnostic methods and treatment protocols in an effort to bridge this chasm. Public health initiatives with an education and awareness focus can also have the ability to influence cyanotic heart disease patient outcomes. Early screening programs must be included in plans, particularly in high-risk populations, in an effort to enable effective diagnosis and treatment. Role of the community health education in minimizing the risk factors for congenital heart disease is also critical. With more cases of cardiovascular diseases being reported across the globe, emphasis on lifestyle modification and preventive approaches is needed in order to reduce the burden of risk posed by these diseases. Besides, ongoing research focused on the genetic and environmental etiology of congenital heart defects will provide insight into possible areas of prevention and treatment. Lastly, collaborative action aimed at ensuring access to healthcare, education, and research is essential in addressing the multifactorial problems of cyanotic congenital heart disease.

CLOSER LOOK

TETRALOGY OF FALLOT AND RELATED DEFECTS

Tetralogy of Fallot (TOF) is a highly common cyanotic congenital heart malformation, which affects approximately 10% of all congenital heart anomalies. TOF is a complex cardiac defect with four key anatomical elements: a ventricular septal defect (VSD), right ventricular outflow tract (RVOT) obstruction (often due to pulmonary stenosis), overriding of the aorta, and right ventricular hypertrophy. These defects as a group result in a right-to-left shunt and decreased oxygenation of the blood to produce cyanosis in affected infants.

The pathophysiology of TOF is a result of abnormal conotruncal septal growth, affecting the relationship of the outflow tracts. The large VSD allows for oxygen-deoxygenated blood mixture, while the pulmonary obstruction at the RVOT results in high right-sided pressures that drive the deoxygenated blood into systemic circulation. The severity of the pulmonary obstruction essentially determines the severity of symptoms.

Clinically, infants with severe pulmonary stenosis may present prematurely with severe cyanosis. Those with milder stenosis may have symptoms not appear until several months of age, when they may have "tet spells"—acute onset of cyanosis, dyspnea, irritability, or syncope due to increased right-to-left shunting secondary to stress or crying. Physical examination is typically dominated by the presence of a harsh systolic murmur secondary to pulmonary stenosis.

Diagnosis is typically confirmed on echocardiography, which easily shows the four defects. Chest X-ray may show a "boot-shaped" heart due to right ventricular enlargement. Cardiac MRI or CT and cardiac catheterization are used for detailed anatomical assessment, especially in complex cases or preoperative evaluation. Surgical correction is the preferred treatment. Complete repair usually involves patch closure of the VSD and relief of obstruction of the RVOT by removing muscle and, if indicated, augmentation of the pulmonary valve or artery. The operation typically is performed early in infancy, but it may be performed at a different point based on the infant's status. In others, especially when the pulmonary arteries are too small, a palliative operation like a Blalock-Taussig shunt is done to augment pulmonary blood flow until repair is possible.

Late outcomes following surgical repair are generally good but need lifelong follow-up. Complications can include pulmonary valve regurgitation, residual RVOT obstruction, arrhythmia, and right ventricular dysfunction. Reoperation or catheter-based therapy will be necessary in some individuals later in life.

Several defects are closely related to TOF and may be considered part of the TOF spectrum. These include:

1. **TOF with Pulmonary Atresia:** A more severe form where the pulmonary valve is completely closed, often requiring staged surgical repair and use of conduits.
2. **TOF with Major Aortopulmonary Collateral Arteries (MAPCAs):** Where abnormal vessels supply the lungs, requiring complex surgical planning.
3. **Double Outlet Right Ventricle (DORV):** Both great arteries arise from the right ventricle, sometimes resembling TOF anatomically and functionally.

References

1. Abulimiti, K., Ma, Z., Abudureheman, A., Aizezi, Y., Abudunaiyimu, S., Shi, L., Bolatihan, B., et al. (2025). Retrospective analysis of clinical characteristics and surgical treatment of congenital heart disease complicated by infective endocarditis from 2009 to 2023. *The Heart Surgery Forum.* https://www.semanticscholar.org/paper/f7d401a2d7fe26be9f408b1ecd7286aaed1b0e8d (accessed on 15th July 2025).

2. Ahamd, B., Ashraf, R., Naseem, C., Ullah, K., Ali, S., & Raza, M. (2025). Correlation of multidetector computed tomography and transthoracic echocardiography in the diagnosis of congenital cyanotic heart diseases. *Kashf Journal of Multidisciplinary Research.* https://www.semanticscholar.org/paper/6db9f9c10e40161f26cef9aeee2dd9b5f263a3de (accessed on 15th July 2025).

3. Albisetti, M., Tartakovsky, I., Halton, J., Bomgaars, L., Chalmers, E., Mitchell, L. G., Luciani, M., et al. (2024). Dabigatran for treatment and secondary prevention of venous thromboembolism in pediatric congenital heart disease. *Journal of the American Heart Association: Cardiovascular and Cerebrovascular Disease, 13.* https://www.semanticscholar.org/paper/562608203bc2f3f9976a80db00a0b4904a4c2f6d (accessed on 15th July 2025).

4. Alsaied, T., Aboulhosn, J., Cotts, T. B., Daniels, C. J., Etheridge, S. P., Feltes, T. F., Gurvitz, M., et al. (2020). Coronavirus disease 2019 (COVID-19) pandemic implications in pediatric and adult congenital heart disease. *Journal of the American Heart Association, 9.* https://doi.org/10.1161/jaha.120.017224 (accessed on 15th July 2025).

5. Amin, P., Ahmed, I., Hussain, A., Omair, M., Lashari, A. A., & Tayyab, M. (2024). Anesthetic management of a patient with Tetralogy of Fallot for cesarean section. *Pakistan Armed Forces Medical Journal.* https://www.semanticscholar.org/paper/b0944dfa02baaad96a4c767fda1b5f1c61316359 (accessed on 15th July 2025).

6. Areias, J., Areias, M., Castro, M., Freitas, D., et al. (2013). A cohort study on psychosocial adjustment and psychopathology in adolescents and young adults with congenital heart disease. https://core.ac.uk/download/143405020.pdf (accessed on 15th July 2025).

7. Ashraf, H., Pandya, K., Wack, M. F., & Sawada, S. G. (2019). Complications of pulmonic valve endocarditis in repaired tetralogy of Fallot. *Journal of Cardiovascular Echography, 29*, 123–123. https://doi.org/10.4103/jcecho.jcecho_17_19 (accessed on 15th July 2025).

8. Atiq, M., & Humayun, K. N. (2008). Clinical profile and outcome of cyanotic congenital heart disease in neonates. https://core.ac.uk/download/47257387.pdf (accessed on 15th July 2025).

9. Batra, A. S., Silka, M., Borquez, A., Cuneo, B., Dechert, B., Jaeggi, E., Kannankeril, P. J., et al. (2024). Pharmacological management of cardiac arrhythmias in the fetal and neonatal periods: A scientific statement from the American Heart Association: Endorsed by the Pediatric & Congenital Electrophysiology Society (PACES). *Circulation.* https://www.semanticscholar.org/paper/bad527fd1dc2a7925238441497bb9e574decfd6d (accessed on 15th July 2025).

10. Baumgartner, H., De Backer, J., Babu-Narayan, S. V., Budts, W., Chessa, M., Diller, G. P., Lung, B., et al. (2020). 2020 ESC guidelines for the management of adult congenital heart disease. *European Heart Journal, 42*, 563–645. https://doi.org/10.1093/eurheartj/ehaa554 (accessed on 15th July 2025).

11. Bokulich, N. A., Ellis, C. L., Elumalai, J., Haapanen, L., et al. (2013). Probiotic administration in congenital heart disease: A pilot study. https://core.ac.uk/download/323071651.pdf (accessed on 15th July 2025).

12. Calcinotto, A., Kohli, J., Zagato, E., Pellegrini, L., Demaria, M., & Alimonti, A. (2019). Cellular senescence: Aging, cancer, and injury. *Physiological Reviews, 99*, 1047–1078. https://doi.org/10.1152/physrev.00020.2018 (accessed on 15th July 2025).

13. Chau, A. K. T., Cheuk, D. K. L., Cheung, Y. F., Choi, Y., et al. (2004). Parents' understanding of their child's congenital heart disease. https://core.ac.uk/download/37881538.pdf (accessed on 15th July 2025).

14. Cullen, S., Deanfield, J., Fteropoulli, T., Newman, C., et al. (2013). Quality of life of adult congenital heart disease patients: A systematic review of the literature. https://core.ac.uk/download/9982967.pdf (accessed on 15th July 2025).

15. Cyran, S. E., & Geskey, J. M. (2011). Managing the morbidity associated with respiratory viral infections in children with congenital heart disease. https://core.ac.uk/download/pdf/8693930.pdf (accessed on 15th July 2025).

16. Diller, G. P. (2009). Pathophysiologic correlates of exercise intolerance in adults with pulmonary hypertension and congenital heart disease. https://core.ac.uk/download/17294714.pdf (accessed on 15th July 2025).

17. Duman, D., & Karpuz, D. (2024). Current follow-up results of cyanotic congenital heart diseases detected during pregnancy in a specific region. *Journal of Contemporary Medicine.* https://www.semanticscholar.org/paper/ff2dc2effac05a93308ebd6831533acf68037bea (accessed on 15th July 2025).

18. Eilers, L., Kyle, W. B., Allen, H. D., & Qureshi, A. M. (2021). Patent ductus arteriosus. *Pediatrics in Review, 42*, 632–634. https://doi.org/10.1542/pir.2020-004564 (accessed on 15th July 2025).

19. Fedorczak, A., Kruk, B., Mazurek-Kula, A., Kępczyński, Ł., & Stawerska, R. (2025). Resistance to thyroid hormone in a boy with a severe, complex, congenital heart defect (CHD) requiring multiple cardiac surgeries—Whether and how to prepare child for the surgery. *Journal of Clinical Medicine, 14.* https://www.semanticscholar.org/paper/2f6593d629b64ff845bce5da2f6b7d7d0745aa3f (accessed on 15th July 2025).

20. Ghasemi Shayan, R., Fatollahzadeh Dizaji, M., & Sajjadian, F. (2025). Surgical and postoperative management of congenital heart disease: A systematic review of observational studies. *Langenbeck's Archives of Surgery, 410.* https://www.semanticscholar.org/paper/d066cd7407e9a298270437d31e8635f9fc7db5e6 (accessed on 15th July 2025).

21. Harvey, D. C., Verma, R., Sedaghat, B., Hjelm, B. E., Morton, S. U., Seidman, J. G., & Kumar, S. R. (2023). Mutations in genes related to myocyte contraction and ventricular septum development in non-syndromic tetralogy of Fallot. *Frontiers in Cardiovascular Medicine, 10.* https://doi.org/10.3389/fcvm.2023.1249605 (accessed on 15th July 2025).

22. Ilyas, S., Rehman, Y., Hussain, I., Khan, A., Rajput, T. A., & Ali, A. (2021). Emergency department presentation and outcome of children with cyanotic congenital heart diseases. *Cureus.* https://doi.org/10.7759/cureus.17960 (accessed on 15th July 2025).

23. Iolascon, A., Bianchi, P., Andolfo, I., Russo, R., Barcellini, W., Fermo, E., Toldi, G., et al. (2021). Recommendations for diagnosis and treatment of methemoglobinemia. *American Journal of Hematology, 96,* 1666–1678. https://doi.org/10.1002/ajh.26340 (accessed on 15th July 2025).

24. Kaiser, A. E., Husnain, M. A., Alam, L. F., Murugan, S. K., & Kumar, R. (2024). Management of Fallot's uncorrected tetralogy in adulthood: A narrative review. *Cureus, 16.* https://www.semanticscholar.org/paper/b4a346833a8805ff754d1f68e0d23a3efb4d1da7 (accessed on 15th July 2025).

25. Kamal, A. F., Mostafa, F. A. Z., Fakher, W., Soltan, A., & Abdelraouf, M. M. (2024). Cognitive assessment in children with congenital heart diseases after cardiac surgeries. *Pediatric Sciences Journal.* https://www.semanticscholar.org/paper/0b74b57e0a380d1fbf96eb9338343b4790676751 (accessed on 15th July 2025).

26. Khan, M. K. (2025). Management of dental problems in a case of Tetralogy of Fallot. *Journal of Datta Meghe Institute of Medical Sciences University.* https://www.semanticscholar.org/paper/10eebe3a9a884bdf90c58251d1190ccffc5d7efa (accessed on 15th July 2025).

27. Khedewy, A., Abdel Aal, M., & Kassem, M. (2024). Patterns of congenital heart diseases at Sohag University Hospital. *Sohag Medical Journal.* https://www.semanticscholar.org/paper/b5f6fa8ca9f8fd30708ac0438ab6a0265b06a230 (accessed on 15th July 2025).

28. Konstam, M. A., Kiernan, M. S., Bernstein, D., Bozkurt, B., Jacob, M., Kapur, N. K., Kociol, R. D., et al. (2018). Evaluation and management of right-sided heart failure: A scientific statement from the American Heart Association. *Circulation, 137.* https://doi.org/10.1161/cir.0000000000000560 (accessed on 15th July 2025).

29. Kozik, D. (2019). Neurodevelopmental outcomes in pediatric extracorporeal membrane oxygenation. *ASAIO Journal, 66,* 89–90. https://doi.org/10.1097/mat.0000000000001112 (accessed on 15th July 2025).

30. Lim, T. B., Foo, S. Y. R., & Chen, C. K. (2021). The role of epigenetics in congenital heart disease. *Genes, 12,* 390. https://doi.org/10.3390/genes12030390 (accessed on 15th July 2025).

31. Liu, H. C., Chaou, C. H., Lo, C. W., Chung, H. T., & Hwang, M. S. (2022). Factors affecting psychological and health-related quality-of-life status in children and adolescents with congenital heart diseases. *Children, 9,* 578. https://doi.org/10.3390/children9040578 (accessed on 15th July 2025).

32. Martini, S., Beghetti, I., Annunziata, M., Aceti, A., Galletti, S., Ragni, L., Donti, A., et al. (2021). Enteral nutrition in term infants with congenital heart disease: Knowledge gaps and future directions to improve clinical practice. *Nutrients, 13,* 932. https://doi.org/10.3390/nu13030932 (accessed on 15th July 2025).

33. Mehta, L. S., Warnes, C. A., Bradley, E. A., Burton, T., Economy, K. E., Mehran, R., Safdar, B., et al. (2020). Cardiovascular considerations in caring for pregnant patients: A scientific statement from the American Heart Association. *Circulation, 141.* https://doi.org/10.1161/cir.0000000000000772 (accessed on 15th July 2025).

34. Osawa, T., Machino, T., Saji, M., Sumita, Y., Kanaoka, K., Kawamatsu, N., & Ishizu, T. (2024). Risk factors of 30-day mortality following cardiac surgery in adults with congenital heart disease: Analysis from the Japanese registry. *European Heart Journal.* https://www.semanticscholar.org/paper/17b5a8af059c65f4f1503b288f345efe16f11e92 (accessed on 15th July 2025).

35. Patel, K., Lin, T. K., Clark, J., Ceneviva, G., Imundo, J. R., Spear, D., Kunselman, A. R., et al. (2024). Randomized trial of pulsatile and nonpulsatile flow in cyanotic and acyanotic congenital heart surgery. *World Journal for Pediatric & Congenital Heart Surgery, 16*, 329–337. https://www.semanticscholar.org/paper/0af5d7074b16cbb13308f76aaa44a9abb55102bd (accessed on 15th July 2025).

36. Rabbani, G. M. (2025). A case report of a 10-month-old child diagnosed with tricuspid valve atresia. *Medicine Today.* https://www.semanticscholar.org/paper/bb04204cfe9741001fd8460bde1d26d1ae12d24f (accessed on 15th July 2025).

37. Román-Rodríguez, A., Silva-Lago, R., Gallego-Sánchez, J. A., Silva-Ramos, L., & Díaz Rodríguez, D. R. (2025). An unusual congenital heart disease, Pentalogy of Fallot. *South Health and Policy.* https://www.semanticscholar.org/paper/eef60911a75ad6c0c79ce3c91f73fa693569b2ca (accessed on 15th July 2025).

38. ST-Amour, P. (2015). Impacts of prenatal ultrasound on morbidity and mortality of cardiac pathologies in pediatrics. https://core.ac.uk/download/84058610.pdf (accessed on 15th July 2025).

39. Stout, K., Daniels, C. J., Aboulhosn, J., Bozkurt, B., Broberg, C. S., Colman, J. M., Crumb, S. R., et al. (2018). 2018 AHA/ACC guideline for the management of adults with congenital heart disease: A report of the American College of Cardiology/American Heart Association Task Force on Clinical Practice Guidelines. *Circulation, 139.* https://doi.org/10.1161/cir.0000000000000603 (accessed on 15th July 2025).

40. Talwar, S., Subramaniam, K. G., Bhende, V. V., Krishnakumar, M., & Pathak, H. (2025). The legacy of innovation: A comprehensive review of eponymous procedures in thoracic, congenital, and pediatric heart diseases. *Cureus, 17.* https://www.semanticscholar.org/paper/f73c9a2d8bce52ef95fd45450abf2d921e428669 (accessed on 15th July 2025).

41. Walker, K., Specht, I., Hjortdal, V., Christesen, H., Heitmann, B. L., Santorelli, G., West, J., et al. (2025). Circulating 25-hydroxyvitamin D levels during pregnancy and risk of congenital heart diseases: Multivariable and Mendelian randomization analyses using 3 birth cohorts. *Journal of the American Heart Association.* https://www.semanticscholar.org/paper/a6c7826711b19d9edf64e08b434a2f13e9cfebb2 (accessed on 15th July 2025).

42. Yang, W., Chen, I., & Lu, W. (2021). International commercial air transport of the child with severe cyanotic congenital heart disease. *Journal of Pediatrics and Child Health, 58.* https://www.semanticscholar.org/paper/16a15d588ceb7c680dbbc17220662eca0805b99c (accessed on 15th July 2025).

43. Yogi, R. N., Awasthi, S. R., Mandal, A. K., Shahi, K., Thani, K., & Pradhan, S. (2025). Delayed diagnosis of tricuspid atresia: A case report. *Journal of Nepal Medical Association.* https://www.semanticscholar.org/paper/e06bdb58c94cc096393205e168be3c6cf8339f12 (accessed on 15th July 2025).

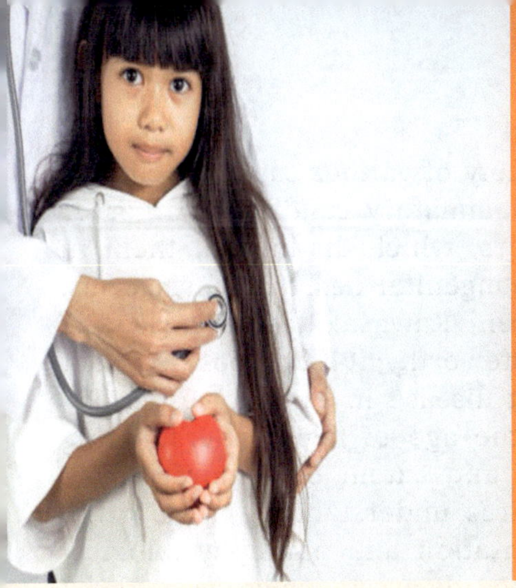

Chapter 8

ACQUIRED HEART DISEASES IN CHILDREN

Contents

Introduction

The prevalence of acquired heart diseases (AHD) in children is a serious public health problem, dwarfed by that of congenital heart diseases. AHD is a diverse group of cardiac disorders that manifest after birth due to various factors, including infections, rheumatic fever, and lifestyle behaviors. Unlike congenital heart diseases, which are congenital, AHD can manifest at any age, making early detection and treatment problematic. It is critical to know the epidemiology of AHD because delayed presentation usually leads to severe complications and increased mortality. For instance, in Nigerian pediatric research, myocarditis and dilated cardiomyopathy were the most common forms of AHD, and more diagnostic and therapeutic efforts are required to diagnose and treat these conditions in children (Daniels et al., 2014). Therefore, growing awareness of AHD brings to the fore the importance of early diagnosis in being able to salvage young lives. Apart from the sheer health implications, AHD has the tendency to cause a great deal of distress among caregivers and families. The signs can be mild or extensive, and differential diagnosis is further complicated. Clinical presentation in most children will be non-specific or mild, with repeated episodes of respiratory infection and failure to thrive, without any specific conditions that are typically encountered in primary care clinics. The lack of a clear presentation will likely result in delayed diagnosis, which may make the disease more severe and affect health outcomes negatively. Research has established that the early detection and effective diagnosis of symptoms play a vital role in the prevention of AHD-related complications (Sreeman et al., 2017). As acquired heart disease spreads variably globally, public health measures and education programs have to be tailored to equip healthcare professionals with the necessary tools to diagnose and cure these disorders effectively. The prevalence of AHD in children parallels more universal epidemiological trends influenced by local healthcare practices and environmental factors. In the majority of developing countries, such as Nigeria, AHD prevalence is increasing significantly, presenting special challenges to healthcare systems that perhaps are not equipped to offer complete cardiac care. The escalating incidence of conditions like rheumatic heart disease in various geographical regions necessitates re-examination of existing healthcare policies and investment in cardiac care units. Moreover, patterns of AHD distribution underscore the need for preventive interventions and public health interventions to reduce risk factors for cardiovascular diseases, including childhood infections (Daniels et al., 2014). By promoting awareness and early diagnosis, we hope to decrease the prevalence of AHD and improve overall cardiovascular outcomes in children globally.

Definition of Acquired Heart Diseases

Acquired heart diseases are those which arise in childhood after birth and are not of congenital nature. These diseases can be the result of a variety of various causes, including infections, inflammatory conditions, or other extrinsic factors, which distinguish them in nature from congenital heart malformations. Among children, Kawasaki disease (KD) is particularly noteworthy; it is the most frequent acquired heart disease in children, especially those below the age of five. Understanding the definition and extent of acquired heart diseases requires understanding of both the clinical presentation and pathophysiological process of these diseases, which are often a cause of such complications as coronary artery injury. Efforts at standardization of treatment and diagnosis procedures for acquired diseases like KD demonstrate the necessity for modifying healthcare practice and indicate the importance of early identification and intervention towards the management of pediatric acquired heart disease (N/A, 2023). The presentation of acquired heart diseases in children can be extremely variable, usually depending on the etiological factors present. Diseases such as myocarditis, pericarditis, and rheumatic heart disease may arise as significant acquired heart ailments to cause concern to clinicians. All these conditions impair cardiac function and cause severe long-term damage if left untreated. For instance, myocarditis most often follows viral infections leading to inflammation of the heart muscle, whereas pericarditis may occur secondary to infection or autoimmune conditions. Furthermore, rheumatic fever, a complication of untreated streptococcal infection, could initiate chronic heart valve damage. All of these conditions should be strictly followed up and treated with targeted treatments to relieve symptoms and prevent further complications, particularly since it is a crucial year in the formative years of a child's life (Justin et al., 2021). Pediatric acquired heart disease requires multidisciplinary care, integrating cardiology, infectious disease, and at times rheumatology for proper management. Interventions can vary from medications to surgical intervention, depending on the intensity and type of the diagnosis. For example, pediatricians may utilize anti-inflammatory drugs for Kawasaki disease in order to reduce inflammation of the arteries or prescribe echocardiographic surveillance in order to monitor the heart function over a period. As outlined in today's guidelines, a critical element is the formulation of accurate procedures for early diagnosis and treatment of such conditions in order to enhance patient outcomes and reduce morbidity. Ultimately, the accurate characterization and adequate awareness of acquired heart diseases should provide effective healthcare interventions and emphasize the need for ongoing research and education among the pediatric cardiology community (N/A, 2023) (Figure 8.1).

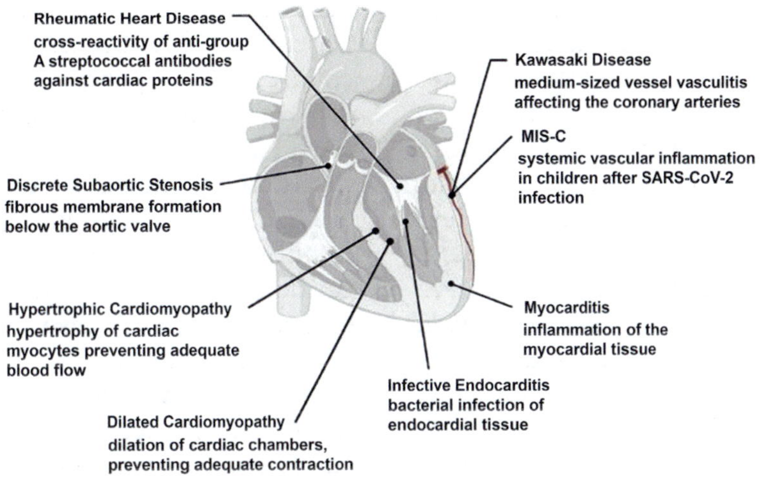

Figure 8.1. Overview of acquired pediatric heart disease.

Source: https://www.researchgate.net/figure/Overview-of-acquired-pediatric-heart-disease-Acquired-pediatric-heart-diseases-can-arise_fig1_353482574.

Importance of Studying Heart Diseases in Children

One of the key aspects to understanding acquired heart diseases in children relates to an active health approach. Investigations on these diseases not only lead to prompt detection and treatment but also to the development of comprehensive guidelines on management. A case in point is screening for lipids in all children that provides a platform for preventing long-term cardiovascular disease outcomes. This screening is particularly critical in children with chronic diseases predisposing them to premature atherosclerosis, indicating the relevance of certain healthcare interventions. National policies emphasize the aspect that children with certain cardiac diseases need to be offered additional early screening for early detection and treatment of risk factors that may have permanent effects on their overall long-term health condition (Berger et al., 2022). Thus, the greater priority for preventive care and knowledge of heart diseases is required to ensure future good health for this risk group. Further, the importance of studying heart diseases extends beyond individual health, affecting public health vision more generally. Evidence indicates that the majority of children with acquired heart disease present with multiple complications affecting their quality of life. Some determinants, like the incidence of chronic diseases, the impact of invasive procedures, and even the socioeconomic determinants of health, could exacerbate these conditions. Conditions such as cardiomyopathy are most frequently identified with higher rates of comorbidities in children and therefore need extensive research in their risk factors and mechanisms. Identification of such correlations supports the development of specialized interventions, as well as training caregivers and medical professionals on the necessity of exercising keen observation and bespoke management tools to cater to the exact requirements of children suffering from heart diseases (Baalaaji, 2022). It improves the effectiveness of allocating resources towards uncovering these complex medical conditions, which contributes to positive health outcomes for affected children. Finally, the studies of heart diseases among children are crucial to advancing treatment and rates of survival. Pediatric cardiology previously learned less than adult cardiology, and there were gaps in treatment for children. With increased research and focus on acquired heart diseases, significant advances have been developed in therapies and interventions that benefit children. By studying these conditions, the efficacy of treatment for different interventions can be measured, paving the way for evidence-based interventions tailored to the individual physiological characteristics of children. Moreover, having information regarding the results of long-term effects of therapies used in this population is important to ensure survival as well as quality of life following recovery. Therefore, a focused emphasis on the study of pediatric heart ailments remains central to the development of a healthcare system that prioritizes the longevity and well-being of such affected people (Berger et al., 2022).

8.1. Types of Acquired Heart Diseases

Acquired heart disorders of children are many conditions that have not been present at birth but evolve over time depending on a number of factors including infections, metabolic disorders, and environmental issues. Among these, rheumatic heart disease is a major one. This develops after an infection of the throat caused by *Streptococcus*. The immune response can lead to inflammation of the heart valve with long-term consequences if left undiagnosed early. A study asserts despite a better quality of medical care, rheumatic fever continues to be prevalent in low socioeconomic regions, necessitating preventive approaches that focus on early identification and treatment of pharyngeal infections. Similarly, Kawasaki disease, a disease acquired in life, occurs predominantly among children who are under the age of five years and can lead to inflammation of coronary arteries. Early treatment is required to prevent life-threatening cardiovascular complications of these diseases, highlighting the importance of attentive monitoring of child health. Dilated cardiomyopathy is a significant other category of acquired heart diseases characterized by inefficient pumping of blood by the hearts since the left ventricle is enlarged. It can lead to congestive heart failure, arrhythmias, and sudden cardiac death if left untreated. This disorder has a variety of etiologic factors, including viral infection and toxins, complicating diagnosis and treatment. Pediatric cardiologists advocate thorough evaluation to identify occult causes and choose appropriate therapies. New therapies, including drugs and, in some cases, heart transplantation, are applicable to improving results in affected children. An understanding of the multidetermined etiology of dilated cardiomyopathy acknowledges the paramount role of research and education in enhancing the range of management options available to these patients. Myocarditis, or heart muscle inflammation typically resulting from viral infections, is also a similarly critical type of acquired heart disease in children. This condition may present with varied symptomatology, ranging from complaints of mild chest pain to devastating heart failure. Early echocardiography and cardiac MRI diagnosis is crucial to ascertain the severity of myocarditis and to guide appropriate management. Proper public health measures to prevent viral infections are of utmost necessity, as certain pathogens have been linked with outbreaks of myocarditis among children. Additionally, family and community awareness of the symptomatology and signs will ensure prompter intervention, aiming for improved prognostic outcomes among affected children. Integrated care using multidisciplinary teams, as is true for other acquired heart disorders, is central to long-term improvement in health in children that are faced by these conditions.

8.1.1. Rheumatic Heart Disease

Rheumatic heart disease (RHD) is a life-threatening manifestation of rheumatic fever, itself a consequence of untreated streptococcal pharyngitis. The autoimmune process may result in inflammation of the heart valves and chronic damage, particularly in children. Because of its association with poverty and inadequate health systems, RHD disproportionately affects children living in low- and middle-income countries, where early detection and effective antibiotic prophylaxis against streptococcal infection are generally suboptimal. Its occurrence among children in these groups highlights a priority public health issue, warranted by greater alertness and preventive measures directed toward decreasing its effect. The effects of RHD extend beyond the clinical environment, as it could also have significant social and economic consequences for infected families and communities, taking into consideration the associated healthcare costs and decreased quality of life for affected children. The course of RHD is variable in the clinic but more often valvular heart disease, heart failure, and cardiovascular complications. Since RHD is a progressive disorder, children develop signs such as fatigue, dyspnea, and arrhythmias, which can significantly impair their physical performance and well-being. The pathophysiologic process involves the formation of antibodies against cardiac tissue, followed by chronic inflammation and scarring of the heart valves. Prevention remains the cornerstone of RHD management, as secondary prophylaxis with antibiotics can substantially reduce the incidence of recurrent rheumatic fever in at-risk individuals (Figure 8.2).

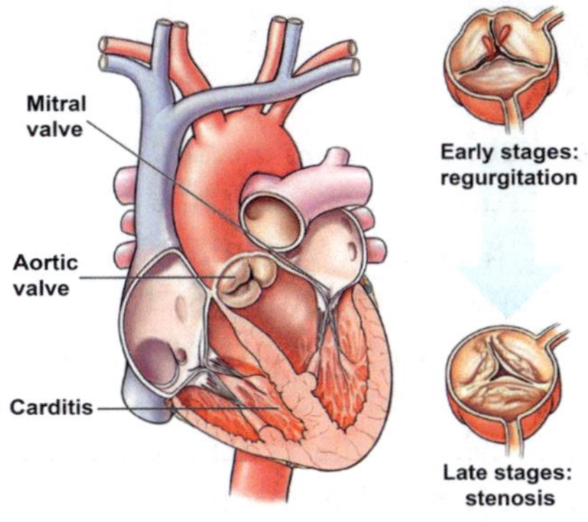

Figure 8.2. Rheumatic heart disease.

Source: https://my.clevelandclinic.org/-/scassets/images/org/health/articles/rheumatic-heart-disease.jpg.

However, poor access to healthcare and poor education regarding the disease are forcing delayed treatment and poor health outcomes. Closing these gaps in the guise of community education and improved healthcare infrastructure is important in reducing the burden of RHD on affected populations. Research into rheumatic heart disease identifies rising interest in precision medicine approaches that will aim to improve diagnostics and treatments tailored to the individual patient's special needs. While therapeutic approaches remain sparse, progress in knowledge regarding the genetic and environmental contributions towards RHD is pivotal in ensuring tailored intervention. Precision medicine incorporation endeavors to streamline guidelines for treatment, with the long-term aim of enhanced management regimens and outcomes in children with RHD. The need to delineate high-risk individuals early, according to research, is thought to have a universal role in ensuring the alleviation of harmful effects on the disease. However, effective utilization of such measures is contingent on overcoming existing healthcare disparities and harmonization of efforts among medical practitioners, researchers, and policy-makers. Consistent with recent reviews, it is critically important to continue integrating precision medicine into global health programs in a bid to effectively combat rheumatic heart disease (Khan et al., 2024; Marhaba et al., 2025).

8.1.2. Kawasaki Disease

Kawasaki disease (KD) is a critical and emerging problem of pediatric cardiology, the most frequent acquired cardiac illness of children, and particularly of children less than five years of age. It is an etiologic unknown vasculitis that is characterized by prolonged fever, conjunctivitis, rash, and lymphadenopathy and, unless treated, will generate severe cardiovascular complications. In fact, approximately 25% of untreated KD children develop coronary artery aneurysms, a condition that can result in future morbidity or mortality. Awareness of the clinical presentation and early diagnosis of KD is thus crucial because children who have symptoms must realize that they must seek immediate medical attention to prevent complications arising from coronary artery involvement, and also emphasizing the need for clinicians' awareness for early detection of the disease (Jone et al., 2024) (Figure 8.3).

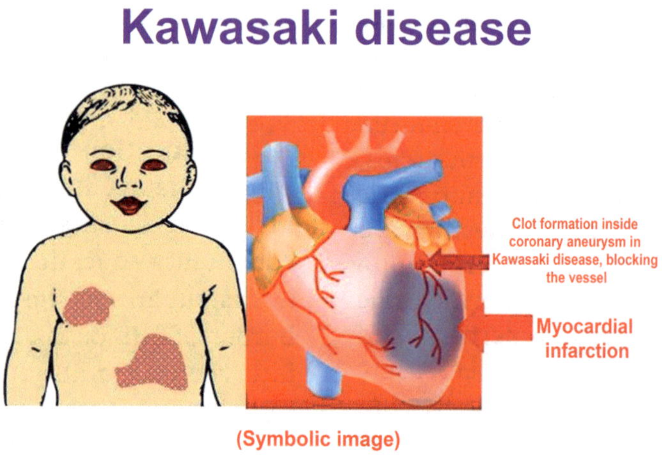

Figure 8.3. Manifestations of Kawasaki disease.

Source: https://johnsonfrancis.org/professional/awasaki-disease-and-coronary-involvement/.

Quick and effective treatment of Kawasaki disease typically includes intravenous administration of immunoglobulin (IVIG), which has been shown to reduce the risk of cardiovascular complications significantly. Use of the therapy has lowered the incidence of coronary artery aneurysms from 25% to around 4% in treated patients. But it does not stop there; long-term follow-up and ongoing monitoring is the essence. Children with Kawasaki disease require regular cardiovascular assessment (i.e., imaging studies) to monitor stenosis or thrombosis. Regular medical management (e.g., potential lifelong thromboprophylaxis) is important in cardiovascular risk management and giving a benefit of quality of life for these children (Jone et al., 2024). Despite improvement in treatment and imaging diagnostics, some aspects of ignorance regarding appropriate management and follow-up techniques for children with Kawasaki disease remain. As the science unfolds, there is an important need for clinicians to be updated with the latest available therapeutic strategies and practices, in order to optimize results in these at-risk patients more effectively. This entails the detection of at-risk patients who may require more intensive upfront treatment protocols. With advancements in novel anti-inflammatory medications and anticoagulant therapy, clinical practice guidelines must be revised to reflect their perceived risks and benefits so that optimal management of Kawasaki disease and its complications is ensured in children (Malska et al., 2024) (Figure 8.4).

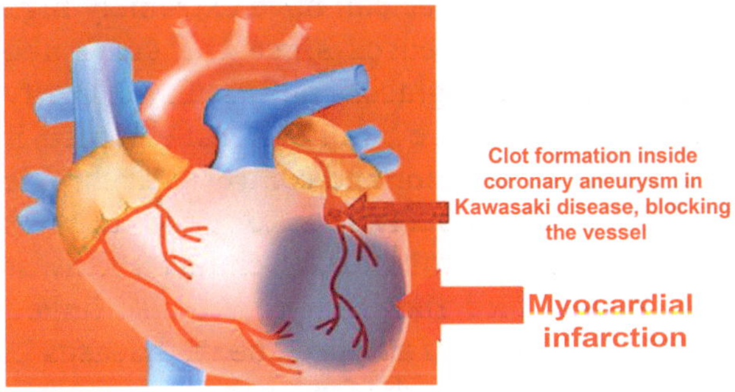

Figure 8.4. Diagrammatic representation.

Source: https://johnsonfrancis.org/professional/kawasaki-disease-and-coronary-involvement/.

8.1.3. Infective Endocarditis

Infective endocarditis, a condition involving inflammation of the inner heart lining, is increasingly being understood as a significant illness among the pediatric population, and particularly that with congenital heart disease. The relative rarity of infective endocarditis in healthy children presents in stark contrast to increased frequency in subjects with previous heart disease, which calls for early detection in order to administer optimal therapy. *Streptococcus viridans* and *Staphylococcus aureus* remain the most frequent causative organisms. The clinical presentation of this disease can be catastrophic, often leading to valvular insufficiency, heart failure, or emboli within the systemic circulation, potentially causing death if untreated. Furthermore, while most children affected by the condition can be seen to have a favorable outcome with early diagnosis and treatment, those with pre-existing cardiac anomalies are at far greater risk, underlining the need for ongoing surveillance and preventive efforts in this high-risk group (Jung et al., 2014). The role of healthcare environments in the evolution of new infective agents, such as extended-spectrum β-lactamase-producing *Klebsiella pneumonia* (ESBL-KP), contributes to the challenges in managing infective endocarditis in children. Surprisingly, the prevalence of ESBL-KP infective endocarditis remains low but with high morbidity and mortality. Risk of infection is also further increased in hospitalized children, particularly those who undergo invasive procedures or compromised immune systems. The distinctive characteristics of ESBL-producing organisms require a re-shaping of clinical practices and guidelines for treatment. Pediatricians and health-care providers must be vigilant in the management of these pathogens, especially in the case of health-care-associated infective endocarditis, to make accurate diagnosis and maximize management (Jung et al., 2014) (Figure 8.5).

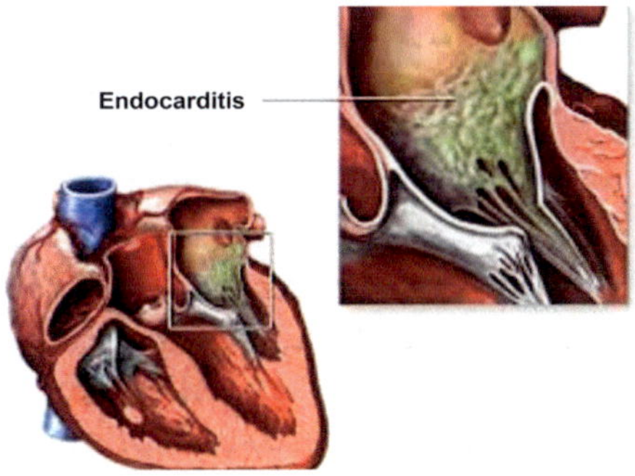

Figure 8.5. Endocarditis.

Source: https://encrypted-tbn0.gstatic.com/images?q=tbn:And9GcRthYlXp-76QtK_IP9HvBgfZ5c5djngMZr37Q&s.

Lastly, familiarity with treatment regimens for infective endocarditis in the pediatric arena must be achieved in order to optimize patient outcomes. Current treatment regimens typically involve intravenous antibiotic therapy over a long term and, in some cases, valve replacement by surgery of infected valves. For the emerging pathogenic patterns of bacteria like *Klebsiella pneumoniae*, treatment regimens must be designed to effectively treat resistant organisms, which could include directed carbapenems. With ongoing research, keeping abreast of current best practice in management of infective endocarditis is crucial, especially as new pathogens emerge and infective complications in children with comorbid conditions arise. Sensitive and informed education of healthcare workers will be the key to reducing incidence and mortality from this serious acquired cardiac disease in children (Edgar et al., 2001).

8.2. Causes and Risk Factors

The intimate interaction of environmental factors and the pathogenesis of acquired heart disease in children must not be overstated. Children are particularly vulnerable to chronic health effects of environmental toxins and pollutants; such exposures may have profound effects on cardiovascular health over the long term. For instance, there have been correlations noted between air quality degradation, such as increased airborne particulate matter, and the occurrence of diseases like Kawasaki disease, an acquired heart disease. Also, developing bodies in children are more susceptible to these environmental insults, which can result in the build-up of a variety of cardiovascular risk factors. This underscores the need for environmental health programs to be a priority among policymakers and healthcare workers because protection measures can reduce such risks and achieve better health outcomes for children (Justin et al., 2024). Apart from the environment, pre-existing medical conditions like diabetes contribute significantly to the prevalence of acquired heart diseases in children. Diabetes mellitus is not just a metabolic disorder; it triggers a cascade of medical complications that includes cardiovascular risks. Hyperglycemia or increased blood glucose affects the immune system and renders a person susceptible to infections such as pneumonia, which secondarily affects cardiovascular morbidity. In children, undiagnosed diabetes can have extremely high risks for heart diseases since the combined effects of increased glucose on vascular integrity and inflammation are bound to ensue. Hence, it is necessary to monitor and control such chronic conditions continuously so as to reduce the risk of heart diseases in suffering children (Anwar et al., 2024). Diet and lifestyle are also linked with the induction of acquired heart diseases in children. Poor diet, in the form of overindulgence in processed food and sugar, accompanied by inactivity, is a key cause of obesity rates rising and with it associated cardiovascular disease. Early formation of bad habits sets the stage for long-term health consequences, including hypertension and dyslipidemia, which are robust predictors of heart disease. School programs that encourage healthy eating and frequent physical activity among children are major prevention measures. Through intervention of these modifiable risk factors, there is a possible decrease in the incidence of acquired heart diseases in subsequent generations, inducing better total cardiovascular health (Justin et al., 2024).

8.2.1. Genetic Predispositions

Genetic susceptibility plays an important role in the pathogenesis of acquired heart ailments in children, typically combined with environmental factors. Children with a history of coronary artery disease (CAD) in the family have been reported to be at increased risk of developing these conditions, demonstrating the role of hereditary influences. For instance, research established that children of individuals diagnosed with CAD have greater levels of serum lipoprotein(a) and overall cholesterol compared to same-aged peers without a corresponding family history, which is an indication of a direct connection between genetic risk and CAD risk factors (Saxena et al., 2025). This finding is highlighted by the necessity for regular tests in children who have a family history of heart disease, both to monitor for potential health issues and to act preventatively before problems arise. Furthermore, the intricate interplay of genetic predispositions and the actual causes of cardiovascular disease demands a thorough study of specific biological markers. Recent research of microRNAs (miRNAs) shows their potential as important regulators of the development of heart condition, especially in the pediatric population. The short RNA molecules are involved in a variety of regulatory processes, such as gene expression associated with heart disease. The ability of these molecules to control cell proliferation, differentiation, and apoptosis shows that genetically mediated variations in miRNA profiles could be an important aspect of vulnerability to heart disease (Pas et al., 2024) (Figure 8.6).

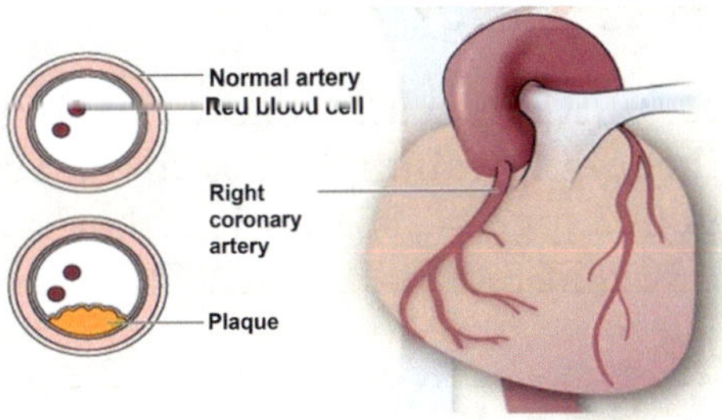

Figure 8.6. Coronary artery disease (CAD).

Source: https://www.maxlab.co.in/categoryimage/1667374386.jpg.

Therefore, the study of how such genetic markers interact with environmental determinants can provide more information on the etiology and pathogenesis of acquired heart diseases and provide avenues for diagnostic and therapeutic innovation. In addition, the interdependence of genetics and lifestyle factors makes it imperative that acquired heart disease in children be addressed through an integral approach. Environmental influences, such as diet, physical exercise, and exposure to pollutants, can exacerbate the effect of genetic tendencies. As a rising pattern of sedentary lifestyles among children, interaction between genetic risk factors and unhealthy living conditions becomes dangerously concentrated. According to studies, sedentary lifestyle compounded by genetic tendency significantly heightens the danger of acquiring cardiovascular disease at a young age (Saxena et al., 2025). Therefore, promoting health awareness for the heart in terms of lifestyle modification and individualized interventions, particularly among risk groups, becomes a necessity. It not only decreases the short-term burden of genetic vulnerabilities but also promotes long-term cardiovascular health in children.

8.2.2. Environmental Influences

The environmental determinants of secondary heart diseases in children are a complex interplay of multiple determinants. Among the salient considerations is air quality, or the impact of air pollutants such as particulate matter, nitrogen dioxide, and sulfur dioxide, which can exacerbate pre-existing cardiovascular diseases or are causative agents. Studies have shown that children who have been exposed to contaminated air are liable to develop inflammatory responses that will condition them to cardiovascular issues. Widespread exposure to these harmful chemicals over an extended period of time interferes with normal cardiovascular development and function, such that it is vital that there be effective policies for monitoring and improving the quality of air. Reducing air pollution is vital, not just to protect the children's present well-being but also to provide a healthier atmosphere that will sustain their later cardiovascular well-being. Socioeconomic status (SES) is another crucial determinant of the environment that affects children's frequency of acquired heart diseases. Children with lower SES have several adversities, including limited healthcare access, poor nutrition, and minimal physical activity. These conditions have the potential to cause conditions such as hypertension and obesity, which are proven risk factors for heart disease. The disparities in the provision of health resources may expose vulnerable groups to higher cardiovascular diseases at a young age. For instance, studies show that diet improvement and physical activity interventions among disadvantaged groups lead to significant reductions in cardiovascular disease risk factors in children, thereby reaffirming the implication of a supportive environment in avoiding such diseases. In addition, psychosocial environments, including family and stress, can potentially have a significant effect on children's heart health.

Excess stress in the household or community can be uncovered through behavior problems and negative coping mechanisms such as inactivity and poor nutrition, which contribute to developing heart disease risk. Children under stress are more susceptible to high blood pressure and other cardiovascular complications, as research shows. Healthy settings with supportive families to adopt healthy lifestyles can lead to better health. Intercepts aimed at managing psychosocial stressors and encouraging healthier lifestyles can be part of reducing the prevalence of acquired heart conditions in children. Community support infrastructure needs to be built to create a system supportive of better physical and mental health and welcoming of healthier future opportunities for children.

8.2.3. Infections and Inflammatory Responses

The pathogenesis of acquired heart disease in children, primarily through disorders such as Kawasaki disease (KD) and multisystem inflammatory syndrome in children (MIS-C), revolves around interaction between infections and inflammatory processes. KD is a significant pathophysiologic challenge since it is an expression of systemic vasculitis with direct involvement of the coronary arteries. The pathogen associations with infectious agents have been under vigorous examination, demonstrating how immune responses against these pathogens initiate ferocious inflammatory processes that lead to irreversible cardiac complications.

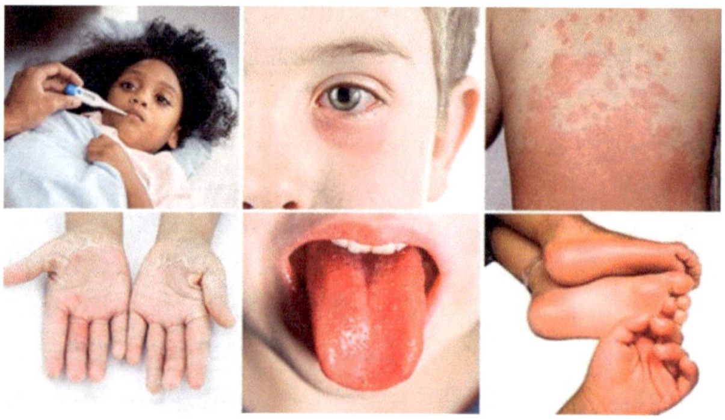

Figure 8.7. Multisystem inflammatory syndrome in children (MIS-C).

Source: https://childrenswi.org/-/media/chwlibrary/newshub/2020/covid-19-pims/pims900v3.jpg?h=286&w=500&hash=C73C33C94115C3FED5A95B8EF14A971E.

Despite the mysterious nature of KD's particular etiologic stimuli, the observation that the common infections often precede the disease has accentuated the central role of infectious pathogens in initiating the inflammatory cascades to acquired heart disease in predisposed children (Wang et al., 2022). The emergence of MIS-C in the context of the COVID-19 pandemic has further compounded the complexity of infection in cardiovascular inflammation. The novel syndrome has common clinical features with KD, raising fundamental questions regarding the mechanisms and pathophysiology underlying both of these inflammatory conditions. While KD was recognized decades earlier as the principal cause of acquired disease of the heart in children, MIS-C more recently demonstrates an extremely severe inflammatory reaction against SARS-CoV-2 (Figure 8.7).

The acute presentation and aggressive course of MIS-C suggest that the underlying immuno-inflammatory process may be predictive of significant cardiovascular involvement, with prompt medical intervention necessary to forestall sequelae (McCrindle et al., 2020). Both illnesses highlight the critical intersection between infectious pathogens and inflammatory pathways in the pathogenesis of target cardiovascular complications in children. Understanding the biological underpinnings of the immune response in KD and MIS-C might provide much-needed clarity on their pathophysiology as well as potential treatments. Immunologic studies reveal that these diseases may be linked with increased activation of both innate and adaptive immunity, resulting in the vascular endothelial dysfunction and subsequent cardiac injury. The sophistication of these immuno-inflammatory pathways is matched by the complexity of balancing immune activation due to infection and the risk of harmful systemic inflammation. Researchers are studying genetic susceptibility and environmental factors that could potentially interact with infectious stimuli, perhaps to trigger KD and MIS-C. With more knowledge of these interactions, health professionals can give more effective prevention and treatment strategies to reduce the rate of acquired heart diseases in children linked to infection (McCrindle et al., 2020; Wang et al., 2022).

8.3. Symptoms and Diagnosis

Acquired heart disease-associated symptoms in children must be recognized, as early diagnosis affects outcomes. A few of these suggestive symptoms are chest pain, syncope, and palpitations, which need careful assessment. Children may also present with nonspecific complaints of fatigue, dyspnea, or exercise intolerance. These symptoms may frequently be mistakenly attributed to secondary benign causes, leading to delay in diagnosis. Clinicians should be highly suspicious, particularly when such symptoms are chronic or progressive. Other symptoms, such as cyanosis, blue discoloration of the skin, and edema, can also provide critical clues. These findings should be supplemented by an excellent history and physical examination to aid in proper guidance of the further diagnostic workup. Accurate diagnosis of acquired heart disease in children is a multi-faceted exercise combining elements of clinical astuteness and advanced imaging modalities. Initial assessment is frequently performed with non-invasive methods, for instance, echocardiography, allowing detection of structural abnormalities or functional disturbances within the heart. ECGs can be employed in carefully chosen cases to assess electrical activity and rhythm, uncovering potential arrhythmic problems indicative of underlying pathology. Besides, laboratory exams, including blood work to evaluate markers of cardiac strain or inflammation, can be necessary. Using all these diagnostic tests builds an integrated description of the child's cardiac condition and aids in the differentiation between acquired disease and congenital cardiac defects (King et al., 2017). Treatment regimens can vary according to the diagnosis, but a consistent focus on symptom management and monitoring for potential complications must be maintained. In situations of diagnosing arrhythmias or heart failure, medication such as beta-blockers or diuretics is employed in order to decrease the symptoms and improve the patient's quality of life. More serious conditions can involve surgeries to correct structural defects or to insert devices that ensure improved cardiac function. In addition, persistent monitoring and refinement of therapeutic strategies are necessary because the clinical evolution in children can evolve over time. Therefore, integration among pediatric cardiologists, family medicine specialists, and families is necessary to optimize outcomes and acquire a proper vision of the child's health over the course of time, especially during adolescence (Abrahamian et al., 2008) (Figure 8.8).

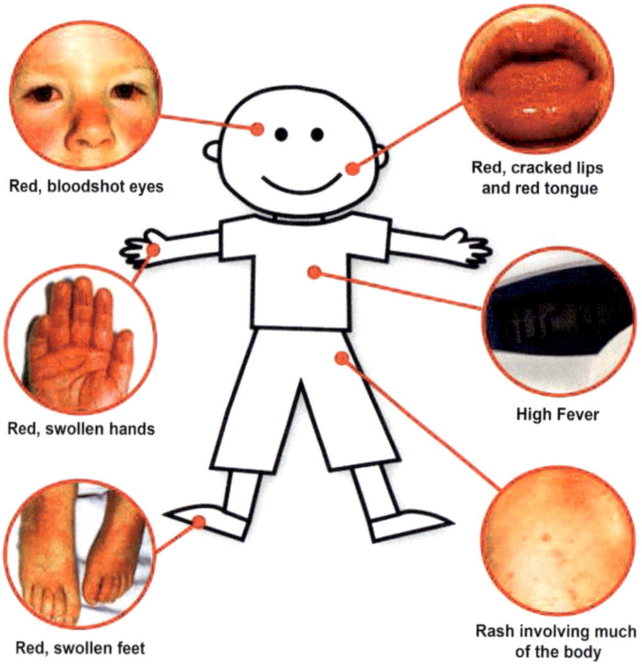

Figure 8.8. Kawasaki disease symptoms.

Source: https://www.kawasakikidsfoundation.org/wp-content/uploads/symptoms_kawasaki-disease-1.jpg.

8.3.1. Common Symptoms in Children

Identification of nonspecific general symptoms in children with acquired heart disease is crucial for timely diagnosis and treatment. Children can present a wide range of nonspecific symptoms that can readily be confused with other conditions. Fatigue, for instance, is a frequent complaint among children with heart disease, and the children present diminished levels of energy during activities previously well tolerated. In addition, breathlessness or shortness of breath during breathing can be experienced, particularly when undergoing physical activities or even when resting in severe cases. Such signs and symptoms not only affect the child's day-to-day life but can also lead to long-term developmental delays. In this respect, the discovery of such early warning signs is essential for effectively addressing acquired heart diseases and providing children with the appropriate support within the right timeline. Furthermore, palpitations and chest pains are common presentations among children with acquired heart diseases, further complicating diagnosis. Palpitations may manifest as irregular heart rhythms, giving rise to worry in both the parents and children. Chest pains, though less commonly associated with heart disease in children, need to be thoroughly investigated because they may indicate cardiovascular abnormalities underlying them (e.g., rheumatic heart disease). The association of rheumatic fever, which typically presents with elevated inflammatory markers, with rheumatic heart disease (RHD) also makes symptomatology more complex. As has been reported in recent studies, the progressive presentation of symptoms by RHD tends to contribute to delayed diagnosis, highlighting the need for intense cardiovascular examination in children showing such symptoms (Hüseyin et al., 2024). In addition to physical symptoms, psychological presentations can also present among children with acquired heart disease. Depression and anxiety are not uncommon as children deal with the realities of having a chronic illness. Ongoing physician visits, possible surgeries, and lifestyle modifications can create an increased level of distress. Additionally, social stigma associated with heart disease can discourage children from participating in typical peer interactions, reinforcing feelings of isolation. This psychological dimension calls for a multidisciplinary approach to the management of acquired heart diseases, which not only addresses bodily well-being but also addresses emotional and social well-being. Taking a look at the entire perspective of a child's health, healthcare workers are better placed to enable the overall management of acquired heart diseases (Naizihijwa et al., 2024) (Figure 8.9).

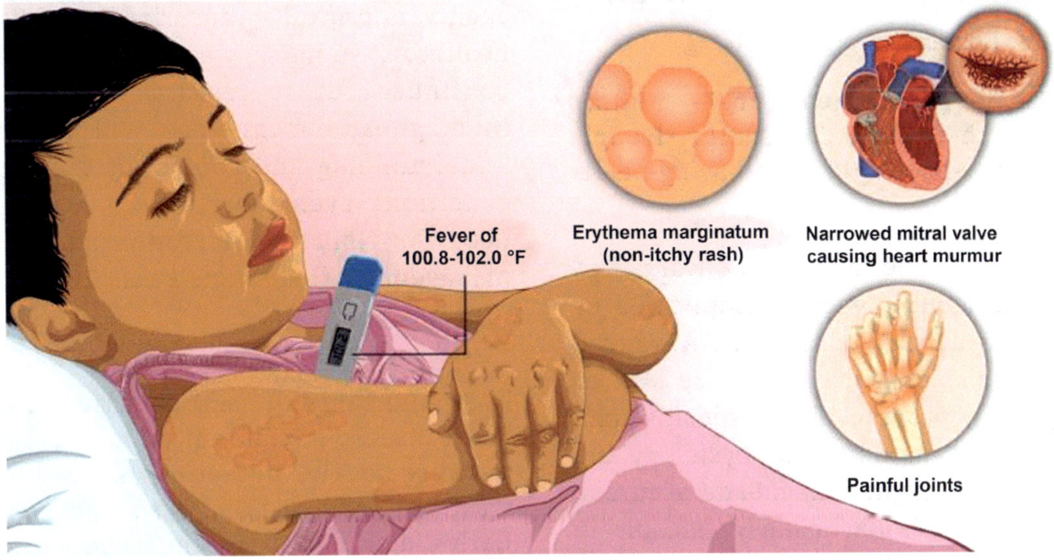

Figure 8.9. Symptom of rheumatic heart disease (RHD).

Source: https://cdn.storymd.com/optimized/OoYe2gcMoG/original.png.

8.3.2. Diagnostic Tests and Procedures

In diagnosis of acquired heart disease in children, correct diagnostic tests and interventions are essential for accurate identification and treatment. Initial evaluations typically begin with a complete history and physical, which provide useful information regarding potential cardiac defects. Subsequent non-invasive tests such as electrocardiograms (EKG) and echocardiograms are most often used. The EKG analyzes the electrical activity of the heart, identifying arrhythmias or hypertrophy, and echocardiography pictures heart structures and functions with sound. Both procedures are greatly beneficial not only for diagnosis but for observing the progression of heart disease in children as well. By utilizing these tests at the outset, clinicians are able to establish a baseline for comparison and tailor treatment interventions according to the specific needs of each child (Figure 8.10).

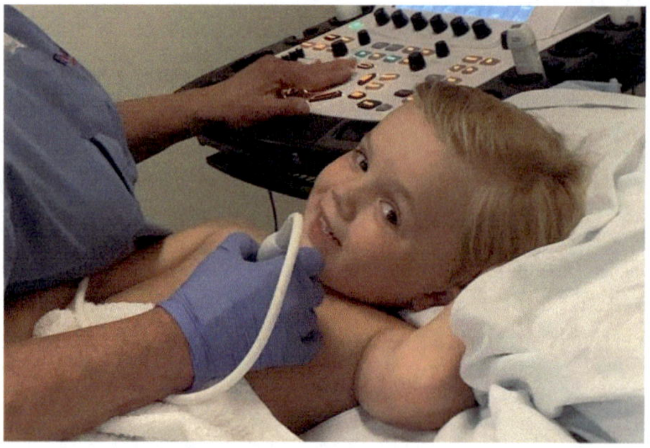

Figure 8.10. Echocardiogram test.

Source: https://www.heart.org/-/media/Images/Health-Topics/Congenital-Heart-Defects/Survivor-photos/Jackson-having-heart-test.jpg?sc_lang=en.

Further diagnostic tests can be warranted if initial assessment suggests complicated or atypical cardiovascular conditions. Advanced imaging technologies, such as cardiac MRI or CT angiography, provide highly specific data regarding cardiac anatomy and physiology and are able to afford higher diagnostic accuracy. These modalities are particularly valuable in the context of acquired heart disease occurring secondary to systemic infections or inflammatory disorders. For example, in infective endocarditis, visualization of vegetations or abscesses on these imaging modalities helps guide therapeutic interventions. In addition, laboratory studies such as biomarkers and cultures have the ability to identify infectious pathogens that may be the etiology of cardiac conditions, such as viral myocarditis or post-infectious states such as *Francisella tularensis* infection in the context of transplantation cases, showing the severity of diagnostic processes in pediatric cardiology (Annambhotla et al., 2019). In addition, integration of multi-disciplinary approaches in diagnostics is also essential in addressing integrated care in children with acquired cardiac diseases. Multidisciplinary teamwork of pediatric cardiologists, radiologists, and infectious disease specialists allows for consideration of all the aspects of a child's overall well-being. For instance, determining the epidemiology of infection carriers like *Coxiella burnetii*, which have complicated histories within many settings, can inform febrile illness prevention measures that can precipitate cardiac dysfunction. Early recognition through diagnostic testing, such as serological tests or PCR methods for infectious agents, is critical in ensuring a child's overall health. As we manage acquired heart diseases, continued future research and innovation in diagnostic technology will enhance our understanding and control of these complex conditions even more, which highlights the need for vigilant observation and innovative management (Benkirane et al., 2014).

8.3.3. Importance of Early Detection

The importance of early detection of acquired heart disease in children cannot be overstated because early detection indeed impacts treatment outcomes and the patient's prognosis. Early diagnosis and screening allow clinicians to apply effective interventions that can alleviate symptoms, improve quality of life, and even save lives. It is particularly important due to the complexity of heart diseases, whether they have a component of genetics or environmental exposure, which usually renders their pathogenesis more complex. With proper recognition of the unique condition that a child suffers from, doctors are able to design treatment courses that address each patient's specific requirements, which eventually leads to greater prospects of successful control. Furthermore, advances in medical technology and genetics are ever more clearly playing a deciding role in optimizing diagnostic accuracy, underlining the value of early detection as a means of maximizing tailoring of therapy to specific cases and increasing efficacy and lifespan in patients (Reemtsen et al., 2017). Beyond its role in maximizing treatment efficacy, early detection is critical for reducing the long-term morbidity of acquired heart disease in children. Children suffering from conditions such as congenital heart disease or arrhythmias can potentially be provided with monitoring and preventive treatment that would normalize their health dangers. For instance, early intervention can prevent severe complications such as heart failure or pulmonary hypertension that are experienced in untreated conditions. The early identification of risk factors, including underlying comorbidities like congenital heart disease or chronic respiratory disease, allows medical practitioners to create preventive treatment strategies. Through research, which has proved this to be the case, children with early RSV infection and underlying cardiac disease are at greater risks; thus, early identification can lead to a more extensive control and better long-term health conditions (Bakir et al., 2014). Secondly, early diagnosis encourages an informed and active approach to health care among families and communities. Since parents know their child's heart ailment from early childhood, they can make educated choices regarding lifestyle adjustments, nutrition, and activity restrictions that may prove to be crucial in adapting to the disease. Education concerning the impact of early diagnosis will enable the family to recognize symptoms early, for a quicker reaction to future health issues. This forward-looking intervention not only benefits the child's present health but can also create lifelong habits, including a healthier cardiovascular system. Through encouraging frequent screenings and campaigns on conditions acquired heart diseases, society can significantly enhance early detection rates, to the advantage of children and the healthcare system overall (Reemtsen et al., 2017).

8.4. Treatment Options

Treatment of acquired heart disease in children is often a multi-faceted treatment strategy with pharmacologic and non-pharmacologic intervention. Early diagnosis is crucial, as delay can have a deleterious effect on the prognosis. Therapeutic intervention in children with acquired heart diseases can be anticoagulants, anti-inflammatory agents, and immunosuppressive drugs, especially if autoimmune etiology is suspected. For instance, the child patient diagnosed with maternal antibody circulation diseases may require early intervention so as not to experience complications due to congenital heart block. The practice is in line with the new practices that ensure active management strategies that are specifically tailored to the condition of the individual child to ensure optimized health outcomes and access to the necessary interventions in good time (King et al., 2017). In some cases, most prominently those of congenital block heart or structural problems complicating and therefore exacerbating a condition, surgery is necessary. Children with serious conduction defects or other problems will require a pacemaker implanted, especially when in danger of life-threatening harm from a misbehaving heartbeat. Surgical intervention based on empirical data has been developed with a view to providing the maximum possible benefit with minimum risk, thus laying more stress on the development of therapy guidelines. The interventions are for not only managing the acute presentation of heart disease but also for maximizing long-term quality and functional ability of the child with acquired heart disease (Buyon et al., 2003). In addition, integrating cardiac rehabilitation programs as part of acquired heart disease management is becoming widely accepted as a core component of worldwide care. These programs offer personalized exercise routines, dietary counseling, and psychosocial support, all aimed at promoting cardiovascular health and overall well-being among pediatric patients. Evidence shows that an interdisciplinary approach, involving lifestyle modification alongside traditional medical therapy, can significantly reduce morbidity and enhance recovery. Kids are most responsive to such interventions since they can greatly impact longer-term trajectories of health. Treatment options thus should not only be limited to drugs or surgery but also to a broad array of strategies allowing for lifelong management of health (King et al., 2017).

8.4.1. Medical Management and Medications

Effective medical management and treatment with drugs play critical roles in the treatment of acquired heart diseases among children, and they can come about through a variety of causes including infection, systemic disease, and habits. The pediatricians are required to conduct comprehensive assessments to determine the precise etiology of each child's condition of the heart since these guides treatment regimens. Evidence-based practice advises that individualized treatment plans be developed, with regard to the child's individual clinical presentation, potential comorbidities, and home life. For instance, children with congenital heart diseases may require medications such as ACE inhibitors or beta-blockers to manage heart failure symptoms, whereas others may require anticoagulants to prevent thromboembolic complications, highlighting the importance of a tailored therapeutic approach according to each patient's requirements and clinical scenario (Marilyn et al., 2022). Besides, it is important to monitor children undergoing treatment for heart diseases with accuracy. Pediatric cardiologists need to regularly monitor the effectiveness of drugs given and change doses based on that to prevent side effects and maximal therapeutic benefit. This is specifically relevant in the pediatric population, where body metabolism of medication varies significantly from that in adults. Moreover, drugs used in the management of cardiovascular diseases in children should consider the risk of growth and developmental impact; therefore, pediatric pharmacists play a critical role in counseling towards an adequate medication regimen. Joint care from pediatricians, subspecialists, and pharmacists is necessary to ensure coordinated and uncomplicated care to benefit the children during their treatment process (François et al., 2019) (Figure 8.11).

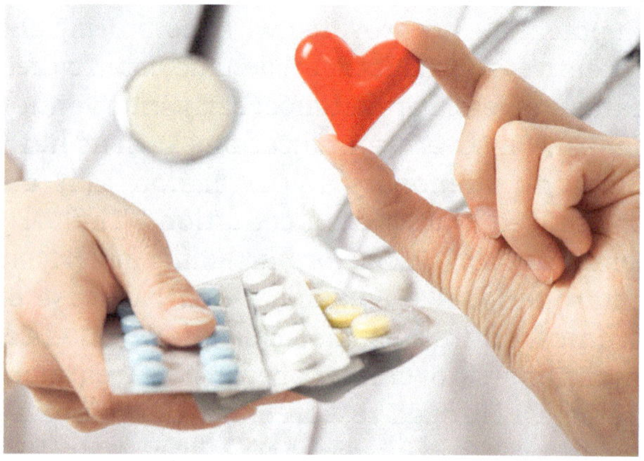

Figure 8.11. Medications used to treat heart conditions in children.

Source: https://external-content.duckduckgo.com/iu/?u=https%3A%2F%2Fwatsonshealth.com.ph%2Fwp-content%2Fuploads%2F2021%2F07%2Fshutterstock_340527668.jpg&f=1&nofb=1&ipt=76a0f0a6fbb90e73d543186490ae512e1f77909d249bbdcabadb91224619555e.

Besides pharmacological interventions, non-pharmacologic interventions also have an important role to play in the efficient management of acquired heart diseases in children. Lifestyle modifications, including food habits, physical activity, and control overweight, are integral components of comprehensive care. Education of families about heart disease, following medication, and detection of signs that require urgent help is required in order to maintain good long-term results. Educational materials and support groups can empower families and children alike as they navigate the intricacies of heart disease management. Ultimately, a multidisciplinary method with medical management, medication adherence, lifestyle change, and family involvement will foster better outcomes and better quality of life for children with acquired heart diseases (François et al., 2019).

8.4.2. Surgical Interventions

Surgical interventions play a critical role in the management of acquired heart disease in children, particularly when nonsurgical interventions are inadequate. Children's patients typically present with unique anatomical and physiological conditions, which necessitate individualized surgical strategies based on the specific requirements of individual cases. Unlike cardiac surgery in adults, where attention is placed on relatively more homogeneous conditions, surgical treatment of congenital heart disease in children requires profound understanding of the maturing anatomy. The complexity of such cases brings to fore the importance of skilled surgical teams who have the ability to function under changing physiological conditions of young children. Care teams must also anticipate the occurrence of complications and involve a multidisciplinary system that includes the services of cardiologists, anesthesiologists, and critical care experts, thereby enhancing patient outcomes and minimizing the risks associated with surgical interventions. After surgical repair of congenital heart disease, children typically have to be closely observed during postoperative management since their chances of complication development are high. Findings indicate that surgical approaches, especially open-heart surgery, can result in high hospital-acquired infection rates as opposed to minimally invasive techniques. The rate of purulent-septic infections, for instance, is comparatively high in children exposed to open-heart surgery, based on a comparison study of over 500 clinical records. These infections can protract significantly the length of recovery, leading to unnecessary morbidity and necessitating prolonged intensive care monitoring (Figure 8.12).

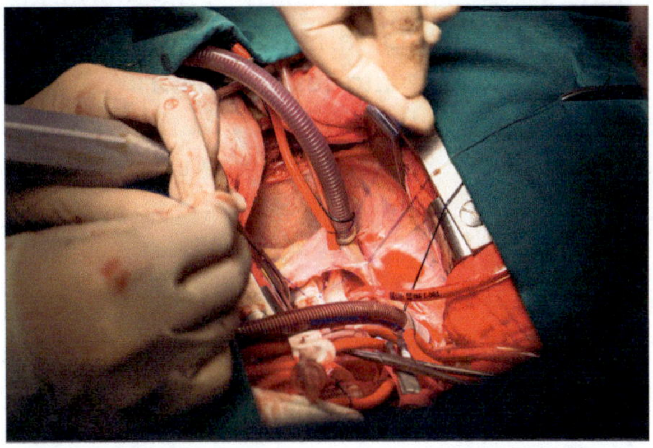

Figure 8.12. Surgical interventions play a crucial role in managing acquired heart disease in children.

Source: https://www.thetransmitter.org/wp-content/uploads/2019/10/Congenetial844.jpg.

Moreover, the use of artificial lung ventilation in surgery is also a new risk, and meticulous surgical planning as well as postoperative management are necessary to avoid complications and optimize the possibility of recovery in these vulnerable groups (Kudryavtseva et al., 2021). Apart from the health results of surgical treatment of acquired heart disease in children, there are psychosocial connotations that spread to family and caregivers. Extended surgical procedures have a tendency to induce tension and stress among families, and hence need an integrated support system that addresses emotional and logistical support demands. Parental education and psychological counseling contained within family-focused models of care are critical in addressing the complex recovery process. Furthermore, disparities in access to high-level pediatric cardiac care exacerbate these conditions since limited resource families can be unable to access required surgical services. This inequality has to be tackled, and it will require policy reform activism and investment in pediatric healthcare infrastructure. Ultimately, a holistic approach with regard to the emotional, physical, and social dimensions of care will enhance recovery and lead to improved long-term outcomes for children suffering from acquired heart diseases (Talwar et al., 2025).

8.4.3. Role of Lifestyle Changes and Rehabilitation

Treatment of acquired heart diseases in children necessitates an interdisciplinary approach with emphasis on the crucial role of lifestyle modification and rehabilitation. Understanding etiology of the conditions highlights the need to control modifiable risk factors. Initiation of lifestyle modification, such as dietary improvement and physical activity enhancement, lies at the core of effective disease control. Also, physical rehabilitation programs directed at children can contribute significantly towards physical and psychological well-being. Apart from providing improved cardiovascular fitness, these programs also enhance the sense of responsibility among young patients towards health and hence reduce comorbidities in the future. Rehabilitation strategies must be multicomponent in the sense that they integrate medical treatment with proper behavioral interventions. For instance, family nutrition education has been proven to improve the eating habits of children who are at risk of heart disease. This intervention is particularly important in multiethnic communities where the health condition may be influenced by ethnic food habits. Specialists must promote healthy consumption via culturally targeted interventions since some ethnic populations become increasingly vulnerable to complications like obesity and diabetes risk in connection with heart disease. Study indicates early education regarding nutrition is paid back with long-term dividends and the avoidance of undesirable health consequences (Szczepura et al., 2011). Inclusion of regular physical activity in acquired heart disease children is also crucial. Physical activities should be enjoyable and tailored to the interests and capacities of the child so that they are sustainable. Rehabilitation, along with body recovery, also involves emotional resilience, as the social sphere of the diseases may prove difficult for children to overcome. To achieve maximum outcomes, medical professionals must employ multidisciplinary approaches with cardiologists, dietitians, psychologists, and physical therapists. Such combinations permit comprehensive treatment of the illness on both physiological and psychological aspects, facilitating a smoother recovery towards healthy adulthood (N/A, 2014). By placing maximum emphasis on lifestyle modification and rehabilitation, it is possible to enhance the quality of living and future health prospects of children with acquired heart diseases to a large degree.

8.5. Long-Term Effects and Complications

Acquired heart diseases in kids can potentially bring long-term complications and effects that can critically impair their quality of life and overall health condition. Among the central problems is the development of coronary artery lesions, particularly in Kawasaki disease (KD), which is similarly extremely prevalent in children. Studies indicate that early treatment and diagnosis can minimize severe complications, but continued follow-up of patients who have had KD is essential to ascertain present risks. Serial echocardiograms are typically recommended to assess cardiac function and detect complications if they arise later. Proper management protocols are emphasized in newer guidelines to provide standard care in a way that healthcare personnel are adequately prepared to deal with possible long-term sequelae so that, ultimately, morbidity related to KD can be reduced and improved survival rates can be achieved in the affected children (N/A, 2023). Besides that, children with acquired heart diseases can also face ongoing psychological and emotional stress. The weight of having a chronic illness, coupled with the physical limitation brought about by heart disease, can lead to anxiety, depression, and social isolation. A treatment approach that addresses this dual physical and emotional impairment includes mental health interventions besides medical care. Research has established that children with chronic conditions given psychosocial intervention exhibit better adaptation and coping strategies, thus making a real case for integrated models of care. Thus, making sure the child is not only given healthy medical care but also psychological care becomes the need of the hour to address the entire scope of challenge brought about by acquired heart diseases (Kenneth et al., 2004). Lastly, the long-term effects of acquired heart diseases extend beyond immediate health outcomes to affect education and economic development as these children transition into adulthood. Chronic health challenges can lead to higher school absenteeism, affecting educational attainment and future employment opportunities. In addition, additional health care costs associated with chronic disease management can impose significant financial pressures on families, thereby affecting their overall socioeconomic status. It is important to understand that such children are at risk of lifelong consequences, and hence active healthcare policy fulfilling both short-term medical as well as long-term supportive requirements is needed. Early intervention and extended care can significantly alter the trajectory of health results so that children afflicted with acquired heart diseases can have productive lives despite the condition, thus reducing long-term socioeconomic consequences related to such diagnoses (N/A, 2023).

8.5.1. Potential for Chronic Heart Conditions

The susceptibility to chronic cardiovascular diseases in children, particularly those with a history of acquired cardiovascular diseases, pose significant long-term health complications. There is evidence that sickness in children, including infections and inflammatory disease, causes cardiovascular morbidity that continues into adulthood.

For instance, such chronic diseases like rheumatic fever and Kawasaki disease, which predominantly affect children, lead to permanent scarring of heart valves and coronary arteries. Also, sepsis prevalence, as observed in studies, shows that it is a significant burden of heart-related morbidity in children. With about 48.9 million new sepsis cases in 2017 globally, and its association with heart dysfunction, knowledge of the connection is crucial in the administration of children's health (Kristina et al., 2020) (Figure 8.13).

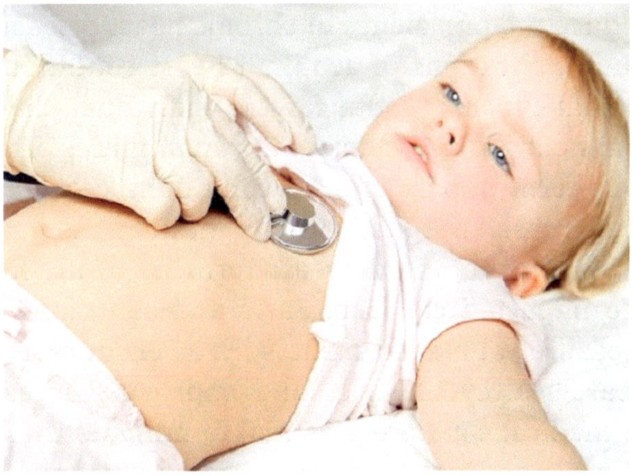

Figure 8.13. Potential for chronic heart conditions in children.

Source: https://www.hackensackmeridianhealth.org/-/media/project/hmh/hmh/public/healthu/heart-disease-children.jpg.

Early detection and prompt interventions are very essential to prevent the escalation of these acute illnesses into chronic cardiac diseases in adult life. The underlying reason for the causation of chronic cardiac disorders in children is the combination of genetic susceptibility with the environmental pressures. Children with congenital cardiac disease or a family history of cardiovascular disease are at increased risk of developing chronic illness after any acute periods of heart stress. Furthermore, obesity in childhood, inactivity, and dietary poor lifestyle factors increase the risk of cardiovascular disease. Increased awareness and adherence to guidelines, such as those of health agencies, can lead to enhanced prevention and management in high-risk groups. It is critical that the healthcare providers remain vigilant as their clinical acumen based on the latest evidence and recommendations immediately will determine the health outcomes of the children (François et al., 2019).

The personalized care accommodates prevention as well as treatment of already established complications, ultimately aiming to reduce the prevalence of chronic heart disease. The implications of acquired heart conditions are far-reaching, both for the individual child and healthcare systems and communities. The long-term impact of such conditions can lead to increased hospitalization, continued medical management, and decreased quality of life for the impacted children. Early and coordinated measures of management, such as encouraging heart-healthy lifestyles and improving access to medical care, are essential to mitigate these risks. In addition, additional research is greatly needed on the long-term effects of childhood infections and acquired cardiac disease on cardiovascular health.

The convergence of clinical practice, public health action, and robust research remains essential in fighting this public health issue effectively and sustainably. By giving prevention and early intervention policies high priority, the risk of chronic heart diseases can be reduced, which in turn will contribute to better health outcomes for generations to come.

8.5.2. Impact on Physical Activity and Quality of Life

The physical activity effects of acquired heart diseases on children are severe, frequently appearing in terms of physiological and psychological dimensions. Such children frequently experience limitations in engaging in physical activities that are otherwise typical of their respective age group. As a result, they generally have poor endurance and increased susceptibility to fatigue, which limits their participation in sport and recreational activities. These limitations not only prevent their physical development but also add to feelings of loneliness and frustration since they compare themselves with others. Additionally, illness stigma can further compound the emotional cost, contributing to a decline in overall quality of life.

Thus, the ability to be fully active physically is not only key to the maintenance of physical health in such children but also to the development of emotional well-being in them. Quality of life for children with acquired heart diseases can be significantly affected by both physical limitations caused by the condition and by emotional challenges. Such children can have their day-to-day activity, like play and social interactions, severely cut short owing to their illness.

With physical activity lowered in performance, children can fall victim to a lack of human relationships, which is so important at the age of development. The reluctance to play actively may be due to fear of overstrain or that they will get their symptoms provoked because of heart disease (Figure 8.14).

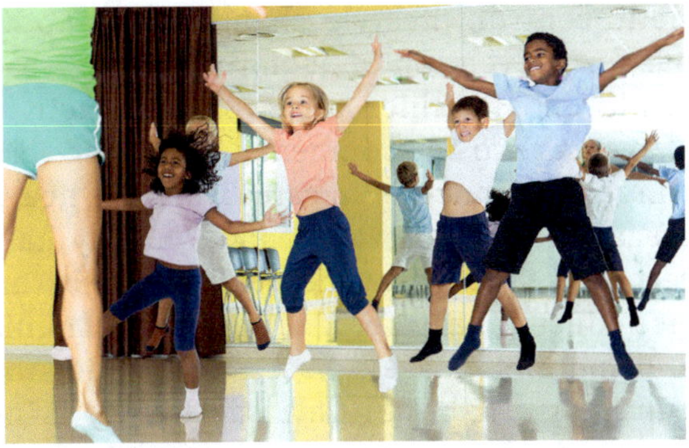

Figure 8.14. Impact of acquired heart disease on the physical activity levels of children.

Source: https://www.ideafit.com/wp-content/uploads/2021/04/Fit-Kids.jpg.

Thus, this stress can lead to a cycle of less activity and poorer mental health. In the quest to deal with these intricate issues, it is essential that caregivers, educators, and healthcare professionals collaborate to provide a setting in which safe physical activity engagement is facilitated and thereby aim for enhancement in physical and psychological dimensions of quality of life. Individualized interventions addressing the unique needs of children with acquired heart disease are necessary to improve their level of physical activity and quality of life. Exercise programs should be individually tailored by healthcare providers so that they not only compensate for limitations imposed by the child's condition but also allow progressive and safe engagement in physical activities. Also, encouraging participation in group activities, i.e., exercise classes or adapted sports, can encourage social interaction, which can increase emotional resilience. The group work can help improve the isolation and loneliness that are often associated with these children. By establishing a competitive-free environment where physical work is central, healthcare professionals can come a long way in improving the overall life of children suffering from acquired heart diseases (N/A). Also, with the understanding of these conditions' depth, treatment is able to be fully completed so that children are able to live an active and full life with their conditions (Abrahamian et al., 2008).

8.5.3. Psychological Effects on Children and Families

Psychological impact of acquired heart disease in children extends far beyond the initial medical issue. Families are faced with heightened anxiety and emotional distress as they navigate the complexities of their child's health condition. Parents may be made to feel helpless and anxious, particularly in the face of the uncertain prognosis that often accompanies heart disease. Children, nonetheless, can also suffer from depression or anxiety as they cope with limitations that accompany their condition. Such emotional distress is capable of deranging family relationships, with support systems liable to strain. Emotional responses of family members play a crucial role in deciding how children adapt to their diagnoses, illustrating the interconnectedness of psychological health and the family organization. Both families and children adapt their coping strategies to the nature of treatment and diagnosis. Parents attempt to institute normalcy in the midst of chaos created by hospitalization and medical consultations. Nevertheless, their ability to provide a stable and supportive environment can be derailed by their own emotional instability. The kids are able to mirror this fear in their actions, avoiding social activity or becoming overly reliant on their caretakers. The European Society of Cardiology guidelines advocate that health practitioners ought to consider the psychosocial viewpoints of care during treatment planning for pediatric patients (Silvia et al., 2015). The integration of psychological care into medical treatment can play a pivotal role in improving both mental health status and overall quality of life in such children and their families. Frequent and open communication cannot be overstated enough in its contribution to preventing the psychological effect of heart disease on families. Frequent open communication allows families to discuss their fears, concerns, and expectations, which can foster resilience and understanding. Parents can be strong too by raising issues regarding their child's health, facilitating emotional expression, and validating feelings. Moreover, interaction with support groups or counselors who specialize in pediatric chronic illness can prove to be very useful for both children and parents. The ESC guidelines emphasize the significance of psychiatric evaluation in pediatric cardiology interventions (Elliott et al., 2014), a sign that there is more recognition of the connection between psychological and physical well-being. Ultimately, intervention on the psychological component of heart disease is essential to ensuring the holistic treatment of affected children and families.

8.6. Prevention Strategies

For proper prevention against the rise of acquired heart diseases in children, prevention programs have to take a multifaceted approach. Identification and treatment of chromosomal defects early in life have been recognized as central to mitigating against the risk of sudden cardiac death (SCD). The majority of acquired heart diseases usually arise from genetic disorders inherited and can be controlled with early intervention. The identification of these risks, combined with appropriate screenings and genetic counseling, can significantly improve health status in high-risk children. Procedures such as echocardiography are also important for detecting structural defects, allowing for prevention as well as, where necessary, early surgery. Therefore, an integrated model with focus on early detection and management can effectively minimize the pediatric burden of acquired heart diseases, highlighting the importance of proactive healthcare. Apart from genetic control, lifestyle changes are another pillar for prevention of acquired heart disease in children. Healthier diets, physical activity, and exposure to environmental toxins can serve an important function in cardiovascular health. Increasing the rate of childhood obesity has a direct consequence on heart disease risk and hence educational interventions within families and communities are a necessity. Besides this, a culture for habitual physical activity is not only conducive to weight control but also enhances cardiovascular fitness. Communities and schools can collaborate to develop programs encouraging active play and physical exercise, which are key in shaping a future generation that is healthier. These programs can reduce risk factors of cardiovascular diseases, with especial attention to the central importance of prevention through lifestyle modification. New research on the function of microRNAs (miRNAs) in cardiovascular health offers a new direction for the creation of novel prevention interventions.

MiRNAs are identified as having the power to regulate gene expression responsible for many cardiovascular ailments, including congenital heart disease, arrhythmias, and cardiomyopathies. Identification of the involved miRNAs could provide novel diagnostic markers capable of identifying children with higher vulnerability to heart conditions. Adding miRNA profiling to routine medical screening, clinicians would have the ability to better direct intervention strategies towards life-style adjustments and genetic counseling on the basis of individual risk profiles. As research goes on, the utility of miRNAs as biomarkers can potentially improve early diagnosis and treatment regimens for acquired cardiac conditions, ultimately revolutionizing prevention strategies and benefits to health in children with risk, encouraging proactive rather than reactive handling of cardiovascular conditions in pediatrics (Pas et al., 2024; Salzillo et al., 2024).

8.6.1. Importance of Regular Health Check-Ups

Regular health check-ups play a central role in the early detection and management of acquired heart diseases in children. The frequent examinations create the platform upon which doctors can monitor cardiovascular health, identify risk factors, and pick any abnormalities that are likely to emerge with time. One of the outstanding attributes of such check-ups is the incorporation of technology, such as wearable sensors, which are capable of offering real-time information linked to a child's physiology and activity. Through the use of such technologies, clinicians are in a better position to assess a child's cardiovascular condition outside a hospital and thereby have a better overall perspective. Additionally, the earlier identification of potential issues can lead to interventions on time, tailored management plans, and long-term advantages for children at risk of heart disease (Vijayan et al., 2021). Thus, regular health check-ups not only safeguard cardiovascular health but also enhance the well-being of children with such problems. Regular health check-ups have another significant benefit in that they provide healthcare professionals the opportunity to educate families regarding heart health and living styles. These consultations assist the health workers in discussing the significance of nutrition, exercise, and other factors that can assist in maintaining the overall cardiovascular well-being of the child. Families, when they are aware of the potential consequences of poor living lifestyles, i.e., no exercise or unhealthful eating habits, take preventive care. Moreover, parents being aware of the family risk factors of heart diseases can motivate them to be proactive and vigilant in taking their children to the medical practitioner at the first sign of symptoms. For instance, the parents of children with a history of heart disease in the family must emphasize routine check-ups as a preventive measure to detect any sign of acquired heart diseases early (Machhi et al., 2020). Hence, such appointments allow families to make informed decisions that essentially help their child's heart health. Apart from early diagnosis and education, regular health check-ups establish a continuous relationship between families and healthcare providers that is required for managing acquired heart diseases. This extended relationship helps healthcare professionals deliver personalized care and support specific to each child's situation. Follow-up on a regular basis can also allow medical practitioners to assess the effectiveness of therapy regimens, change drugs, or prescribe further treatment when needed. In addition, such interaction can create trust and confidence between families and provide impetus for parents to adhere to medical advice and follow up with experts when needed. Consequently, the creation of a foundation of chronic care enhances the possibility of positive health consequences as children become more conscious of the importance of maintaining their heart health throughout their lives (Vijayan et al., 2021). Lastly, regular check-ups for health are a significant part of the overall management of acquired heart disease in children to the detriment and benefit of immediate and long-term health trajectories.

8.6.2. Vaccination and Infection Control

In the case of acquired diseases of the heart in children, vaccination plays a crucial role in managing infection, significantly reducing the incidence of the conditions that can lead to cardiovascular outcomes. Vaccination against diseases such as rheumatic fever can be employed to lower the global burden of rheumatic heart disease (RHD), a major origin of acquired heart disease among younger populations, most especially in low- and middle-income countries. Prevention of the initial streptococcal infections that cause RHD will prevent long-term health effects of the disease. Thus, improving vaccination programs is essential to safeguard children's cardiovascular health. Apart from individual benefits, wider implications of vaccination include herd immunity and prevention of spread of preventable infections in populations. Proper infection control practices within the healthcare setting are also required to encompass the risk of acquiring heart disease linked with infectious processes. HAIs may complicate pre-existing cardiovascular conditions or induce new instances of acquired heart ailments in vulnerable children. As a measure to curb the spread of pathogens that may complicate the health status of a child, hospitals are capable of implementing stringent infection prevention and control practices. The design of the health care facilities must prioritize infection control principles as the setting affects HAI rates. Understanding the dynamics of transmission on which exogenous- and endogenous-sourced HAIs function is critical in the formulation of interventions intended to protect pediatric patients upon hospital admission. This multifaceted approach facilitates an improved health care environment that ultimately contributes towards the overall goal of cardiovascular maintenance and enhancement in children. Moreover, bringing together vaccine approaches with aggressive infection control measures can yield huge dividends, particularly for vulnerable children in risk of contracting heart diseases. Proper diagnosis and treatment of streptococcal infections can be achieved through vaccination programs along with them, thus preventing ensuing complications that affect long-term cardiac health. Employment of periodic echocardiography screenings among asymptomatic children in endemic regions demonstrates the value of early detection and intervention efforts towards RHD. By integrating these screening programs with benzathine penicillin prophylaxis, health systems can prevent the formation of latent RHD ahead of time and minimize the impact of associated complications. As pediatric infectious diseases are evolving, increasingly there is a demand for clinicians and researchers to appeal the case for updated guidelines that outline the dynamics of vaccination and infection control measures in safeguarding cardiovascular health among children (Ali, 2022; Vos et al., 2024).

8.6.3. Education and Awareness Programs

Education and health awareness programs play a critical role in the control and prevention of acquired heart diseases among children. The interventions are focused on educating parents, caregivers, and healthcare providers on the risk factors associated with heart diseases and thereby embracing preventive health practices. Education programs can deliver critical information through community health outreach, workshops, and the internet concerning nutrition guidance, exercise, and routine medical examinations. Such awareness not only prepares families with the ability to recognize early signs of heart disease but also emphasizes the need for preventive care, bringing the rate of such conditions down. By making the resources accessible and creating supportive environments that encourage heart-healthy behavior, education and awareness programs form a core support in the arena of pediatrics cardiology. In particular, focused community-based interventions can well address the unique needs of at-risk children for acquired heart diseases. These interventions focus on high prevalence communities and employ culturally relevant materials and strategies to reach diverse populations. For instance, education on the impact of processed-food diets, lack of physical activity, and tobacco exposure can be complemented with lively activities such as food demonstration cooking or physical activity mobilization projects. These also allow for the potential to create collaborative networks that bring schools, local health agencies, and voluntary groups together in order to enhance the reach and influence of the campaign. By promoting community spirit regarding heart health, education of this type can incite action on a population level, having a dramatic effect upon the health of children and making long-term changes to lifestyles. Furthermore, integrating education and awareness programs within schools is particularly relevant as children spend the majority of their day at school. Adding heart health education will not only capture students' attention but also promote early learning and personal responsibility. Physical education, nutrition education, and even health fairs can build an educational climate that prioritizes heart health. Collaborating with local healthcare professionals to provide screening and workshops can also enhance school education efficacy. This coordinated strategy functions to normalize dialogue regarding heart health so that children can acquire knowledge of the threats and take responsibility for their heart health early in their lives. This has been emphasized in research as required in the endeavor to enhance against rising incidence of acquired heart disease among children, necessitating ongoing investment in awareness campaigns (Bayapareddy et al., 2024; Lam, 2022).

SUMMARY

The increasing prevalence of acquired heart diseases among children calls for an extensive understanding of their etiology and appropriate management principles. Socioeconomic status, access to health care, and genetic predispositions play significantly influencing roles on outcomes. Rheumatic heart disease (RHD), for instance, remains common in some populations due to the inappropriate treatment of streptococcal infections. Recognition of HLA class II alleles that impart increased risk as well as resistance to rheumatic fever highlights the role of genetic factors in disease susceptibility and dictates preventive intervention of an individualized nature. Recognition of such genetic markers also provides for better screening techniques, allowing clinicians to identify susceptible individuals before irrevocable complications are established and thereby improving public health status overall. Combining these findings into clinical practice is essential in reducing the burden of acquired heart conditions in children. Advances in diagnostic imaging and monitoring have also changed the approach to acquired heart conditions in pediatric patients. Utilizing real-time imaging techniques, including those employing Compressed Sensing, allows accurate assessment of ventricular function without the need for breath-holding, which can be challenging in children. Research confirms the feasibility of these techniques, which allow for rapid data collection—potentially shortening the time needed for MRI scans significantly, as can be attested by the comparison between accelerated imaging and traditional methods (Hughes et al., 2018). Not only does this technology improve the comfort of patients, but also accurate diagnosis and prompt treatment. The inclusion of such advanced imaging technology in the routine clinical practice will enhance our understanding of cardiac performance in children with acquired heart disease so that medical professionals can design more effective treatment plans. Lastly, resolution of acquired heart diseases among children requires a multidisciplinary approach with genetic research, refinement in diagnostic methodology, and improved access to healthcare. Interdisciplinary partnerships among physicians, researchers, and public health professionals play a critical role in assisting in the effective screening programs and education measures. Raising awareness of the risks of uncontrolled infection and inherited susceptibility, we can enable the population to battle effectively against the diseases. Apart from this, continued study of the pathophysiology of acquired heart disease and development of new therapeutic strategies will continue to gain from decreased diagnoses and improved quality of life among infected children. From these considerations, it is imperative that intervention be directed towards prevention and cure in order to gain a healthy future generation (Eglite et al., 2003).

The terrain of acquired heart diseases in children can be drastically shaped by their own vulnerabilities, specifically in contemplating the impact of treatment of other serious illnesses like cancer. For example, children receiving cytotoxic chemotherapy have a much-increased risk of life-threatening infection from neutropenia, a frequent adverse reaction to such treatment. Neutropenia occurs when the bone marrow reduces neutrophil production, crucial white blood cells that combat infection. The discovery that febrile episodes in neutropenic patients demand the immediate empirical antibiotic treatment has altered clinical practice, and priority is given to the acute need for individualized approaches to pediatric oncology that also consider potential cardiac complications. Thus, the understanding of these dynamics not only identifies the broader significance of chemotherapy among children but also the necessity of watchful observation for cardiac health through treatment regimens (Pizzo, 2019). To cure congenital heart conditions (CHD) that can develop into acquired ones, advancements in imaging technologies such as cardiovascular magnetic resonance (CMR) have become imperative for pediatric cardiology. CMR offers a non-invasive technique to quantify cardiac structure and function, which is especially useful for CHD children in whom serial evaluation is required over their growth. In addition to being a diagnostic tool, CMR is employed to directly influence clinical decision-making and management strategies, providing an integrated description of the anatomical and functional status of the heart. As imaging technologies become more accessible and continue to improve, clinical cardiologists must integrate CMR findings not only into primary diagnosis of acquired heart diseases but also into follow-up treatment plans and protocols in order to optimize outcomes (Buechel et al., 2015). Clinical implications for diagnosis of acquired and congenital heart disease in children necessitate an interdisciplinary process across healthcare specialties. Because pediatricians, cardiologists, and oncologists work in a synergistic relationship to observe and treat children who have acquired heart disease, cross-specialty communication becomes even more critical. In specific cases, information gained from immunology and infectious diseases physicians can be beneficially useful in deciphering the possible manner in which secondary illnesses may develop after chemotherapy or cardiac surgery. Through integrating data from these various fields, medical professionals can design comprehensive information plans to address the complicated risks associated with acquired heart disease so that every child receives an evenly balanced and efficient course of treatment based on his or her unique health profile. This consolidated approach is pivotal in preventing complications and improving long-term health status in children with the condition.

CLOSER LOOK

PEDIATRIC HYPERTENSION AND ITS CARDIAC EFFECTS

Childhood hypertension, once uncommon, has become increasingly recognized with the rise in the prevalence of obesity and better screening techniques for blood pressure. Children's hypertension is blood pressure at or above 95th percentile for age, sex, and height and can be primary (essential) or secondary to conditions like renal disease, endocrine disorders, or cardiovascular disease. While secondary hypertension tends to occur more frequently in younger children, primary hypertension tends to occur more frequently in teenagers, especially obese teenagers or teenagers with a family history of hypertension.

Diagnosis of child hypertension must be measured with precise blood pressure, using the appropriate cuff size and repeated on multiple visits. Ambulatory blood pressure monitoring (ABPM) is often used to confirm the diagnosis and screen for white coat hypertension or masked hypertension.

Hypertension in children, particularly if left undiagnosed or poorly controlled, has potentially severe cardiac consequences. The most significant and common is left ventricular hypertrophy (LVH), a consequence of the increased load placed on the heart due to elevated systemic pressure. LVH is an adaptive response that may progress to diastolic dysfunction and, in long-standing or severe cases, systolic dysfunction. Echocardiography is used to quantify left ventricular mass and geometry, and LVH has been associated with increased cardiovascular risk in adults.

In addition to LVH, hypertensive children may also have arterial stiffness, endothelial dysfunction, and carotid intima-media thickness, which are markers of early atherosclerosis. Vasculature alterations raise the risk for future cardiovascular events and highlight the importance of earlier diagnosis and treatment.

Another concern is diastolic dysfunction, where the left ventricle is less compliant and cannot fill as well, with consequent increased left atrial pressures. This will eventually cause heart failure symptoms unless treated. Although overt heart failure in childhood hypertension is unusual, subclinical cardiac function changes will be overlooked without specific evaluation.

In more aggressive or severe forms of pediatric hypertension, such as those related to renal parenchymal disease or aortic coarctation, cardiac damage is deeper. Chronic hypertension can lead to concentric hypertrophy, fibrosis of the myocardium, and increased cardiac load, further impairing cardiac function and increasing the risk of cardiovascular complications.

Treatment of pediatric hypertension involves a combination of lifestyle modifications and drug therapy. Weight reduction increased physical activity, low-sodium diet, and avoidance of tobacco and alcohol are the pillars of lifestyle modification. Antihypertensive medications like ACE inhibitors, angiotensin receptor blockers (ARBs), beta-blockers, calcium channel blockers, and diuretics need to be used, especially in secondary hypertension or when there is target organ damage.

Repeated follow-up with observation of blood pressure and echocardiographic evaluation is necessary for assessing the efficacy of treatment as well as for reversing or preventing cardiac damage. Prompt treatment may lead to LVH regression and improvement of vascular function.

References

1. Abrahamian, F. M., Moran, G. J., & Talan, D. A. (2008). Diagnosis and management of pneumonia in the emergency department. https://core.ac.uk/download/323062323.pdf (accessed on 15th July 2025).
2. Ali, S. (2022). Rheumatic heart disease control: The time for a paradigm shift. *Sudanese Journal of Pediatrics, 22*(2), 125–130. https://www.semanticscholar.org/paper/7849822beb7225eed128238e1e3196caed3ef6b0 (accessed on 15th July 2025).
3. Annambhotla, P., Asad, S., Aslam, S., Basavaraju, S. V., et al. (2019). *Francisella tularensis* transmission by solid organ transplantation, 2017. https://core.ac.uk/download/323070878.pdf (accessed on 15th July 2025).
4. Anwar, S., Alhumaydhi, F., Rahmani, A., Kumar, V., & Alrumaihi, F. A. (2024). A review on risk factors, traditional diagnostic techniques, and biomarkers for pneumonia prognostication and management in diabetic patients. *Diseases, 12.* https://www.semanticscholar.org/paper/00e1d365b30b08ed50aa75e644680ddd179c48f5 (accessed on 15th July 2025).
5. Baalaaji, M. A. R. (2022). Invasive candidiasis in children: Challenges remain. *Indian Journal of Critical Care Medicine.* https://www.semanticscholar.org/paper/1a7c51d7fa56d355b8028d8078e6104f079c7ac9 (accessed on 15th July 2025).
6. Bakir, J., Castellano, V., Gentile, Á., Grobaporto, M., et al. (2014). Respiratory syncytial virus: Clinical and epidemiological pattern in pediatric patients admitted to a children's hospital between 2000 and 2013. https://core.ac.uk/download/159292401.pdf (accessed on 15th July 2025).
7. Bal, H. I., Türkyılmaz, İ., Kayalı, Ş., & Kılıç, A. (2024). Subtle myocardial effects of rheumatic heart disease in children are revealed earlier with two-dimensional speckle tracking echocardiography. *The Turkish Journal of Pediatrics, 66*(3), 346–353. https://www.semanticscholar.org/paper/5de76438786b1ef605d5d43c085ad0236fa6570d (accessed on 15th July 2025).
8. Bashshur, R. L., Doarn, C. R., Frenk, J., Kvedar, J. C., & Woolliscroft, J. O. (2020). Telemedicine and the COVID-19 pandemic, lessons for the future. *Telemedicine Journal and e-Health, 26,* 571–573. https://doi.org/10.1089/tmj.2020.29040.rb (accessed on 15th July 2025)
9. Bayapareddy, N., Zahrani, Y., Alqahtani, H. E. M., Mamilla Mugaiahgari, B. K., Viswanath Reddy, L. K., Asif, S. M., Almoyad, M. A. A., et al. (2024). Examining the prevalence of congenital anomalies in newborns: A cross-sectional study at a tertiary care maternity hospital in Saudi Arabia. *Children, 11.* https://www.semanticscholar.org/paper/6e4986ba29f3522a75346ec86cdc87282d9c8fd5 (accessed on 15th July 2025).
10. Benkirane, A., Benslimani, A., Corwin, A., Omezzine-Letaief, A., Rekiki, A., Znazen, A., et al. (2014). Epidemiology of *Coxiella burnetii* infection in Africa: A OneHealth systematic review. https://core.ac.uk/download/20480149.pdf (accessed on 15th July 2025).
11. Berger, J., Faerber, J., Chen, F., Lin, K. Y., Brothers, J., & O'Byrne, M. (2022). Adherence with lipid screening guidelines in children with acquired and congenital heart disease: An observational study using data from the MarketScan Commercial and Medicaid Databases. *Journal of the American Heart Association: Cardiovascular and Cerebrovascular Disease, 11.*

https://www.semanticscholar.org/paper/5b8f8df9c6324aa18131980036546dd10dff2489 (accessed on 15th July 2025).

12. Bull, M. J., Trotter, T. L., Santoro, S. L., Christensen, C. K., & Grout, R. W. (2022). Health supervision for children and adolescents with Down syndrome. *Pediatrics, 149.* https://doi.org/10.1542/peds.2022-057010 (accessed on 15th July 2025).
13. Buyon, J. P., Duncanson, L. J., Friedman, D. M., Glickstein, J., et al. (2003). A review of congenital heart block. https://core.ac.uk/download/46602900.pdf (accessed on 15th July 2025).
14. Corsello, G., Falsaperla, R., Parano, E., Pavone, P., Praticò, A. D., Rizzo, R., Ruggieri, M., et al. (2016). Congenital muscular dystrophy: From muscle to brain. https://core.ac.uk/download/286528712.pdf (accessed on 15th July 2025).
15. Daniels, Q., Sadoh, E. W., & Uzodimma, C. C. (2014). Childhood acquired heart disease in Nigeria: An echocardiographic study from three centers. https://core.ac.uk/download/478289365.pdf (accessed on 15th July 2025).
16. Eglite, J., Gardovska, D., Shantere, R., Sochnevs, V., et al. (2003). HLA class II associations with rheumatic heart disease among clinically homogeneous patients in children in Latvia. https://core.ac.uk/download/pdf/3405302.pdf (accessed on 15th July 2025).
17. Elliott, P., Anastasakis, A., Borger, M. A., Borggrefe, M., Cecchi, F., Charron, P., Hagège, A., et al. (2014). 2014 ESC guidelines on diagnosis and management of hypertrophic cardiomyopathy. *European Heart Journal, 35,* 2733–2779. https://doi.org/10.1093/eurheartj/ehu284 (accessed on 15th July 2025).
18. Hughes, M., Kowalik, G. T., Mortensen, K. H., Muthurangu, V., et al. (2018). Real-time assessment of right and left ventricular volumes and function in children using high spatiotemporal resolution spiral bSSFP with compressed sensing. https://core.ac.uk/download/195312244.pdf (accessed on 15th July 2025).
19. International Labour Office, Bureau of Statistics. (2004). *Statistics on the Employment Situation of People with Disabilities: A Compendium of National Methodologies.* https://core.ac.uk/download/5129420.pdf (accessed on 15th July 2025).
20. Jaeggi, E. T., & Suter, S. (2001). [Clinical presentation, diagnosis and management of inflammatory heart diseases in childhood]. *Therapeutische Umschau. Revue Thérapeutique, 58*(2), 87–93. https://www.semanticscholar.org/paper/2cf5fdefb9fdcdf1e605d9dded7befcd666dca0d (accessed on 15th July 2025).
21. Jone, P., Tremoulet, A., Choueiter, N., Dominguez, S. R., Harahsheh, A. S., Mitani, Y., Zimmerman, M., et al. (2024). Update on diagnosis and management of Kawasaki disease: A scientific statement from the American Heart Association. *Circulation.* https://www.semanticscholar.org/paper/e5bfcb90a1431fdaa571bcb0fe2bdf515646eb58 (accessed on 15th July 2025).
22. Jung, H., Ha, Y., Kim, D., Park, J., Kang, C., Chung, D., Park, S., et al. (2014). Native valve endocarditis due to extended spectrum β-lactamase producing *Klebsiella pneumoniae. The Korean Journal of Internal Medicine, 29,* 398–401. https://www.semanticscholar.org/paper/82f2db67381a8955e7e8857c9ddd04ce8cc8244e (accessed on 15th July 2025).
23. Khan, M. H., Ahsan, A., Mehta, F., Kanawala, A., Mondal, R., Dilshad, A., & Akbar, A. (2024). Precision medicine in congenital heart disease, rheumatic heart disease, and Kawasaki disease of children: An overview of literature. *Cardiology in Review.* https://www.semanticscholar.org/paper/77b9f91bcbe63d3ee3613764e5f4f9930021e181 (accessed on 15th July 2025).

24. King, J., Lehrnbecher, T., Pana, Z. D., Steinbach, W. J., et al. (2017). Recognition and clinical presentation of invasive fungal disease in neonates and children. https://core.ac.uk/download/131024549.pdf (accessed on 15th July 2025).

25. Kudryavtseva, L. G., Lazarkov, P. V., & Sergevnin, V. I. (2021). Comparative assessment of risk of development of purulent septic infections in children after open and closed cardiac operations for congenital diseases. *Medical Alphabet.* https://www.semanticscholar.org/paper/e313df6a0918540e87a1044e34968c40f938f23b (accessed on 15th July 2025).

26. Lam, D. (2022). World Lung Day 2022—Lung health for all. *Respirology, 27,* 810–811. https://www.semanticscholar.org/paper/d526c41df71006c778cd6469f69afc1b6563c018 (accessed on 15th July 2025).

27. Mach, F., Baigent, C., Catapano, A. L., Koskinas, K. C., Casula, M., Badimón, L., Chapman, M. J., et al. (2019). 2019 ESC/EAS guidelines for the management of dyslipidemias: Lipid modification to reduce cardiovascular risk. *European Heart Journal, 41,* 111–188. https://doi.org/10.1093/eurheartj/ehz455 (accessed on 15th July 2025).

28. Machhi, J., Herskovitz, J., Senan, A. M., Dutta, D., Nath, B., Oleynikov, M., Blomberg, W. R., et al. (2020). The natural history, pathobiology, and clinical manifestations of SARS-CoV-2 infections. *Journal of Neuroimmune Pharmacology, 15,* 359–386. https://doi.org/10.1007/s11481-020-09944-5 (accessed on 15th July 2025).

29. Majani, N. G., Koster, J. R., Kalezi, Z., Letara, N., Nkya, D. A., Mongela, S., Kubhoja, S., et al. (2024). Spectrum of heart diseases in children in a national cardiac referral center Tanzania, Eastern Africa: A six-year overview. *Global Heart, 19.* https://www.semanticscholar.org/paper/69ef90527c0c7fb79584b1ab78129fe520562abd (accessed on 15th July 2025).

30. Malska, A., Kurilyak, O., Nakonechna, L. M., Klymyshyn, Y., Stogova, O., Raad, T., & Rudenko, N. (2024). Features of diagnosis of incomplete Kawasaki disease in young children. A clinical case of Kawasaki disease with the formation of giant coronary artery aneurysms. *Child's Health.* https://www.semanticscholar.org/paper/1842a293a47a3f7cffa9bc29c992cb7e5864b152 (accessed on 15th July 2025).

31. Marhaba, A., Gul, J., Jan, M. A., Karim, S. A., Waqas, M., & Ikram, M. (2025). Prevalence and management of congenital heart diseases in Pakistan: A comprehensive cross-sectional study. *Journal of Health, Wellness and Community Research.* https://www.semanticscholar.org/paper/741b3fd6c7928a9675f3187a8ba53483f7a9a1fc (accessed on 15th July 2025).

32. McCrindle, B., & Manlhiot, C. (2020). SARS-CoV-2-related inflammatory multisystem syndrome in children: Different or shared etiology and pathophysiology as Kawasaki disease? *JAMA.* https://www.semanticscholar.org/paper/efbc8e17fe8ed15fb31d6590aa4d2dc875873321 (accessed on 15th July 2025).

33. Murray, C. J. L., Ikuta, K. S., Sharara, F., Swetschinski, L. R., Aguilar, G. R., Gray, A. P., Han, C., et al. (2022). Global burden of bacterial antimicrobial resistance in 2019: A systematic analysis. *The Lancet, 399,* 629–655. https://doi.org/10.1016/s0140-6736(21)02724-0 (accessed on 15th July 2025).

34. Musana, K. A., Yale, S., Mazza, J., & Reed, K. (2004). Practical considerations to influenza vaccination. *Clinical Medicine & Research, 2*(4), 256–259. https://www.semanticscholar.org/paper/a6017056a37ef59dd7b835b186fb582ea4a4786f (accessed on 15th July 2025).

35. Pasławska, M., Grodzka, A., Peczyńska, J., Sawicka, B., & Bossowski, A. (2024). Role of miRNA in cardiovascular diseases in children—Systematic review. *International Journal of Molecular Sciences, 25.* https://www.semanticscholar.org/paper/7edec4460a52808b076fe69f454355300a5e0283 (accessed on 15th July 2025).

36. Pizzo, P. (2019). Management of patients with fever and neutropenia through the arc of time. *Annals of Internal Medicine, 170*, 389–397. https://www.semanticscholar.org/paper/230391e07a5738835a59c2f1a9997846bf05c34b (accessed on 15th July 2025).

37. Priori, S. G., Blomström-Lundqvist, C., Mazzanti, A., Blom, N., Borggrefe, M., Camm, A. J., Elliott, P., et al. (2015). 2015 ESC guidelines for the management of patients with ventricular arrhythmias and the prevention of sudden cardiac death. *European Heart Journal, 36*, 2793–2867. https://doi.org/10.1093/eurheartj/ehv316 (accessed on 15th July 2025).

38. Reemtsen, B., Finn, J. P., Alejos, J., Touma, M., Halnon, N., Nelson, S. F., et al. (2017). A path to implement precision child health cardiovascular medicine. https://core.ac.uk/download/323077346.pdf (accessed on 15th July 2025).

39. Rudd, K. E., Johnson, S. C., Agesa, K. M., Shackelford, K. A., Tsoi, D., Kievlan, D., Colombara, D. V., et al. (2020). Global, regional, and national sepsis incidence and mortality, 1990–2017: Analysis for the Global Burden of Disease Study. *The Lancet, 395*, 200–211. https://doi.org/10.1016/s0140-6736(19)32989-7 (accessed on 15th July 2025).

40. Salzillo, C., La Verde, M., Imparato, A., Molitierno, R., Lucà, S., Pagliuca, F., & Marzullo, A. (2024). Cardiovascular diseases in public health: Chromosomal abnormalities in congenital heart disease causing sudden cardiac death in children. *Medicina, 60.* https://www.semanticscholar.org/paper/2ea7ce72d6c06fe55f2371702a5e36f24076f095 (accessed on 15th July 2025).

41. Saxena, R., Mehrotra, M., Mehrotra, V., Singh, A., & Saxena, S. (2025). Assessment of serum lipoprotein (a) and total cholesterol in children of CAD parents. *International Journal of Clinical Biochemistry and Research.* https://www.semanticscholar.org/paper/5beb6889c40d5aa4d4762b13a3e8777eb0f0c41d (accessed on 15th July 2025).

42. Sreeman, N. (2017). Study on spectrum of heart diseases in children aged 1 month to 12 years. https://core.ac.uk/download/235661353.pdf (accessed on 15th July 2025).

43. Szczepura, A., Bhopal, R., Cappuccio, F. P., Connor, M., Duke, V., Foster, C., Hawthorne, G., et al. (2011). Nutrition in an ethnically diverse society: What are some of the key challenges? https://core.ac.uk/download/44180.pdf (accessed on 15th July 2025).

44. Talwar, S., Bhende, V. V., Krishnakumar, M., Tandon, K., & Patel, P. R. (2025). Is surgery for congenital heart defects in neonates, infants, and children more challenging and demanding than surgery for acquired heart defects in adults? *Cureus, 17.* https://www.semanticscholar.org/paper/9bb3735cac3b263a8f5717c33b31c009c4b62ca2 (accessed on 15th July 2025).

45. Tretter, J. T., & Jacobs, J. (2021). Global leadership in pediatric and congenital cardiac care: "Coding our way to improved care: an interview with Rodney C. G. Franklin, MBBS, MD, FRCP, FRCPCH". *Cardiology in the Young, 31*, 11–19. https://www.semanticscholar.org/paper/69f51d3829904f495469f7a321ef3d37a037b61c (accessed on 15th July 2025).

46. Valsangiacomo Buechel, E. V., Grosse-Wortmann, L., Fratz, S., Eichhorn, J., Sarikouch, S., Greil, G., Beerbaum, P., et al. (2015). Indications for cardiovascular magnetic resonance in children with congenital and acquired heart disease: An expert consensus paper of the Imaging Working Group of the AEPC and the Cardiovascular Magnetic Resonance Section of

the EACVI. *European Heart Journal Cardiovascular Imaging, 16*(3), 281–297. https://www.semanticscholar.org/paper/095dc586cd508ae48a0fc14d62397921b82809e8 (accessed on 15th July 2025).

47. Vijayan, V., Connolly, J., Condell, J., McKelvey, N., & Gardiner, P. (2021). Review of wearable devices and data collection considerations for connected health. *Sensors, 21*, 5589–5589. https://doi.org/10.3390/s21165589 (accessed on 15th July 2025).

48. Vos, M., Voor in 't Holt, A. F., Severin, J., & van der Schoor, A. S. (2024). Creating synergy: The partnership between infection prevention & control architectural design for a healthier hospital. *Studies in Health Technology and Informatics, 319*, 280–291. https://www.semanticscholar.org/paper/95e0c621a8fb2a93355c90a0f822aae0733400e7 (accessed on 15th July 2025).

49. Wang, Y., & Li, T. (2022). Advances in understanding Kawasaki disease-related immuno-inflammatory response and vascular endothelial dysfunction. *Pediatric Investigation, 6*, 271–279. https://www.semanticscholar.org/paper/6d284018648ea9ab17e6a60580d2cda73d779288 (accessed on 15th July 2025).

50. Zachariah, J. P., Jone, P., Agbaje, A., Ryan, H. H., Trasande, L., Perng, W., & Farzan, S. (2024). Environmental exposures and pediatric cardiology: A scientific statement from the American Heart Association. *Circulation, 149*, e1165–e1175. https://www.semanticscholar.org/paper/5fc70b83a52940c661c4da3eb46d8ca7bad70014 (accessed on 15th July 2025).

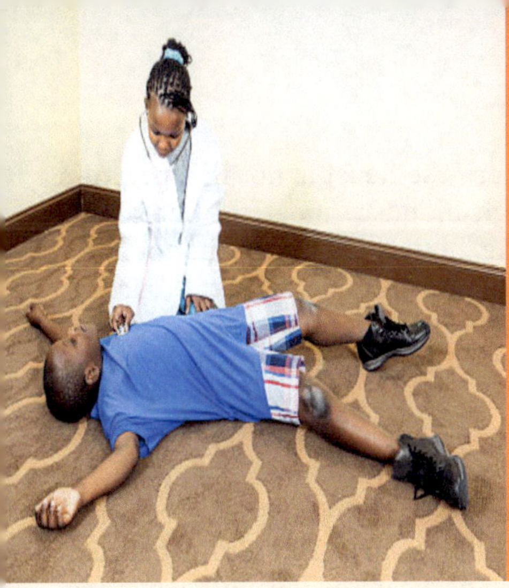

Chapter 9 HEART FAILURE IN CHILDREN

Contents

Introduction

Heart failure in children is a complex and multi-faceted syndrome that needs to be understood and recognized in its totality. Unlike in adults, where heart failure has most frequently been linked with ischemic heart disease, heart failure in children is frequently the result of congenital heart lesions, cardiomyopathies, and other systemic conditions. Presentation in children can be uncharacteristic, leading to misdiagnosis or delayed treatment. This makes the situation more complicated because of children's various developmental levels, necessitating individualized diagnostic and management methods. Emerging research emphasizes the need for early detection and treatment because early therapeutic intervention might significantly maximize outcomes. Knowledge about the unique etiology of heart failure in children forms the foundation for both health care providers and families to collaborate in managing this life-altering disorder. The implication of heart failure extends beyond the physical limitations that impact children with the disease; there are immense psychosocial implications as well. Children with heart failure typically remain anxious, isolated, and scared, impacting not only their but also their family members' quality of life. Further, the role of the caregivers is very important since they need to handle complex care plans while providing emotional support as well. This interconnection between medical care and psychological wellness highlights the need for balanced treatment strategies that factor both physical and emotional health. Programs aimed at these factors such as the iPad-Enhanced Shared Care Intervention for Partners (iSCIP) have succeeded in enhancing self-management and inter-personal communication between patients, caregivers, and healthcare workers. By prioritizing these areas, we can create an environment with resilience and adaptability for children with heart failure. With ongoing research, increased emphasis is being placed on novel interventions to improve the outcome of care in pediatric heart failure. The use of technology, such as mobile health applications, is facilitating patient management by enhancing communication and self-monitoring capabilities. These interventions are also being fashioned to not only educate children and caregivers regarding the disease but also empower them in the process. For instance, a study comparing the iSCIP—a patient- and caregiver-involving intervention—demonstrates its effectiveness in improving self-management and communication of care preferences. With the growing pediatric population becoming increasingly diverse, it is imperative that health professionals embrace such transitions and prioritize initiatives that reinforce the medical and psychosocial dimensions of care for pediatric patients with heart failure, ultimately building improved health outcomes and quality of life.

Definition of Heart Failure in Children

Diagnosis of heart failure in children is also intricate and requires an understanding of the involved physiology and also the clinical presentation of the condition. Heart failure is a condition where the heart is not in a position to pump enough blood to meet the metabolic demands of the body, which can happen for numerous reasons like congenital cardiac abnormalities, cardiomyopathies, and acquired cardiac diseases. Children are not like adults, wherein they have different signs according to their growing body and systems. This calls for a delicate evaluation of the child's development stages and how heart failure affects their physical and psychosocial health. Heart failure in children can also occur in the form of tachypnea, fatigue, and failure to feed, thereby complicating the diagnosis and treatment of this condition further (Shaigany et al., 2020).

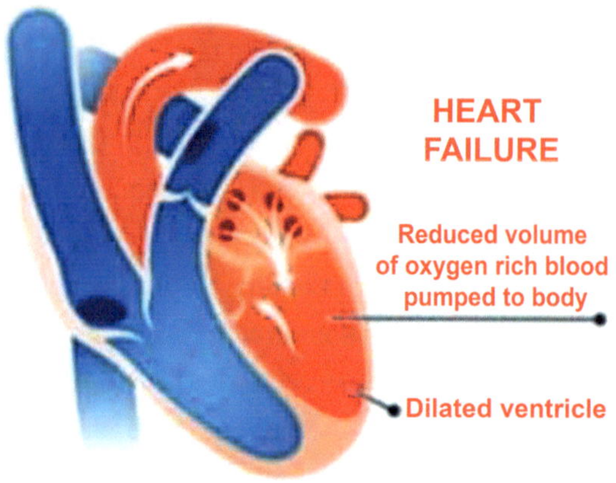

Figure 9.1. Heart failure in children.

Source: https://external-content.duckduckgo.com/iu/?u=https%3A%2F%2Fimage.slidesharecdn.com%2Fheartfailureinchildren-240711090826-ddec5a85%2F85%2FHeart-failure-in-children-AND-ITS-MANAGENMT-pptx-4-638.jpg&f=1&nofb=1&ipt=6d900345799f3d4951378768c9cfcb077add15c28ebdea01be3586917352bee5.

Heart failure in children is incredibly difficult to diagnose because of similar symptomatic manifestations of other diseases in children. While adult heart failure shows distinct clinical presentation, children can only show nonspecific presentation such as failure to grow or intolerance to exercise. Moreover, as a result of the continuous maturation of the pediatric cardiovascular system, compensatory physiological mechanisms start to become capable of concealing the severity of heart failure, and late presentations become frequent. This necessitates a reliance on many diagnostic modalities, including echocardiography, to successfully detect cardiac dysfunction. Apart from that, acute versus chronic heart failure classification is vital in management because chronic heart failure progresses over years while acute ones emerge overnight, at times even requiring urgent medical intervention (Clyde et al., 2016) (Figure 9.1).

The implications of pediatric heart failure extend beyond the cardiology clinic to affect the overall quality of life and long-term health status of the child. Families can also wrestle with the psychological and emotional demands of managing a chronic illness in an infant. Understanding the definition of heart failure in this context is essential for the planning of individualized treatment plans. Management often involves a multidisciplinary approach which may include medication, lifestyle counseling, and ongoing monitoring to be adjusted to the evolving needs of the child. It is also important for healthcare practitioners to include families in shared decision-making, making decisions about treatment to match the individualized needs and circumstances of the child, yet fostering hope and resilience in the context of challenges posed by heart failure (Shaigany et al., 2020).

Importance of Studying Pediatric Heart Failure

The growing incidence of heart failure in children poses the necessity for a comprehensive study of its cause and implications. Studies of heart failure in children provide valuable insight into the unique cause and pathophysiology of this group that may be significantly different from those of adults. Congenital heart disease (CHD), for instance, is prevalent among children and presents unique clinical challenges. It is essential to understand such differences so that one can design age-appropriate treatment modalities and interventions. Furthermore, the prevalent prevalence of hypertension among young people, as proven by Agabiti-Rosei et al. (2016), again emphasizes the importance of its existence in the progression of heart failure. By studying these factors, healthcare professionals can better individualize preventive interventions, therapy, and education designed to reduce the incidence of heart failure among children. Also, pediatric heart failure has an impact that extends beyond its clinical significance, spilling over into the psychological and social lives of children. Children with heart failure are typically faced with chronic illness stressors that might disrupt their emotional development and social adaptation. Evidence shows that failure to manage these psychosocial problems will exacerbate the condition and affect long-term health. Being proponents of an integrative model for pediatric medicine, there is a need to consider the various aspects of heart failure in pediatric patients. This will enable physicians to make appeals for interventions and resources that not only improve clinical outcomes but also their overall well-being as individuals and families. By such an outlook, the importance of pediatric heart failure research comes across as an interdisciplinary process dynamically integrated into the general healthcare environment. Methodological advancements in pediatric heart failure assessment have further highlighted the importance of this research. Advances in technology, such as noninvasive monitoring devices that employ near-infrared spectroscopy (NIRS), enable researchers to understand more deeply the physiological response to exercise and recovery in children with heart disease, writes Danduran et al. (2012). Advances make possible early detection and intervention, which are most critical in the management of the complications arising from heart failure among children. Secondly, it can promote remarkable advancements in treatment policies and guidelines, further closing the gap between adult and pediatric cardiovascular management. In all, a concerted effort on pediatric heart failure not only improves clinical practice but also informs public health strategies to reduce the occurrence and severity of heart ailments in children (Figure 9.2).

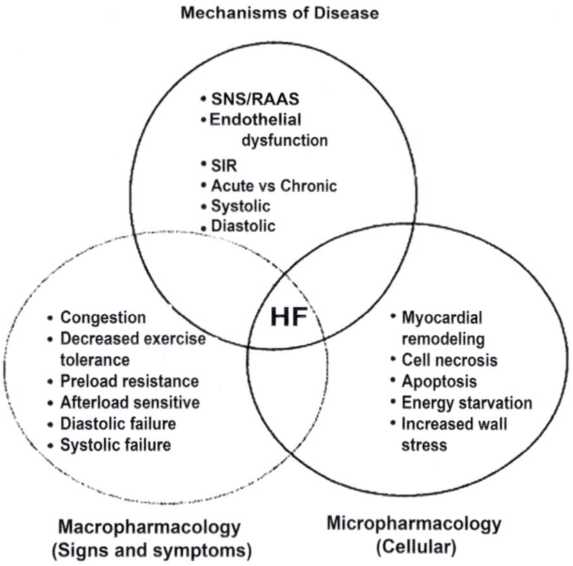

Figure 9.2. In this model, the proposed paradigms have been placed into three major groups that intersect to define the heart failure syndrome.

Source: https://www.sciencedirect.com/science/article/pii/S1058981300000485.

9.1. Causes of Heart Failure in Children

Heart failure in children can be due to many underlying etiologies that need prolonged clinical assessments. Congenital heart malformations are one of the major reasons for heart failure because structural defects disrupt usual dynamics of blood flow across the heart. Some malformations, such as ventricular septal malformations or aortic coarctation, can cause workload on the heart, which, if not managed, ultimately results in heart failure. Besides, cardiomyopathy, an illness of the heart muscle, also leads to heart failure in children. Conditions such as dilated cardiomyopathy tend to present with no easily discernible etiology, though they may have a genetic, viral, or toxic etiology. Recognition of the causative factors is vital in order to create a proper treatment regimen appropriate to the specific needs of each child, thereby maximizing clinical benefits. The second leading cause of heart failure in children is the existence of diastolic dysfunction. While usually characteristic of adults, particularly with heart failure with preserved ejection fraction (HFpEF), this condition also exists in children. Diastolic dysfunction is defined as the impaired filling of the heart due to the structural or functional impairment of the left ventricle, which thus impairs cardiac output. Although less frequent than in adults, diastolic dysfunction diagnosis in children is likewise difficult. A number of variables, including pulmonary hypertension, have been identified as potential causative variables in children and complicate the clinical scenario typically. Given that diastolic dysfunction is also able to induce congestive heart failure when systolic function is intact, identification and knowledge of its importance by the pediatric population are essential for intervention and treatment at an early stage (Quennelle et al., 2023). Last but not least, drug therapy interaction with physiological feedback mechanisms among children is very effective in deciding the course of heart failure progression. As an example, increased plasma renin activity (PRA) levels have come under investigation, particularly among children with heart failure. Data show that infants with heart failure tend to have increased PRA levels, which again increase after administration of angiotensin-converting enzyme inhibitors (ACEi). These findings suggest a complex physiological response that may impact the clinical course of children with heart failure. The physicians ought to be attentive towards the dynamic fluctuations in PRA levels and its implications in forecasting prognosis and treatment response. Proper knowledge of the delicacies of such physiological markers will eventually assist the healthcare providers to deliver best-fit care strategies to this vulnerable population (Steichert et al., 2023) (Figure 9.3).

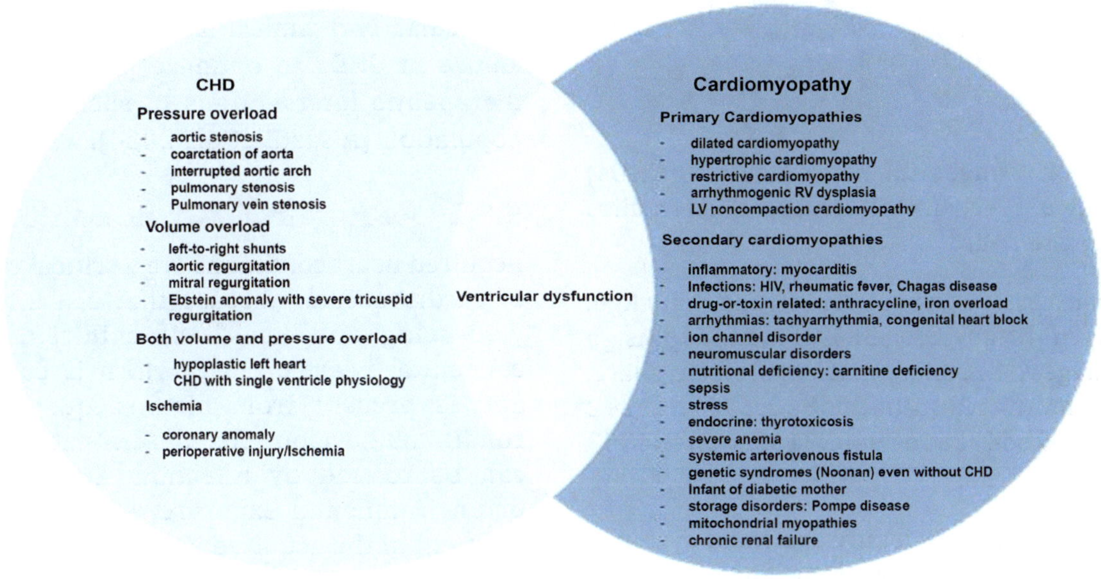

Figure 9.3. Common causes of heart failure in children—the relationship of ventricular dysfunction to CHD and cardiomyopathy.

Source: https://www.mdpi.com/2227-9067/5/7/88.

9.1.1. Congenital Heart Defects

Congenital heart defects (CHDs) are a spectrum of cardiac structural abnormalities, which can have a major impact on pediatric health, including heart failure. The defects hamper normal blood flow and can result from genetic or environmental insults during fetal development. Studies indicate that CHD is present at a rate of 1 in 100 among live births, and thus it is crucial to have a clear understanding of their etiology and clinical relevance. Heart failure secondary to CHDs usually presents as the result of ventricular dysfunction, volume overload, or pressure overload. Pediatric cardiologists are thus faced with the dilemma of management that must differ from adults because of the different physiological status of children. It is vital to know the mechanisms behind to improve outcomes and requires continued research on common and uncommon congenital abnormalities precipitated by heart failure in children (Alsaadi et al., 2024). Congenital cardiac malformations are usually treated with surgery, which results in further complications including inflammation and organ failure. One of the most significant complications of corrective surgery of CHDs is the use of cardiopulmonary bypass, an intervention required to obtain a bloodless field of surgery (Figure 9.4).

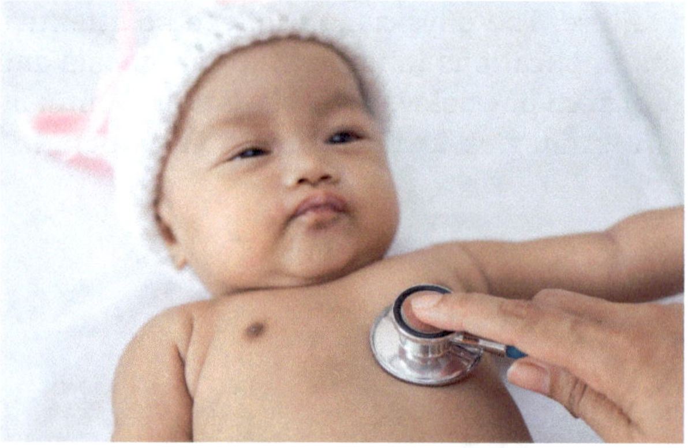

Figure 9.4. Congenital heart defects (CHDs) represent a spectrum of structural anomalies affecting the heart.

Source: https://external-content.duckduckgo.com/iu/?u=https%3A%2F%2Fmedlineplus.gov%2Fimages%2FCongenitalHeartDefects_share.jpg&f=1&nofb=1&ipt=b4d0d860c5117ddb29260341bfd97bd47031d8948391a8afb5f4848538eaef3e.

However, this procedure can cause systemic inflammatory responses that aggravate the condition of the child, including the development of acute kidney injury. Studies have proven that renal replacement therapy can be an effective treatment of postoperative complications in pediatric patients. Particularly, the use of renal replacement therapy along with routine surgical treatment has been effective in stabilizing patients after heart surgery, considering the intricate interaction between surgical recovery and organ function (Artyom et al., 2024). Furthermore, the long-term effects of congenital heart malformations extend beyond the acute postoperative condition and impact the lifelong well-being of the affected children. Children, however, are usually presented with a large number of comorbidities like developmental delay and psychological disorders complicating their overall medical condition. These caregivers would hence present with characteristic presentations of heart failure markedly deviating from the adult type necessitating the creation of a special way of clinical evaluation and treatment. It is imperative to adopt a multidisciplinary model of care that includes cardiologists, surgeons, nutritionists, and psychiatrists to cater to the diverse needs of such patients. There is a need for the future research to continuously investigate the genetic, molecular, and clinical factors related to heart failure in CHDs to optimize preventative and therapeutic interventions in such a high-risk population (Alsaadi et al., 2024).

9.1.2. Acquired Heart Conditions

Acquired heart conditions are a critical category of cardiovascular disease that can affect the well-being and health of children. Unlike congenital heart disease, which is congenital and is present from birth, acquired heart conditions develop after the neonatal age and can be caused by infection, autoimmunity, or environmental exposure. Among the most frequent of the acquired conditions in children, myocarditis, endocarditis, and cardiomyopathy are among the most frequent. Myocarditis, in the majority of cases from viral infection, can lead to inflammation of the heart muscle and ultimately to compromised cardiac function. With the acute onset of heart failure in these cases, parents and healthcare providers alike need to be vigilant about early indicators to provide on-time intervention that can radically alter outcomes and minimize long-term complications of the heart. Thus, it is important in pediatric cardiology to appreciate the intricacies of acquired heart conditions, especially as they impact the potential for heart failure in children. Adding complexity to the situation is the role of systemic diseases, such as autoimmune diseases, which can lead to specific cardiac complications. Lupus and rheumatic fever are some examples of diseases that can cause an increased risk of cardiac issues, such as pericarditis or valvular heart disease, which will further deteriorate the already weak health of a child's heart. The long-term inflammation caused by these conditions will trigger changes in the structure of cardiac tissue and thus predispose manifestations of heart failure. This association leads to the need for interdisciplinary care that involves not only cardiovascular implications, but also the overall health of the child. Their management will have to be carried out by cardiologists and pediatricians in collaboration, with the inference being that interdisciplinary treatment is essential in the management of acquired heart disease to avoid risks of heart failure in children. The epidemiologic patterns of acquired heart conditions also mirror the significance of regional health issues, as seen through those of Chagas disease. Predominantly affecting children in endemic areas, the parasitic illness may lead to chronic heart failure by inducing cardiac tissue and conduction system injury. Of particular note in Latin America, the burden of Chagas disease is more than a function of its direct clinical effect since it can result in life-long cardiac complications in infected children. Furthermore, the World Health Organization and Centers for Disease Control and Prevention emphasize the importance of targeted public health interventions to reduce the burden of this neglected tropical disease, which remains endemic in most countries. Treating these acquired heart conditions not only requires medical progress and resources but also preventive care attention. Combined, understanding the causes of acquired heart conditions is important to reduce heart failure prevalence in children, hence promoting healthier futures for those who are vulnerable.

9.1.3. Genetic Factors and Syndromes

Genetic factors are of extreme significance in the etiology of heart failure in children, particularly by way of occurrence of congenital heart diseases (CHDs) and syndromes rendering these patients susceptible to cardiovascular sequelae. Congenital heart disease develops due to heterogeneous genetic abnormalities, either inherited or de novo mutations. In a study at Bangabandhu Sheikh Mujib Medical University, it was discovered that a high percentage of CHD children had associated genetic disorders (i.e., Down syndrome in 8% of CHD cases). This underlines the need for early genetic evaluation and careful clinical evaluation in children with heart failure symptoms. Through the early detection of genetic predispositions, medical clinicians can institute specific interventions that can reduce morbidity and mortality from heart failure resulting from congenital defect. Additionally, certain syndromes such as Noonan syndrome and other genetic mutations have been linked with poor cardiac outcomes, affecting the prognosis of affected children.

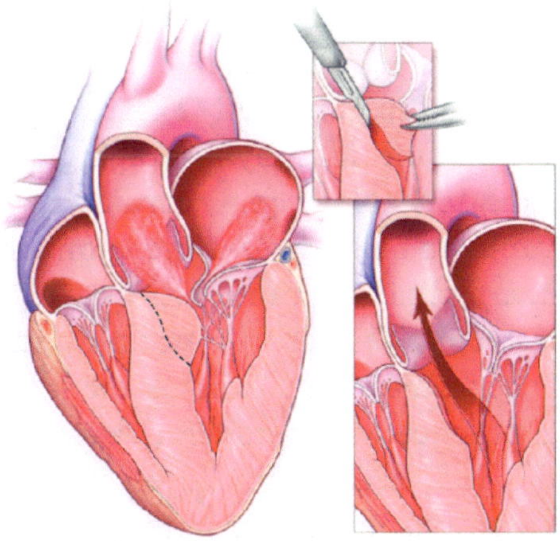

Figure 9.5. Cross-section of a heart with hypertrophic obstructive cardiomyopathy (HOCM), with reduced left ventricular outflow and mitral regurgitation.

Source: https://www.researchgate.net/profile/Frank-Halfwerk/publication/383663764/figure/fig1/AS:11431281283997032@1729075804524/Cross-section-of-a-heart-with-hypertrophic-obstructive-cardiomyopathy-HOCM-with-reduced.png.

A study involving children with hypertrophic obstructive cardiomyopathy (HOCM) showed that the genetically mutated individuals had poorer prognoses following the surgery compared to those not genetically mutated. Genetic mutations here were responsible for a number of complications, including heart failure and malignant ventricular arrhythmias, particularly following surgeries for repair of structural anomalies (Figure 9.5).

The link of some genetic syndromes with the nature of cardiac manifestations mandates tailored treatment. This can include preoperative assessment and genetic counseling to better inform families about the risk of their child's condition. Genetic influences are not only pointing to associations but also enlightening us on interventions that are potentially capable of halting the deterioration of heart failure in children. For instance, tailored treatment planning based on the patient's genetic predisposition (e.g., the extent of left ventricular hypertrophy) can potentially exert a significant influence on outcomes. By leveraging advances in imaging technology (e.g., cardiac computed tomography to build three-dimensional models of the heart) clinicians can identify specific areas of hypertrophy that are prognostic indicators of poor outcomes. This enables them to tailor surgical practice and postoperative care to meet the individual needs of children with genetic predispositions or syndromic presentation. Finally, the integration of genetic information into the management of children can lead to enhanced monitoring, individualized therapies, and improved survival in children at risk for heart failure.

9.2. Symptoms and Diagnosis

The clinical presentation of heart failure in children is occasionally subtle and frequently merges with other childhood conditions, and therefore correct diagnosis is challenging. Common symptoms are non-specific and may present as fatigue, poor feeding, and failure to thrive in toddlers and infants. Such signs are easily misattributed to be symptoms of normal growth or common childhood illnesses. Also, as younger children below two years typically have presentations that resemble respiratory infections, this can conceal the actual diagnosis of dilated cardiomyopathy (DCM) or acute myocarditis (Ahmed et al., 2023). Proper evaluation should then be done in these scenarios, with careful monitoring of vital signs and an accurate clinical history to exclude heart failure due to other common illnesses in children. Diagnostic modalities are a crucial key to diagnosing heart failure and the etiologies thereof in children. Electrocardiograms (ECGs), echocardiography, and, if necessary, cardiac magnetic resonance imaging (MRI) are the crucial tools that allow clinicians to visualize cardiac structure and function. In addition, thorough assessments must include electrocardiographic monitoring and family history assessment, particularly in arrhythmogenic cardiomyopathy, which may have hereditary components (Ahmed et al., 2023) (Figure 9.6).

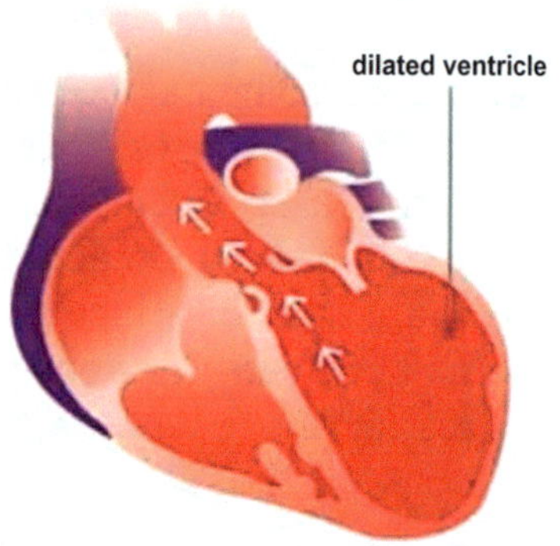

Figure 9.6. Dilated cardiomyopathy.

Source: https://external-content.duckduckgo.com/iu/?u=https%3A%2F%2Futhealtheasttexas.com%2Fsites%2Fdefault%2Ffiles%2Fbasic_page_files%2FUTHET_CHF_FB_012020.jpg&f=1&nofb=1&ipt=4424499769c93782ffd42af1b62d9bab0f1c9a190ba1760945c5e53361d16ab3.

Regrettably, presentations of heart failure in children are not uniform, thus necessitating a broad differential diagnosis that includes other cardiac conditions, respiratory illness, and metabolic diseases. There needs to be an educated and systematic diagnostic approach to enable timely treatment and intervention. Molecular genetic testing has emerged as a useful tool in the diagnostic process for pediatric heart failure, particularly conditions predisposed to genetics. It provides valuable insight into the pathogenic processes occurring in individual cardiomyopathies, which may impact management and prognostication in affected children. In arrhythmogenic cardiomyopathy, for instance, identification of genetic mutations can aid in the identification of those at risk for severe disease and guide therapeutic intervention (Alekseeva et al., 2025). Since classical clinical findings are often masked or unclassical, the addition of genetic testing to routine examinations helps highlight the need for multi-dimensional evaluation protocols that integrate clinical, electrocardiographic, and genetic information. By employing such a multi-modal diagnostic process, physicians are more likely to detect and treat in children heart failure.

9.2.1. Common Symptoms of Heart Failure in Children

Heart failure among children is manifested through a set of serious symptoms that impact the quality of life of the child and require immediate medical attention. Shortness of breath, or dyspnea, is a typical symptom through which heart failure manifests. Dyspnea may manifest itself through increased shallow breathing and has been documented to be accompanied by wheezing or cough. Physical activity or even rest can lead to respiratory distress signs in children based on the severity of their condition. One interesting fact is that infants and small children may present with an increase in the breathing rate without the capacity to communicate their pain, hence being crucial for effective management. Prompt recognition of these signs is extremely critical because it can significantly improve outcomes as well as prevent further deterioration of cardiac function (Chopra et al., 2020). Fatigue is an extremely common symptom of heart failure in the child, and it manifests usually as decreased tolerance to exercise. Parents would observe that the child becomes tired earlier in games or sports that used to be tolerated, a sign that something has gone wrong with the child's cardiovascular system. Lethargy and decreased energies for play may also indicate that the child is shouldering the debilitating effects of impaired cardiac output. This fatigue may also present in the form of irritability or non-responsiveness, again contributing to the clinical syndrome. Those children with heart failure can display an abnormally high level of sleepiness or a lack of energy when compared with age-peers, for which careful assessment by carers is warranted (Dolhnikoff et al., 2020) (Figure 9.7).

Infants	Toddlers
Growth failure Persistent tachypnea Hepatomegaly Respiratory distress	Respiratory distress Poor appetite Decreased activity Hepatomegaly
School Age	**Adolescents**
Fatigue Exercise intolerance Poor appetite Hepatomegaly Orthopnea	Chest pain Dyspnea Pain abdomen, nausea/vomiting Hepatomegaly Orthopnea

Figure 9.7. Common signs and symptoms of heart failure in children.

Source: https://www.researchgate.net/figure/Common-signs-and-symptoms-of-heart-failure-in-children_tbl2_326045798.

In addition, heart failure can manifest as serious nutritional issues in children, most commonly as a failure to thrive or poor feeding. Feeding is impaired in infants and toddlers, who show signs of weakness with bottle-feeding or breast-feeding. In addition to providing too few calories, this exacerbates their cardiovascular symptoms, creating a vicious circle of decreasing heart function and nutrition. Growth measurements such as weight and length can fall below percentiles consistent with normal expectations, indicating a critical need for additional evaluation and intervention by healthcare providers. An appreciation of these symptoms is indispensable to the development of an integrated model of treating pediatric heart failure, particularly the close monitoring and early nutrition (Chopra et al., 2020).

9.2.2. Diagnostic Tests and Procedures

Diagnosis of cardiac failure in children should be carried out in a careful manner with the application of various methods of diagnosis tests and procedures for accurate evaluation. In the initial evaluation, a comprehensive clinical history and physical examination of the symptoms such as dyspnea, fatigue, and edema are commonly done. Electrocardiogram (ECG) is a simple investigation applied in initial evaluation, which identifies arrhythmias and structural anomalies. Furthermore, echocardiography is a cornerstone of diagnosis, and it provides precise visualization of cardiac anatomy and function. This imaging with this method enables the assessment of left ventricular function, which is vital in the assessment of systolic and diastolic dysfunction. These diagnostic procedures are combined, clearing the way for a complete examination of the etiology and severity of heart failure in children, ultimately culminating in the proper selection of therapeutic interventions. In more complex cases, further studies can include advanced imaging and laboratory studies in an attempt to detect underlying causes of heart failure. Cardiac MRI offers excellent resolution of myocardial tissue properties and is particularly useful for the diagnosis of infiltrative diseases, congenital defects, or cardiomyopathies responsible for the illness of the child (Figure 9.8).

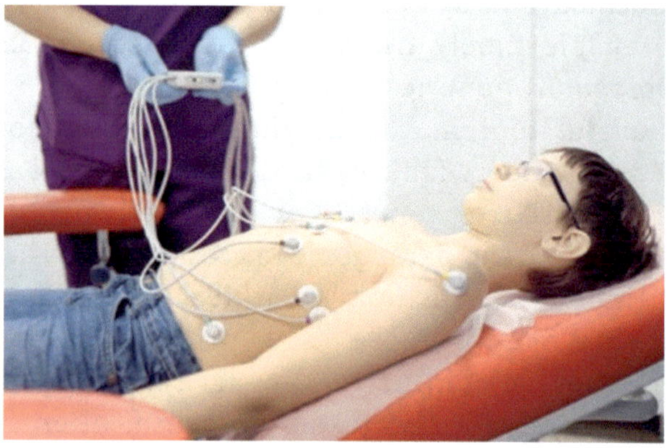

Figure 9.8. Echocardiography serves as a cornerstone in the diagnosis.

Source: https://www.shutterstock.com/image-photo/child-under-ecg-test-doctor-260nw-2498030281.jpg.

Secondly, serum biomarkers such as B-type natriuretic peptide (BNP) could provide valuable information about the heart's stress level and level of fluid overload. Lastly, these advanced diagnostic tests and procedures are critical in risk stratification and guiding therapeutic maneuvers in the child with heart failure. An approach in multiple dimensions allows physicians to adequately tailor management plans and ultimately patient outcomes in the high-risk group. Also, worth mentioning is the psychological impact that diagnoses of heart failure have on the children and families, which can be felt in terms of stress and anxiety in undergoing the treatments and management. In the process of performing these intricate diagnosis procedures, medical professionals must also keep in mind the emotional condition of the patient. Evidence shows that complications of post-acute treatment, such as psychiatric disorders, may negatively impact children's health-related quality of life (HRQOL), as indicated by other chronic diseases' research on their topic (Bilzer et al., 2002). Thus, open communication with families about the diagnostic process can facilitate a supporting environment. Furthermore, incorporating mental health services into care is an essential part of comprehensive patient care, which is important in chronic disease care such as heart failure and in optimizing healthy outcomes for children with such conditions (Lyons et al., 2009).

9.2.3. Challenges in Diagnosing Heart Failure in Pediatric Patients

Diagnosis of heart failure in children represents a unique challenge that stems from the intrinsic similarities between children and adults. Whereas symptoms of heart failure in adults are well established and known, children are likely to present with atypical presentations that are easily misinterpreted. Symptoms such as irritability, poor feeding, and failure to thrive are non-specific and may overlap with many other medical conditions and therefore complicate the diagnostic process. Furthermore, pediatric patients might be less able to describe their symptoms clearly, which further obscures the clinical picture. As such, clinicians are left with a reliance on very careful history and physical exam, but this also underscores the necessity of a high index of suspicion in adolescents with vague complaints. The application of diagnostic testing also that is typically used in adults is a tremendous obstacle for children when it comes to diagnosing heart failure. Techniques such as electrocardiograms and echocardiograms may have to be adapted to suit the unique anatomy and physiology of the pediatric population. For example, interpretation of echocardiographic findings in children needs consideration of age-based norms, which could be significantly different from normal adult values. Additionally, the limited availability of pediatric specialists and diagnostic laboratories may result in such appropriate assessments being delayed, resulting in subsequent delays in significant treatment interventions. This is exacerbated by the fact that children's heart failure tends to be multifactorial so that congenital heart disease, infection, and cardiomyopathy all can have overlapping presentations, so diagnosis is commonly subtle and occasionally multidisciplinary. In addition to that, there is also an emotional and psychological element to diagnosing heart failure in children, in that the implications of such a diagnosis are wide-reaching for both patient and his or her family. Parents feel confused by the complexity of caring for a child with a heart condition and may feel stressed and anxious as a result. This can be compounded by limited knowledge or misinformation about pediatric heart failure, so strong communication between family members and healthcare providers is paramount. Parents need to be informed in a clear, understandable way about their child's illness and their treatment options. It is through this aspect that clinician education becomes so important, with experts becoming increasingly aware of the insidious presentation of heart failure in children so that the likelihood of early and proper diagnosis and management becomes a reality, consequently resulting in improved outcomes (Larry et al., 2015; Nuha et al., 2022).

9.3. Treatment Options

The treatment of heart failure in pediatric patients should be accomplished cautiously and on an individual basis to allow for the variable etiologies and clinical courses of the condition. The administration of diuretics for symptom relief of fluid overload is a frequent pharmacologic intervention, as are the administration of angiotensin-converting enzyme (ACE) inhibitors, beta-blockers, and, in select patients, inotropes to increase cardiac output. The selection of these medications is greatly significant in view of the less well-characterized pathophysiology of heart failure in children, which could greatly differ from adults. As elaborated in contemporary literature, there is a keen desire to investigate various clinical phenotypes concerning heart failure in children in greater detail, leading to more individualized treatment protocols keeping in view the unique requirements of such patients (Pascual et al., 2020). In addition to pharmacotherapy, non-pharmacologic interventions are essential to the overall treatment of heart failure in children. These can include diet modifications, increased monitoring of fluid consumption and weight, and altered physical activity that is timed according to the child's tolerance. The education of caregivers and families is also essential to effective control of childhood chronic heart disease. The availability of a multidisciplinary team of pediatric cardiologists, nutritionists, and nurses promotes an environment of patient-centered care. With such an interdisciplinary facility, tighter control over treatment regimens and quicker responses to changes in the health status of the child can be anticipated. New therapeutic options are likely to become available in the near future, particularly as medical technology and pharmacological innovations continue to impact pediatric cardiology practice (Abela et al., 2004). In severe heart failure, where traditional therapy is not yielding satisfactory results, more complex interventions such as mechanical circulatory support or heart transplant may be utilized. Complex devices including ventricular assist devices (VADs) are life-saving for children listed for heart transplantation and who are stabilizing in heart function support. However, judicious patient selection for such modalities is necessary, balancing benefit against risk. Also, long-term outcomes in these patients are a specific research interest as clinicians attempt to deliver optimal outcomes to children with catastrophic cardiac conditions. Evolving in the treatment paradigm for pediatric heart failure is that future care will be driven by the potential to individualize therapy according to patient profiles and to modify strategies accordingly based on emerging evidence (Pascual et al., 2020) (Figure 9.9).

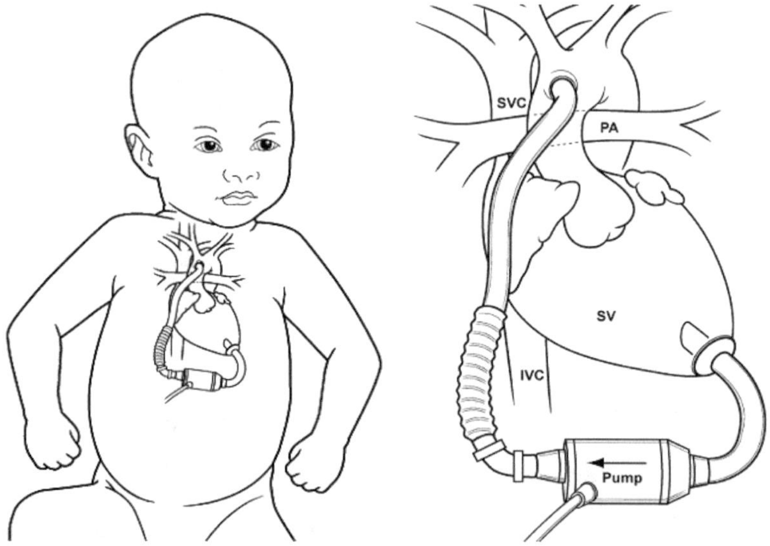

Figure 9.9. Ventricular assist devices.

Source: https://biomed.drexel.edu/labs/biocirc-lab/images/VAD1.png.

9.3.1. Medical Management and Medications

Effective medical treatment of children with heart failure is characterized by a multi-disciplinary strategy that involves the careful selection and utilization of multiple drugs. Relief of symptoms in addition to optimization of cardiovascular function is one of the primary goals of treatment. Diuretics, which help reduce fluid overload, and angiotensin-converting enzyme (ACE) inhibitors, which cause vasodilation and afterload reduction, with a consequent augmentation of cardiac output, are the most frequently employed drugs. In children, the titration of such drugs is important as their physiological uptake may be very different from adults. Also, beta-blockers can be initiated to control heart rate and enhance myocardial function. Side effects have to be constantly monitored by the medical staff and dosages adjusted accordingly in order to balance therapy optimally for each child as an individual (AUTHOR_ID N et al., 2020). Moreover, pharmacologic therapy extends beyond symptom management. Pharmacologic agents such as digoxin can have a primary role in enhancing contractility and attaining rate control in children with specific forms of heart failure. New drug introduction, including neprilysin inhibitors, is a rapidly growing area of pediatric heart failure treatment. The drugs not only improve hemodynamics but are also involved in neurohormonal modulation, essential for long-term therapy. Of particular interest, the synergy of these therapies should be reviewed and adhered to as a matter of regular protocol on the basis of evidence-based guidelines, emphasizing interdisciplinary cooperation among medical professionals. Clinical practice guidelines, such as the European Society of Cardiology (ESC), are continuously formulated and revised, guaranteeing that new evidence impacts treatment of heart failure in children (Williams et al., 2018). Finally, excluding pharmacological treatment, total medical care involves life-style modification and family teaching. Pre-education of families about diet limitations, activity levels, and the necessity of following drug regimens is critical. Engagement of a multidisciplinary team involving cardiologists, nutritionists, and social workers can further enhance drug adherence and quality of life in such children. Follow-ups in repeat visits are essential to monitor the child's response to treatment and adjust treatment strategies accordingly. With an interdisciplinary collaboration between health fields, medical treatment of heart failure in children can lead to an improved outcome, whereby such vulnerable patients get effective as well as holistic treatment (AUTHOR_ID N et al., 2020).

9.3.2. Surgical Interventions

Surgical intervention plays an important role in the management of heart failure in children, particularly when medical therapy is not adequate. Of the several surgical procedures available nowadays, heart transplantation stands as the definitive form of treatment for end-stage heart failure. Although the lack of donors at present limits its usage, efforts to utilize VADs and PAB are increasingly being made. VADs address the short-term needs by assisting pediatric patients' hearts pumping function in the short term until transplantation, thereby improving pediatric patients' quality of life. Transitioning from the treatment of medicine to surgical intervention is a sensitive issue that considers the child's specific condition, development patterns, and recoverability, which serves to illustrate the complicity of the treatments for heart failure in pediatric patients. In patients with dilated cardiomyopathy (DCM), evidence of greater recognition of procedures such as pulmonary artery banding has been reported, which potentially can improve cardiac function. PAB can correct the hemodynamic state by lowering the left ventricular load and favor functional recovery. This is particularly applicable to younger patients, who are potentially more sensitive to regenerative therapy. Recent studies report that nearly 80% of infants with LV-DCM are able to realize significant improvements in the aftermath of PAB, even if they fail the criteria for urgent heart transplantation. These observations imply the need for research into new surgery techniques, as they may make the practice of management strategies change from providing palliative care solely to therapies that aim for curative outcomes (Schranz et al., 2019) (Figure 9.10).

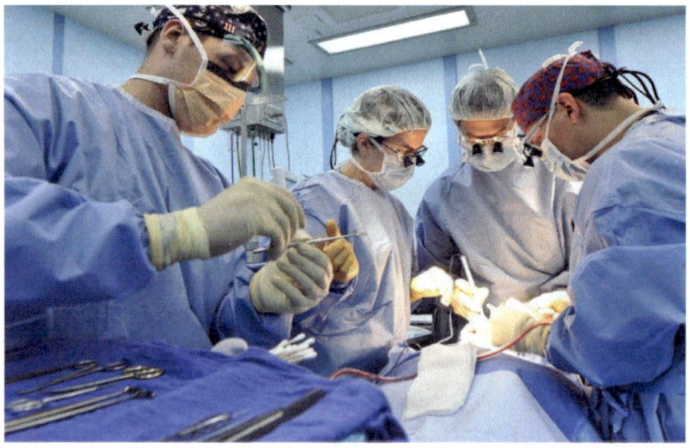

Figure 9.10. Surgical interventions play a vital role in the management of heart failure in children.

Source: https://external-content.duckduckgo.com/iu/?u=https%3A%2F%2Fstorage.googleapis.com%2Faims-edu%2Fimages%2F000%2F001%2F016%2Flead%2Funnamed%2520(43).jpg&f=1&nofb=1&ipt=b3a6f58fcde34633768f858e524d90b8a8a4051164391ee441b683b6af1c701a.

Moreover, the success of surgical procedures rely on an effective perioperative management plan for which multidisciplinary coordination among pediatric cardiologists, surgeons, and nursing staff is needed. Appropriate treatment is not only necessary to manage the short-term danger of surgery but also to attain the best long-term results in young patients recovering from heart failure. In addition, ongoing research into the molecular underpinnings of success in surgery, particularly with regard to PAB-related procedures, holds much potential for improved outcomes in this field in the future. Through reduction of the technical defects in the procedure and coordination with other therapies, healthcare workers can significantly improve the outlook for children suffering from heart failure, ultimately moving toward a paradigm change in therapy strategies that considers emerging medical knowledge and technological improvements (Gregory et al., 2020).

9.3.3. Role of Lifestyle Changes and Rehabilitation

Multidisciplinary management of heart failure in children particularly underscores the central role of lifestyle changes and rehabilitation. Dietary modification, heightened physical activity, and psychological support form the core of improved overall health status. Facilitating healthier lifestyle adaptation in families enables healthcare workers to produce a measurable impact on quality of life and disease course of the child. Studies reveal that structured rehabilitation programs, particularly those tailored for pediatric patients, effectively provide counseling of exercise regimes and diet choices, with the potential to improve self-management and symptom control of heart failure. As advocated by comprehensive reviews, focusing children at the forefront of the care process fosters a more personalized response, with treatment protocols being informed by their needs and preferences, thereby solidifying improved adherence to lifestyle recommendations (Vigni et al., 2024). Rehabilitation is also core not only for physical recovery but also for promoting emotional and psychological strength. Children who are afflicted with heart failure also have to bear a significant amount of stress and anxiety associated with their illness. A rehabilitation program should therefore not only address the physical load of heart failure but should have psychological counseling as well to enable them to cope. Several studies emphasize the necessity for psychological counseling, wherein the scope is there to achieve significant improvement in mental health and general well-being. In creating successful rehabilitation programs, health care providers are able to create a supportive environment that encourages self-reliance in young patients, permitting them to adapt necessary life changes and adhere to treatment regimens (Adiwinata et al., 2024). This integrated approach ultimately leads to reduced hospitalizations and improved long-term outcomes for pediatric heart failure. Rehabilitation interventions and lifestyle changes need to be integrated to achieve optimal management of childhood heart failure but remain a challenge due to the lack of awareness and access to these programs. The majority of families lack sufficient awareness of the need for lifestyle change or the potential benefits of rehabilitation programs. Inadequate awareness would result in less-than-ideal utilization of existing facilities and loss of treatment gains. Enhancement of patient education and extension of community-based activities for the facilitation of such actions can make families more actively engaged. Moreover, multi-disciplinary teams like nurses and rehabilitation professionals play key roles in making compliance with such necessary life adjustments feasible. By providing families with robust education and being backed by individualized rehabilitative plans, healthcare systems are able to enhance the prognostication of children with heart failure, resulting in a better quality of life (Vigni et al., 2024).

9.4. Impact on Quality of Life

Its impact on the quality of life in children is equally extensive, not just affecting their physical condition but also emotional and social well-being. Pediatric heart failure can lead to a variety of physical symptoms such as fatigue, shortness of breath, and reduced exercise capacity that directly interfere with the potential of a child to undertake normal activities.

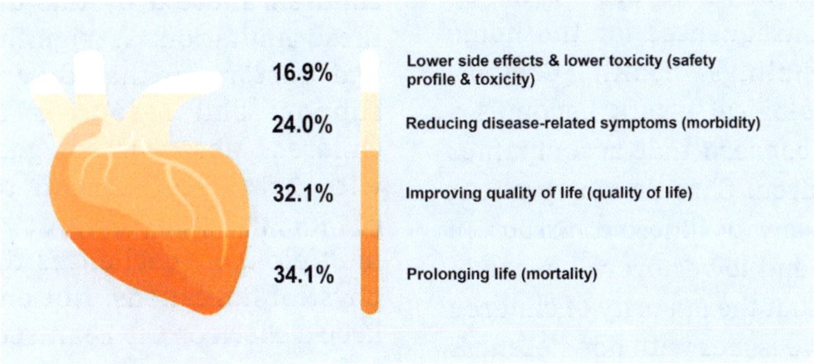

Figure 9.11. The impact of heart failure on the quality of life in children.

Source: https://external-content.duckduckgo.com/iu/?u=https%3A%2F%2Fwww.vintura.com%2Fwp-content%2Fuploads%2F2022%2F11%2FVintura-report-Heartfailure-Importance-of-outcomes-new-treatments.jpg&f=1&nofb=1&ipt=4289d19971dda83787f5c5d0a7bb2b6f006ef1f64daad4bcc144f8dbe262627b.

Since such children normally face limitations in physical activity, they are deprived of meaningful social interaction and play – always integral factors of children's development. Moreover, the chronic nature of heart failure normally requires regular visits to physicians and hospitalization, which can amplify the sense of loneliness in ill children. As already established by studies on post-discharge outcomes for other diseases, chronic limitations and symptoms significantly influence the emotional and psychological well-being of children suffering from heart failure (Chopra et al., 2020) (Figure 9.11).

Social interactions dramatically alter for children who are diagnosed with heart failure. Their condition creates feelings of inadequacy or anxiety because they may not be able to keep pace with those children who don't have similar health ailments. The subsequent stigma and social isolation can fuel a vicious circle of loneliness and decreased self-esteem, which adversely affects their overall lifestyle. Apart from that, children's relationship with their parents may be tense; caregivers experience emotional distress themselves due to their child's condition and the inherent ambiguity of caring for heart failure. Longitudinal study of long-term health consequences emphasizes that such emotional burdens do not only affect the individual but also are borne by the parents, with consequences for the home environment and siblings' health (Gregory et al., 2018). Psychological health becomes a focus of increasing concern that accompanies heart failure in children. Chronic worry about having to live with a serious illness can result in depression, anxiety, and lower overall sense of well-being. It is said that the majority of children with heart failure have issues with hopelessness and worry about their future, which further impinges on them being able to function in day-to-day tasks. Extensive analysis has indicated that these psychological factors positively relate to negative physical consequences, creating a feedback loop potentially exacerbating both psychological and physical well-being. Systems of continued care such as counseling and peer support can provide essential emotional respite and enhance resilience. Their creation is necessary not just for the promotion of healthier coping strategies but also for the improvement of the quality of life in the vulnerable younger patients (Chopra et al., 2020).

9.4.1. Physical Limitations and Daily Activities

Impact of heart failure on children extends far beyond clinical manifestations and requires close examination of physical impairment that arises from disease. Children with heart failure usually experience reduced cardiovascular capability that constrains them in becoming healthy children in a normal way of living. Daily routines normally welcomed activities, such as frolicking with peers, sports activity, or even education, become overwhelming and exhausting for such children. Such exhaustion not just hinders their physical development but also impacts their social interaction, leading to further emotional and psychological consequences. Significantly, a deprivation of these vital experiences can result in children becoming isolated and depressed, significantly affecting the quality of life in such children affected by this disease. Recognizing these limitations is significant for caregivers and doctors so that they can offer effective support and resources to such impacted children. Moreover, the guardians of children with heart failure tend to have significant responsibilities towards looking after the multiple daily challenges that arise from such physical limitations. Not only do they need to keep a check on the health condition of the child but also offer assistance in day-to-day activities that may prove physically demanding for the child. Task-oriented activities like dressing up, bathing, and even cooking can prove to be hindrances, necessitating increased physical attention from caregivers. This burden can lead to physical and emotional stress for caregivers, who might already be dealing with the exigencies of maintaining their own health and wellness. Additionally, as evidenced in studies reporting on the experience of caregivers, it's evident that caregiving has a significant impact on the emotional health, social relationships, and lifestyles of the individuals who fill this role. This means that caregivers should be afforded ample education and information on pediatric heart failure, which in turn will result in better health for both parties (Curtis et al., 2017). Furthermore, community health intervention must be sensitive to the insistent needs of children with heart failure and their families, particularly in relation to the integration of rehabilitative interventions into everyday life. Community nurses play an important part in ensuring that case management models are responding to the multiplexed needs of long-term heart illness, for example, children with heart failure (Gray et al., 2010). These models facilitate not only medical management but also frame towards maximizing everyday functioning with structured care and education for families. Through empowering caregivers with knowledge and practical tools and by encouraging collaboration among healthcare professionals, the weight of physical disability can be lightened. As families are more and more exposed to holistic resources, opportunities for empowering children to engage constructively with their everyday lives increase, ultimately resulting in more independence and a general improved quality of life.

9.4.2. Psychological Effects on Children and Families

The psychological impact of heart failure on the child and family is profound and intricate, extending beyond clinical diagnosis to appear in emotional and social forms. Heart failure children are often exposed to a mix of psychological stressors including withdrawal from social activities, depression, and anxiety. The persistent condition impacts their way of life, interfering with school, play, and social relationships, leading to feelings of isolation. Families are also psychologically stressed, anxious and stressed over their child's health outcomes. Such dual stress can be potentially stressful to family relationships as parents struggle to manage the physical constraints of their children and then try to cope with their emotional response. In some cases, the lack of available support systems can even increase such perceptions, enabling families to manage the heart failure stressors independently. Thus, psychological interventions are part of holistic care for children and their families. Understanding psychosocial family dynamics in families managing a child's heart failure is essential to building right support strategies. Parents are usually laden with guilt, helplessness, and frustration, particularly when faced with limited information regarding treatment possibilities or care strategies. This psychological burden can lead to a decline in the health of parents, subsequently impacting the emotional health of the child. Siblings also suffer from neglect or psychological damage as a result of excessive focus and concern for the afflicted child. Parents can also experience practical stress while dealing with complicated medical procedures, imposing economic strain and escalating stress. Therefore, the most significant step to mitigate the psychological burden on families clinically associated with chronic illness such as heart failure is to enable open communication among family members and include external support systems, such as counseling. The psychosocial impact of chronic illness in children also involves school activities and social integration, further complicating the development picture. Educational complications arise when children suffering from heart failure frequently absent themselves from school due to doctor's consultations or hospital admissions, and thereby fall behind their peers at school. The resulting stress that ensues harms their self-esteem and could also result in behavior problems, as the inherent instability of their condition could cause them to develop an insecurity in life. Moreover, such children will also gain stigma or misunderstanding from others, which also enhances feelings of anxiety and social withdrawal. Therefore, it is essential that schools adopt inclusive approaches and provide appropriate accommodations. Moreover, the common experiences of children with chronic illnesses underpin the need for support programs specifically tailored for developing psychological resilience and coping skills in this high-risk category so as to improve the overall outcomes of children and their families receiving heart failure treatment (Behera et al., 2024; Siyotula et al., 2024).

9.4.3. Long-Term Health Outcomes

The long-term physical effects of children with heart failure extend and are multifaceted, touching virtually every aspect of their life. Heart failure in childhood can lead to long-term physical restriction because defective cardiac function can discourage participation in regular activities, such as physical education and active sports. Later in life, they can find it difficult to maintain proper cardiovascular well-being, which relates to the establishment of early-onset obesity and other metabolic disturbances. Also, the psychological consequence of having a chronic illness can manifest as depression or anxiety, exacerbating their physical impairment and hindering social development. Knowledge of such consequences is important for developing interventions specifically aimed at improving quality of life and functioning in children with heart failure. Furthermore, secondary consequences from heart failure in children carry over to school and social functioning. Many kids with heart failure suffer from cognitive deficits that include tasks such as executive function and memory, which are both brought about by their illness itself and also by the psychological distress thereof. Such cognitive deficits will impact their performance at school, and hence, it will not be easy for them to keep up with their peers. A stigma usually comes with chronic diseases (such as heart failure), isolating children further socially, which can result in challenging relationships and peer activity (Figure 9.12).

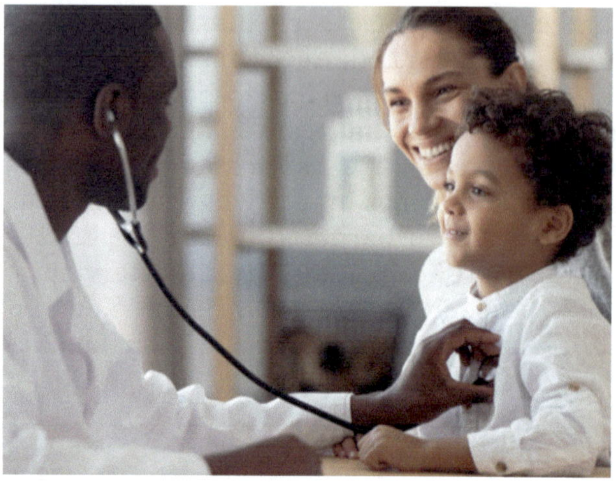

Figure 9.12. The long-term health outcomes for children.

Source: https://www.mcri.edu.au/images/impact/az/Childhood_heart_disease/A-Z_heart_health_1_resized.png.

Consequently, it is essential to address the educational and social dimensions alongside medical care to provide balanced care and management of heart failure in children. Long-term health conditions of children with heart failure need an integrated care model with ongoing medical management, psychological support, and educational support. Diligent follow-up and assessment can identify increasing issues early, thereby facilitating early interventions that minimize complications and enhance overall health. Cardiologists, pediatricians, mental health professionals, and teachers must collaborate to facilitate this, encouraging a multidisciplinary approach that addresses the diverse needs of these children. Support groups and community services can empower families, providing them with the resources and information they require to navigate the complexities of heart failure. A holistic strategy that incorporates physical, emotional, and educational support is paramount to optimizing long-term health for children with heart failure (Chopra et al., 2020; Rebecca et al., 2019).

9.5. Current Research and Advances

Current advancements in research regarding heart failure in children are directed towards a crucial shift in acknowledging the root mechanisms contributing to the condition. Detailed research observed that conditions like obesity and congenital cardiac defects are at high risk of greatly elevating the possibility of heart failure in children. As observed, obesity is capable of producing a chain of metabolic and cardiovascular complications, which ultimately burden a child's cardiac function. Ectopic adipose tissue has been suspected by scientists to exacerbate inflammation in the cardiovascular system and consequently lead to toxic cardiac remodeling. Progress in this area is significant as it illuminates prevention and intervention strategies, particularly in vulnerable groups. Thus, the elimination of obesity by virtue of public health programs may be one key strategy in the prevention of heart failure in children, underlining the significance of interdisciplinary strategies in pediatric cardiology and metabolic medicine (Sattar et al., 2020). Moreover, evolution in imaging modalities and the discovery of biomarkers has taken a fundamentally different approach to diagnosing heart failure in children. In the past, diagnosis also relied significantly on invasive methods and personal judgment, which were risky and cumbersome in children. Modern imaging methods like cardiac MRI and echocardiography have enhanced our capacity to visualize cardiac morphology and function non-invasively, enabling us to make earlier and more accurate diagnoses. More recently, new biomarkers like B-type natriuretic peptide (BNP) and N-terminal proBNP (NT-proBNP) have provided us with objective indices that indicate the severity of heart failure. These innovations not only facilitate timely intervention but also facilitate enhanced monitoring of therapeutic response and prognosis. As with further advances in the area, incorporation of such diagnostic progress into the clinical practice will be critical towards improved outcomes in children with heart failure (Rebecca et al., 2019). Research in therapeutic strategies also promises with emerging new pharmacologic interventions that are tailored for children. Historically, pediatric treatment protocols have been taken from adult guidelines with repeated supervision of the unique physiological and pathophysiological characteristics of the pediatric population. Research has been focused on optimizing existing drugs and exploring new drug classes that target heart failure in children specifically better. The use of angiotensin-converting enzyme (ACE) inhibitors, beta-blockers, and the more recent agents such as sacubitril/valsartan in pediatric patients has been encouraging thus far to enhance cardiac function and quality of life. Gene therapy and regenerative medicine approaches, including stem cell transplant, have been explored as potential future avenues. These advances illustrate the commitment to making age-specific, effective care planning, ultimately for reducing pediatric heart failure morbidity and mortality (Sattar et al., 2020).

9.5.1. Innovations in Treatment Approaches

The management of heart failure among children has undergone drastic advancements, particularly with the utilization of advanced pharmacological treatments aimed at improving cardiac function. The traditional therapies have largely been confined to the utilization of diuretics and angiotensin-converting enzyme (ACE) inhibitors, which while beneficial, fail to bring an end to the etiology of heart failure among children. More recent studies have put a larger focus on the use of newer agents, including angiotensin receptor-neprilysin inhibitors, that are promising to enhance outcomes in these young patients. These advances align with overall trends in the management of adult heart failure, where multidisciplinary approaches have led to dramatic advances in management strategies.

By adopting such innovative pharmacological therapies, pediatric cardiologists can better individualize treatment regimens that address the multifaceted requirements of children with heart failure, enhancing better long-term health outcomes. Beyond the innovations in pharmacology, the emergence of new non-pharmacologic therapies is also revolutionizing the specialty of heart failure therapy in children. Equipment such as continuous hemodynamic monitoring and the utilization of mechanical circulatory support devices such as ventricular assist devices (VADs) have begun to play a central part in treating advanced cases of pediatric heart failure. Such equipment has the potential to provide temporary support for the failing heart, either facilitating potential recovery of the heart or facilitating the pathway to heart transplantation. As has been observed in KorHF III research, which compares present acute heart failure management, an understanding of the long-term impacts of such interventions is essential. Being able to quantify the manner in which advanced devices improve the survival and quality of life of patients is a significant development in the treatment of heart failure in the pediatric patient, connecting treatment pathways with the specific needs of the individual patient and clinical complexity (Yoon et al., 2024). But another area where innovation is making significant inroads is individualized management of children with heart failure, particularly through genetic and biomarker research. As genomics has progressed, clinicians are now in a better position to identify inheritable susceptibility to cardiac dysfunction, which consequently determines treatment strategies based on the individual's genetic makeup. Furthermore, new biomarker profiles for the severity and prognosis of heart failure allow for better monitoring of the patient's condition. With this approach, timely therapeutic plan adjustments are possible and clinical outcomes can be optimized. Although much of this is yet in its formative stages, the promise of joining genetic insight to the practice of clinical care holds forth the possibility of a new era of personalized care in pediatric cardiology. As reflected in the imperative of reporting on and analyzing the efficacy of treatment in varying pediatric populations, such advancement highlights the shift toward more cutting-edge and specific treatment strategies in managing heart failure in children (Yu et al., 2023).

9.5.2. Ongoing Clinical Trials and Studies

Current clinical studies and research are accountable for advancing the condition of the understanding and treating of heart failure in children. Because of how different pediatric heart failure is from that of adults, constant research is being carried out to identify certain therapies and interventions. Most multicenter research studies are determining the effectiveness of various medications like diuretics, beta-blockers, and angiotensin-converting enzyme inhibitors, which have been found helpful in the treatment of this condition. In addition, trials aimed at novel therapy modalities such as gene therapy and stem cell transplant aim to provide new hope for children with congenital heart disease or end-stage cardiac illness to recover. Results of these studies can potentially redesign standard care regimens, improve patient outcomes, and provide a very individualized care to children with heart failure. Along with this, some ongoing trials are using remote monitoring technologies to better manage and communicate patients with healthcare professionals and relatives. The trials will evaluate the feasibility of using telehealth solutions to monitor for symptoms, medication adherence, and patient overall well-being. By integrating data analytics and artificial intelligence into clinical practice, investigators anticipate better early detection of complications and improved optimized treatment plans tailored to the specific needs of each patient. These methods are especially important because they hold the promise of easing some of the logistical constraints that come with standard outpatient care. As healthcare systems grow to meet the complexities of pediatric heart failure, the results of these studies could ensure the integration of technology-based solutions, leading to a new paradigm in care delivery. Other trials, in the wake of the ongoing COVID-19 pandemic, are studying the impact of viral infections on child heart failure. Findings indicate that children with underlying cardiac conditions are likely to have increased risks for viral diseases, such as COVID-19. Studies aim to examine the long-term effects of COVID-19 on cardiovascular outcomes in children, as well as assess potential protective factors and adaptive care approaches. By taking a closer look at the interplay between heart failure and viral infections, these research studies will contribute to the overall body of knowledge required to develop whole-person care practices for this high-risk patient population. The results of these types of studies are significant to clinical decision-making and ensuring child heart failure patients are given adequate treatment in case of international health crises like the one currently taking place (Chopra et al., 2020; Naicker et al., 2020).

9.5.3. Future Directions in Pediatric Cardiology

As pediatric cardiology continues to develop in the future, focus is directed more towards enhancing intervention techniques and device technology to effectively treat heart failure among children. Recent advancements have introduced new transcatheter procedures with immense potential to treat congenital heart defects, which are prevalent among children. For example, developments such as transcatheter pulmonary valve replacement and ductal stenting for ductal-dependent lesions have revolutionized the practice of treatment, allowing procedures to be performed with less invasiveness and shorter recovery periods. However, despite these developments, there remains variability of care across centers, highlighting the need for standardized guidelines. Joining registries and multicenter studies could cast positive illuminations on best practices and help optimize the treatment protocols of pediatric interventional cardiology to compensate for the alarming discrepancies in management practice and results across medical centers (Shibbani et al., 2025). Further illuminations of surgical procedures will also play a critical role in the future of pediatric cardiology, in particular for surgical interventions for heart valve diseases. Ross procedure, which has been found to be of potential value in aortic valve replacement, is increasing following good long-term outcomes in specific patient populations. Class IIb recommendations noted by the American College of Cardiology (ACC) and European Society of Cardiology (ESC) indicate the success of the procedure, especially among young patients receiving aortic valve replacement. With the evolution of surgical techniques and preoperative patient selection by pediatric specialists, ongoing investigations may also bring minimally invasive strategies and tissue engineering technologies. Due to the unique physiological development of children, these innovations could enhance not just immediate surgical outcomes but also long-term quality of life for children with heart failure (Galzerano et al., 2024). In addition to procedural and surgical creativity, pediatric cardiology will more and more rely on personalized medicine to tailor treatment for the unique requirements of an individual patient. Pharmacologic treatment in the form of drugs specially designed for the pediatric population is necessary, as drugs available for use today are not formulated to meet children's needs, leading to less-than-optimal heart failure care. Genomics offer an attractive avenue for the determination of distinct biological markers that can be utilized to guide therapy, potentially enabling targeted interventions that address the underlying drivers of heart failure rather than its symptoms. In reference to precision medicine, pediatric cardiology has the potential to substantially improve outcomes and minimize complications associated with conventional therapy. This cohesive strategy blending cutting-edge technology, innovation, and tailored treatment protocols will certainly reassign the future of pediatric cardiology and lead to better control over heart failure among children.

9.6. Support Systems and Resources

Proper support systems and resources are essential in the management of heart failure among children because these systems, in most cases, will dictate the degree to which the families are able to handle the complexity of the condition. The emotional, financial, and logistical challenges facing families with children diagnosed with heart failure are often overwhelming, necessitating the provision of effective support systems. Social agencies, healthcare centers, and social workers can provide crucial support services, from emotional counseling to financial assistance programs and educational materials on how to treat heart failure. Studies have found that high-quality support systems can significantly enhance the quality of life of participating children and their families, facilitating enhanced coping and overall health status. As children transition from pediatric care, it is that much more critical to connect them and their families with the proper resources to ensure continuity of care as well as optimal care management (Boggs et al., 2021). The transition between pediatric and adult healthcare services is a milestone challenge for adolescent patients with heart failure. The process entails not only the process of transfer of medical care but also adjustment to the adult health care systems, which may or may not be prepared to meet the peculiar needs of such patients. Ambitious support systems are required to make the process successful; in this context, mentorship programs would be crucial in bridging the gap between pediatric and adult care. Having adult healthcare providers with a history of treating chronic conditions that originated in childhood can facilitate the process of transition. Furthermore, as the healthcare system continues to advance, there is a greater need to identify resources where one can track chronic conditions over the long term, which can enhance an individual's ability to adapt to long-term medical conditions over time (Monica et al., 2020). To more fully optimize care for children with heart failure, clinicians must establish sophisticated, multidimensional resource systems that meet clinical and psychosocial needs. These involve access to advanced medical technology and support services that are supportive of coping with the complexity of pediatric heart failure. For instance, the majority of families benefit from medical technology assistance in which there has been a growing trend where most patients transitioning to care under adults require indwelling medical equipment to maintain their health status (Boggs et al., 2021). Nurses also must give priority to the introduction of education schemes that provide families with the necessary information and skills needed in disease management. By establishing a team culture among patients, families, healthcare providers, and community resources, an integrated and comprehensive care approach is enabled, ultimately reducing morbidity and improving outcomes for children with heart failure.

9.6.1. Role of Healthcare Providers and Specialists

In the complex field of pediatric heart failure, the healthcare professionals and specialists have a very important role in delivering the best possible care. They form an interdisciplinary team of pediatric cardiologists, nurse practitioners, and dietitians who contribute their expertise to the table to deliver the optimal possible results for the patients. Their coordination enables accurate diagnosis, treatment, and long-term support for pediatric patients with heart failure. Involving experts guarantees that therapy is tailored based on the unique physiological and developmental needs of pediatric patients, unlike their adult counterparts. Due to the intricate nature of children's cardiac illnesses, health professionals must refresh their competencies and procedures every now and then to implement new research findings and evidence-based standards for therapy so as to optimize their effectiveness in managing heart failure cases. With this as the context, frequent communication between families and health care providers continues to be a strong driving force towards better health outcomes among children with heart failure. Involving parents and caregivers in care processes ensures compliance with treatment plans and facilitates early detection of potential complications. Education plays an essential role within this collaboration; by giving families the tools and education they require to monitor symptoms and detect warning signals, healthcare providers are empowering families to become an engaged partner within their child's care. Strong family-provider relationships result in a sense of trust building, which has the ability to affect mental and emotional health in children and families positively, a key element in treating pediatric heart failure. Experts also play a central role in ongoing assessment and refining of systems of care uniquely developed for children with heart failure. As illustrated by the illustrations from the Brookings-Dartmouth ACO Pilot Program, successful healthcare models prioritize integrated care with a focus on performance measurement and reporting to strengthen accountability and results (Aricca et al., 2012). Such organizations enable medical care professionals to identify unblemished practices and make changes smoothly, providing families with coordinated and effective care. Here, the integration between independent practices and medical groups is an indicator of the learnt lessons for the formation of accountable care organizations that, in turn, enhances the larger landscape of pediatric healthcare (Aricca et al., 2012). Through these findings, healthcare providers are better positioned to address the complexities of children's heart failure and provide solutions that align with the unique needs of their patients.

9.6.2. Support Groups and Community Resources

Caring for the complexities of heart failure in children needs to involve a multi-faceted care system that goes beyond conventional medicine. Support groups form a vital building block in such a care system, providing emotional support and pragmatic help to families of children fighting with the concomitant challenges of cardiac disease. These groups not only offer a platform for parents and caregivers to share experiences and advice but also introduce an element of community that can soothe loneliness feelings. Based on community nursing projects, the contribution of healthcare professionals in such groups is essential, particularly in formulating tools and resources that benefit child welfare as well as long-term heart care needs. This fusion between support groups and nursing practice enhances overall care delivery effectiveness, allowing families to navigate their own path with greater resilience and understanding (Gray et al., 2010). Community resource use is also required in the holistic management of children with heart failure. Locally based health organizations have family education programs and workshops for enhancing family knowledge in managing disease, nutrition, and emergency preparedness. These facilities provide families with skills that allow them to effectively represent their child's interests. Innovative programs like the iPad-Enhanced Shared Care Intervention for Partners (iSCIP) place greater emphasis on involving patients and caregivers in the discussions of managing health care. Not only does the program focus on self-management skills, but it also identifies the importance of communication among family members and healthcare providers in planning care and managing the palliative pathways of heart failure (Garnier-Villarreal et al., 2018). The use of technology-based tools and resources reinforces this collaborative effort by ensuring that families are guided through comprehensive networks. Furthermore, the effectiveness of support groups and community resources in pediatric heart failure care also includes the emotional and psychological control of the disease. Chronically ill children and their families are usually subjected to stress, anxiety, and fear of health unknowns. These negative effects can be minimized via support groups by providing an avenue for the expression of emotions and coming to a consensus, thus enhancing mental status. Secondly, community resources offer access to mental health professionals who can deliver special counseling and therapy services. Interfacing of various stakeholders, from health professionals to support systems, offers a holistic means of care that addresses physical as well as emotional wellness. This connection imposes the reality that managing heart failure in children requires not only medical expertise but also a strong community base that supports families throughout the journey (Gray et al., 2010).

9.6.3. Educational Resources for Families

The importance of educational materials to families that are suffering from heart failure in their children cannot be overstated. The materials equip family members with the information they require to understand their child's condition and navigate the complexities of their healthcare. Comprehensive educational materials, such as information leaflets, online courses, and support networks, improve communication between health workers and family members. By joining these learning portals, families acquire information about signs and symptoms of heart failure, best management practices, and benefits from following up on treatment regimens. Such knowledge acquisition by families not only enhances the quality of care delivered to children but also empowers families with a sense of agency and capability to become active stakeholders in their child's care process.

This proactive involvement ultimately supports better health benefits and resiliency against chronic illness. In heart failure in children, the role of community nurses is particularly vital. A study by NHS Highland highlights the way in which community nursing can enhance educational dissemination to families, especially in chronic disease care like heart failure (Gray et al., 2010). Nurses are also able to serve as primary educators, providing personalized information to families that addresses specific problems regarding their child's heart condition. By utilizing case management models, community nurses are capable of recognizing and providing needed resources that promote understanding and self-management. This engagement can be in the form of home visits, workshops, or telemedicine care and provides long-term education and support to families that will leave them well-informed about dietary restrictions, drug therapy, and lifestyle modifications critical to the management of heart failure. These programs reinforce the shared nature of common goals toward optimal outcome and restoring the equilibrium of care back to the community. Also important is identification of socioeconomic determinants that influence educational access and health literacy in heart failure-affected families (Kronstadt, 2008). Research shows that a parent's socioeconomic status and continuous health needs have powerful effects on children's education and resources accessible. In heart failure-affected families, educational disparities must be noted to create specific interventions that can provide respective support. Reaching education programs, in contrast, can bridge the gap, offering families not just clinical information but life skills to navigate the challenges of raising a child with a chronic illness. Further, integration with schools and community agencies can enhance educational outreach, and families will no longer have to navigate these complexities on their own. These collaborative activities not only augment health literacy but also enhance resilience, enabling families to better prepare for the multifaceted challenges of caring for heart failure in children.

SUMMARY

Briefly, children's treatment of heart failure is unique in character and calls for a polypragmatic approach to improved outcomes. With the application of various treatment modalities, such as pharmacologic therapies and advanced supportive care, a marked improvement in clinical parameters becomes evident. Specifically, the infusion of levosimendan has been effective in increasing cardiac output in children with various types of heart disease. Thus, for instance, cardiomyopathy children experienced doubling of the ejection fraction following treatment, while with congenital heart disease, there was an 18% increase in the heart contractility following treatment. These findings point to the importance of targeted therapies that address the individual pathophysiological processes of heart failure in children and thus lead to improved quality of life and survival. Besides, the addition of technological innovation and evidence-based care in pediatric heart failure treatment can offer enhanced care provisions. Continuous positive airway pressure (CPAP) may be significant in children presenting with coexistent respiratory conditions that exacerbate the signs of heart failure. CPAP's ability to reduce hospital length of stay and improve the primary respiratory interventions can simultaneously reduce some of the burden on the cardiovascular system. Although direct effects on heart failure parameters also need to be investigated further, the interplay between ideal respiratory control and cardiac health demonstrates an interdisciplinarity of first significance to holistic pediatric care. It demonstrates that optimization of respiratory function may play an ancillary but important part in the management of heart failure. Further research into pediatric heart failure and novel therapeutic approaches is required to enhance our understanding and treatment of this illness. Current studies establish the efficacy of such medications as levosimendan and necessitate a broad investigation of their long-term efficacy and safety. The absence of undesirable side effects reported in children who used this medication validates the potential of integrative therapies in this high-risk population. Subsequent research must study the outcomes of innovative techniques, such as the application of CPAP for co-morbid conditions, which can better address treatment regimens. Ultimately, an integrated approach that combines pharmacologic innovation and support therapies will be the key to maximizing outcomes in children with heart failure, giving their youth patients the best care they can receive based on the unique needs of each child.

Congestive heart failure among children is a multifaceted and complicated condition that is associated with the interplay between various anatomical and physiologic factors. The etiology of heart failure in children should be understood as it could be the result of congenital heart disease, cardiomyopathy, or inflammation. Presentation of heart failure among children can be different from that of adults, and thus diagnostic and management strategies should be tailored accordingly. Symptoms such as fatigue, inability to eat, and nonthriving are more prominent in children, highlighting the need for pediatric-specific diagnostic criteria. Identification of the unique factors is paramount for clinicians to come up with the appropriate management techniques and proper monitoring and intervention. Thus, an acute sensitivity to the underlying causes and their individualistic manifestations is key to managing heart failure in this younger population. Successful management of children with heart failure relies on multidisciplinary teamwork, including cardiologists, pediatricians, nutritionists, and nursing staff to offer holistic care. Treatment regimens typically consist of a combination of drug therapy and lifestyle changes, tailored to individual children's requirements. Drugs can include diuretics, ACE inhibitors, and beta-blockers to optimize cardiac function and minimize symptoms. Apart from medicines, lifestyle change and physiotherapy are also crucial in optimizing overall well-being and quality of life. Regular follow-up visits and monitoring of growth and development are also necessary to evaluate the efficacy of treatment and to rectify the necessary correction. Moreover, education and support from caregivers are essential in ensuring that treatment is followed, and that caregivers are educated to the effect that they are aware of the exacerbation of heart failure symptoms and when and how to see the doctor. The ethical implications of the management of heart failure in children cannot be overlooked because they involve coping with complex decisions about the treatment and quality of life. Healthcare professionals must be vigilant in decision-making with the best interest of the child as the priority and conforming to laid-down guidelines and procedures. As foreseen by the ESC/EAS Guidelines, healthcare professionals not only carry the mandate of therapeutic practice but also consultations with the carers of the patients for the purpose of informed decision-making (François et al., 2019). Education regarding the nature of heart failure and its management is most important to facilitate families making informed decisions regarding treatment and facilitate informed decision-making regarding treatment choice. Additionally, health professionals must be up to date with changing guidelines and recommendations in order to ensure that practice is evidenced based at all times (Habib et al., 2015). This cooperative and informed approach ultimately hopes to improve outcomes and assist with the quality of life for children afflicted with this challenging disease.

CLOSER LOOK

DIFFERENCES BETWEEN ADULT AND PEDIATRIC HEART FAILURE

Adult and children heart failure (HF) is a syndrome of reduced cardiac performance, but its etiology, clinical course, pathophysiology, and treatment diverge greatly between the children and adults. Recognition of these divergences is extremely important for early diagnosis and treatment. Etiology is an important differentiating characteristic. In the adult, heart failure is most commonly due to ischemic heart disease, chronic hypertension, or diabetic/alcoholism/valvular cardiomyopathies. In contrast, pediatric heart failure is due to congenital heart diseases (CHDs), cardiomyopathies, or myocarditis. In the neonate and infant, structural heart diseases such as large ventricular septal defect or hypoplastic left heart syndrome are common causes. In older children, dilated cardiomyopathy and post-viral myocarditis are leading contributors. Pathophysiology is likewise heterogeneous. Adult HF is typically classified as heart failure with reduced ejection fraction (HFrEF) or preserved ejection fraction (HFpEF), with the former being more common. Pediatric heart failure is, however, more commonly associated with volume overload from shunts or pressure overload from outflow tract obstruction and produces a blend of systolic and diastolic dysfunction. In addition, due to developmental differences, the infant's immature myocardium has less contractile reserve and increased afterload sensitivity so that they are more prone to heart failure under stress.

Clinical presentation is age-specific. Presentations in adults are classic and include symptoms such as fatigue, exertional dyspnea, orthopnea, and peripheral edema. In children, especially infants, presentation can be subtle or nonspecific—poor feeding, failure to thrive, tachypnea, hepatomegaly, irritability, and excessive sweating during feeds are characteristic features. Older children can present with reduced exercise tolerance or abdominal pain due to hepatic congestion. In both groups, diagnosis is a combination of clinical assessment, imaging, and laboratory studies. Echocardiography is required in order to evaluate cardiac structure and function. Adults possess BNP and N-terminal pro-BNP as well-established markers for diagnosis and monitoring of HF. These biomarkers are used in children, too, but age-related heterogeneity limits their specificity and requires cautious interpretation. Management strategies differ with varying etiology of the disease and response to drugs. In adults, evidence-based usual therapies such as ACE inhibitors, beta-blockers, mineralocorticoid receptor antagonists, and diuretics are the cornerstone of HF therapy with large clinical trial evidence. In children with HF, there are fewer randomized trials and some treatments are more or less directly extrapolated from adult guidelines. ACE inhibitors and diuretics are the most commonly used medications, while beta-blockers and ARNI (angiotensin receptor-neprilysin inhibitors) are used more cautiously due to limited pediatric experience. Mechanical support and cardiac transplantation are reserved for end-stage HF in both cohorts but typically necessitate long-term support in children until an appropriate donor is identified.

Prognosis is also variable. Adult HF is a progressive and highly fatal condition, whereas children with reversible causes like myocarditis may return to normal. Yet, others with advanced cardiomyopathies or complex congenital heart disease might need to be cared for throughout their lives and have recurrent interventions.

References

1. Abela, J. C. (2004). General practice. https://core.ac.uk/download/46601885.pdf (accessed on 15th July 2025).
2. Adiwinata, S., Poetra, B., Lampus, N., Joseph, V. F. F., Jim, E. L., & Rampengan, S. (2024). Comprehensive cardiac rehabilitation in elderly patients with heart failure: Age is just a number? *European Journal of Preventive Cardiology.* https://www.semanticscholar.org/paper/a29043abf11786c49de7165429dc926b60340e03 (accessed on 15th July 2025).
3. Agabiti-Rosei, E., Cruickshank, J. K., Dominiczak, A., et al. (2016). 2016 European Society of Hypertension guidelines for the management of high blood pressure in children and adolescents. https://core.ac.uk/download/46165193.pdf (accessed on 15th July 2025).
4. Ahmed, Y., & Heidemann, S. (2023). Early diagnosis of acute myocarditis or dilated cardiomyopathy in children younger than 2 years. *Pediatric Emergency Care, 39*, 751–754. https://www.semanticscholar.org/paper/aa89191605b001936c9f60d3c56802c2c0e19e12 (accessed on 15th July 2025).
5. Akinyemi, K. (2016). Pulmonary hypertension in adolescents with sickle cell disease. https://open.bu.edu/bitstream/2144/14612/10/Akinyemi_bu_0017N_11712.pdf (accessed on 15th July 2025).
6. Alekseeva, D., Kofeinikova, O. A., Kostareva, A., Vershinina, T., Kovalchuk, T., Fedotov, P., Pervunina, T., et al. (2025). Clinical and genetic patterns of arrhythmogenic cardiomyopathy in children after heart transplant or on the heart transplant waiting list. *Russian Journal of Woman and Child Health.* https://www.semanticscholar.org/paper/30661bf6dfd77e0ee81d4bd4f3fead751ebcda17 (accessed on 15th July 2025).
7. Alsaadi, S. O., Fagihi, A. H., Alfaifi, A. Y., Sayd, A. S., Juraybi, A. M., Alshammari, S. R. H., Alharbi, S. S., et al. (2024). Pharmacological interventions to mitigate immunodeficiency in children with congenital heart defects: A review article. *Egyptian Journal of Chemistry.* https://www.semanticscholar.org/paper/8ceb7259b33699ed65f9bcb4d7aea2caa8fb29f9 (accessed on 15th July 2025).
8. Baddour, L. M., Wilson, W. R., Bayer, A. S., Fowler, V. G., Tleyjeh, I. M., Rybak, M. J., Baršić, B., et al. (2015). Infective endocarditis in adults: Diagnosis, antimicrobial therapy, and management of complications. *Circulation, 132*, 1435–1486. https://doi.org/10.1161/cir.0000000000000296 (accessed on 15th July 2025).
9. Behera, M., Jena, R., & Sethy, S. (2024). Psychosocial assessment of thalassemia major patients in adolescent age group. *Blood.* https://www.semanticscholar.org/paper/c33f80e27628a0bce7432c2f11fb7ec3c28745ff (accessed on 15th July 2025).
10. Bilzer, M., Ehrentraut, S., Gerbes, A. L., et al. (2002). Psychiatric and psychosocial outcome of orthotopic liver transplantation. https://core.ac.uk/download/16432271.pdf (accessed on 15th July 2025).
11. Boggs, E. F., Foster, C., Shah, P., Goodman, D., Hall, M., & Garfield, C. (2021). Trends in technology assistance among patients with childhood onset chronic conditions. *Hospital Pediatrics.* https://www.semanticscholar.org/paper/6c35361f1ec2c8033388f5490525499bc3fec2c1 (accessed on 15th July 2025).

12. Casals Pascual, C., Cominetti, O., Hoffman, F., et al. (2020). Identification of a novel clinical phenotype of severe malaria using a network-based clustering approach. https://core.ac.uk/download/322680513.pdf (accessed on 15th July 2025).

13. Chopra, V., Flanders, S. A., O'Malley, M., Malani, A. N., & Prescott, H. C. (2020). Sixty-day outcomes among patients hospitalized with COVID-19. *Annals of Internal Medicine, 174*, 576–578. https://doi.org/10.7326/m20-5661 (accessed on 15th July 2025).

14. Curtis, H. S. (2017). Exploring the effects of caring for congestive heart failure patients on caregiver well-being: A descriptive study. https://core.ac.uk/download/84120596.pdf (accessed on 15th July 2025).

15. Danduran, M. J., Dixon, J. E., & Rao, R. P. (2012). Near infrared spectroscopy describes physiologic payback associated with excess postexercise oxygen consumption in healthy controls and children with complex congenital heart disease. https://core.ac.uk/download/213086415.pdf (accessed on 15th July 2025).

16. Dolhnikoff, M., Ferranti, J. F., Monteiro, R. A. A., Duarte-Neto, A. N., Gomes-Gouvêa, M. S., Degaspare, N. V., Delgado, A. F., et al. (2020). SARS-CoV-2 in cardiac tissue of a child with COVID-19-related multisystem inflammatory syndrome. *The Lancet Child & Adolescent Health, 4*, 790–794. https://doi.org/10.1016/s2352-4642(20)30257-1 (accessed on 15th July 2025).

17. ElSayed, N. A., Aleppo, G., Aroda, V. R., Bannuru, R. R., Brown, F. M., Bruemmer, D., Collins, B. S., et al. (2022). 2. Classification and diagnosis of diabetes: *Standards of Care in Diabetes—2023. Diabetes Care, 46*, S19–S40. https://doi.org/10.2337/dc23-s002 (accessed on 15th July 2025).

18. Emelyanchik, V. S., Spichak, Y. Y., Teplov, P. V., Ilinykh, K., Cheremisina, A., Ivanitsky, E. A., Mosyakin, N., et al. (2021). Experience of levosimendan using in young children with functional class IV heart failure. *Pediatric. Journal Named After G.N. Speransky, 100*, 201–204. https://www.semanticscholar.org/paper/28b2901944711df2d92036790ae11c05ae809fdc (accessed on 15th July 2025).

19. Feinstein, B., Frum, C., Miller, P. C., et al. (1963). Mothers of children with congenital heart defects: The effects of ethnicity and education on perceptions, attitudes and feelings; (Implications for social work practice). https://open.bu.edu/bitstream/2144/4161/2/Feinstein_1963_web.pdf (accessed on 15th July 2025).

20. Galzerano, D., Kholaif, N., Al Amro, B., Al Admawi, M., Eltayeb, A., Alshammari, A., di Salvo, G., et al. (2024). The Ross procedure: Imaging, outcomes and future directions in aortic valve replacement. *Journal of Clinical Medicine, 13.* https://www.semanticscholar.org/paper/7830dc123b1e789e0c83393b400702d16d232551 (accessed on 15th July 2025).

21. Garnier-Villarreal, M., Sebern, M., Sebern, M. J., et al. (2018). Does an intervention designed to improve self-management, social support and awareness of palliative-care address needs of persons with heart failure, family caregivers and clinicians? https://core.ac.uk/download/213085991.pdf (accessed on 15th July 2025).

22. Gray, C. M., James, B., Lauder, W., et al. (2010). Developing community nursing practice: Promoting case management and skill enhancement to support shifting the balance of care. https://core.ac.uk/download/110605.pdf (accessed on 15th July 2025).

23. Habib, G., Lancellotti, P., Antunes, M. J., Bongiorni, M. G., Casalta, J. P., Del Zotti, F., Dulgheru, R., et al. (2015). 2015 ESC guidelines for the management of infective endocarditis. *European Heart Journal, 36*, 3075–3128. https://doi.org/10.1093/eurheartj/ehv319 (accessed on 15th July 2025).

24. Ivkin, A. A., Balakhnin, D., & Mikhailova, A. (2024). Successful correction of transposition of the great vessels using extracorporeal methods in an infant aged 52 days: Case report. *Complex Issues of Cardiovascular Diseases.* https://www.semanticscholar.org/paper/6a3b101d5f2ba43b64fd3dfc6cc7cf1a0df66b4e (accessed on 15th July 2025).

25. Kronstadt, J. (2008). Health and economic mobility. https://core.ac.uk/download/71351768.pdf (accessed on 15th July 2025).

26. Lemmon, M. E., Truog, R., & Ubel, P. (2020). Allocating resources across the life span during COVID-19—Integrating neonates and children into crisis standards of care protocols. *JAMA Pediatrics.* https://www.semanticscholar.org/paper/a24c958324dc63542d56f0cbdc3e80023d38565f (accessed on 15th July 2025).

27. Li Vigni, M., Meucci, B., Gambone, F., & Giordano, V. (2024). The impact of nurse-led education on quality of life in patients with heart failure during cardiac rehabilitation: A review of the literature. *European Heart Journal Supplements.* https://www.semanticscholar.org/paper/bf575c5d43bfec3e67132e60f41ec1c9d116b867 (accessed on 15th July 2025).

28. Liu, S., Hua, X., Zhao, Y., Mo, H., Chen, X., Wang, W., Li, Y., et al. (2024). Left ventricular posterior wall hypertrophy leads to poor prognosis of hypertrophic obstructive cardiomyopathy in children: A cohort study. *International Journal of Surgery (London, England), 111*, 771–780. https://www.semanticscholar.org/paper/68776af3614c66a5dc6d9691461fe7d23c54c17c (accessed on 15th July 2025).

29. Lyons, B., Tolbert, J., & Perry, M. (2009). In pursuit of affordable health care: On the ground lessons from families in Massachusetts. https://core.ac.uk/download/71347986.pdf (accessed on 15th July 2025).

30. Mach, F., Baigent, C., Catapano, A. L., Koskinas, K. C., Casula, M., Badimón, L., Chapman, M. J., et al. (2019). 2019 ESC/EAS guidelines for the management of dyslipidemias: Lipid modification to reduce cardiovascular risk. *European Heart Journal, 41*, 111–188. https://doi.org/10.1093/eurheartj/ehz455 (accessed on 15th July 2025).

31. Naicker, S., Yang, C. W., Hwang, S. J., Liu, B. C., Chen, J., & Jha, V. (2020). The novel coronavirus 2019 epidemic and kidneys. *Kidney International, 97*, 824–828. https://doi.org/10.1016/j.kint.2020.03.001 (accessed on 15th July 2025).

32. Quennelle, S., & Bonnet, D. (2023). Pediatric heart failure with preserved ejection fraction. A review. *Frontiers in Pediatrics, 11.* https://www.semanticscholar.org/paper/1ab47d264558b0d5881961ea8408a12b6821602d (accessed on 15th July 2025).

33. Roth, G. A., Abate, D., Abate, K. H., Abay, S. M., Abbafati, C., Abbasi, N., Abbastabar, H., et al. (2018). Global, regional, and national age-sex-specific mortality for 282 causes of death in 195 countries and territories, 1980–2017: A systematic analysis for the Global Burden of Disease Study 2017. *The Lancet, 392*, 1736–1788. https://doi.org/10.1016/s0140-6736(18)32203-7 (accessed on 15th July 2025).

34. Roth, G. A., Mensah, G. A., Johnson, C. O., Addolorato, G., Ammirati, E., Baddour, L. M., Barengo, N. C., et al. (2020). Global burden of cardiovascular diseases and risk factors, 1990–2019. *Journal of the American College of Cardiology, 76*, 2982–3021. https://doi.org/10.1016/j.jacc.2020.11.010 (accessed on 15th July 2025).

35. Sattar, N., McInnes, I. B., & McMurray, J. J. V. (2020). Obesity is a risk factor for severe COVID-19 infection. *Circulation, 142*, 4–6. https://doi.org/10.1161/circulationaha.120.047659 (accessed on 15th July 2025).

36. Schranz, D., Recla, S., Malčić, I., Kerst, G., Mini, N., & Akintuerk, H. (2019). Pulmonary artery banding in dilative cardiomyopathy of young children: Review and protocol based on the current knowledge. *Translational Pediatrics, 8*, 151–160. https://doi.org/10.21037/tp.2019.04.09 (accessed on 15th July 2025).

37. Shaigany, S., Gnirke, M., Guttmann, A., Chong, H. L., Meehan, S., Raabe, V., Louie, E., et al. (2020). An adult with Kawasaki-like multisystem inflammatory syndrome associated with COVID-19. *The Lancet, 396*, e8–e10. https://doi.org/10.1016/s0140-6736(20)31526-9 (accessed on 15th July 2025).

38. Sherman, E. (2019). Review of Chagas disease and treatment obstacles to eradication. https://core.ac.uk/download/213464293.pdf (accessed on 15th July 2025).

39. Shibbani, K., & Kenny, D. (2025). Updates in interventional cardiology in children with cardiac disease. *European Journal of Pediatrics, 184.* https://www.semanticscholar.org/paper/c75b1f7c4368bc723fac2deed22456d2a1a2dca1 (accessed on 15th July 2025).

40. Siegel, R. L., Miller, K. D., & Jemal, A. (2019). Cancer statistics, 2019. *CA: A Cancer Journal for Clinicians, 69*, 7–34. https://doi.org/10.3322/caac.21551 (accessed on 15th July 2025).

41. Siyotula, T., Barrell, J., Manning, K., Thomson, M. D., et al. (2024). The state of pediatric deceased-organ donation at a South African tertiary public-sector hospital: A 14-year analysis. *South African Medical Journal = Suid-Afrikaanse Tydskrif vir Geneeskunde, 114*(3b), e1330. https://www.semanticscholar.org/paper/494537bf503db623a6d541c6846309486d846719 (accessed on 15th July 2025).

42. Steichert, M., Cawello, W., Breur, J., Male, C., de Wildt, S. D., & Läer, S. (2023). 23 Plasma renin activity in young children with heart failure: Influence of age, disease and ACE inhibitor treatment. *Archives of Disease in Childhood, 108*, A8–A8. https://www.semanticscholar.org/paper/b967b64682f7de468b9841c456ab7a979b9b1da9 (accessed on 15th July 2025).

43. Tang, G., Lin, J., Zhang, Y., & Shi, Q. (2021). The effects and safety of continuous positive airway pressure in children with bronchiolitis: A systematic review and meta-analysis. *Journal of Tropical Pediatrics, 67*(2). https://www.semanticscholar.org/paper/af085ea9408f6f172ca8bd8a1872415e94a0de20 (accessed on 15th July 2025).

44. Ullah, M. A., Mamun, S., Saha, H., & Al-Miraj, A. (2025). Incidence and pattern of congenital heart disease in children: An observational cross-sectional study. *International Journal of Research in Medical Sciences.* https://www.semanticscholar.org/paper/ea1329372c9c07105edf14bc5b16d3846ab4cccb (accessed on 15th July 2025).

45. Van Citters, A. D., Larson, B. K., Fisher, E. S., Nelson, E. C., Gbemudu, J. N., Kreindler, S. A., & Shortell, S. M. (2012). Norton Healthcare: A strong payer-provider partnership for the journey to accountable care. https://core.ac.uk/download/71358697.pdf (accessed on 15th July 2025).

46. Van Citters, A. D., Larson, B. K., Fisher, E. S., Nelson, E. C., Wu, F. M., Gbemudu, J. N., Kreindler, S. A., et al. (2012). HealthCare Partners: Building on a foundation of global risk management to achieve accountable care. https://core.ac.uk/download/71358347.pdf (accessed on 15th July 2025).

47. Wei, P. F. (2020). Diagnosis and treatment protocol for novel coronavirus pneumonia (Trial Version 7). *Chinese Medical Journal, 133*, 1087–1095. https://doi.org/10.1097/cm9.0000000000000819 (accessed on 15th July 2025).

48. Williams, B., Mancia, G., Spiering, W., Agabiti Rosei, E., Azizi, M., Burnier, M., Clement, D. L., et al. (2018). 2018 ESC/ESH Guidelines for the management of arterial hypertension. *European Heart Journal, 39*, 3021–3104. https://doi.org/10.1093/eurheartj/ehy339 (accessed on 15th July 2025).

49. Yancy, C. W., Jessup, M., Bozkurt, B., Butler, J., Casey, D. E., Colvin, M., Drazner, M. H., et al. (2016). 2016 ACC/AHA/HFSA Focused update on new pharmacological therapy for heart failure: An update of the 2013 ACCF/AHA guideline for the management of heart failure. *Circulation, 134.* https://doi.org/10.1161/cir.0000000000000435 (accessed on 15th July 2025).

50. Yoon, M., Kim, E. J., Han, S., Park, S. M., Kim, I. C., Cho, M. C., Ahn, H., et al. (2024). The third nationwide Korean Heart Failure III registry (KorHF III): The study design paper. *International Journal of Heart Failure, 6*(2), 70–75. https://www.semanticscholar.org/paper/bb6ce213a963ad9de93c520ade7095b1e8ffe106 (accessed on 15th July 2025).

51. Yu, G. I., Kim, D., Sung, J., Jang, E., Yu, H., Kim, T. H., Pak, H., et al. (2023). Impact of frailty on early rhythm control outcomes in older adults with atrial fibrillation: A nationwide cohort study. *Frontiers in Cardiovascular Medicine, 9.* https://www.semanticscholar.org/paper/a7e7926043608792bd667cf5e90b0ca643e39c9b (accessed on 15th July 2025).

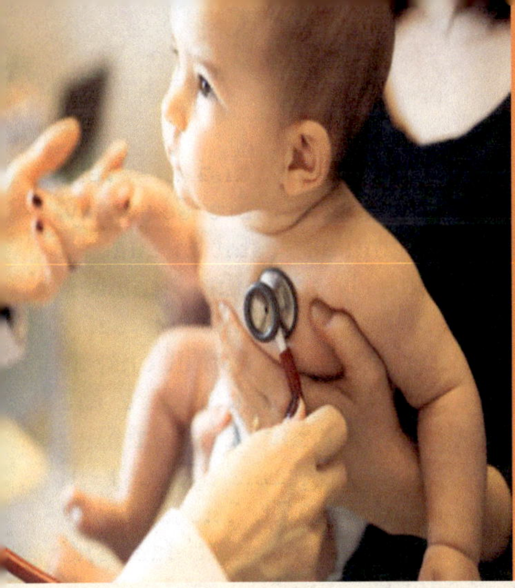

Chapter 10
PEDIATRIC ARRHYTHMIAS

Contents

Introduction

Pediatric arrhythmias are complex and heterogeneous and present particular challenges in pediatric health. The term is used to denote a range of abnormal cardiac rhythms that can have a profound impact on the cardiovascular system and overall health of children involved. Pediatric arrhythmias may be managed as a consequence of congenital defects, structural cardiac defects, or acquired illnesses, and their presentations tend to be highly variable in clinical and severity relevance. Early identification and correct management of the conditions are vital, as they are likely to result in significant morbidity and mortality if left untreated. Existing literature supports the call for early intervention, particularly among children, as required in a number of clinical studies that suggest responding to this essential field of pediatric care, thus requiring further study in this field (Gamayunov et al., 2025). In the last few decades, diagnostic imaging and monitoring techniques have seen some stunning advancements, which have significantly enhanced the detection and management of pediatric arrhythmias. Clinicians now more frequently employ cutting-edge devices such as electrocardiograms and newer imaging modalities to properly diagnose these conditions. These advancements not only help to detect arrhythmias but also permit the formulation of targeted therapeutic measures, from drug therapy to more complex interventions. Lastly, incorporation of a multidisciplinary team of pediatric cardiologists and electrophysiologists and other healthcare professionals is required to optimize treatment outcome. Such an integrative approach signals a heightened realization of the complementary interaction between technological advancement and clinical practice, as emphasized through current advancements in this area (Helman et al., 2024). Irrespective of such advancements, some issues remain in managing pediatric arrhythmias. A critical issue is under-detection of arrhythmias in the pediatric population, often due to atypical symptomology that masks the disorder. Other treatment response is also variable from child to child, and an individualized approach of management for considering patient variability is needed. Long-term outcome of arrhythmias and their interventions need to be studied in the future to determine best practices that will deliver maximum benefits in the high-risk group. By gaining a more profound understanding of pediatric arrhythmias, clinicians are better able to build on their clinical skills, ultimately leading to enhanced care and improved results for the children in question.

Definition of Pediatric Arrhythmias

Pediatric arrhythmias are a significant area of study in the area of pediatric healthcare, and they are characterized by irregular heart rhythms that occur due to malfunction of the heart's electrical system. They exist either as tachycardias, in which the heart rate is too fast, or bradycardias, in which the heart rate is significantly slower. The prevalence of such disorders among children warrants complete evaluation and management to prevent potential complications, including syncope and, in severe cases, sudden cardiac death. More seriously, certain types of arrhythmias result in sudden cardiac death, particularly in young athletes. This also underlines the importance of early detection and treatment of such conditions, as the changing guidelines well underscore the importance of healthcare providers learning to interpret electrocardiograms (ECGs) in children (Aagaard et al., 2017). The etiology of pediatric arrhythmias may be multi-factorial with underlying congenital and acquired causes. Congenital arrhythmias are usually linked with genetic conditions that affect the heart's structure and conduction pathways, some such conditions being Long QT syndrome and Wolff-Parkinson-White syndrome. Acquired arrhythmias, on the other hand, can result from external causes, such as infections, electrolyte disturbances, or the intake of certain medications.

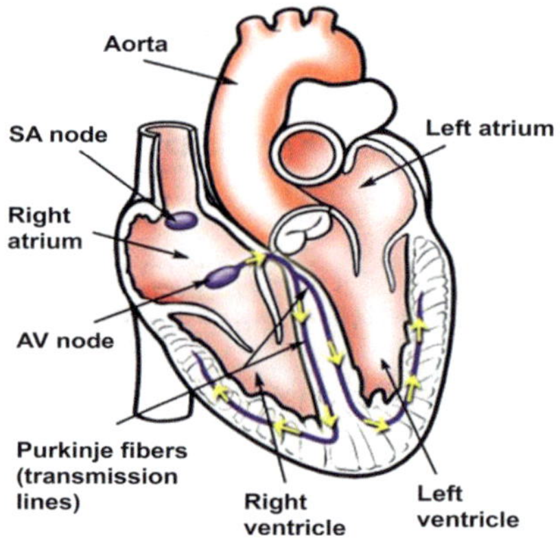

Figure 10.1. A diagram of the normal electrical system pathway inside the heart.

Source: https://my.clevelandclinic.org/-/scassets/images/org/health/articles/14788-pediatric-arrhythmias.ashx.

Understanding these diverse etiologies is significant for customized treatment options and emphasizes the importance of pediatrics that has in-depth knowledge of environmental as well as genetic influences on cardiac health. Such a multi-disciplinary approach also calls for interspecialty collaboration among pediatricians, cardiologists, and geneticists for best care of the children with these conditions (Seita et al., 2013) (Figure 10.1).

Management of pediatric arrhythmias typically requires a judicious response, based on the child's age, overall condition, and character of the arrhythmia identified. Non-invasive tools like ECG monitoring are particularly vital in diagnosis and follow-up after treatment but may be supplemented in severe cases by more invasive tools, such as electrophysiological testing or implantable devices. Pharmacologic interventions also prevail in the treatment regimens, tailored to the underlying etiology of the arrhythmia. Ongoing technological progress and therapeutic advancements continuously alter management strategies, emphasizing the importance of ongoing education among healthcare providers. Because pediatric arrhythmias are a broad group of diseases, healthcare providers should ensure that they are constantly updated with the latest research findings and clinical guidelines to ensure early diagnosis and management (Aagaard et al., 2017).

Importance of Studying Arrhythmias in Children

Arrhythmia in children is a research field of significance due to their anatomical and physiological differences with adults. Children are more likely to have arrhythmias due to congenital heart disease, genetic factors, or drug influence. For instance, the QT interval, which plays an important role in assessing the risk of ventricular tachyarrhythmias, is typically about 450 ms; however, both prolongation and shortening are associated with potentially catastrophic outcomes, such as sudden cardiac death. These need to be familiarized with for proper early diagnosis and management. The ability to identify and classify such arrhythmias not only serves immediate management but also impacts long-term health outcomes for children. Pediatricians and cardiologists, therefore, require expert knowledge in preparation for the complexities of arrhythmia diagnosis prevalent among children. Moreover, knowledge of the mechanisms behind pediatric arrhythmias can provide insights into the necessary treatment strategies. Molecular determination of action potential duration and ensuing risk of long and short QT syndromes is beneficial for the detection of potentially lethal illness in children. For example, there is evidence that arrhythmogenic mechanisms often involve processes like reentry and triggered activity, especially in genetic backgrounds. Disruption of these mechanisms can lead to enhanced clinical markers of risk according to the QT interval, which reflects arrhythmic risk and cardiovascular mortality. Recognition of the arrhythmogenic pathways that separate children from adults enables clinicians to make tailored treatment plans. This focused interest is important in order to avert the worsening of outcomes when arrhythmias are not treated in children. Lastly, the implications for public health and pediatric practice are relevant, with early diagnosis and management of arrhythmias being crucial for substantially changing patient outcome. Among children, undiagnosed cardiac disease highlights the imperative for extensive screening programs that serve to identify the at-risk children. With adequate education and awareness campaigns, clinicians can better recognize the presentation of arrhythmias, and this will be reflected in early referral and management. Implementing strong screening protocols within schools and at pediatric visits is essential to the safety of children's cardiovascular health. Covering research and education for pediatric arrhythmias pays dividends not just to individual patients, but it also works to initiate greater public health standards generally. With each development in this important arena, the pediatric healthcare system becomes increasingly capable of addressing the challenges posed by these potentially life-threatening conditions in children.

10.1. Types of Pediatric Arrhythmias

Pediatric arrhythmias are a diverse class of cardiac disease with irregular heart rhythm from diverse causes. One of the most frequent ones is bradyarrhythmia, where the heart rate is lower than normal, usually appearing in congenital heart disease or as an adverse effect of medication. In infants and young children, the illness may manifest as impaired ability to produce adequate cardiac output that could lead to manifestations like lethargy or feeding intolerance. Tachyarrhythmias, which are abnormally fast heart rates, are represented by supraventricular tachycardia and ventricular tachycardia. Understanding these arrhythmias is essential as they are able to create severe hemodynamic instability and, therefore, intervention is emergently necessary to correct a normal cardiac rhythm and prevent long-term sequelae.

Arrhythmias in children may also be further classified based on their etiology within the heart. Supraventricular arrhythmias, which are located above the ventricles, are a prevalent diagnosis in children and are most often described as palpitations or syncope. In contrast, ventricular arrhythmias that arise from the lower chambers of the heart are possibly more dangerous, particularly in the context of background structural heart disease. These arrhythmias can have catastrophic outcomes like cardiac arrest if not treated immediately. Diagnosis is most commonly a combination of clinical assessment, electrocardiogram monitoring, and sometimes advanced imaging modalities to determine the presence of underlying structural reasons behind the arrhythmia. Management of these disorders requires interdisciplinary collaboration between pediatric cardiologists, electrophysiologists, and emergency care practitioners in order to achieve optimal management for the child. Also important is the consideration of the impact of pediatric arrhythmias on the child's quality of life and process of development. Chronic arrhythmias can interfere with normal day-to-day activities, leading to extra stress on the child and family. Research has indicated that children with arrhythmias are at an increased risk of experiencing anxiety and disruption of social interaction caused by concerns regarding their health (Sulu et al., 2024). Management interventions should, therefore, not only treat the clinical management of the arrhythmia but also include psychological care and parental counseling. By providing a comprehensive treatment approach that addresses the physical and emotional needs of pediatric patients, healthcare providers can significantly improve the overall prognosis and well-being of children with arrhythmias.

10.1.1. Supraventricular Tachycardia (SVT)

Supraventricular tachycardia (SVT) is a frequent arrhythmia in children, with an abnormally rapid heart rate situated above the ventricles. The disease is also represented as paroxysmal attacks, where the heart rate can extend to over 220 beats per minute in infants and to 180 beats per minute in adults. The clinical effect of SVT should not be exaggerated, as untreated episodes might lead to severe complications like heart failure and cardiogenic shock, especially in the young with less perfect cardiac reserve. Early recognition and treatment are crucial to prevent such adverse results. Vagal maneuvers would often be the initial treatment of preference, providing an easy, non-invasive way to return NSR efficiently, particularly in stable patients. Despite being successful, however, these maneuvers are not always successful, and other pharmacological maneuvers come into play (Zachaj et al., 2024). Pharmacological treatment is indicated when treatment of SVT in children is indicated, and adenosine is usually employed as a first-line agent following failed vagal maneuvers. The European Resuscitation Council and the American Heart Association guidelines support this practice, highlighting its effectiveness and safety profile (Figure 10.2).

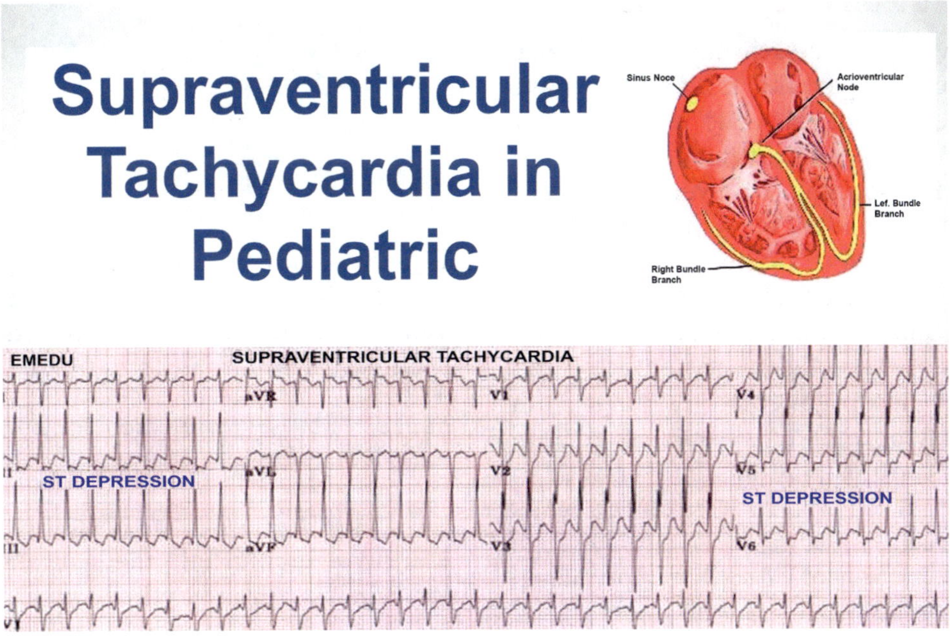

Figure 10.2. SVT in pediatrics.

Source: https://external-content.duckduckgo.com/iu/?u=https%3A%2F%2Fcdn.slidesharecdn.com%2Fss_thumbnails%2Fcardiacarrhythmia-151001035925-lva1-app6892-thumbnail-4.jpg%3Fcb%3D1443674810&f=1&nofb=1&ipt=e074d0ed83eb42a8400e3c4ec864b54a5d3c6a109d86e38841400f371ce9201e.

Adenosine, when administered intravenously, immediately has the ability to re-establish NSR by blocking atrioventricular nodal conduction temporarily. While intraosseous delivery might be utilized in extreme circumstances, that is still comparatively underutilized and further study is required before it can be accepted clinically more broadly. Management programs must consider the unique patient's clinical presentation because underlying pathophysiology can differ markedly. In addition, constant surveillance and readjustment of treatment plans are necessary in order to fight the reoccurrence of SVT effectively (Zachaj et al., 2024). In addition to pharmacological treatments, non-pharmacological therapies also have an equally significant role in the treatment of pediatric SVT. Electrophysiological tests and catheter ablation are now reasonable alternatives, particularly in conditions where medication is insufficient. Efficient utilization of such strategies has markedly improved results in children with recurrent episodes of SVT, especially in patients with symptoms unresponsive to initial intervention. Further, the interaction between SVT and other structural cardiac diseases needs strict assessment and planning since existing pathology makes management approaches complex. Evidence has proven the critical need for vigilant monitoring in pediatric post-operative cardiac settings; arrhythmias, such as SVT, are more common in these cases. Thus, a synchronized, multi-disciplinary process is required to achieve maximized care and enhanced quality of life in infant patients with arrhythmias.

10.1.2. Ventricular Tachycardia (VT)

In children, ventricular tachycardia (VT) also has specific challenges and issues that make it distinct from what happens in adults. VT may occur as a consequence of congenital heart lesions, cardiomyopathy, or even secondary to myocardial ischemia. In pediatric VT, the underlying pathophysiological mechanisms tend to be reentrant circuits or focal triggers that result in uncoordinated electrical activity in the ventricles. The clinical presentation can be extremely heterogeneous, varying from completely asymptomatic attacks in certain children to syncope, palpitations, or even sudden cardiac death in others. Such heterogeneous presentations call for very extensive knowledge of the pathophysiology of VT so that appropriate management modalities can be formulated specifically for the pediatric age group, where interventions need to be tailored to take into account special physiological and psychosocial needs of younger patients. Early detection of VT in children is significant as early management will dictate outcomes.

Diagnostic tests may include electrocardiograms (ECGs), Holter monitoring, and tachyarrhythmia mapping that provide data on the nature and frequency of arrhythmia. They enable clinicians to differentiate between monomorphic and polymorphic ventricular tachycardia, and this is helpful for management. Secondarily, prolonged VT durations can lead to hemodynamic instability and thus the need for immediate medical evaluation. Children who have developed expressions of VT usually need a multi-disciplinary team for management that involves pediatric cardiologists and electrophysiologists familiar with the treatment of arrhythmias to offer a care plan that addresses short-term and long-term health care of the child with ventricular tachycardia (Figure 10.3).

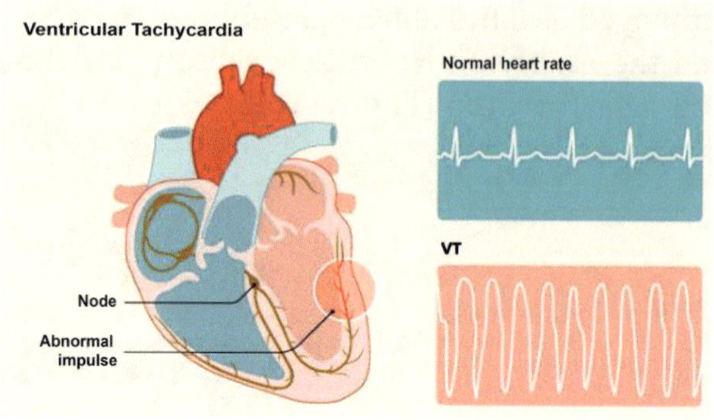

Figure 10.3. Ventricular tachycardia may eventually lead to low blood pressure and ventricular fibrillation, a condition in which the heart beats in a rapid, inadequate rhythm.

Source: https://www.healthline.com/health/ventricular-tachycardia.

Pediatric VT management is complex and involves multiple medical and procedural approaches. Antiarrhythmic medication can be employed to stabilize the cardiac rhythm, but the effectiveness and toxicity profiles need to be carefully weighed, particularly in children. VT refractory or recurrent and unresponsive to medical treatment has traditionally been treated with surgery, but increasing experience with catheter ablation has made it an increasingly attractive alternative, with potentially curative results. But these interventions must be approached with caution due to the risks of anesthesia as well as the intrusiveness of the intervention among children. Lastly, the outcome among children with VT would largely depend on the etiology of the condition, the severity of the symptoms, and the quality of the intervention. As depicted in previous studies, ongoing improvement in therapy and care methods continues to improve outcomes for children suffering from this complex arrhythmia (Abe et al., 2013; Meijboom et al., 2004).

10.1.3. Atrial Fibrillation and Flutter

Atrial fibrillation (AF) and atrial flutter are

significant arrhythmias that, although they are usually characteristic of adults, are increasingly visible among children. The occurrence of these arrhythmias in children can result from a range of pathologies, including congenital heart defects, structural lesions, and previous cardiac operations. In contrast to adults, presentation of AF and flutter in children is usually less typical and may necessitate specialized diagnostic strategies. Specialist imaging techniques and ambulatory monitoring, including Holter monitoring or wearable ECG monitors, can be valuable in detecting these arrhythmias, leading to timely diagnosis and treatment. Pediatric cases have a special nature that necessitates multi-disciplinary treatment involving pediatric cardiologists and electrophysiologists to ensure accurate diagnosis and appropriate management plans. The profile of treating atrial fibrillation and flutter in children is radically different from adults, primarily due to variations in disease etiology and patient physiology. Although pharmacological treatment is typically the first to be used, with beta-blockers and antiarrhythmics, catheter ablation is an appropriate option for more challenging cases. The Pediatric Radiofrequency Registry has demonstrated radiofrequency ablation (RFA) may be safely performed in children, although this is generally reserved for teenagers and older children. Concerns over the efficacy and safety of RFA in children still linger, especially in patients weighing less than 15 kg, due to their heightened risk for complication. As such, extreme care must be taken in weighing the suitability of RFA in infants and toddlers, taking into consideration the nature of the arrhythmias, their clinical impacts, and the potential long-term impacts of such treatments (Blaufox et al., 2005) (Figure 10.4).

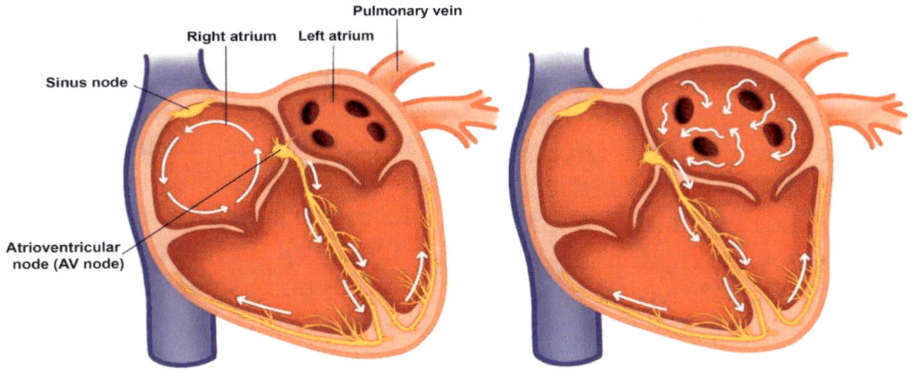

Figure 10.4. Atrial fibrillation and flutter in pediatric patients.

Source: https://external-content.duckduckgo.com/iu/?u=https%3A%2F%2Fucarecdn.com%2Fe39eef98-8185-4032-a394-4359fcbbb2e4%2F-%2Fformat%2Fauto%2F-%2Fpreview%2F3000x3000%2F-%2Fquality%2Flighter%2Fdifference%2520between%2520atrial%2520flutter%2520and%2520atrial%2520fibrillation.png&f=1&nofb=1&ipt=4695d123bcd7a6391fbe8ec0923556a477240e0f6a5137be252cecdc382da069.

Emerging technologies are remodeling the approach for detecting and treating atrial fibrillation and flutter in kids. Traditional tools such as the traditional 12-lead electrocardiogram have worked but were limited in being able to monitor continuously. The progression of wearable ECG technology over the past few years has revolutionized the world of monitoring by providing unobtrusive, real-time data for prolonged periods. These devices add to the diagnostic yield in busy clinic settings and offer a more patient-focused care for arrhythmia (Carlson et al., 2015). With increased utilization of these types of technologies, they have the potential to improve clinician-patient communication, ultimately helping to improve delivery of care and potentially improve outcomes among children with atrial arrhythmias. This paradigm shift is rooted in the focus of the need for ongoing research and adaptation in clinical practice to realize the potential of current technology to effectively diagnose and treat pediatric atrial fibrillation and flutter.

10.2. Causes of Pediatric Arrhythmias

Pediatric arrhythmias have multiple etiologies that are both structural and functional cardiac conditions. Congenital heart defects are among the key etiologic factors since defects may obstruct normal conduction pathways within the myocardium and produce irregular heart rhythms. Arrhythmias like ventricular extrasystoles have been detected in apparently healthy children; however, the rhythm can be a manifestation of underlying structural cardiac alteration that needs assessment. Evidence indicates that such ventricular extrasystoles, while often benign in etiology, can still be concomitant with more significant disorders when related to underlying myocardial disease or channelopathy, as studies that review their incidence in children reveal (Kunigeliene et al., 2025). Hence, good evaluation is central to an understanding of the clinical relevance of any arrhythmias found in children. Besides structural abnormality, genetic mechanisms also play an important role in pediatric arrhythmias. Genetic channelopathies (i.e., cardiac ion channel dysfunction) may result in severe rhythm disturbances and manifest as Long QT Syndrome and Brugada Syndrome. They are usually inherited conditions that present in infancy or childhood with characteristics of abnormal electrocardiogram and susceptibility to fatal arrhythmias. Clinical presentations may be fine and cause challenges in early diagnosis. Moreover, these conditions are usually subject to the need for genetic counseling and cardiogenetic testing, focusing on understanding familial histories when dealing with pediatric arrhythmias. As evidenced by results of recent studies, precise identification and treatment of such conditions provide better outcomes while treating pediatric arrhythmias (Doğan et al., 2024). In addition, outside influences, such as environmental factors and comorbid medical conditions, may increase the occurrence of arrhythmias among children. For example, electrolyte disorders, which commonly result from dehydration or severe illness, can cause cardiac rhythm disturbances. Stimulants and medications, such as caffeine or some over-the-counter medications, also may induce arrhythmic episodes in vulnerable teens. Furthermore, stress and emotional distress are also recognized as potential precipitating causes for arrhythmias, adding further complexity to the management of affected children. While these extrinsic contributors continue to be explored by research, practitioners must adopt a multi-dimensional approach by considering intrinsic and extrinsic factors impacting pediatric arrhythmias in order to provide proper prevention and management strategies.

10.2.1. Congenital Heart Defects

Congenital heart defects (CHDs) represent a heterogeneous category of structural heart anomalies at the time of birth with profound pediatric health and development consequences. They are caused by abnormal development of the heart during fetal life and can affect the walls, valves, or great blood vessels of the heart and cause a diverse array of complications that both are present at birth and in later life. Prevalence of CHDs is nonspecific but are a leading cause of infant and child morbidity and mortality. As illustrated in the context of pediatric arrhythmias, CHDs subject the patient to numerous cardiac issues, such as arrhythmias. Proper diagnosis and early intervention are crucial in the avoidance of long-term sequelae of such defects and in the improvement of patient outcomes. Also, ongoing monitoring and tailored treatment possibilities might enhance the quality of life for children with CHDs by not only repairing their structural heart defects but also their associated rhythm disturbances. The inter-connection between congenital cardiac abnormalities and arrhythmias is intimately intertwined with the pathophysiologic foundation of such defects. Upon surgical repair, which can be needed to restore normal physiological function, the distorted geometry of the hearts and the resulting scarring can offer an environment for arrhythmias. From clinical evidence, the severity of the CHD and the timing of surgery both play a significant role in the probability of developing cardiac arrhythmias following surgery. For instance, children undergoing surgery, particularly the low body weight ones, may experience an increased incidence of these disturbances due to increased hemodynamic stress and alterations in cardiac structure. Arrhythmias may also be varied in their presentation, varying from palpitations to syncope, depending on the degree and duration of the rhythm disturbance and the causative congenital anomaly (Ganea et al., 2023). Recent studies point towards the importance of exploring the genetic etiologies of congenital heart defects, particularly comorbidities like arrhythmias. The genetic defects involving genes like the NAA10 and NAA15 genes have been utilized to account for various neurodevelopmental diseases, showing a connection between genetics, congenital heart disease, and rhythm diseases. As an example, cardiac manifestations such as long QT syndrome and ventricular tachycardia have been described in patients with NAA10-related syndromes. Similarly, some patients with NAA15 variation have been observed to suffer from ventricular septal defects and arrhythmias related to them (Alyssa et al., 2020). These findings emphasize the imperative of incorporating genetic testing and counseling into treatment regimens in patients with congenital heart defect, as this may lead to more tailored treatments and improved prognoses in risk patients who are likely to manifest extensive arrhythmias.

10.2.2. Genetic Predispositions

Understand genetic predispositions is crucial in the management of pediatric arrhythmias, considering that inherited factors contribute to a large extent to the risk of having such conditions. Congenital heart defects (CHDs) that affect approximately 1% of live births usually arise from complex interactions between genetic, environmental, and epigenetic determinants (Reemtsen et al., 2017). Such high prevalence of defects reflects the necessity for further understanding of the genetic mechanisms involved that drive arrhythmias in children. Although new technology in genetic sequencing and research methods has improved our capacity to identify individual variants associated with CHDs, the complex etiology of these diseases complicates the development of an efficient targeted treatment. Continued research into genetic predisposition, beyond improving the specificity of diagnosis, augments the potential for personalized treatments and ultimately better outcomes for the patient. The implications of genetic susceptibility extend beyond the straightforward identification of children at risk; they also emphasize the importance of integrating genetic data into clinical care. From the research, a high percentage of arrhythmias in children is linked to identifiable genetic syndromes or mutations, which necessitates the implementation of a systematic approach to genetic screening (Reemtsen et al., 2017). Using a multi-leveled strategy of phenotypic characterization, molecular genotype/phenotype analysis, and next-generation sequencing technology, clinicians can more precisely outline the range of cardiac anomalies of affected patients. Multi-modal testing can lead to timely intervention and facilitation of more effective management of arrhythmic events. Furthermore, genetic predispositions serve to advise families regarding risk and family patterns, thus preparing them with information required to make informed decisions regarding health care. Despite advancements in the discovery of genetic predispositions for pediatric arrhythmias, there remain significant difficulties. The majority of genetic variants continue to elude classification, thus rendering it difficult to develop precise treatment methods (Reemtsen et al., 2017). Moreover, the identification of genetic presentations of phenotypes continues to be an evolving field, where many cases are likely to go undiagnosed or poorly explained. It is this gap which emphasizes the requirement for extensive coordination between clinicians and genetic researchers to facilitate the establishment of disease models and refinement of diagnostic techniques. By enhancing access to high-quality biological samples from well-characterized patient cohorts, it is possible to enlist a systematic strategy to the genetic topology of pediatric arrhythmias. This integrated paradigm is essential in addressing the unmet challenges of the field and aligning to the future of personalized medicine for childhood cardiovascular disease.

10.2.3. Acquired Conditions and Environmental Factors

The juxtaposition of acquired disease and environmental factors provides an important setting for the understanding of arrhythmias in children. Environmental factors, particularly extreme weather conditions such as heat waves, have been shown to exacerbate existing conditions among children, leading to greater healthcare utilization. Research indicates that record heat events in California have resulted in substantial numbers of pediatric acute care visits, establishing a disturbing correlation between such environmental stressors and well-being among vulnerable populations. Of specific concern are conditions such as heat-related illness and metabolic disorders, which have demonstrated substantial increases with these events, warranting immediate concern regarding how environmental stressors impact cardiac health. Identifying such connections is imperative in developing targeted interventions. These interventions will safeguard children against harmful environmental effects, especially in the context of socio-economic and inequality areas (Ndovu et al., 2025). Apart from this, pediatric arrhythmias may also be influenced by the socio-economic as well as educational context of the neighborhoods that house children. Low-income community children are likely to be overexposed to toxic environmental factors, including pollution and inadequate access to healthcare services. These conditions not only amplify the risks of arrhythmias but also place a larger context within which structural inequality increases health disparities. Geographic studies recognize an evident spatial heterogeneity in health outcomes, particularly in those regions that are dominated by Black, Hispanic, and Pacific Islander inhabitants. The system deprivation and resource limitations of such populations may compound the severity of pediatric arrhythmias and other conditions and necessitate policies addressing environmental and social determinants of health. Such disparities should be addressed to improve pediatric cardiac care and outcomes (Ndovu et al., 2025). Another layer of complexity arises when addressing environmental factor-influenced biological markers and psychological contexts. New research defines the role of brain-derived neurotrophic factor (BDNF) as a potential biomarker for the understanding of pediatric acquired brain injury and its interaction with the environment. BDNF is not only sensitive to physical trauma but also to psychosocial circumstance, implying that both genetic predisposition and extrinsic conditions have a role in the neurobiological processes that shape cardiac health. Measurement of BDNF levels following injury or during stress periods can provide valuable information on neuroplasticity and mechanisms of recovery, reshaping clinical treatment strategies for conditions such as arrhythmias. This awareness indicates the potential of including biological, psychological, and environmental variables in holistic treatment techniques to render greater health gains for children battling arrhythmias' complexity.

10.3. Symptoms and Diagnosis

In pediatrics arrhythmias, symptom recognition is crucial in early diagnosis and intervention. Children may have variable presentation that complicates the clinical presentation. Common presentation, such as palpitations, syncope, and fatigue, may readily be overlooked or misdiagnosed as other benign processes. There are also newer problems, such as myocarditis due to COVID-19 vaccination, that compound arrhythmias in some children. A study presented the reality that 92% of patients who had developed myocarditis following vaccination presented with symptoms like dysrhythmia, among other cardiological issues, necessitating appropriate evaluations among this population to distinguish the many reasons for presenting symptoms (Jain et al., 2021). Practitioners should therefore remain vigilant when attending to non-specific presentations and consider potential underlying arrhythmic conditions. Pediatric arrhythmia diagnosis is greatly reliant on clinical evaluation as well as advanced diagnostic techniques. The initial evaluation of patients is typically a good history and physical exam, with the subsequent use of electrocardiography (ECG) to define abnormal cardiac rhythms. When details of arrhythmias are suspected, echocardiography also plays a significant role in assessment of cardiac function and identification of structural abnormalities and thereby affects the management plan. Herein, retrospective analysis also indicated that these symptoms like fever, cough, and chest pain were most commonly present in relation to acute myocarditis, its arrhythmic complication of which can present (Han-Wu et al., 2017). Early diagnosis and subsequent observation in all such patients are required to monitor for the interventions such as the application of ECMO in critical cases, allowing early intervention for children involved. Post-diagnostic treatment often involves multidisciplinary collaboration in an attempt to personalize treatment regimens aimed at curing arrhythmia as well as its causative factor. Pharmacologic therapy could be utilized in an attempt to stabilize cardiac rhythms or, where necessary, more invasive strategies such as catheter ablation. Close follow-up of patients with a history of myocarditis is essential, with there being the possibility of long-term sequelae such as myopathy or chronic arrhythmias. The findings of previous studies are in favor of strict follow-up, which can lead to good long-term outcomes and improvement of symptoms in most pediatric patients with such disorders (Jain et al., 2021). Through awareness of the interconnectedness of symptoms and application of complete diagnostic methods, clinical professionals are able to effectively treat pediatric arrhythmias and improve patient treatment.

10.3.1. Common Symptoms in Children

In pediatrics arrhythmias, it is essential to have an exhaustive understanding of the common symptoms in children for timely detection and treatment. Palpitations, dizziness, and syncope are often typical signs of cardiac abnormalities. Further, palpitations may be felt as a sensation of a running heart or occasional beats, which can be extremely alarming to children and their parents alike. Concern symptoms worsen on exertion and indicate the likelihood of an underlying arrhythmia. The recognition of these signs at an early stage can enable early referrals to cardiologists, which is pivotal in preventing complications. These children presenting such signs need to be handled with care because the psychosocial interference can also lead to anxiety and fear of physical activity, thereby making it difficult for their general health and well-being. In certain contexts, drug consumption like levothyroxine can cause symptoms that are mimicking arrhythmia and make diagnosis in children even more complicated. More specifically, accidental consumption will lead to mixed presentation ranging from an asymptomatic condition to exhibiting dangerous manifestations like hypertension and tachycardia (Figure 10.5).

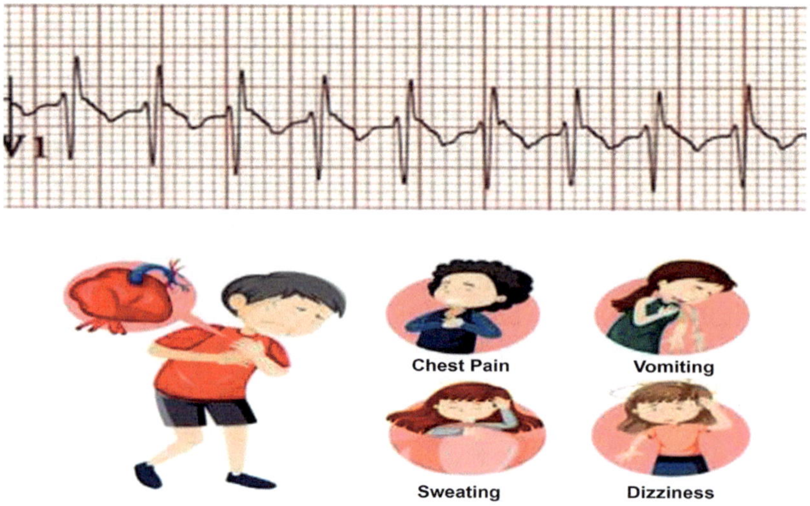

Figure 10.5. Supraventricular tachycardia (SVT) symptoms.

Source: https://www.kauveryhospital.com/nightingale/pediatric-arrhythmia-management/.

In one case, a three-year-old child had impressive changes in blood pressure and heart rate following unintentional levothyroxine ingestion, necessitating medical care. This serves to illustrate how external factors should be considered when evaluating cardiac symptoms in children. Further, vulnerability to arrhythmias increases the need for proper monitoring and educative training of caregivers in identifying early warning signs so that they can acquire prompt medical attention in order to provide pediatric patients with the requisite treatment. Another significant aspect of the evaluation of common symptoms among children understands the implication of drugs such as inhaled selective short-acting β-2 agonists (SABA) employed in treating asthma. Although such medication is essential in alleviating the immediate symptoms and preventing severe asthma attacks, they have been associated with cardiovascular side effects, i.e., a risk of causing supraventricular tachycardia (SVT). The link between SABA usage and arrhythmia development among children is paramount to medical practitioners' consideration. Since SVT is the most common severe dysrhythmia in children, detection of associated symptoms becomes essential in management of accompanying complications. By addressing the requirement for adequate asthma control while maintaining close observation for cardiac side effects, caregivers as well as healthcare professionals can ensure successful cardiovascular as well as respiratory well-being in children.

10.3.2. Diagnostic Tools and Techniques

Childhood arrhythmias need evaluation by an armamentarium of diagnostic modalities and techniques adjusted to the child's unique anatomical and physiological distinctions. Electrocardiogram (ECG) is the gold standard for testing arrhythmias, measuring in real-time the heart's electrical activity. ECG interpretations by children need to be expert because common variations in heart rate and rhythm are unlike adults.' This heterogeneity is especially apparent in children, making it challenging to study arrhythmias in this group. Additionally, ambulatory Holter monitoring is occasionally used for prolonged periods to pick up transient arrhythmias not seen on standard ECG recordings. This technique is extremely useful as it allows one to monitor with the patient's usual activity without interference from attendant noises or room reverberations, thus improving diagnostic sensitivity. Echocardiography is another critical diagnostic tool in pediatric arrhythmia assessment. The non-invasive imaging examination provides detailed structural and functional cardiac data, calling attention to potential underlying etiologies of arrhythmias, such as congenital heart disease or cardiomyopathies. If echocardiogram abnormalities are evident, additional genetic testing may be warranted. For instance, certain hypertrophic cardiomyopathy mutations may have the possibility of predisposing children to arrhythmias, implying that genetic information has to be integrated into standard diagnostic practice (Ali et al., 2017) (Figure 10.6).

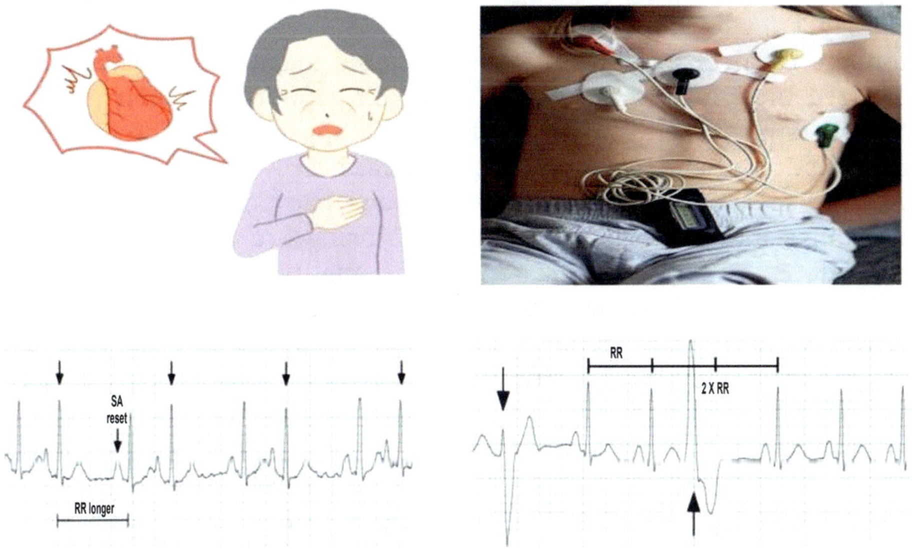

Figure 10.6. Diagnosis of pediatric arrhythmias.

Source: https://www.kauveryhospital.com/wp-content/uploads/2025/05/pad11-768x477.jpg.

Echocardiographic information integrated with clinical history helps to identify risk factors leading to sudden cardiac events, and decisions regarding management and intervention are made accordingly. In complex cases, advanced diagnostic techniques such as electrophysiological testing (EPS) and mapping technologies come into play. EPS enables precise localization of electrical arrhythmia sources, most crucial in determining catheter ablation. This therapy is typically indicated in the case of failure of non-invasive therapies or whenever arrhythmia is moderately endangering sudden cardiac arrest. Furthermore, the application of implantable cardioverter-defibrillators (ICDs) has also grown, particularly in high-risk children (Berto et al., 2017). The capability of these devices to offer life-saving intervention in potentially lethal arrhythmias exists. With ongoing enhancement of these diagnostic instruments and techniques, pediatric arrhythmias can be better managed by clinicians and ultimately improved in outcome and quality of life for these fragile patients.

10.3.3. Importance of Early Detection

Early detection of pediatric arrhythmias cannot be overstressed, as timely intervention can virtually diminish the mortality threat of these conditions. Arrhythmias, a sign of various underlying cardiovascular disorders, pose threats for sudden cardiac death, particularly in children and adolescents who engage in sports activities. The use of screening tools, such as the resting 12-lead electrocardiogram (ECG), is informative of cardiac function and can identify abnormalities that are suggestive of coming arrhythmic events. Since the majority of the hereditary cardiac disorders that lead to sudden cardiac death can be identified through ECG abnormalities, early detection is crucial in formulating anticipatory management strategies to avoid loss of life. Therefore, there is an urgent necessity for improving physician education and training in interpreting ECG results in order to encourage improved screening and diagnosis outcomes among young patients. In addition to raising screening procedures, early detection also guarantees the identification and treatment of congenital heart defects (CHDs), which remain largely unknown among children. CHD affects approximately 1% of live births and remains a leading cause of morbidity and mortality even in high resource care settings. The earliest possible diagnosis is crucial since it paves the way for individualized therapeutic approaches based on genetic and environmental etiologies of such conditions. With a properly designed, multileveled approach combining clinical phenotypic description and sophisticated molecular techniques, healthcare providers are in a position to gain lessons of great value regarding the uniqueness of each patient. Not only does this knowledge direct treatment plans, but follow-up care and monitoring are also enhanced so as to reduce the risk of complications in the future, thus enhancing quality of life in general. The inclusion of early detection strategies in routine pediatric care is facilitated by the need for interdisciplinary collaboration between health professionals, families, and schools. With enhanced sensitivity and understanding of pediatric arrhythmias, the stakeholders are able to enhance their lobbying for screening protocols and early cardiology referral. The ongoing development of guidelines and consensus statements attests to early detection's role in managing these arrhythmias and suggests that such interventions could lead to outcomes that are improved. Parallel with technological and research progress, increased promotion of early diagnosis can transform pediatric cardiology and finally reduce patient risk and slow the rate of avoidable cardiac events in children (Aagaard et al., 2017; Reemtsen et al., 2017).

10.4. Treatment Options

In the management of pediatric arrhythmias, treatment varies significantly based on the nature of the arrhythmia and the underlying cause. Among these treatments, catheter radiofrequency ablation (RFA) has been a leading intervention, especially for arrhythmias like supraventricular tachycardia (SVT), which are common among children. While RFA has proven effective and safe as a form of therapy within pediatric patients, there remains a great consideration in the case of very young patients, particularly those below 15 kg, who are at higher risk for the development of complications. With the combination of this risk factor and the technical challenge of performing RFA within smaller hearts, there is reluctance to implement this type of therapy within very young children. As such, physicians must thoughtfully weigh the potential benefits of RFA against the risks, considering the natural history of participating arrhythmias and the individualized situation of specific patients (Blaufox et al., 2005). Pharmacologic interventions are also highly engaged in the management of pediatric arrhythmias, particularly when there is an emergent need for intervention. In fetal tachycardia, the administration of antiarrhythmic medications could be instrumental in the prevention of complications such as congestive heart failure or fetal hydrops. The drug treatment must nevertheless be determined with consideration for various factors, such as gestational age, ventricular rates, and tachycardia duration. Although there might be a spontaneous resolution in selected situations, expectant management is not as favorable compared to treatment, especially when there is severe fetal distress. Although pharmacological agents may poorly transfer through the placenta, their timely administration is essential in stabilizing the fetus's hemodynamic status, emphasizing the importance of individualized drug choice (Meijboom et al., 2004). Aside from RFA and medication, complete management of pediatric arrhythmias may also require non-invasive measures, including lifestyle modifications and ongoing monitoring. These are pivotal in managing less severe or less urgent arrhythmic illnesses, where the most important aim is to maintain a normal heart rhythm and overall well-being. In others, especially those with episodic symptoms or well-controlled illness, vigilant monitoring may suffice, limiting the need for invasive procedures or long-term medication. Education in symptom recognition and healthy living can also empower families and patients, encouraging an active approach to managing arrhythmias. Lastly, management of children with arrhythmias should be a multidisciplinary strategy, uniting families, pediatric cardiologists, and allied health staff, to guarantee that the chosen treatment is the best response for the child's personal medical needs and circumstances (Figure 10.7).

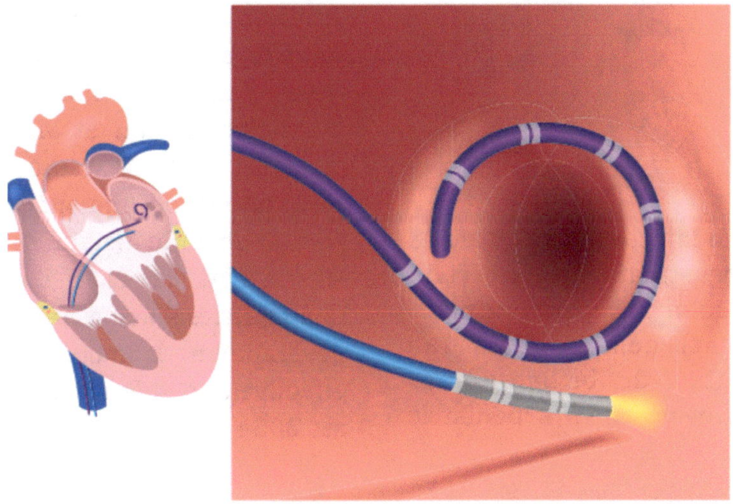

Figure 10.7. Radiofrequency ablation (RFA) of pediatric arrhythmias.

Source: https://www.drkarthigesanclinic.com/wp-content/uploads/2023/06/Types-of-Arrhythmias-Treated.jpg.

10.4.1. Medications for Arrhythmia Management

The management of pediatric arrhythmias is more or less drug based and greatly influences the clinical course in these children. Antiarrhythmic drugs are typically categorized into a series of classes to target various types of arrhythmias. For instance, drugs in Class I, such as sodium channel blocking drugs, can be beneficial for the management of supraventricular and ventricular tachycardias. On the contrary, Class II medications, being beta-blockers, play a crucial role in controlling heart rate and symptomology in inappropriate sinus tachycardia. Prescription of such medications is an age, co-morbidities, and side effects-dependent function. Thus, therapeutic regimens have to be tailored in individual cases to obtain optimal therapeutic outcomes as well as to prevent complications of arrhythmia management. In addition to the usual antiarrhythmic drugs, newer agents have come into play, providing different approaches to treating multifactorial arrhythmias in children (Figure 10.8).

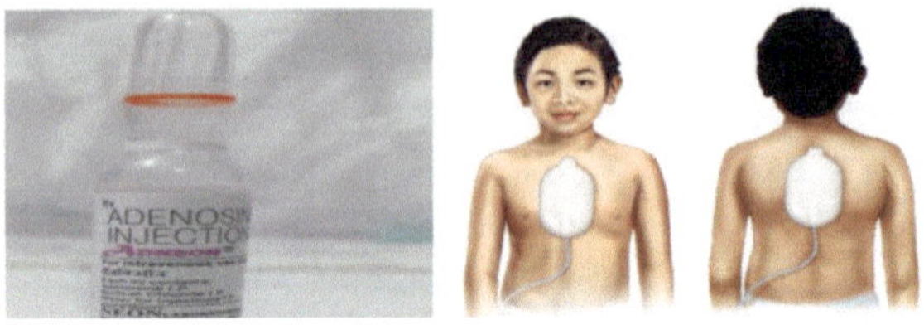

Figure 10.8. Adenosine injection (left) used as a first-line pharmacologic treatment for certain pediatric supraventricular tachyarrhythmias. The illustration (right) demonstrates the appropriate placement of defibrillator pads for synchronized cardioversion in a pediatric patient.

Source: https://www.kauveryhospital.com/nightingale/pediatric-arrhythmia-management/.

Agents such as flecainide and propafenone, typical of the Class IC antiarrhythmics, have been found useful for the control of atrial fibrillation and atrial flutter in well-selected pediatric patients. In most instances, however, the use of these agents is preceded by critical review of the child's cardiac status and risk-to-benefit consideration for the likelihood of proarrhythmic action. Most important, drug effect and tolerance in the patient need to be checked repeatedly, and follow-up visits at regular intervals must be carried out to titrate the doses as the child grows or his/her clinical status alters. Multidisciplinary therapy becomes all the more important based on the intricacies of pharmacological treatment in pediatric patients with arrhythmias. Furthermore, electrophysiological testing, including transesophageal electrophysiological testing (TEEPS), continues to be valuable in determining the effectiveness of antiarrhythmic therapy. TEEPS provides data on arrhythmia inducibility and aids in the explanation of a child's specific arrhythmic disease and guides treatment. These types of diagnostic tests have also been reported to be highly negative predictive values, and they enhance predictive value regarding recurrence rates of tachycardias, which can direct management in the future (Manickavasagam et al., 2022). Furthermore, inclusion of these studies in practice facilitates adjustment of pharmacotherapy to make it person-specific instead of using a one-size-fits-all strategy. This change is particularly relevant in pediatrics since it normalizes for growth and development to make medication management effective and safe for children (Hiranrattana et al., 2024).

10.4.2. Non-Pharmacological Interventions

Non-pharmacological treatments have significant contributions in the management of pediatric arrhythmias as an adjunct to pharmacotherapy. In children, non-pharmacological treatments are especially vital given the side effects associated with the prolonged use of medications. Methods such as electrophysiological studies and catheter ablation have been highly appreciated as treatments for various forms of arrhythmias in cases where drug therapies are inappropriate or even inadequate. In particular, catheter ablation targets focal arrhythmogenic spots in the heart with improved arrhythmia control and without the concomitant burden of long-term medication therapy. This inclusion of non-pharmacological treatments contributes to the composite treatment paradigm so that individualized care plans are formulated for every pediatric patient with arrhythmias with the goal of better clinical outcomes and quality of life. Another critical point is the contribution of education programs as a non-drug intervention in the pediatric arrhythmia management. Through education programs, families and patients can be empowered with knowledge that will allow them to understand their condition, encourage compliance with treatment regimens, and recognize worsening arrhythmia signs. Education programs can be designed to target a variety of areas, including lifestyle modification, participation in supervised activities, and triggers that can evoke arrhythmias. By giving children's families this information, medical professionals not only help the patient take ownership of their health but also provide precious emotional support in an otherwise chaotic medical environment. In this way, the application of instructional strategies has the use of teaching strategies in the practice of caring for pediatric patients with arrhythmias firmly planted in line with best practices in child health care. Furthermore, the implementation of technology-mediated interventions is an innovative move towards the non-pharmacological management of child arrhythmias (Figure 10.9).

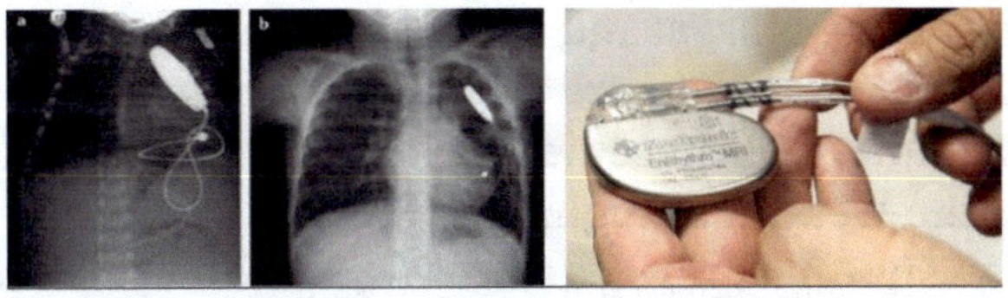

Figure 10.9. Pacemaker implantation if chronotropic incompetent and refractory to medications.

Source: https://www.kauveryhospital.com/wp-content/uploads/2025/05/pad8-768x218.jpg.

Interventions can include telehealth for routine monitoring or mobile applications aimed at tracking symptoms and medication adherence effectively. Technology allows real-time monitoring of the heartbeat of the child, enabling prompt adjustment in the management strategy. These platforms can also serve as a link between healthcare providers and families to enable seamless communication regarding the health of the child. Through the application of technology, not only can healthcare systems reinforce patient participation but also promote proactive management of arrhythmias in kids. In the end, such non-pharmacological interventions lead to improved clinical outcomes and play a very useful role in the context of overall care required for pediatric patients suffering from arrhythmias, substantiating the adoption of diverse modes of treatment in clinical practice, as highlighted in relevant literature (Dakhel et al., 2024; Kim et al., 2024).

10.4.3. Surgical Options and Catheter Ablation

The treatment of pediatric arrhythmias will often involve surgical intervention and catheter ablation as fundamental components of therapy in instances where drug therapy is ineffective. Procedures may include the creation of a surgical lesion to stop abnormal electrical circuits, while sophisticated procedures employ the generation of catheter ablation to specifically target and eliminate arrhythmogenic areas of the heart. Catheter ablation, for example, has become an integral component of the treatment regimens due to its minimally invasive nature, hence allowing for accurate diagnosis and treatment of arrhythmias, both supraventricular and ventricular. With the utilization of transesophageal electrophysiologic studies, physicians are in a better position to decipher such arrhythmias, and this enables them to devise personalized treatment regimens to children, particularly in terms of the special physiological factors in this age bracket (Benson et al., 1995). Catheter ablation has transformed the practice of pediatric arrhythmia management. The procedure depends on advanced mapping technology to identify abnormal electrical pathways within the heart and apply precise energy to stop these arrhythmias. Thus, catheter ablation not only mitigates symptoms but also addresses the pathophysiological substrate. A growing amount of work also recognizes the efficacy and safety of catheter ablation in children, with over 90% cure rates for certain arrhythmias (Aguinaga et al., 2019). This is a shift in paradigm that indicates focus on proper diagnosis with electrophysiological studies, which can match well with the subsequent ablation procedure, achieving maximum outcome and minimal complications with surgery. In addition, application of catheter ablation in pediatric patients is directed by evolving guidelines and best practices based on comprehensive research and clinical experience. Recent consensus documents have reaffirmed the value of implementing a systemic approach to patient selection with an emphasis on individual risk stratification based on the patient's specific arrhythmia type, age, and comorbid disease. The advancement in catheter technologies and techniques has also widened the arena for electrophysiologists to carry out ablation safely and effectively in children. Catheter ablation has not only emerged as an alternative treatment, but in most cases, the treatment of choice for curing complex arrhythmias in children, opening doors toward more patient-centered and advanced management paradigms in pediatric cardiology (Aguinaga et al., 2019).

10.5. Long-Term Management and Follow-Up

For pediatric arrhythmias, long-term follow-up and management are the key to ensuring the best outcome in the patient. The conditions need a general plan with frequent monitoring, medication, and immediate interventions if necessary. Arrhythmia patients can have varying degrees of presentations, and the presentation can shift during development. An individualized follow-up schedule is thus necessary to assess the effectiveness of any treatment used initially. This includes evaluating the need for dose adjustment of the drugs according to growth and development, and evaluating the need for ablation procedures in some cases, particularly in those who undergo recurrent supraventricular tachycardia. An active follow-up protocol enables medical professionals to manage any complications or changes in the arrhythmia pattern more effectively in a timely manner, which is extremely crucial because such diseases can leave lasting impacts on heart health. Furthermore, whether or not to continue treatments such as radiofrequency ablation (RFA) in children is beset with unique challenges and considerations. As safe as it has been shown to be for the treatment of certain arrhythmias, RFA carries inherent risks, particularly for young kids or those under 15 kg. In light of the reluctance to recommend such procedures among the population, clinicians must objectively weigh the risk against the benefit while taking into account patient-specific factors during decision-making. According to the current evidence, complications of RFA can potentially be even more severe in patients with congenital heart disease, calling for careful selection and long-term follow-up. Regular evaluation of the patient's clinical presentation, description of the tachycardia, and general state of health must be done to determine the best time and necessity of any intervention upon return visits (Blaufox et al., 2005). Long-term follow-up extends beyond clinical assessment; it also addresses psychosocial concerns relevant in pediatric patients and their families (Figure 10.10).

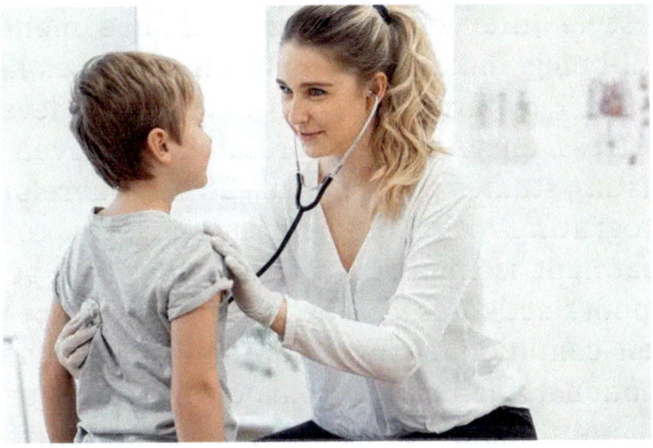

Figure 10.10. Long-term management and follow-up are critical for ensuring optimal patient outcomes.

Source: https://external-content.duckduckgo.com/iu/?u=https%3A%2F%2Fwww.indiancrestpeds.com%2Fwp-content%2Fuploads%2F2023%2F11%2FPediatric-Arrhythmia.jpg.webp&f=1&nofb=1&ipt=81721dc90766670ecd46892540bb69ec7498bdc023dac16b6eeb87d5a542ac47.

Children with arrhythmia may experience emotional and psychological concerns relating to the condition, which require a holistic management plan that considers these challenges. Parent and guardian involvement in educational interventions for the etiology of the arrhythmia, management, and lifestyle adjustments can encourage enhanced compliance with management strategies and patient outcomes. Also, the employment of organized communication among multidisciplinary teams like cardiologists, rehabilitation teams, and nurses can be advantageous in managing both medical and emotional issues of the patients. As recent recommendations identify, coordination of care activities within multidisciplinary teams is likely to optimize the treatment of pediatric arrhythmias with particular emphasis being laid on high-strength care during long-term follow-up (Aickin et al., 2019).

10.5.1. Importance of Regular Monitoring

Regular monitoring is essential in the management of pediatric arrhythmias as it allows medical professionals to rapidly identify changes in the status of a child that may indicate deteriorating arrhythmias or arising complications. Children with known arrhythmic conditions receive regular follow-up appointments with electrocardiograms (ECGs) to look for any arrhythmia attacks that are not immediately symptomatic. This proactive approach is not only essential for catching any abnormalities early but also to proper management of long-term treatment regimens. By constantly monitoring heart rhythm and function, healthcare providers can intervene by making timely adjustments in medications or interventions, which avoids the risk of severe consequences from prolonged arrhythmias. Regular interaction between healthcare providers, patients, and families produces a healthy environment that facilitates compliance with treatment regimens and the best cardiovascular care. Routine monitoring covers the needs of more than short-term treatment schedules because it involves assessing drug impact and potential side effects. Pediatric patients, for example, may react differently to medication than adults, so special care must be given in their treatment plan. As highlighted in the literature, corticosteroids, which are commonly used in most pediatric conditions, highlight the extreme significance of careful monitoring to prevent side effects like iatrogenic Cushing's syndrome, which has far-reaching consequences on a child's growth and well-being (Rai, 2025). Continuous observation not only facilitates early identification of such complications but also supports logical prescribing trends, where medications are titrated based on the fluctuating needs of the child. Monitoring, thus, represents an invaluable component in the prevention of pharmacological intervention risks during pediatric arrhythmia management. Moreover, repeated monitoring plays a pivotal role in determining the efficacy of both non-pharmacological as well as pharmacological interventions. For instance, in children requiring electrophysiological interventions, such as catheter ablation for arrhythmias, continuous evaluation is crucial in determining the efficacy and safety of the intervention (Dakhel et al., 2024). During this time, hospital staff are able to assess recovery, manage acute post-procedure complications, and adjust care plans if required. Children will quite often have idiosyncratic physiological reactions to arrhythmias, and so individual monitoring is essential to ensure that any emerging issues are addressed early. Overall monitoring strategies thus not only enhance the therapeutic efficacy but also make an extremely valuable contribution towards optimizing the overall prognosis and quality of life for such pediatric patients with arrhythmias.

10.5.2. Lifestyle Modifications for Affected Children

Lifestyle modification is crucial in the management of pediatric arrhythmias to improve the health of children and their families with these conditions. Encouraging a stable routine that involves regular physical exercise can improve cardiovascular health as well as symptoms mitigation of anxiety and depression that typically accompany chronic illnesses. Research has proven that after arrhythmia detection, adding exercise regimens into organized patterns of activity to a child's state fosters better cardiac function and overall fitness. This is critical considering the evidence shown decreased ability for exercise in children with congenital heart defects and therefore a requirement for specialist training to ensure children can safely engage in physical activity. Incorporating activity that enhances cardiovascular conditioning can overcome the constraints imposed by arrhythmias and increase overall well-being, thus resulting in an active life that is enjoyable as well as safe for such children. In addition, the psychological effects of pediatric arrhythmias necessitate lifestyle interventions that enhance mental well-being. Children with chronic illnesses like Long QT Syndrome (LQTS) have higher levels of stress, anxiety, and depression, as proven in existing studies (Conlin et al., 2012). Therefore, integrating psychological support in total treatment is important. Counseling and peer support activities can help the child adapt to their condition, ensure adaptability, and foster emotional stability. This collaborative care model not only manages the physical symptoms of arrhythmias but also addresses the psychosocial factors that play a significant role in children's quality of life. The inclusion of mental health professionals as members of the pediatric cardiac care team can ensure that the emotional needs of children are met, fostering an approach to health that considers the whole person, including physical and psychological health. Finally, nutrition lifestyle modification is a key element in the management of pediatric arrhythmias. A heart-healthy diet rich in fruits, vegetables, whole grains, and lean protein can have a very significant impact on the cardiovascular system and health. Effective nutrition education can help enable households to choose foods favoring cardiac wellness while avoiding processed dinners that are full of sodium and sugar and contribute to worsening arrhythmia conditions. Given the increasing presentation of childhood obesity, especially in children with congenital heart disease, early education about healthy eating habits can mitigate future health effects. Additionally, home environment support for a healthy lifestyle aware of meal planning and physical activity can enhance children's adherence to such lifestyle changes. Lastly, an interrelated approach through physical exercise, psychosocial support, and nutritional education becomes inevitable for the proper management of pediatric arrhythmias and allowing these children to lead healthy and productive lives (Cervi et al., 2016).

10.5.3. Psychological Support for Patients and Families

Pediatric arrhythmia care is not only the medical management of the conditions but also the psychological counseling of patients and their families. Psychological distress has been noted to impact the patients' well-being who are diagnosed with chronic diseases like arrhythmias. Families are apprehensive and concerned when faced with the complexity of their child's health issues as well. To offer psychological assistance can enhance enhanced coping abilities, enhance family communication, and result in more effective treatment adherence. Through the use of a multi-dimensional intervention of counseling services, family education, and support groups, healthcare professionals can some of the psychological burdens associated with these medical diagnoses. This holistic care has the potential to generate a situation where families are empowered to become more involved in their child's care, ultimately producing better results. In the case of certain conditions, including those caused by genetic flaws or structural cardiac defects, the emotional effect can be staggering. For example, families struggling with a diagnosis such as Tuberous sclerosis complex (TSC), which frequently occurs in association with arrhythmias, will have specific psychological issues to contend with. The complicated nature of TSC, as documented in the literature, is a sign of the necessity for early monitoring and regulation of both the physical symptoms as well as the associated neuropsychiatric conditions that are prone to enhance family distress. As per the new recommendations, the management of these psychological factors with certain interventions can potentially augment the quality of life and coping strategies of families remarkably, and hence emphasize the very crucial necessity of integrating psychological care into pediatric cardiology practice (Northrup et al., 2021). Moreover, the impact of extrinsic stressors, i.e., global occurrences like the COVID-19 pandemic, has heightened the need for comprehensive psychological support in pediatrics. Families with pediatric arrhythmias who are dealing with them can have their emotional burdens worsened by external disease fear like COVID-19, which will lead to feelings of fear and isolation on the part of their children's health. Medical management is not just the responsibility of healthcare providers, but they also need to include resources that target these fears. These interventions like telehealth counseling and Internet support groups have become valuable resources for families in such difficult situations, helping to reduce the psychological effects of both chronic illness and unexpected life stress. Lastly, psychological well-being is treated as a part of the overall care while treating pediatric arrhythmias (Machhi et al., 2020).

10.6. Current Research and Advances

Current studies of pediatric arrhythmias highlight the need for increased pharmacological management in children. While impressive progress in cardiology has been seen in the guise of handling adult congenital heart disease (ACHD), pediatric populations have a unique set of challenges due to the uniqueness of their developmental needs. The existing literature highlights that the management of arrhythmias in children remains more empirical and reliant on a greater number of times on an incomplete understanding of the optimal pharmacotherapy for their age and physiological status. As discussed by Ladouceur et al. (2023), there is still a significant knowledge gap in the long-term effects of cardiac pharmacotherapy in the pediatric patient, particularly regarding safety and efficacy. On top of that, progress in interventional techniques holds promise for decreasing complications associated with arrhythmias, but more research needs to be done in order to develop in-depth guidelines based on evidence and focused on outcome improvement of pediatric treatment. Recent research on anticoagulant therapies also contributes to the emerging picture of treating pediatric arrhythmias. Since current anticoagulants have proven effectiveness as well as risk, especially that of major bleeding complications, there is an urgent need to explore other approaches that minimize such risks. Exploration of inhibitors of coagulation factor XIa (FXIa) has emerged as more prominent and promising, as reviewed by Xia et al. (2023). These inhibitors may be therapeutically advantageous with reduced bleeding events, a point of special significance in children who may have to be treated for arrhythmias for extended periods. The clinical trials in progress to assess efficacy and safety of FXIa inhibitors portend a paradigm-shifting shift in anticoagulant therapy that may be beneficial in the pediatric population. As this research progresses, the implications for pediatric cardiology are profound, with potential enhancement of both safety and quality of life for pediatric patients with arrhythmias. Where technology convergence meets pediatric arrhythmias exhibits as vast a frontier of research as there is now. Wearable tech and telemedicine allow for real-time monitoring of cardiac rhythms, enabling timely intervention as well as data collection. These innovations allow for a more personalized approach to the treatment of pediatric arrhythmias, particularly in remote patient evaluation, thus reducing the hassle of repeated hospital visits. The integration of digital health solutions can also facilitate clinicians to identify patterns and triggers of arrhythmias specific to pediatric patients. The intersection of clinical intuition and technology can most probably bring about breakthrough interventions that are tailored to individual patient needs, a significant leap from standard pediatric arrhythmia treatment. The more advanced science becomes, the more incorporation of such advancements is capable of dramatically enhancing the models of treatment and thus contributing to the improvement of long-term outcomes for children with potential arrhythmia.

10.6.1. Innovations in Diagnostic Technology

The diagnostic technology has significantly enhanced detection and care for pediatric arrhythmias. The focus of the technology is on the use of sophisticated imaging techniques such as cardiac magnetic resonance imaging (MRI) and echocardiography. These modalities provide superior anatomical and functional measurements, enabling clinicians to more effectively visualize involved cardiac structures associated with arrhythmias. With the introduction of three-dimensional modeling, there can be sophisticated preoperative planning, which is extremely crucial in the case of congenital heart diseases. With the incorporation of such imaging in the traditional diagnostic equipment, medical professionals are able to come up with more accurate diagnoses, leading to personalized therapy, which improves the outcome in pediatric patients with arrhythmias (Das et al., 2025) (Figure 10.11).

In addition to imaging equipment, the integration of artificial intelligence (AI) in the diagnosis systems has revolutionized pediatric cardiology. AI algorithms can review vast amounts of information and make inferences on patterns that may escape human eyes, thereby enhancing the diagnostic capabilities for most arrhythmic conditions. For instance, AI systems today are more adept at recognizing subtle irregularities on electrocardiograms (ECGs) and correlating them with clinical data to generate predictive reports. The technology not only streamlines the diagnostic process but also aids clinicians in planning treatment by sharing evidence-based suggestions. As a result, AI technologies are setting new standards for accuracy in pediatric diagnostics, ultimately resulting in improved patient care outcomes in cases of arrhythmia (Alharbi et al., 2024). The ongoing advance of diagnostic technology in pediatric arrhythmias is also evident through the development of wearable devices and remote monitoring systems. These technologies allow for ongoing physiological monitoring, enabling clinicians to track patients beyond clinical environments. Wearable devices have the capacity to identify arrhythmias in real-time, triggering alerts to families as well as medical practitioners about impending problems before they develop further. This transition towards early health management allows for timely interventions and improved quality of life in children with these conditions.

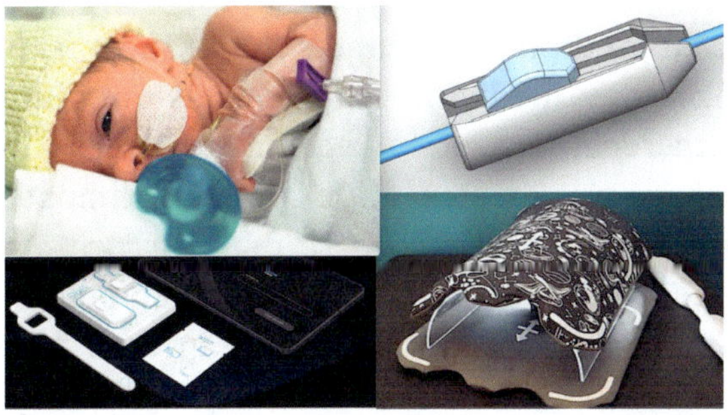

Figure 10.11. Five winning pediatric cardiology medical devices recognized for innovation in a medical device competition.

Source: https://www.dicardiology.com/sites/default/files/Congenital_heart_new_devices.jpg.

In addition, smooth integration of telemedicine platforms allows for real-time transmission and consultation of data, and crucial information becomes easily accessible. With increased developments and penetration, these technologies can possibly reshape the existing scenario of pediatric arrhythmia management toward improved monitoring and more personalized care strategies (Das et al., 2025).

10.6.2. Emerging Treatment Modalities

New therapies for pediatric arrhythmias have generated great interest over the last few years, precisely due to advances in technology and enhanced knowledge of pathophysiology related to them. Traditional therapy approaches include drug treatment and ablation with a catheter that have been the mainstays of treatment. These are lacking for complex conditions with unique anatomical and electrophysiological complexities in children. Emerging technologies, such as advanced imaging techniques and complex electrophysiological mapping, enable clinicians to more clearly visualize arrhythmogenic substrates, thus enabling tailored intervention methods. The application of such complex technology is crucial to achieving improved outcomes for children with arrhythmias, especially in those who have non-ischemic cardiomyopathy, where standard methods could be limited (Aănciulescu et al., 2025). Accompanied by advanced imaging, new treatment methods such as SBRT are becoming more widely recognized in the context of pediatric arrhythmias. Although previously utilized in oncology, secondary application for SBRT is currently on the cutting block for its potential use in changing arrhythmogenic foci without the need for invasiveness. With precise radiation targeting, the modality provides little collateral injury to nearby healthy cardiac structures, a particular concern in the sensitive physiological landscape of children. Though still in its infancy of experimentation, the integration of SBRT has the potential to revolutionize the approach to the management of arrhythmia, especially in instances where conventional intervention poses higher risk. As science advances, the use of these modalities in the clinic holds promise for deep impact on the safety and efficacy of pediatric arrhythmia management (Aănciulescu et al., 2025) (Figure 10.12).

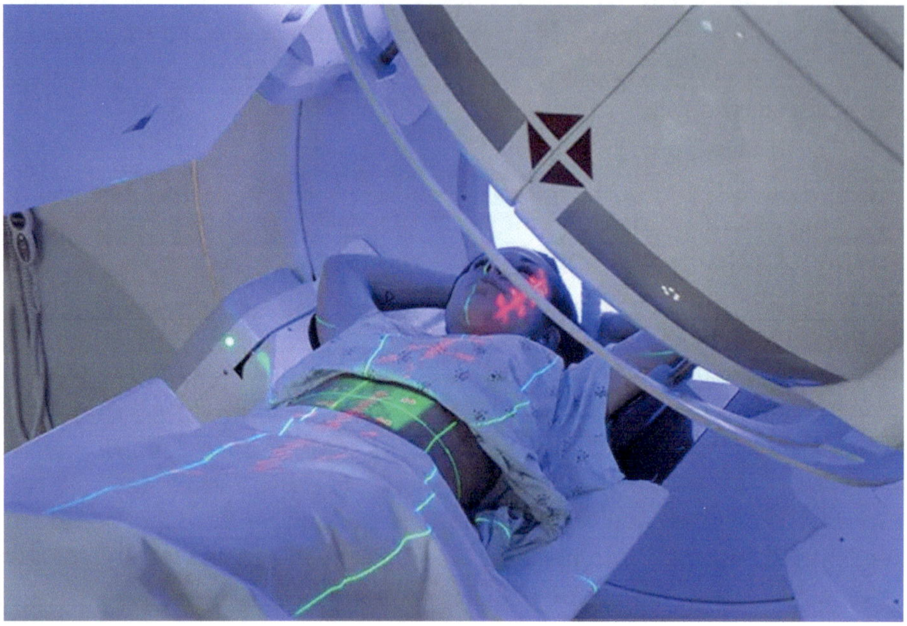

Figure 10.12. Stereotactic body radiation therapy.

Source: https://assets.clevelandclinic.org/transform/LargeFeatureImage/cbdbe4aa-fe0e-4c9f-acb9-096c2468f323/650x450-Safety-of-Metastasis-Directed-SBRT-and-Concurrent-Pazopanibin-Pediatric-Sarcoma_jpg.

Moreover, artificial intelligence (AI) in pediatric arrhythmias management is increasingly being highlighted, offering unparalleled promise for precision medicine. AI platforms are able to analyze gigantic volumes of data from electronic health records to help recognize patterns that exceed conventional analysis. This can potentially enhance risk stratification for arrhythmogenic conditions, predictive value of outcomes from therapy, and personalized care plans according to the specific needs of children. Furthermore, AI has the potential to enhance catheter guidance during ablation procedures for the purpose of enhancing intervention accuracy in addition to reducing procedure times and complications. These developments herald a move toward more data-based practice in the management of pediatric arrhythmias that will pave the way for yet more innovative treatments.

10.6.3. Future Directions in Pediatric Cardiology

With pediatric cardiology progressing further, unprecedent progress is anticipated in diagnosing and managing pediatric arrhythmias. One of the avenues that promise to make breakthroughs is the incorporation of sophisticated imaging techniques and artificial intelligence in handling arrhythmias. Future studies have promised potential improvements in using machine learning algorithms to enhance diagnostic accuracy, particularly between arrhythmia types in children. This advance in technology will be focused on improving risk stratification and individualizing treatment plans based on integrating genetic, phenotypic, and clinical data. Advances of this nature are especially critical when considering the wide array of arrhythmic presentations and responses to treatment in children. Keeping technology at the forefront allows future studies to fill gaps that presently abound and offer standardized approaches that basically improve outcomes in this high-risk group. No less important is the development of less invasive, interventional approaches for treating pediatric arrhythmias. Advances in catheter-based interventions for ablation of arrhythmogenic foci will increasingly become prominent, enabling safer and more effective treatment of conditions conventionally warranting open surgery. The manufacture of pediatric-specific devices to perform these interventions is important in order to meet the unique anatomical and physiological requirements of children, as current devices are mostly inadequate in fulfilling such demands. Additionally, multicenter registry experience can also derive very valuable information on how well these new devices and techniques work in a broad population as highlighted in recent literature. Such data not only inform clinical care, but they are also utilized to standardize care protocols so that arrhythmia patients are treated with the most recent care compatible with their individual health needs (Shibbani et al., 2025). Finally, comprehensive focus on pediatric patients with arrhythmia will be paramount in future pediatric cardiology directions. This includes the management of psychosocial problems, familial support, and follow-up treatment after the long term to improve quality of life with medical treatment. Streamlining of care pathways will demand cardiologists, electrophysiologists, psychologists, and primary care physicians to get together and come up with a merged model of care. Emphasizing studies on successful early interventions, risk factors, and long-term outcomes will be essential in building a more effective and integrated approach to pediatric cardiology in the future. The future research holds the potential to develop evidence-based practice and guidelines that continue to enhance both the clinical and psychosocial outcomes in child patients, with promises for the coming years of a more complex understanding of pediatric arrhythmias (Park et al., 2025).

SUMMARY

The completeness of any extensive examination of pediatric arrhythmias demands a multi-faceted view of the intricacy of diagnosing and treating the conditions. Pediatric arrhythmias, in that they may manifest themselves in various guises and levels, challenge clinicians to remain sharply aware of the unique physiological differences present between children and adults. Although there has been advancement in interventional therapy such as radiofrequency ablation (RFA), there has also been a conservative approach, especially to smaller patients who are at a higher risk for procedural complications. Hence, there has to be a fine balance between the benefit of proper treatment and the level of risk from intervention, particularly in patients with a weight of less than 15 kg, for whom the frequency of tachycardias such as supraventricular tachycardia (SVT) is significantly high (Blaufox et al., 2005). Furthermore, interplay between medical management and interventional methods supports the provision of individualized modalities of care in children. Children do present some unique challenges, including their inability to describe symptoms in a clear manner, which can slow diagnosis and treatment and hence increase the risk of severe consequences. When treating arrhythmias, pediatric practitioners are presented with the double challenge of selecting the most appropriate intervention while considering the long-term impact of treatment on a child's still-developing cardiovascular system. As suggested by variable responses to drug therapies, an integrated approach combining education, continuous monitoring, and active symptom management can lead to improved patient outcomes (Blaufox et al., 2005). Thus, continuous adjustment and innovation in treatment techniques are integral aspects of improving care in children with arrhythmias. Setting sights on the future, it is equally significant that ongoing research seeks to advance a deeper understanding of efficacy and safety of various therapeutic modalities for pediatric arrhythmias. Advances in technology and procedural ability, as in studies using animal models and new ablation techniques, hold promise for optimizing therapeutic interventions. The effective and safe application of new methods, such as those outlined in recent literature on muscular ventricular septal defects, proves the merits of developing tailored solutions to pediatric heart disease. In the future, our clinical approaches need to be based on solid evidence and a sound grasp of the specific physiological and psychological needs of pediatric patients. This will facilitate the creation of consolidated treatment paradigms, ultimately contributing towards higher rates of success and improved quality of life in pediatric arrhythmias.

Pediatric arrhythmias require an integrated integration of various key concepts that cut across both practice and education frameworks. Pediatric arrhythmias, or irregular heart rhythms, are benign or life-threatening. The high incidence of pediatric arrhythmias supports the necessity for heightened awareness and appropriate diagnosis by practitioners. Recent advances in diagnostic technology, such as ECG and wearable monitoring devices, have improved immensely in early detection of such irregularities. Furthermore, competency-based education among healthcare providers is imperative; clinicians ought to be proficient in diagnosis and management of pediatric arrhythmias according to accepted guidelines. This serves to highlight the importance of synchronizing education efforts with clinical practice to prepare potential practitioners more effectively to deliver high-quality care with focus on the unique needs of pediatric patients (Sukal-Moulton et al., 2025). In practice, effective management of pediatric arrhythmias is dependent upon employing organized assessment methods. Through the development of a standardized protocol for diagnosis, medical professionals can ensure that they use a structured process when diagnosing and treating such conditions. Such protocols must be evidence-based and include the most up-to-date practices to provide an adequate overview of each patient's presentation and signs. Additionally, using a movement system diagnosis model, encouraged in modern physical therapy literature, can further understanding and communication across interdisciplinary teams. The framework focuses on the discovery of functional impairments and adaptations of interventions based on the same, which is essential in maximizing the care of pediatric patients (Cobb et al., 2025). An understanding of the interrelatedness of movement systems and cardiovascular well-being is central, as it highlights the compounded nature of care in pediatrics, in which several factors can make arrhythmia presentations. The journey towards improved pediatric arrhythmia management also involves continued education and professional development along the healthcare continuum. Healthcare professionals must be provided with regular training programs that assist them in keeping pace with evolving practices and technology in pediatric cardiology. Emphasis on reflective practices such as portfolio-based assessment will motivate healthcare professionals to become intensively involved in their learning processes, and hence become more competent in managing pediatric arrhythmias. These portfolios may also function as active critical thinking and reflection tools, enabling clinicians to effectively deal with the complexities of patient care. Finally, the synergy of robust training, standardized examinations, and reflective practices offers a foundation for enhancing pediatric arrhythmia clinical outcomes, which helps child patients adhere to the optimal care possible in accordance with their specific needs (Sukal-Moulton et al., 2025).

CLOSER LOOK

SINUS TACHYCARDIA

Sinus tachycardia is a common arrhythmia in children characterized by an elevated heart rate with a normal sinoatrial (SA) node origin as the inherent pacemaker of the heart. It is generally considered to be a physiologic response and not a primary cardiac illness, but it may on occasion be a reflection of underlying pathology. In sinus tachycardia, there is increased heart rate with normal rhythm, and P waves on the ECG maintain normal axis and morphology (Figure 10.13).

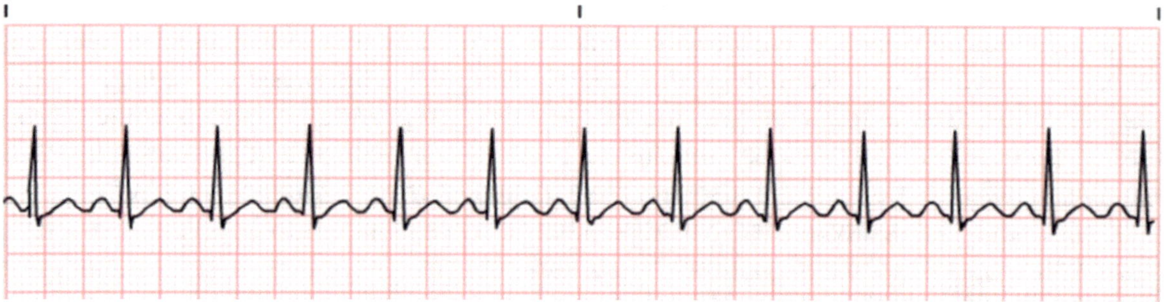

Figure 10.13. Electrocardiogram (ECG) showing sinus tachycardia, characterized by a regular rhythm with a heart rate greater than 100 beats per minute, upright P waves before each QRS complex, and consistent PR intervals. This pattern typically indicates a physiologic response to conditions such as fever, dehydration, or anxiety.

Source: https://external-content.duckduckgo.com/iu/?u=https%3A%2F%2Fwww.protrainings.com%2Fblog%2Fwp-content%2Fuploads%2F2020%2F06%2Fsinus-tach.jpg&f=1&nofb=1&ipt=2b510010f58a2f26050efa41d5dd7bc0aa54649586ed0689456a49471772470c.

The normal pediatric heart rate varies by age. Infants, for instance, can have resting rates between 120 and 160 bpm, while teenagers and children of a more advanced age typically have rates between 70 and 110 bpm. Sinus tachycardia is diagnosed when the rate exceeds the child's established upper limit of normal for age, often secondary to pathologic or physiologic stimuli.

Causes of sinus tachycardia in children are broad and usually non-cardiac in origin. Frequent causes are physiological and consist of fever, pain, anxiety, exercise, and excitement. In infants and toddlers, agitation or crying can also cause transient tachycardia. Pathological causes include dehydration, anemia, hypoxia, hypovolemia, sepsis, hyperthyroidism, and drug effects (e.g., stimulants, bronchodilators, or anticholinergics). Sinus tachycardia may also be a compensation for heart failure or shock, where cardiac output is preserved.

Clinical presentation of sinus tachycardia depends on its etiology and the child's age. The majority of children are not symptomatic, especially if it is physiological tachycardia. Some others may feel palpitations, dizziness, tiredness, or chest discomfort. Most of these symptoms, however, play second fiddle to manifestations of the underlying illness—like fever, respiratory distress, or dehydration. Unlike pathological arrhythmias, sinus tachycardia should normally correct once the underlying precipitant has been addressed.

Diagnosis is typically clinical and made with ECG, where a normal P wave precedes each QRS complex, a constant PR interval, and an unchanging rhythm are found. The rate is elevated but typically changes with exertion or position—differentiating from supraventricular tachycardia (SVT), which often has an abrupt onset and fixed rate without alteration by exertion. Sinus tachycardia also does not have the "P wave dissociation" or reentrant circuit morphologies of other arrhythmias.

Treatment of sinus tachycardia is directed towards the cause of it and not at decreasing the heart rate in itself. Antipyretics can be given for fever, fluids for dehydration, oxygen in hypoxia, and treatment of infection. Even if the cause is not evident, then investigation in the form of blood tests, imaging, or Holter monitoring may be performed. Antiarrhythmic drug or beta-blocker is rarely indicated unless the sinus tachycardia is symptomatic and prolonged, or in the presence of an associated inappropriate sinus tachycardia syndrome, a rare condition in children.

Prognosis is generally excellent, especially when the etiology is reversible or transient. Sinus tachycardia by itself does not typically lead to subsequent long-term cardiac sequelae in children, although persistent or unexplained tachycardia may necessitate additional cardiology evaluation.

References

1. Aagaard, Baggish, A., Ackerman, A., Anderson, A., La Gerche, A., Pelliccia, A., Antzelevitch, C., et al. (2017). International criteria for electrocardiographic interpretation in athletes: Consensus statement. https://core.ac.uk/download/287649657.pdf (accessed on 15th July 2025).
2. Abe, Ackerman, A., Alexander, A., Amin, A., Krahn, A., Leenhardt, A., Anttonen, A., et al. (2013). HRS/EHRA/APHRS expert consensus statement on the diagnosis and management of patients with inherited primary arrhythmia syndromes. https://core.ac.uk/download/pdf/81940605.pdf (accessed on 15th July 2025).
3. Aguinaga, L., Al-Khatib, S. M., Anter, E., Berruezo, A., et al. (2019). 2019 HRS/EHRA/APHRS/LAHRS expert consensus statement on catheter ablation of ventricular arrhythmias: Executive summary. https://core.ac.uk/download/225127007.pdf (accessed on 15th July 2025).
4. Aickin, R., Andersen, L. W., Atkins, D. L., Aziz, K., et al. (2019). 2019 international consensus on cardiopulmonary resuscitation and emergency cardiovascular care science with treatment recommendations: Summary from the basic life support; advanced life support; pediatric life support; neonatal life support; education, implementation, and teams; and first aid task forces. *(no journal provided)*
5. Alharbi, N., & Alharbi, A. S. (2024). AI-driven innovations in pediatric dentistry: Enhancing care and improving outcome. *Cureus, 16.* https://www.semanticscholar.org/paper/99b9e05e9119a8279f70abe581bd186510165f17 (accessed on 15th July 2025).
6. Aumann, R., Hinterseer, M., Kozlik-Feldmann, R., Lang, D., et al. (2008). Creation of ventricular septal defects on the beating heart in a new pig model. https://core.ac.uk/download/16432659.pdf (accessed on 15th July 2025).
7. Benson, D. W., Deal, B. J., Samson, R. A., Strasburger, J. F., et al. (1995). Comparison of transesophageal and intracardiac electrophysiologic studies in characterization of supraventricular tachycardia in pediatric patients. https://core.ac.uk/download/pdf/82819249.pdf (accessed on 15th July 2025).
8. Blaufox, A. D. (2005). Catheter ablation of tachyarrhythmias in small children. https://core.ac.uk/download/pdf/86243.pdf (accessed on 15th July 2025).
9. Bouma, B. J., & Mulder, B. J. M. (2017). Changing landscape of congenital heart disease. *Circulation Research, 120*, 908–922. https://doi.org/10.1161/circresaha.116.309302 (accessed on 15th July 2025).
10. Carlson, S. K., Chang, P. M., Doshi, R. N., Fung, A., et al. (2015). Electrocardiographic patch devices and contemporary wireless cardiac monitoring. https://core.ac.uk/download/77002540.pdf (accessed on 15th July 2025).
11. Cervi, E. (2016). New applications of cardiopulmonary exercise testing and training in pediatric heart disease. https://core.ac.uk/download/76520310.pdf (accessed on 15th July 2025).
12. Chan, Y. W. F., Keung, W., Tse, G., Yan, B. P., et al. (2017). Electrophysiological mechanisms of long and short QT syndromes. https://core.ac.uk/download/77416285.pdf (accessed on 15th July 2025).
13. Cobb, L., Shane, K. A., McGee, P. N., Nesbit, C., Brennan, E., Moore, J., Girolami, G., et al. (2025). Movement system diagnosis: A consensus-based position for pediatric movement

specialists. *Pediatric Physical Therapy, 37*, 257–264. https://www.semanticscholar.org/paper/b162c6657554bf20b186c2b0642e9a62f9023953 (accessed on 15th July 2025).

14. Conlin, E. (2012). Attention to psychosocial concerns related to LQTS: A survey of medical providers. https://core.ac.uk/download/234121837.pdf (accessed on 15th July 2025).

15. Czachor, A., Grelewicz, O., Haber, M., Juśkiewicz, J., et al. (2024). Cardiovascular risks of methylphenidate in children with ADHD. https://core.ac.uk/download/620863915.pdf (accessed on 15th July 2025).

16. Dakhel, A., Alsharekh, N., Alqeaid, F., Alkholaif, A., Alharbi, S., Alzaydi, M., Alkholaif, A., et al. (2024). Current trends and challenges in the management of pediatric arrhythmias in Saudi Arabia: A comprehensive review of pharmacological and non-pharmacological approaches during 2024. *International Journal of Medicine in Developing Countries.* https://www.semanticscholar.org/paper/82a9490efd0166ee23c44c96feb808b47b989477 (accessed on 15th July 2025).

17. Das, S., & Das, D. (2025). The dawn of a new era in congenital heart surgery: Decadal innovations and future prospects. *International Journal of Scientific Research.* https://www.semanticscholar.org/paper/53197206334383066c856b5e21f74508dc365ae0 (accessed on 15th July 2025).

18. Doğan, E., Ergin, F., Beyter, M., Kaşıkçı, G. K., Ön, Ş. Ş., Ay, O., Levent, R., et al. (2024). Arrhythmias in children undergoing orthotopic heart transplantation. *Frontiers in Cardiovascular Medicine, 10.* https://www.semanticscholar.org/paper/2a7891a73130aa1b75e4f0b571bf46e6ccd1537c (accessed on 15th July 2025).

19. Gamayunov, R., Snetkov, A., Pleskushkina, A., & Ishkinyaev, I. D. (2025). The effectiveness of puncture therapy for sacral aneurysmal bone cysts in kids and teenagers. A concise overview of the available research. Presentation of clinical cases. *N.N. Priorov Journal of Traumatology and Orthopedics.* https://www.semanticscholar.org/paper/d8579a61c567a266614ea3f5dfb8a30713b8e790 (accessed on 15th July 2025).

20. Ganea, G., Cinteză, E., Filip, C., Iancu, M. A., Balta, M., Vătășescu, R., Vasile, C., et al. (2023). Postoperative cardiac arrhythmias in pediatric and neonatal patients with congenital heart disease—A narrative review. *Life, 13.* https://www.semanticscholar.org/paper/b94eba84627e4b42582303924f49ae84df18e81d (accessed on 15th July 2025).

21. Helman, S., Riek, N., Sereika, S., Olsen, R., Gaynor, J., Lisanti, A., & Al-Zaiti, S. (2024). Abstract 4141460: Exploring novel data-driven clustering methods for uncovering patterns in longitudinal neonatal postoperative temperature measurements. *Circulation.* https://www.semanticscholar.org/paper/59bd4832da5d3c8d0da96ab27e1ea9b2515409cd (accessed on 15th July 2025).

22. Hinge, D. V., Raizada, M., Gomase, S., Khapekar, S., & Javvaji, C. K. (2025). Unintentional levothyroxine ingestion by a child: A case report. *Cureus, 17.* https://www.semanticscholar.org/paper/86121496c826af4085ef6ee0f32146c2d1e79463 (accessed on 15th July 2025).

23. Hiranrattana, A., Fitzgerald, R., Kehoe, A., Heckler, G., Gilbert, C., Katwa, U., & Maski, K. (2024). 0849 Characterization of patient referrals to ED/inpatient admission from an outpatient pediatric sleep center. *SLEEP.* https://www.semanticscholar.org/paper/1cb14c2ab23cb120d5a3a0906ab5a38ddbb1d54c (accessed on 15th July 2025).

24. Jain, S., Steele, J., Fonseca, B., Huang, S., Shah, S., Maskatia, S. A., Buddhe, S., et al. (2021). COVID-19 vaccination–associated myocarditis in adolescents. *PEDIATRICS, 148.* https://doi.org/10.1542/peds.2021-053427 (accessed on 15th July 2025).

25. Khan, M. K., Jindal, D., Selvaganesh, S., & Jindal, M. (2025). Effective modalities to manage the failure of dental implants in pediatric patients. *National Journal of Maxillofacial Surgery, 16*, 14–18. https://www.semanticscholar.org/paper/809a3e3a95a91436af318a33775fad82e88c8bbb (accessed on 15th July 2025).

26. Kim, K., Jeong, J. H., & Choi, E. K. (2024). Non-pharmacological interventions for delirium in the pediatric population: A systematic review with narrative synthesis. *BMC Pediatrics, 24.* https://www.semanticscholar.org/paper/887a72d6e86a37fc20c3c5e4f2ef3209b406231a (accessed on 15th July 2025).

27. Kunigeliene, R., Kinciniene, O., Marinskis, G., & Usonis, V. (2025). Predictors of ventricular abnormalities in children with idiopathic ventricular extrasystoles. *Children, 12.* https://www.semanticscholar.org/paper/1e25ad298cd56afed0b558fc82eb71dd6b699c40 (accessed on 15th July 2025).

28. Ladouceur, M., Valdeolmillos, E., Karsenty, C., Hascoet, S., Moceri, P., & Le Gloan, L. (2023). Cardiac drugs in ACHD cardiovascular medicine. *Journal of Cardiovascular Development and Disease, 10.* https://www.semanticscholar.org/paper/037eb0233994da80fad03c8306bec3e61e87b1a9 (accessed on 15th July 2025).

29. Machhi, J., Herskovitz, J., Senan, A. M., Dutta, D., Nath, B., Oleynikov, M., Blomberg, W. R., et al. (2020). The natural history, pathobiology, and clinical manifestations of SARS-CoV-2 infections. *Journal of Neuroimmune Pharmacology, 15*, 359–386. https://doi.org/10.1007/s11481-020-09944-5 (accessed on 15th July 2025).

30. Manickavasagam, A., Patloori, S., Perla, H., Chase, D., & Roshan, J. (2022). Impact of transesophageal electrophysiological study on midterm management of pediatric tachyarrhythmias. *Annals of Pediatric Cardiology, 15*, 453–458. https://www.semanticscholar.org/paper/474c59ba44bf19d5a752321bf708d3a82d9203cf (accessed on 15th July 2025).

31. Marian, A. J., & Braunwald, E. (2017). Hypertrophic cardiomyopathy. *Circulation Research, 121*, 749–770. https://doi.org/10.1161/circresaha.117.311059 (accessed on 15th July 2025).

32. Meijboom, E. J., Oudijk, M. A., & Visser, G. H. A. (2004). Fetal tachyarrhythmia–Part II: Treatment. https://core.ac.uk/download/pdf/86250.pdf (accessed on 15th July 2025).

33. Meijboom, E. J., Oudijk, M. A., & Visser, G. H. A. (2004). Fetal tachyarrhythmia–Part I: Diagnosis. https://core.ac.uk/download/pdf/86258.pdf (accessed on 15th July 2025).

34. N/A. (2007). *Outlook Magazine, Winter 2007.* https://core.ac.uk/download/70380374.pdf (accessed on 15th July 2025).

35. Ndovu, A., Chen, C., Schwarz, L., Lasky, E., Weiser, S. D., & Benmarhnia, T. (2025). Spatial variation in the association between extreme heat events and warm season pediatric acute care utilization: A small-area assessment of multiple health conditions and environmental justice implications in California (2005–2019). *Environmental Health Perspectives, 133.* https://www.semanticscholar.org/paper/6bef7ba232d5d648bbb2be3d5066dac0c6056333 (accessed on 15th July 2025).

36. Northrup, H., Aronow, M. E., Bebin, E. M., Bissler, J. J., Darling, T. N., de Vries, P. J., Frost, M., et al. (2021). Updated international tuberous sclerosis complex diagnostic criteria and surveillance and management recommendations. *Pediatric Neurology, 123*, 50–66. https://doi.org/10.1016/j.pediatrneurol.2021.07.011 (accessed on 15th July 2025).

37. Park, J. S., Park, S. Y., Moon, J. W., Kim, K., & Suh, D. (2025). Artificial intelligence models for pediatric lung sound analysis: Systematic review and meta-analysis. *Journal of Medical Internet Research, 27.* https://www.semanticscholar.org/paper/3d124d272c80f7dbc9c731751c696fc0f7f8255c (accessed on 15th July 2025).

38. Reemtsen, B., Finn, J. P., Alejos, J., Touma, M., Halnon, N., Nelson, S. F., et al. (2017). A path to implement precision child health cardiovascular medicine. https://core.ac.uk/download/323077346.pdf (accessed on 15th July 2025).

39. Ritter, A. L., Berger, J., Deardorff, M., Izumi, K., Lin, K. Y., Medne, L., & Ahrens-Nicklas, R. C. (2020). Variants in NAA15 cause pediatric hypertrophic cardiomyopathy. *American Journal of Medical Genetics Part A, 185*, 228–233. https://www.semanticscholar.org/paper/a249344f5f68bf7af1892457ddc626acb53dc0f6 (accessed on 15th July 2025).

40. Seita, H. M. (2013). Food allergies in pregnant women: A study of prevalence in expecting mothers and association with neonatal outcomes. https://open.bu.edu/bitstream/2144/12219/6/Seita_Helene_2013.pdf (accessed on 15th July 2025).

41. Shibbani, K., & Kenny, D. (2025). Updates in interventional cardiology in children with cardiac disease. *European Journal of Pediatrics, 184.* https://www.semanticscholar.org/paper/c75b1f7c4368bc723fac2deed22456d2a1a2dca1 (accessed on 15th July 2025).

42. Stănciulescu, L. A., Dorobanțu, M., & Vătășescu, R. (2025). Targeting ventricular arrhythmias in non-ischemic patients: Advances in diagnosis and treatment. *Diagnostics, 15.* https://www.semanticscholar.org/paper/55d1a8ec48ae3512a3062113cecee3fba2477030 (accessed on 15th July 2025).

43. Sukal-Moulton, T., Walrath, J., Brossman, H. L., Moerchen, V., Schreiber, J., & Tovin, M. (2025). ePortfolios: A tool to demonstrate ongoing development of competency in pediatric physical therapy. *Pediatric Physical Therapy.* https://www.semanticscholar.org/paper/84aeb24a42a85463be240ebda13a7938526fb489 (accessed on 15th July 2025).

44. Sulu, A., Uner, G., Kosger, P., & Ucar, B. (2024). Does the ST2 level in pediatric heart failure patients correlate with cardiovascular events and mortality? *Children, 11.* https://www.semanticscholar.org/paper/2b403dd63793a16af47d8ecc972239f8495a6951 (accessed on 15th July 2025).

45. Swati Rai, Dr. S. (2025). Steroid-induced rashes and Cushingoid features in a pediatric patient. *International Journal of Pharmaceutical Research and Applications.* https://www.semanticscholar.org/paper/f5a520a72cdcf1fd23a42544d76ec3665f9b72c8 (accessed on 15th July 2025).

46. Tampu, I., Bianchessi, T., Blystad, I., Lundberg, P., Nyman, P., Eklund, A., & Haj-Hosseini, N. (2024). Pediatric brain tumor classification using deep learning on MR images with age fusion. *Neuro-Oncology Advances, 7.* https://www.semanticscholar.org/paper/4b88bb40ec3986a10b8dddb6afeef61da6dd88df (accessed on 15th July 2025).

47. Tchana, B., & Caffarelli, C. (2023). Inhaled short-acting beta agonist treatment-associated supraventricular tachycardia in children: Still a matter of concern in pediatric emergency

departments? *Children, 10.* https://www.semanticscholar.org/paper/2bdced3e79c3ec2874d097cf7592c23c19e40cfa (accessed on 15th July 2025).

48. Treble-Barna, A., Petersen, B. A., Stec, Z., Conley, Y. P., Fink, E. L., & Kochanek, P. (2024). Brain-derived neurotrophic factor in pediatric acquired brain injury and recovery. *Biomolecules, 14.* https://www.semanticscholar.org/paper/a0cad640bbe75b26fffd52942b89547ef882671e (accessed on 15th July 2025).

49. Wu, H. P., Lin, M. J., Yang, W. C., Wu, K. H., & Chen, C. Y. (2017). Predictors of extracorporeal membrane oxygenation support for children with acute myocarditis. *BioMed Research International, 2017,* 1–8. https://doi.org/10.1155/2017/2510695 (accessed on 15th July 2025).

50. Xia, Y., Hu, Y., & Tang, L. V. (2023). Factor XIa inhibitors as a novel anticoagulation target: Recent clinical research advances. *Pharmaceuticals, 16.* https://www.semanticscholar.org/paper/4fc86c26760a950e9c24408776085e1075df8dd8 (accessed on 15th July 2025).

51. Zachaj, J., Kręglicki, Ł., Sikora, T., Moorthi, K., Jaśkiewicz, F., Nadolny, K., & Gałązkowski, R. (2024). Successful intraosseous (IO) adenosine administration for the termination of supraventricular tachycardia (SVT) in a 3.5-year-old child—Case report and literature review. *Healthcare, 12.* https://www.semanticscholar.org/paper/6b364c5460cf903dd91547128153e4eb197fc262 (accessed on 15th July 2025).

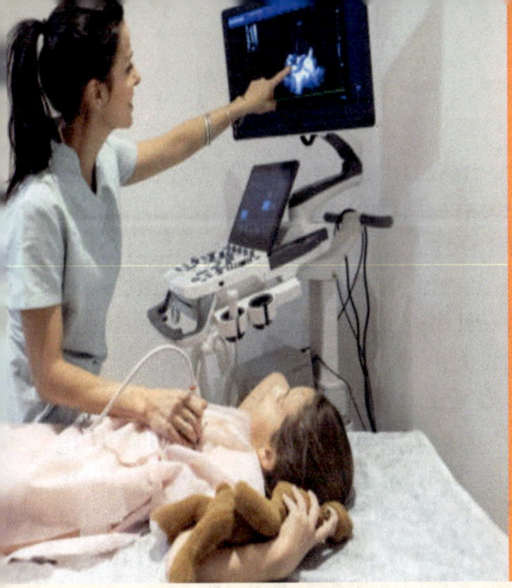

Chapter 11

CARDIOMYOPATHIES IN CHILDREN

Contents

Introduction

The quest for cardiomyopathies in children comes with the complex situation of cardiovascular diseases that afflict young patients. Cardiomyopathies are a heterogenous group of diseases mostly characterized by the structural and functional changes in the myocardium. The diseases range from hereditary diseases to secondary causes and are clinically relevant among the causes of morbidity and mortality in pediatric populations. Recognition that these disorders may manifest early in life and progress rapidly prompts the necessity for early diagnosis and treatment. The heterogeneity of cardiomyopathy presentations necessitates keen awareness of their pathophysiology, particularly given the reality that these diseases can lead to lethal complications if left untreated. Hence, a careful review of the classification, presentation, and treatment is crucial for clinicians and families such that improved outcomes can be achieved. Central to understanding pediatric cardiomyopathies are the aspects of genetics, particularly in disorders characterized as genetic cardiomyopathies. The diseases as a collective entity have significant effects on health due to their predictability for early occurrence and significant complications. As outlined, heterogeneity of the diseases requires advanced model systems to study their mechanisms and develop successful therapies. While traditional animal models have been utilized, they may not be adequate in mirroring human pathologies. Alternatively, generating induced pluripotent stem cells (iPSCs) presents an exciting platform to unravel the underlaying biological mechanisms of these genetic diseases. With the use of iPSCs, researchers have been able to generate patient-specific cellular models that hold the capability to facilitate the study of cardiomyopathies and eventually introduce new therapeutic avenues, thereby bridging the clinic-bench gap. The clinical management of cardiomyopathies in children also has unique challenges that need a multidisciplinary team-based approach. There are a variety of treatment options that can be utilized, from pharmacologic management to surgery, based on the type and severity of cardiomyopathy. An example of such a treatment is surgical myectomy in the event of hypertrophic cardiomyopathy since it has been successful in alleviating symptoms as well as obstruction, as the literature indicates (Barry et al., 2022). Conversely, the spectrum of care must also consider the psychosocial effects of suffering from a chronic illness, with attention to support systems for families and patients. On this foundation, it is evident that long-term research and education are essential in order to facilitate development in the field and enhance quality of life for children suffering from such conditions.

Definition of Cardiomyopathy

Cardiomyopathy is a broad term that describes a large number of myocardium diseases, which may significantly affect its structure and function. The disorders are capable of leading to heart failure, arrhythmias, and other serious complications, particularly in children. Cardiomyopathy is commonly classified based on the specific morphological and functional traits of the heart. The predominant types are dilated, hypertrophic, and restrictive cardiomyopathy, each with distinct diagnostic and therapeutic complexities. Despite the variations, pediatric cardiomyopathy is often linked with genetic origins, where early identification is crucial for the best management and intervention. Understanding the etiology of cardiomyopathies, particularly in children, is significant, as early diagnosis can greatly change clinical courses and therapeutic choices. Genetic causes are the key to the development of cardiomyopathy, with the majority of childhood cases owing to familial conditions. Advanced genetic testing may identify causative variants leading to such disorders to enable more directed management. Family screening, for instance, may identify the relevance of discovered genetic variants through their segregation with the phenotype within familial cases, giving important information to clinicians about the condition of the patient. As discussed, integration of clinical evaluation with genetic data underpins an all-inclusive image of cardiomyopathy. The interaction between patient and clinician enhances the specificity of the diagnosis, particularly in cases in which classical presentations can be overshadowed by identical symptoms, emphasizing the worth of an individualized care approach in treating cardiomyopathies in children (Arbustini et al., 2022) (Figure 11.1).

The effects of cardiomyopathy extend past the acute medical outcomes to include involved children's family dynamics and quality of life. Children who are patients will require ongoing follow-up and potentially have physical activity restrictions, adding emotional weight to an already challenging situation. Further, as more studies are conducted, gaining insight into how and where genetic pre-dispositions meet environmental triggers in pediatric cardiomyopathy can result in more effective treatments. With almost 80% of rare diseases being genetic in origin, addressing the causal issues of cardiomyopathy is a global concern in pediatrics (Abbate et al., 2021). Due to this fact, greater understanding of such relationships is absolutely essential, with the need for continued research and greater clinical protocols in an effort to enhance the quality and lives of children suffering from such diseases.

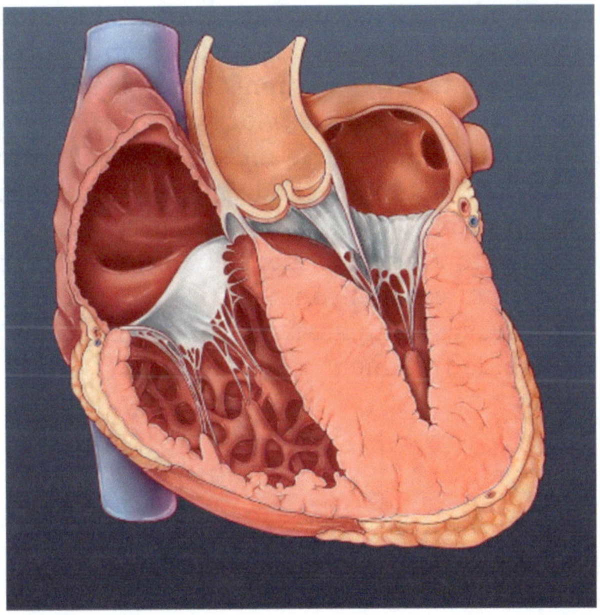

Figure 11.1. Cardiomyopathy.

Source: https://img.lb.wbmdstatic.com/vim/live/webmd/consumer_assets/site_images/article_thumbnails/BigBead/heart-disease-and-cardiomyopathy-bigbead/1800x1200-heart-disease-and-cardiomyopathy-bigbead.jpg.

Importance of Studying Cardiomyopathies in Children

Understanding of the pathologies of cardiomyopathies in children is important for developing more effective diagnostic and therapeutic strategies against such conditions, which might have severe implications if left untreated. Pediatric cardiomyopathy is a multifaceted disease with functional abnormalities of the myocardium that have a profound effect on the overall well-being and quality of life in children. The development of diseases such as dilated cardiomyopathy and hypertrophic cardiomyopathy needs a focused research plan to reveal the environmental and genetic determinants behind their development. Furthermore, research on these diseases explains how cardiovascular failure may present differently in children than in adults, calling for interventions tailored to individuals' requirements. Increased studies and knowledge can lead to groundbreaking discoveries in management strategies, from pharmacologic interventions to surgery, ultimately reducing morbidity and mortality caused by pediatric cardiomyopathies. The effect of cardiomyopathies not only lies in the clinical setting but also on healthcare systems and families. Knowledge about the disease is not only imperative for medical practitioners but also for families dealing with the challenge of pediatric heart diseases. The emotional and financial strain on the family can be high, given that conditions like dilated cardiomyopathy in children can have long-term follow-up and management. As evident in evolving studies, the economic burden of medical care is a prime consideration worldwide, necessitating effective and low-cost interventions. Knowledge on cardiomyopathy can be applied to inform health policy and resource allocation so that children receive appropriate, timely care. Therefore, the research into these conditions is a pre-requisite for promoting educative decision-making in clinical and family-based settings. Recent advances in research have opened up new novel therapy strategies for cardiomyopathies in children, emphasizing the importance of research into these conditions. For example, the research into surgical interventions such as pulmonary artery banding (PAB) has been promising as a groundbreaking treatment for children with conditions such as dilated cardiomyopathy, as demonstrated through auspicious preclinical trials. These findings offer a glimmer of hope towards improved circumstances and are in accordance with this persistent quest for effective management techniques within pediatric populations. Knowledge of such interventions' mechanisms not only helps treatment progress but also benefits the overall field of pediatric heart disease research. As medicine keeps advancing, research into cardiomyopathies in children is a crucial element to ensuring young patients achieve improved health outcomes and quality of life.

11.1. Types of Cardiomyopathies

It is necessary to learn the various types of cardiomyopathies in pediatric cardiology because these may have a huge impact on the development and growth of a child as well as on overall health. Cardiomyopathies are classified into four principal types, and these are hypertrophic, dilated, restrictive, and arrhythmogenic right ventricular cardiomyopathy. Hypertrophic cardiomyopathy, which is abnormal thickening of the heart muscle, leads to obstruction of blood flow and has a genetic component. Conversely, dilated cardiomyopathy is the enlargement and weakening of the walls of the heart, which impairs its ability to pump blood efficiently. In children, early diagnosis and treatment of these types are important as they can present with variable intensity and can have a major impact on the quality of a child's life. Similar to any other medical entity, genetics also plays a significant role in the etiology and progression of cardiomyopathies in children. The genetic variability of the mutations that lead to these diseases complicates their diagnosis and treatment. A clear knowledge of the genes involved can guide treatment and prognosis.

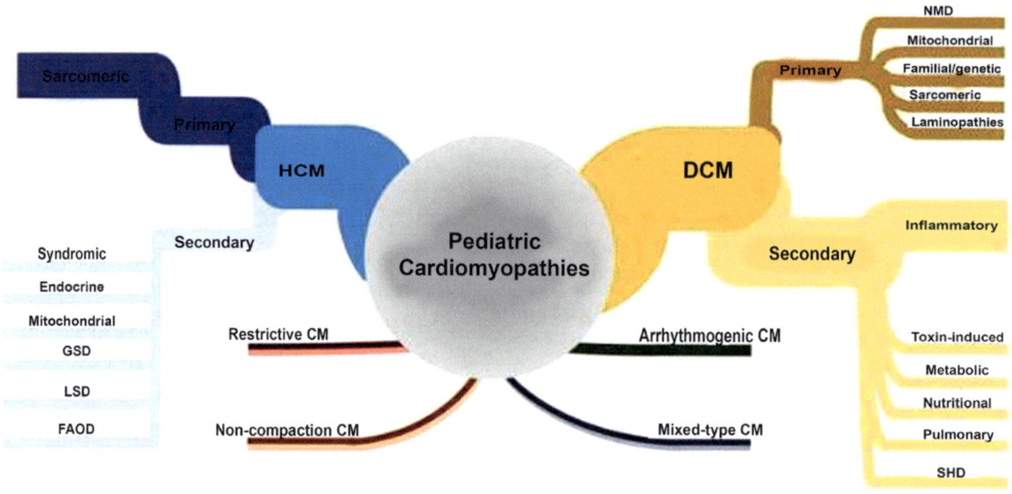

Figure 11.2. Overview of pediatric cardiomyopathy (CM) types. The thickness of the branches reflects the relative prevalence in children, except for the rare cardiomyopathies (restrictive, arrhythmogenic, non-compaction, and mixed-type CMs).

Source: https://www.intechopen.com/chapters/86077.

Genetic testing, for instance, allows clinicians to customize interventions based on a child's individual condition and family background. As discussed in recent conferences, incorporation of personalized medicine in therapy is a promising line, with each pediatric patient being treated with thoroughly individualized therapy according to their unique genetic makeup. Not only does this optimize the efficiency of treatment but also allows for early screening and intervention of families, which are critical components in management of familial cardiomyopathies (Lee et al., 2015) (Figure 11.2).

Additionally, public health measures encouraging cardiac screening for children have grown more robust, especially as such associated dangers as sudden cardiac arrest have grown more evident. Studies have determined that the threat of cardiac events increases with age, particularly for adolescents who participate in high-competitiveness athletics. It is typically recommended that rigorous cardiac screening begin no earlier than age twelve so that its essential basis can be accurately assessed. Besides, children with symptoms of problems or genetic cardiac diseases within their families should come in for immediate medical evaluation. Coordination of screening systems should be put into place to abate risks as well as provide timely intervention for young sportsmen, ultimately encouraging safe participation in sports and physical activity (D'Ascenzi et al., 2024). By knowing the nature of cardiomyopathies and using specialized measures for identification and management, medical professionals can considerably improve the prognosis for children affected by these conditions.

11.1.1. Hypertrophic Cardiomyopathy

Hypertrophic cardiomyopathy (HCM) is a significant problem in pediatric cardiology since it has the potential to lead to serious health issues, including sudden cardiac death. While HCM can be asymptomatic in some children, it is worth mentioning that the disease tends to exhibit many changes in the structure of the heart muscle, which, in turn, compromises the organ's functionality.

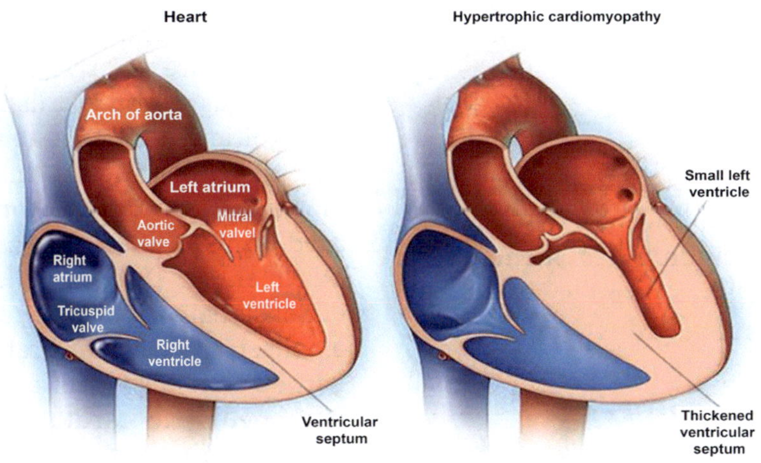

Figure 11.3. Hypertrophic cardiomyopathy (HCM).

Source: https://www.mayoclinic.org/diseases-conditions/hypertrophic-cardiomyopathy/symptoms-causes/syc-20350198#dialogId32405530.

Early detection through regular cardiovascular screenings, like electrocardiograms, is essential to identifying vulnerable children. Young athlete pre-participation screening has gained greater popularity as organizations strive to decrease the occurrence of sudden cardiac events, caused by undiagnosed cardiac disorders like HCM (Biffi et al., 2019). Therefore, the incorporation of systematic screenings into the practices of pediatrics in healthcare ensures an active approach in the safeguarding of young sportspersons participating in competitive sport, identifying any symptoms of hypertrophic cardiomyopathy at the earliest. The genetic etiology of hypertrophic cardiomyopathy also makes its diagnosis and management challenging in children. As a genetic illness, HCM is usually linked to mutations of sarcomere genes responsible for the functioning of heart muscle (Lee et al., 2015) (Figure 11.3).

This genetic heterogeneity also means that the clinical presentation can be very diverse among affected children, making treatment challenging. Knowing the exact genetic mutation involved will help healthcare providers make clear decisions about management and intervention strategies. Recent developments in genetic diagnosis highlight the potential of personalized medicine in pediatric cardiomyopathy. By categorizing risk according to genetics, clinicians can tailor their management for each patient's particular condition and ensure the best possible chance of good outcomes and enable family screening to identify at-risk relatives in order to apply preventive interventions in subsequent generations. Handling of hypertrophic cardiomyopathy in children requires multidisciplinary handling incorporating not only cardiology but also genetics, sports medicine, and family education. Treatment decision-making may involve lifestyle modifications, pharmacological treatment, or, for severe symptoms, surgical intervention such as septal myectomy or alcohol septal ablation. Increased awareness of HCM decreases risk factors of sudden cardiac death, particularly among child athletes. Adequate education of families so that they can make informed decisions about their child's care is critical for effective management (Lee et al., 2015). On a larger scale, the intricacies of hypertrophic cardiomyopathy mandate a multidisciplinary strategy—coupling cutting-edge diagnostics with an emphasis on genetics and strict compliance with prevention strategies—to maximize both quality of life and long-term outcome in the pediatric population.

11.1.2. Dilated Cardiomyopathy

Dilated cardiomyopathy (DCM) is a critical concern in pediatric cardiology, impairing the heart's pumping ability and leading to heart failure. DCM is characterized by enlargement and weakened contraction of the heart muscle, which is best described in the left ventricle. DCM may be due to a variety of factors such as gene mutations, infection, and exposure to toxins in children. Of particular interest is that presentation of DCM in children is often discordant from one taking place in adults, presenting typically in young and otherwise well patients. Early recognition and diagnosis are crucial to proper management; symptoms such as fatigue, failure to thrive, and respiratory distress may be suggestive of this significant condition. Recognition of the unique pathophysiology and clinical presentation of dilated cardiomyopathy in children is crucial for clinicians treating cardiomyopathies in this population. The treatment of DCM in children remains multi-dimensional and needs a personalized approach, emphasizing the identification of specific cardiac pathophysiology. This approach is consistent with pediatric cardiology guidelines, which endorse precision medicine where the cause of the cardiomyopathy is identified to enable cause-directed therapy whenever possible. Present management is most likely to involve pharmacologic therapy with angiotensin-converting enzyme inhibitors, beta-blockers, and diuretics. In addition, in severe cases of DCM, there is a potential for the need for mechanical device or transplantation as a last resort. Existing literature suggests that management of pediatric cardiomyopathy should also treat the concurrent clinical environment, thereby necessitating individualized care plans that account for the unique situations and cardiovascular complication risk factors of each child (Bogle et al., 2023) (Figure 11.4).

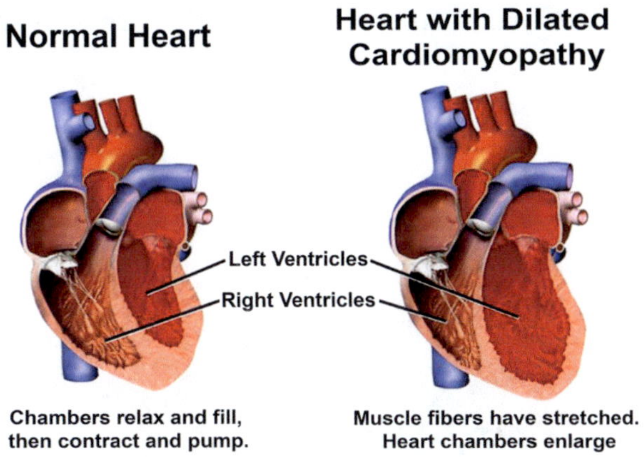

Figure 11.4. Dilated cardiomyopathy (DCM).

Source: https://www.cidg.org.nz/patients-families/cardiac-inherited-diseases/dilated-cardiomyopathy-dcm/.

Further, the management of dilated cardiomyopathy in children is also faced with various challenges, particularly in light of recent global public health issues such as the COVID-19 pandemic. During such periods, the congenital heart disease (CHD) community has devised measures to ensure the safety and continuity of care for affected children who, in most cases, require timely interventions. Limited resources and elevated risks of infection necessitate a triage approach to the prioritization of the sickest patients. When working in these confines, ongoing investigation into the epidemiology, treatment, and outcome of pediatric DCM remains an importance. This focus will not only improve acute care but also guide future treatment protocols, so children with dilated cardiomyopathy receive the optimal treatment despite general systemic limitations (Elizabeth et al., 2020).

11.1.3. Restrictive Cardiomyopathy

Restrictive cardiomyopathy (RCM) is a relatively uncommon but significant disorder within the spectrum of pediatric cardiomyopathies, accounting for approximately 2.5% to 3% of children with cardiomyopathies. It is characterized by a rigid myocardial wall that hinders proper filling of the heart during diastole, leading to elevated filling pressures and signs of heart failure. Children who have been diagnosed with RCM are more likely to experience poor outcomes, with an elevated mortality rate, and studies indicating that nearly 50% of the affected individuals can die within two years of diagnosis. The etiology of RCM is extremely varied in age and geography, with underlying causes varying from genetic susceptibility to idiopathic causes, including disease states such as endomyocardial fibrosis, indicating the diversity of this entity in children (Nguyen et al., 2025). The diagnosis of restrictive cardiomyopathy involves an amalgam of clinical picture, electrocardiogram, and echocardiographic imaging. Pediatric patients may present with signs of exercise intolerance, fatigue, and signs of heart failure, simulating other cardiac or systemic illnesses. Proper and early diagnosis is mandatory because timely treatment has a significant impact on outcome. Point-of-care ultrasound (POCUS) has emerged as a great diagnostic tool, enabling medical professionals to examine cardiac functions and structures directly and within seconds. Interestingly, RCM is usually unnoticed or misdiagnosed due to its non-specific presentation; therefore, heightened awareness among clinicians is paramount in achieving early identification and intervention (Tanwar et al., 2025) (Figure 11.5).

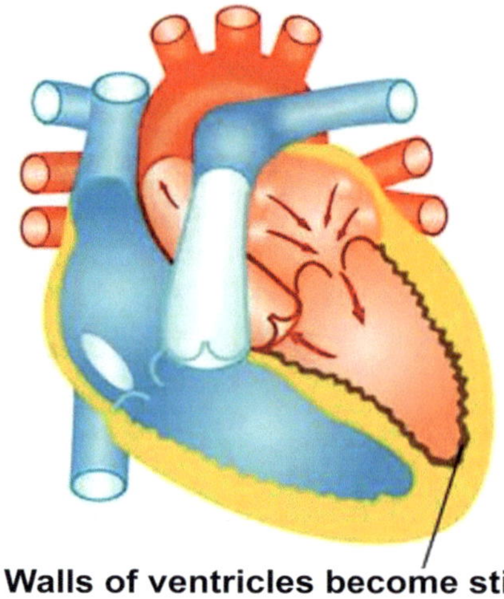

Figure 11.5. Restrictive cardiomyopathy.

Source: https://pulse-cardiology.com/wp-content/uploads/2020/04/Types-of-Cardiomyopathy.jpg.webp.

Management strategies of restrictive cardiomyopathy in children are largely symptomatic and with focus on symptom relief of heart failure and improving the quality of life. Pharmacological strategies may include the use of diuretics to manage fluid overload, as well as drugs that can increase cardiac output. However, in the case of severe disease with failure of conventional therapies, more invasive treatments such as heart transplantation may be performed. The risks of severe cardiac failure in the pediatric populations require ongoing research into new therapies and preventive measures for potentially reversible causes of RCM. With increased clinical understanding regarding pediatric cardiomyopathies such as their pathophysiology and treatment, it is essential to recognize restrictive cardiomyopathy as a priority research and clinical activity to provide optimal patient outcomes (Nguyen et al., 2025).

11.2. Causes and Risk Factors

Understanding the causes and risk factors of cardiomyopathies in children is critical to accurate diagnosis and treatment. Genetic factors are one of the most significant factors in the etiology of the conditions. Dilated cardiomyopathy (DCM), for example, can be caused by several genetic mutations that weaken heart muscle function, which could be inherited generationally or sporadically. Research shows the complex interaction between acquired factors and inherited genetic differences, implying that while some children inherit some mutations that predispose them to cardiomyopathy, others can develop symptoms induced by acquired factors, such as infection and toxins exposure. This dualism underscores the necessity for continued research into the genetic processes that lead to DCM and other forms of cardiomyopathy, with an eye to integrative analysis of these diseases (Arnăutu et al., 2024). In addition to genetic factors, certain demographic and environmental components are also significant in the presence of cardiomyopathies among children. These cardiac conditions could be affected by age, gender, and ethnicity with respect to rates of susceptibility. For instance, boys are more likely to be diagnosed with cardiomyopathies compared to girls, which implies that the biological differences may be the cause of the variation. Additionally, familial clustering of cardiomyopathy cases points towards shared environmental exposures and hereditary predispositions. Furthermore, viral infections such as myocarditis have also been identified as precipitates for DCM among children. Infections can provoke inflammation and damage to cardiac tissue, enhancing inherited genetic susceptibility. Recognition of such environmental and demographic factors is thus critical in the initial diagnosis and treatment of risk children who are to develop cardiomyopathies (Arnăutu et al., 2024). The significance of identifying the causative factors and risk factors of cardiomyopathies transcends individual case identification; it reveals the necessity of area-specific screening and patient-specific treatment protocols. Early detection with genetic testing can be revolutionary, allowing for individually tailored management plans based on unique genetic profiles. Children with cardiomyopathy due to a known genetic etiology may be advantaged by increased monitoring and even preventive treatment aimed at retarding disease progression. Furthermore, the recognition of multiple phenotypic expressions linked to gene mutations allows for improved risk stratification of relatives who may also be at risk. With the intricacies behind cardiomyopathies being better unveiled by research, incorporating genetic data into clinical practice has not only the potential to improve the treatment outcomes of affected children but also to enhance familial risk stratification and guidance (Arnăutu et al., 2024) (Figure 11.6).

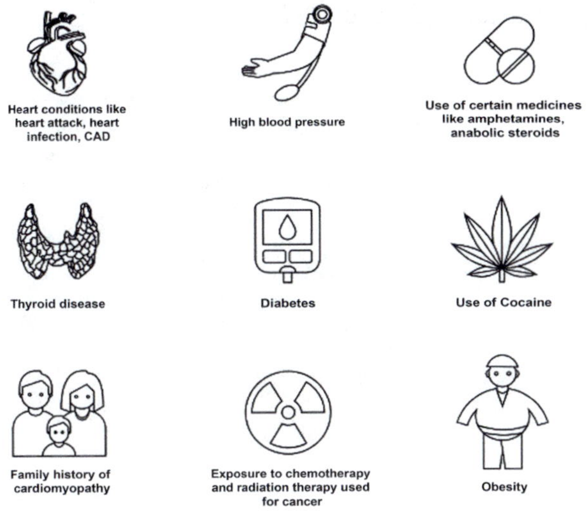

Figure 11.6. Risk factors for cardiomyopathies.

Source: https://external-content.duckduckgo.com/iu/?u=https%3A%2F%2Fas1.ftcdn.net%2Fv2%2Fjpg%2F04%2F82%2F14%2F66%2F1000_F_482146647_3d6aOr1E9FfY2kQv3IYsSA7WqOWUBOoM.jpg&f=1&nofb=1&ipt=6572dfdbb15ae1122370ecc0a064fd773f23aa58cc124ac62af925d5268054ed.

11.2.1. Genetic Predispositions

It is critical to assess the genetic predispositions in the diagnosis of cardiomyopathies in children because the condition has an element of heredity that decides the causation and progression of the disease. Mutations in genetic material, such as sarcomeric proteins, have been linked to various forms of cardiomyopathy and highlight the significance of family history and genetic testing in affected patients. Research has indicated that heightened awareness of such mutations leads to early diagnosis and treatment, significantly altering patient outcomes. By identifying genetic markers that predispose some cardiomyopathies, clinicians can offer tailored preventive strategies and therapeutic interventions in accordance with the patient's need for more targeted treatment. Moreover, exploring these genetic roots can also serve to illuminate the public health implications of cardiomyopathies more broadly, and buttress the call for continued research into this area. In kids, genetic vulnerabilities to cardiomyopathies often necessitate careful family screenings because most such diseases are inherited in autosomal dominant or recessive manner. Disease states such as dilated cardiomyopathy and hypertrophic cardiomyopathy usually become apparent at the childhood age, demanding worries over the genetic risk to siblings and future generations (Figure 11.7).

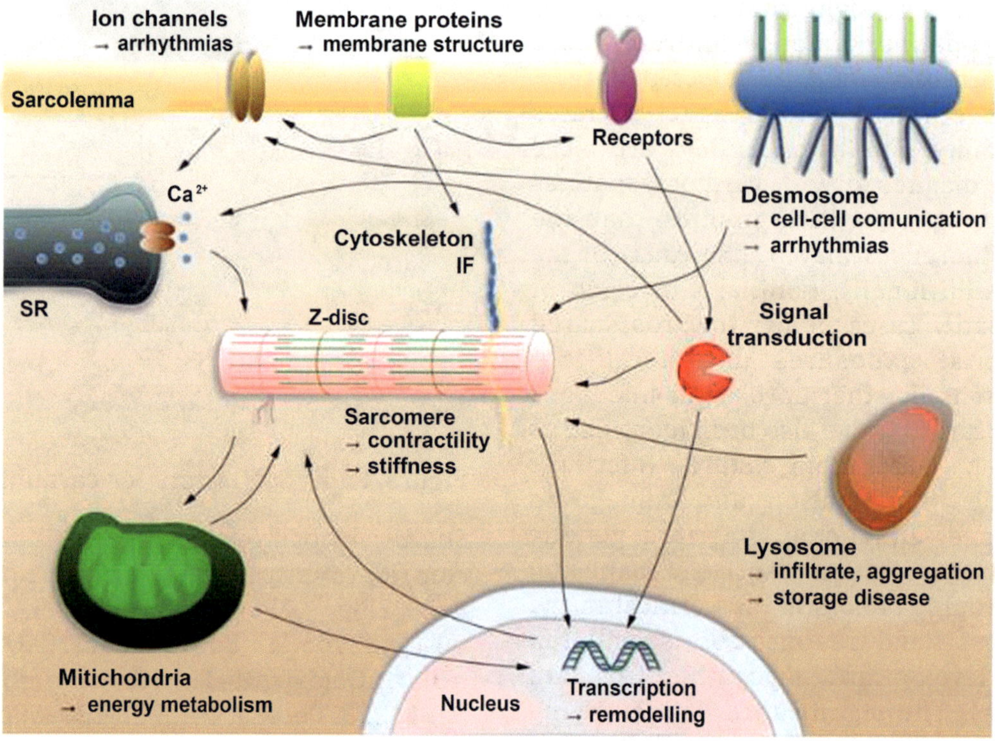

Figure 11.7. Cellular compartments affected by genetic mutations causing cardiomyopathy in children. Arrows indicate interactions between different compartments altered in the presence of mutations (e.g., sarcomeric mutations leading to energy depletion and altered transcription).

Source: https://www.intechopen.com/chapters/86077.

The discovery of important genetic markers will also be helpful in determining how environmental influences further interact with susceptibilities at the genetic level, therefore giving a detailed picture of disease initiation. Research indicates that the existence of some genetic profiles might predispose children not just to cardiac conditions but also to comorbidities, making it harder to treat and manage them. Therefore, efficient communication of genetic risks and implications plays a significant role in the formulation of informed decision-making among families carrying the burden of hereditary cardiomyopathies. With rapid advancements in technology, greater emphasis is laid on the integration of genetic counseling with the care of children suffering from cardiomyopathies. Providing access to genetic testing among families may help in the earlier diagnosis and preventive measures that can change the course of the disease. Through the detection of high-risk individuals at an early stage, clinicians can initiate lifestyle modifications or screen asymptomatic siblings for the emergence of symptoms. In addition, understanding the genetic basis of such disorders can result in research on focused therapies, which may pave the way for therapy advancement. Ironically, despite the promise of a genetic predisposition's information to more effectively manage patients, it creates ethical dilemmas of discrimination as well as anxiety within families. Therefore, discussion of genetic predisposition in cardiomyopathies needs to be mindful of psychosocial implications for children and families as they navigate this complex landscape (Caio et al., 2019; Zeppenfeld et al., 2022).

11.2.2. Environmental Influences

Environmental determinants play a crucial role in the causation of cardiomyopathies among children. Prenatal exposures like maternal health, socioeconomic status, and housing situation play a major role in the causation of acquiring cardiovascular disease. For instance, maternal determinants like age and educational accomplishment have been shown to co-vary with the health status of newborns, wherein older maternal age and lower educational levels are both related to higher risk of circulatory system abnormalities in offspring. This emphasizes the importance of addressing optimal control of environmental factors affecting maternal health to enhance normal pregnancy and reduce possible risk factors related to cardiomyopathies in offspring. Interventions for maternal health can therefore lead to improved cardiac prognosis in pediatric groups, a testament to the interconnectedness of child cardiology and societal determinants. Additionally, research is emphatic regarding the role of birth pattern as an environmental determinant of cardiomyopathies. Evidence shows that conditions like low birth weight and occurrences of asphyxia during delivery significantly increase the probability of contracting circulatory system diseases in children. Specifically, low birth weight carries a relative risk of 2.26 for circulatory disease death, while asphyxia at varying points during delivery is also a significant reason for unfavorable outcomes. The findings indicate that measures to eliminate issues with prenatal care and delivery itself must be taken if risks related to cardiomyopathy development are to be minimized. Appreciation of the role of these variables enables health practitioners to identify vulnerable infants early enough to allow early intervention for enhancing their cardiovascular development and health. In addition, the field of environmental effect is broader than prenatal and birth and includes lifestyle and social milieus in which children grow up. Environmental determinants such as accessibility of proper nutrition, access to exercise, and exposure to toxins affect the cardiovascular health of children. For instance, poorer socioeconomic kids can be weighed down with concerns like no exposure to healthy foods or safe areas to play, which raise the risk of obesity and its subsequent cardiac conditions. \

Longitudinal research has indicated that lifestyle in early childhood, according to one's environmental situation, can influence cardiac health in long-term manners. Therefore, interventions in the community that focus on improving resource access and quality lifestyle choices can become major determinants of reducing the incidence of cardiomyopathies, underscoring the heterogeneity of environment factors influencing the cardiac health of children.

11.2.3. Associated Medical Conditions

The coexistence of cardiomyopathies in children with their associated medical conditions is an evolving situation that must be paid close attention to. The majority of children presenting with cardiomyopathies also present with accompanying health conditions, which can significantly influence the clinical management and prognosis of the underlying cardiac condition. For instance, diseases such as congenital heart disease, hypertension, and arrhythmias are frequent comorbidities in cardiomyopathy, commonly rendering both its diagnosis and management difficult. The concomitant existence of these interrelated medical conditions demonstrates the necessity of a multidisciplinary team to address the multifaceted nature of care, such as pediatric cardiology, genetics, and various other specialties. Ultimately, an intelligent understanding of the interrelatedness between these disorders enables treating practitioners to develop more productive individualized treatment regimens to meet the unique needs of each unique individual pediatric patient. One such concerning aspect of cardiomyopathy in children is that the risk of having associated genetic diseases, which have a propensity to aggravate cardiac conditions, exists. Duchenne Muscular Dystrophy and Friedreichs Ataxia are the syndromes that have been recognized to have a very high correlation with cardiomyopathies, leading to deterioration of the functioning of the heart. The interplay of genetic predisposition and cardiomyopathy etiology may not only lead to compromised cardiac performance but can also manifest with other clinical concerns, such as neurological involvement. In the context of such association, it is highly advisable that physicians refer genetic counseling and testing within affected families, especially when a child comes with idiopathic cardiomyopathy. By recognizing and being familiar with these genetic disorders, clinicians are able to present preventive management approaches that may improve general patient outcomes. Furthermore, mitochondrial dysfunction is an extremely relevant but oftentimes overlooked associated medical disorder in pediatric cardiomyopathy. Primary mitochondrial dysfunction can primarily manifest as cardiac disease and result in dilated or hypertrophic cardiomyopathy in children. This association is meant to highlight the importance of clinicians remembering to consider mitochondrial etiologies when evaluating cardiomyopathy patients, especially if other organ systems are involved. For example, some patients will present with symptoms of myopathy or neurologic impairment along with their cardiac symptoms, complicating diagnosis and treatment. The complexity of mitochondrial disorders, as exemplified by the pathologic observations of biventricular fibro-adipose replacement, underscore the susceptibility of the heart's first exposure to TSFM dysfunction (Bonnen et al., 2019). Translating this into clinical practice can give rise to improved patient outcomes via early detection and well-managed intervention protocols that encompass the multifactorial nature of pediatric cardiomyopathies.

11.3. Symptoms and Diagnosis

During the diagnosis of cardiomyopathies in children, identification of symptoms is crucial to ensure effective diagnosis and management. The children acquire a variety of signs, which are mistaken for typical children's conditions, such as chest pain, shortness of breath, or tiredness. The signs may be deceptive because they may be a sign of mild conditions, making early detection challenging. In asymptomatic patients, subtle changes on an electrocardiogram (ECG) or abnormal findings on a transthoracic echocardiogram may be the first indication of an underlying condition since these diagnostic investigations are important in detecting evidence of structural heart disease in the young. Absent from regular screening, underlying cardiomyopathies may lead to more severe complications like fatal arrhythmias, which emphasizes the importance of comprehensive clinical evaluation and diagnostic imaging (Mariucci et al., 2024). Challenging for the diagnosis in children is compounded by the multiplicity of forms and nonspecific clinical presentations. Dilated cardiomyopathy, for instance, typically presents with findings characteristic of heart failure, such as retardation of growth and intolerance to exercise. Superimposed upon age-related developmental phases in the early childhood years, this renders an easy diagnosis impossible. Pediatricians and cardiologists must remain vigilant in evaluating complete patient histories and performing complete clinical examinations to detect abnormal results, such as cardiomegaly on chest X-rays or obvious ECG abnormalities. Additionally, advanced diagnostic procedures such as cardiac magnetic resonance imaging and molecular genetic tests, whilst helpful in making an absolute diagnosis, are not utilized on a routine basis in practice. Thus, the challenge continues to balance needs for advanced diagnostic equipment with their availability in pediatric cardiology (Kauk et al., 2024) (Figure 11.8).

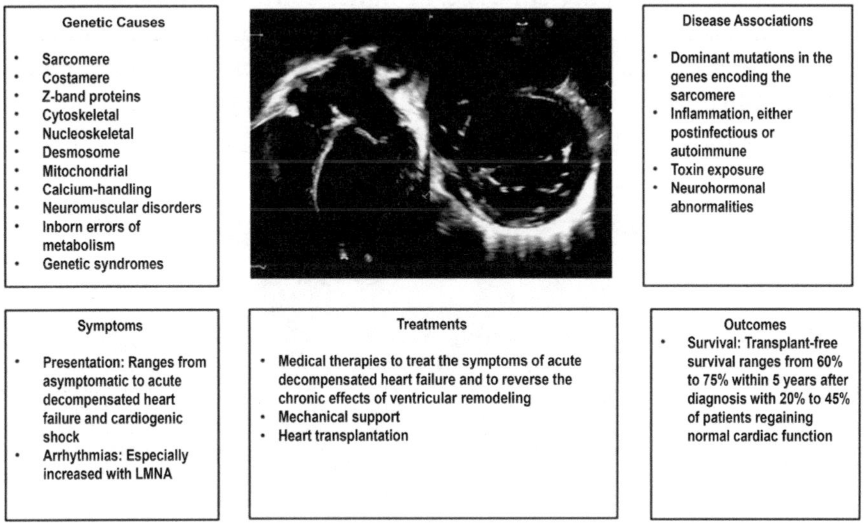

Figure 11.8. Dilated cardiomyopathy. End-diastolic apical 4-chamber (left) and parasternal short-axis end-diastolic (right) views of the left ventricle in a patient with severe dilated cardiomyopathy.

Source: https://www.ahajournals.org/doi/10.1161/circresaha.116.309386.

Early diagnosis of cardiomyopathies is crucial to reduce the risk of dire outcomes, including sudden cardiac death, even in asymptomatic children. The frequency of such a devastating outcome in pediatric dilated cardiomyopathy patients underscores the need for early intervention, with reported rates of sudden death ranging from 1.5 to 4%. Identification of the manifestations that express cardiac stress, i.e., cardiac chamber hypertrophy or cardiac repolarization abnormality on ECG, is important in high-risk populations, especially in athletes. Therefore, a strategy that encompasses multifaceted diagnostics using the integration of clinical examination data and imaging data is essential. Effective management, including careful follow-up and possibly therapeutic intervention, can improve worldwide prognoses and quality of life in affected children, which makes awareness and ongoing research in this cardiology subspecialty important (Kauk et al., 2024).

11.3.1. Common Symptoms in Children

Common indications of cardiomyopathies among children should be identified for early treatment and diagnosis. The symptoms tend to express themselves in a very subtle way, tending to go unnoticed or mistaken for common childhood disease. Fatigue is a common complaint that tends to occur during physical exertion. Unusual effort, like easily getting winded when playing, is a clue that the heart is having a hard time keeping up with the body's needs. A persistent cough or wheeze can be a sign of fluid accumulation in the lungs, making the clinical picture more complex. These presentations are of great vigilance to the parents and healthcare professionals, as early detection is one of the variables that could enhance the prognosis of children with cardiomyopathies, which are also at risk of severe complications if undetected and left untreated. Apart from this, children with cardiomyopathies could also present with palpitations which are alarming to the child and to the caretakers. The majority of these arrhythmias can be mistaken to represent normal stress or anxious reaction which is usual in younger children. However, when these episodes occur on a regular basis or are accompanied by other symptoms like dizziness or syncope, they are entitled to immediate medical attention. This is particularly true in the context of the dangerous consequences of unrecognized illness; sudden cardiac death is an achievable outcome due to omitted cardiomyopathy (Mariucci et al., 2024). Recognition of patterns within these symptoms, for instance, whether they recur or coincide with physical exertion, may lead healthcare practitioners to prioritize further investigation, including echocardiography and electrocardiography (Figure 11.9).

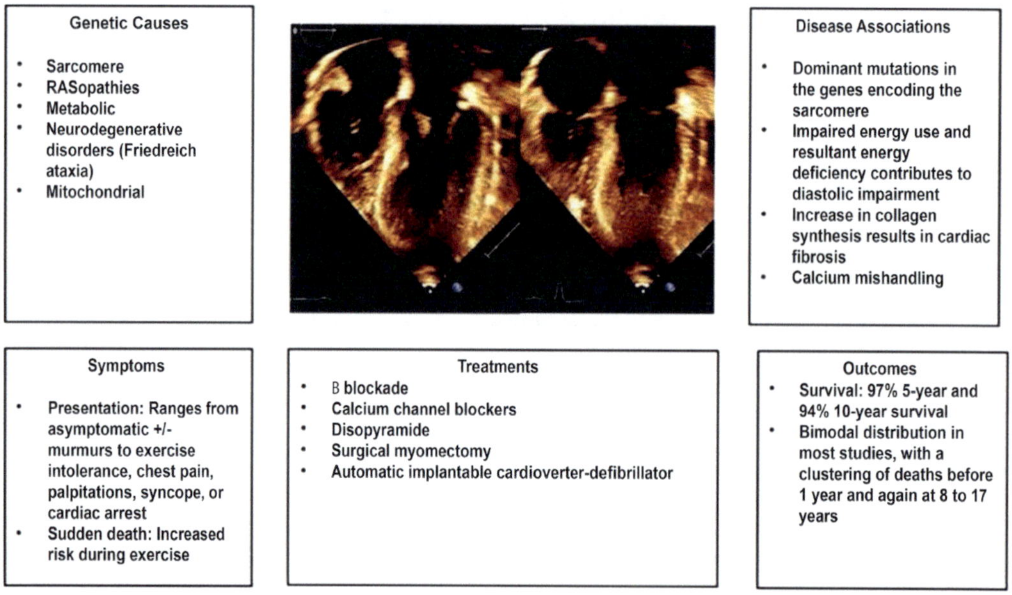

Figure 11.9. Hypertrophic cardiomyopathy. End-diastolic (left) and end-systolic (right) apical 4-chamber views of the left ventricle in a patient with severe hypertrophic cardiomyopathy.

Source: https://www.ahajournals.org/doi/10.1161/circresaha.116.309386.

Another sign of great significance to look out for in children who may have cardiomyopathy is growth retardation, which indicates underlying cardiac dysfunction. Kids that have heart failure are neither gaining weight nor growing as they ought, something generally attributed to the body's compromised capacity to circulate blood sufficiently (Kauk et al., 2024). This symptom is particularly disconcerting since it strikes at the very heart of childhood development, affecting physical health and psychosocial function. In the absence of treatment, growth disturbances can lead to long-term effects, including development delay and decreased quality of life. As such, healthcare providers must remain alert for indicators of failure to thrive as well as other common cardiomyopathy symptoms. Employing a holistic approach to assessing these children aids in the formulation of effective treatment plans according to their unique needs.

11.3.2. Diagnostic Tests and Procedures

The diagnosis of cardiomyopathies in children needs a robust panel of investigative procedures and interventions that can accurately diagnose the condition and inform clinical care. Among the most visible diagnostic modalities is echocardiography, which generates real-time images of heart structure and function. The non-invasive method allows clinicians to assess the size of cardiac chamber, wall motion, and global hemodynamics. In light of the diverse presentations of cardiomyopathies, echocardiography is often complemented by electrocardiograms (ECGs) in order to evaluate the electrical activity of the heart.

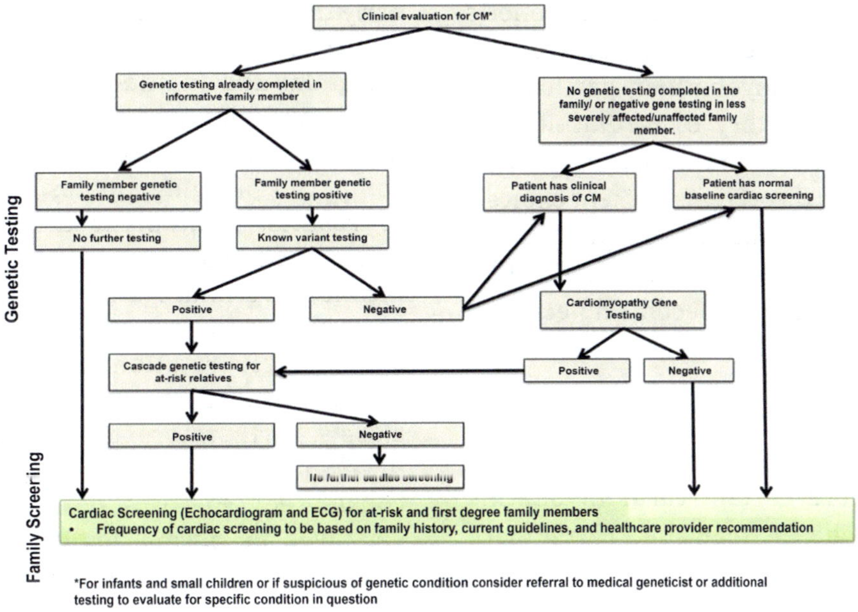

Figure 11.10. Genetic testing algorithm for pediatric cardiomyopathy.

Source: https://www.ahajournals.org/cms/10.1161/CIRCRESAHA.116.309386/asset/676b944c-aaf6-4255-9d12-e3ec0d34b268/assets/graphic/855fig05.jpeg.

The diagnostic tests are highly beneficial in the identification of arrhythmias classically associated with cardiomyopathies, facilitating early treatment that can improve patient outcomes. In more complex cases, additional imaging studies can be utilized to further investigate cardiac morphology and function. Cardiac magnetic resonance imaging (MRI), for example, gives the accurate anatomical information and is able to discriminate between a number of cardiomyopathies. It is important as it can assess the features of myocardial tissue, isolating ischemic from non-ischemic cause of heart disease. Cardiac catheterization can be performed as an adjunct imaging technology to these technologies. This technique not only allows for pressure measurement within the heart chambers but also allows direct visualization and biopsy of myocardial tissue when necessary. That it can do endomyocardial biopsies is particularly helpful in inflammatory cardiomyopathy suspects, where histology can guide therapy (Freixa-Benavente et al., 2023). Laboratory investigations play a similarly important role to diagnosis in children with cardiomyopathies. Blood work testing for such markers as B-type natriuretic peptide (BNP) is also of further supportive diagnostic utility, indicating the intensity of heart failure. Genetic testing is more and more being recommended in children with cardiomyopathies, particularly if there is a family history of cardiac illness. Identification of genetic mutations may carry prognostic value and direct management choices, such as screening of relatives and prevention. In other patients, invasive methods like endomyocardial biopsy can become a necessity in circumstances where other diagnostic examinations and methods are not decisive, particularly when rejection is to be excluded in the case of post-transplant individuals, or in situations where certain cardiomyopathic conditions are to be distinguished (Breinbjerg et al., 2021). Overall, these examinations and interventions form the primary framework that should underpin the effective management of pediatric cardiomyopathies (Figure 11.10).

11.3.3. Challenges in Diagnosing Cardiomyopathies in Pediatric Patients

Diagnosis of cardiomyopathies in children poses a special set of challenges, the majority of which are due to the varied and often non-specific nature of presentation of heart disease in children. Unlike adults, children exhibit a greater variability in presentation, added to further by the incidence of overlapping conditions such as congenital heart defect. This heterogeneity is most typically accountable for a delay in the diagnosis because medical practitioners may be confusing signs of cardiomyopathy with benign gastrointestinal or respiratory symptoms. These diagnostic difficulties are particularly relevant in the acute setting, where a speedy and proper appraisal is critical. Pediatric heart failure, a common clinical presentation of cardiomyopathy, may be presenting with age-related patterns that make standardized diagnostic criteria less relevant. Thus, clinician experience and knowledge of these pitfalls are important towards maximizing early treatment and detection results. Moreover, pediatric patients' anatomical and physiological variations add additional diagnostic challenges. They have miniaturized cardiac structures and distinctive hemodynamic profiles, which might complicate imaging studies and interpretation of results. Equipment that has been well established in adults might yield inaccurate or inconclusive findings in children. The reliance on echocardiography, for instance, needs skilled interpretation, since mild structural changes can be missed if not scrutinized very closely. Furthermore, the effects of growth and development on heart function also have to be considered; what is abnormal in an adult may very well be normal for infants and children. This complexity demands a multidisciplinary approach to diagnosis, with extensive clinical evaluation, advanced imaging techniques, and genetic analysis when necessary (Moeinipour et al., 2025). Beyond specific clinical problems, psychosocial problems can interfere with accurate diagnosis and proper management of cardiomyopathies in children. The emotional and psychological burden that comes with a diagnosis of cardiomyopathy can lead to anxiety and stress that might impair compliance with medical recommendations. The parents can either miss or miss-read the signs because of the usual chaos involved in caring for a child with chronic illness. In addition, specialized pediatric care may not be readily available in some areas, and thus evaluations by pediatric cardiologists who have the requisite expertise to navigate the intricacies of childhood heart diseases can be delayed. As many cases of pediatric cardiomyopathy can be attributed to genetic etiology, understanding the impact is crucial (Lee et al., 2025). Better education for healthcare providers and increased awareness in parents can encourage earlier recognition and intervention, finally improving the prognosis for the children.

11.4. Treatment Options

In discussing treatment for cardiomyopathies in children, it is necessary to consider an individualized approach that is oriented to the specific type and severity of the disease. Drug treatments are often the first line of treatment and can include drugs designed to regulate symptoms, improve cardiac function, and prevent complications. For instance, beta-blockers and ACE inhibitors are also routinely used to relieve workload on the heart and to facilitate the improvement of obstructive hypertrophic cardiomyopathy-related symptoms. The drug efficacy, though, can vary widely in pediatric patients, necessitating careful monitoring and adjustment by experts in pediatric cardiology. Family engagement is important in this kind of situation because informing them about the condition and how the treatment is placed within it can enhance compliance and health results. In more serious cases where children have recurrent symptoms despite optimal medical management, surgical treatment can be necessary. The myectomy remains a viable treatment for hypertrophic cardiomyopathy, against which it has proven capable of reducing mechanical obstructions as well as improving quality of life. As this operation has become one of the safest open-heart operations with perioperative mortality falling to 0.6%, it is increasingly regarded as a viable therapeutic option in children with significant left ventricular outflow obstruction. Of particular significance, studies have shown that more than 90% of patients experience impressive symptom relief following surgery, improving them to more functional classes, and this is particularly vital for active lifestyles that are prevalent in children (Barry et al., 2022).

Referral for surgical intervention should, therefore, involve consultation among healthcare providers, patients, and families to determine informed consent and to harmonize risk and benefits adequately. In addition to this, there are novel treatment protocols that overlap with traditional methods and are increasingly playing a role in the specialty of pediatric cardiology. These include some of the following protocols such as gene therapy and using new negative inotropic agents focusing on targeting the pathophysiological pathways of cardiomyopathies. As more knowledge is acquired in the genetic etiology of cardiomyopathies in children, personalized medicine approaches come into perspective. These forms of treatments can also bring hope to children with genetic variation that standard therapies cannot fully address. Continuous research and the development of new therapies cannot be overstated, as breakthroughs here can potentially improve patient outcomes in the long run and reduce the burden of cardiovascular disease on a global scale (Gregory et al., 2020). Engaging families in discussions regarding these new therapies is necessary because it establishes a common ground conducive to navigating the challenges of treating with several options (Figure 11.11).

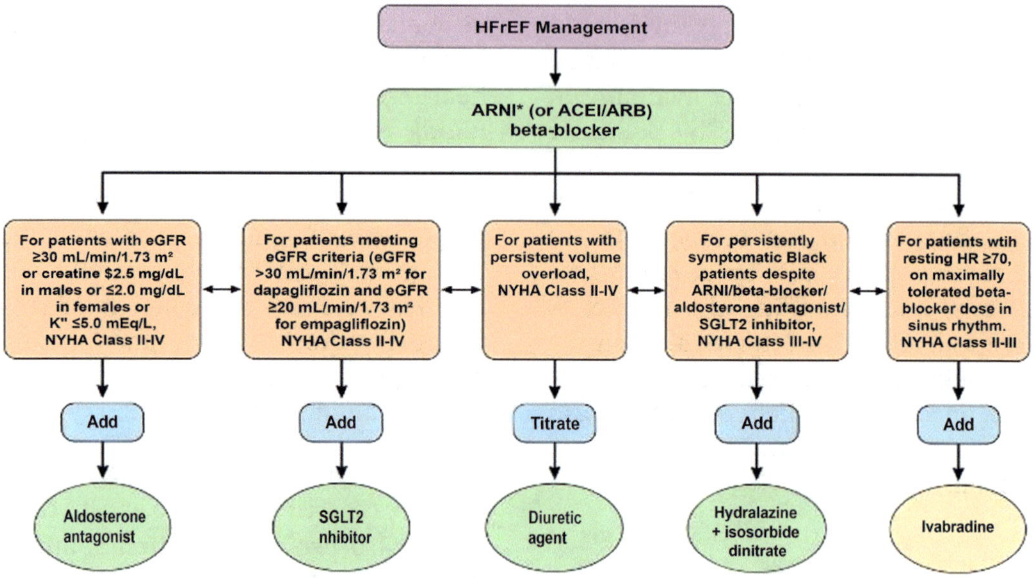

Figure 11.11. The most recent revision of American College of Cardiology/AHA treatment algorithms for treating adults with HF and reduced left ventricular ejection fraction.

Source: https://www.ahajournals.org/doi/10.1161/CIR.0000000000001151.

11.4.1. Medications and Their Roles

The role of drugs in the management of cardiomyopathies in children is diverse and critical to the improvement of patient outcomes. For conditions such as dilated cardiomyopathy, pharmacological treatment aims at enhancing cardiac function, hemodynamics, and symptom relief. These drugs include angiotensin-converting enzyme (ACE) inhibitors, beta-blockers, and diuretics, which serve the purpose of reducing fluid overload and reducing the cardiac workload. These treatments can be significantly influenced by the underlying genetic basis of the specific cardiomyopathy. Understanding the molecular pathways that lead to different forms of cardiomyopathy is relevant, as tailored pharmacologic approaches may be helped with enhanced treatment outcomes in children. This need for personalized treatment also underscores the need for ongoing genetic research, which informs the most effective treatment course in affected children (Arnăutu et al., 2024). Part of the evolving picture of pharmacotherapy in pediatric cardiomyopathies is also the promise of new treatments, including potentially using disease-modifying drugs that target the pathophysiologic mechanism. New studies have identified genetic variations that predispose young children to cardiomyopathies like familial hypertrophic cardiomyopathy, and this has created the need for treatment with specific therapies. Medications that have the potential to directly alter genetic expressions or enhance the cellular response could fundamentally transform the treatment of these children. With advances in the understanding of cardiomyopathies, including the integration of adjunctive therapy like lifestyle modifications and holistic care protocols, becomes increasingly significant. This integrated approach not only targets cardiovascular health but overall well-being in children who have such disorders (Arnăutu et al., 2024). In management of pediatric cardiomyopathy, consideration must be taken for drug therapies' long-term consequences. Continuous monitoring of medication effectiveness and potential side effects comes into focus, especially with the peculiar physiological changes that occur in childhood. Medications must be brought in and adjusted gradually as children grow up, and so do their hearts. Such continuous assessment is the way to minimize risks associated with treatment, understanding that children's metabolisms may metabolize drugs differently from adults. As scientists continue to learn about the path of cardiomyopathies, there is also hope that the treatments are more accurate and effective, ultimately improving the prognosis for the pediatric population. Interventions directed towards both drug optimization and genetic screening hold promise for the management of these complex disorders and therefore quality-of-life enhancement in such children and their families.

11.4.2. Surgical Interventions

Surgical interventions are crucial in the management of cardiomyopathies in children, particularly when medical therapy is not sufficient. Of all the surgical interventions that may be utilized, septal myectomy and heart transplantation are remarkable. Septal myectomy, primarily utilized for hypertrophic obstructive cardiomyopathy, allows the resection of obstructive muscle, relieving symptoms from left ventricular outflow tract obstruction. Through an increase in blood flow, the intervention positively improves the functional capacity and quality of life of a child to a significant level. Furthermore, the decision to proceed with such interventions is usually made following a proper evaluation of the clinical condition of the child, coupled with the probable benefits against the associated risks with surgery, including infection or the need for further procedures. Heart transplantation is another life-saving surgical procedure in children with end-stage cardiomyopathies, most notably dilated cardiomyopathy, which can progress to heart failure and other fatal conditions. Transplantation is performed after the identification of carefully selected candidates whose prognosis on medical care is unfavorable (Figure 11.12).

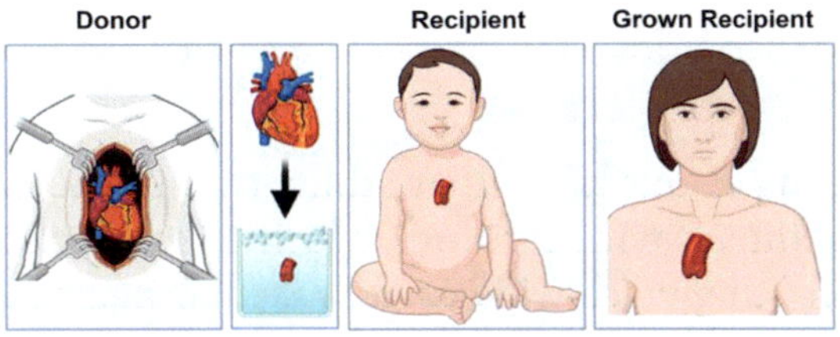

Figure 11.12. Partial heart transplantation as a method to provide growing valves to children.

Source: https://www.researchgate.net/figure/Partial-heart-transplantation-as-a-method-to-provide-growing-valves-to-children-Figure_fig1_364378090.

Availability of donor hearts is a significant concern, and child recipients have longer waited times because fewer appropriate donors exist. Successful transplant can lead to dramatic improvement in cardiac function and quality of life. Results following transplant are usually favorable but involve ongoing immunosuppressive therapy to prevent organ rejection, adding yet another layer of complexity to management. In addition to corrective surgery, interventional techniques such as catheter-based interventions have been developed as potent treatment modalities for chosen types of cardiomyopathies in children. These minimally invasive techniques can be employed to correct arrhythmias associated with cardiomyopathies or provide palliation with definitive surgery later. Interestingly, catheter ablation has been found to be effective for symptom control and incidence of arrhythmic occurrences, particularly relevant in the pediatric age group where the maintenance of quality of life is of greatest concern. The inclusion of such cutting-edge operations within the therapeutic protocol is a testament to the evolving advancement of cardiology practice, promoting a tailored approach taking into account the unique growth demands of children suffering from cardiomyopathies.

11.4.3. Lifestyle Modifications and Management

Talking about lifestyle modification in the care of children with cardiomyopathies is crucial in promoting worldwide cardiovascular health and quality of life. Dietary management is also key, as healthy eating habits with fruits, vegetables, whole grains, and lean proteins aid in healthy energy levels and optimal heart function. Most specifically, increasing dietary fiber and fluid intake will diminish gastrointestinal issues often associated with chronic disease, continuing to illustrate the multimodal process involved in the management of cardiomyopathies and their sequelae. The addition of regular physical exercise is also significant, not only in the improvement in cardiovascular wellness, but overall well-being as well. These lifestyle modifications have long-established advantages, not only to physical well-being, but also in the ability to cope psychologically, an aspect of growing significance for children with chronic illness. By taking a holistic approach, addressing overall modifications, as opposed to isolated factors, healthcare providers can best equip families to promote healthier habits toward enhanced cardiomyopathy control. In addition, management of lifestyle factors such as stress, sleep hygiene, social support is also important in the overall care of children with cardiomyopathy. Stress is very negative on heart health, and cardiomyopathic children may require counseling regarding coping mechanisms for management of anxiety and emotional issues. Encouraging effective communication within families helps to establish supportive relationships in which children feel free to express their concerns. Disturbances of sleep, which can exacerbate the cardiovascular diseases, must also be regulated by proper sleep hygiene training. Regularity of sleep and sleeping environment for the child with cardiomyopathies are required to facilitate restorative sleep. The integration of these lifestyle changes not only assist in the control of symptoms but also instill a stronger psychosocial framework as a whole, which is paramount in assisting the child to adjust and live with their health challenges. Finally, education and follow-up are essential components in the successful treatment of cardiomyopathies in children. Parents, caregivers, and children themselves need to be informed about the character of the disease, the treatment that is accessible, and the impact of lifestyle choices on health. Cooperation with health care workers, including nutritionists, physical therapists, and psychologists, creates a multidisciplinary group that aids in adherence to lifestyle changes. For instance, Drastal et al. (2025) puts emphasis on lifestyle adjustments in the management of dyslipidemia that may be used for children with cardiomyopathies in the context of cardiovascular risk. Pan et al. (2025) puts emphasis on continuous research and education in streamlining management protocols for pediatric patients as well. By placing emphasis on education and continued support, healthcare professionals can promote genuine interaction with families, ultimately creating improved health results in treating cardiac disease.

11.5. Prognosis and Long-Term Outcomes

Prognosis and long-term prognosis of cardiomyopathies in children are central problems, particularly as these conditions significantly influence the health and quality of life of a child. Dilated cardiomyopathy (DCM) is most especially the most prevalent in children, defined by worsening heart failure and multiple comorbidities. One long-term prognosis in children with DCM study revealed large percentages of chronic disease, such as all-cause mortality and need for heart transplants, especially among non-echocardiographic recovery children. With a mean follow-up of close to 15 years, data demonstrated that early pharmacologic therapy, such as the use of beta-blockers, significantly alleviated these side effects and reduced the mortality risk among affected children, with the importance of early medical management in improving survival rates and quality of life emerging (Navarro et al., 2024). Hypertrophic cardiomyopathy (HCM) adds another level of complexity in terms of long-term outcome and prognosis in the child population. The genetic underpinnings of HCM and penetrance variability in children make careful surveillance and individualized management of paramount importance. Children with HCM are at significant risk of developing severe complications, including fatal arrhythmias and sudden cardiac death. Importantly, the onset age and certain underlying genetic determinants largely predict these outcomes, hence necessitating an efficient evaluative model for early detection and longitudinal surveillance. Cardiac magnetic resonance (CMR) imaging is a central imaging modality in this context, and the clinician's ability to assess myocardial morphology, function, and even initial fibrotic changes that may be linked to disease progression, thus informing prognosis and treatment (Tessa et al., 2024). Ultimately, long-term prognosis in children with cardiomyopathies underscores the importance of tailored clinical management and ongoing multidisciplinary care. Research shows that survival and outcomes for health are significantly improved in children who are given regular cardiac evaluations and ongoing follow-up throughout their development. Additionally, whereas some patients might show spontaneous recovery, others need ongoing medical care and perhaps surgical intervention, including heart transplantation, to improve their results. Therefore, the understanding of the far-reaching courses of cardiomyopathies in children not only highlights the importance of early intervention but also how long-term health care strategies can adapt to changing pediatric patients' requirements and eventually help to bring about better prognostic outcomes within this vulnerable group (Navarro et al., 2024; Tessa et al., 2024).

11.5.1. Factors Influencing Prognosis

The prognosis of cardiomyopathies in children depends on a number of factors including the etiology of the disease, the severity of the disease at presentation, and the age of presentation of the child. Various types of cardiomyopathies such as hypertrophic, dilated, and restrictive cardiomyopathy have various prognoses depending on their presentation and the age of presentation. For instance, youngsters with hypertrophic cardiomyopathy may present with variable features ranging from mild symptoms to potentially lethal arrhythmias. Prompt identification with screening in at-risk groups may significantly alter the natural history of the disease, emphasizing the importance of early intervention for the improvement of functional and mortality results. In addition to etiology and severity of cardiomyopathy, patient-related factors such as genetic predisposition and comorbid illness play a critical role in determining prognosis. Genetic mutations underlying cardiomyopathy have not only implications for clinical presentation but also for treatment response and long-term outcome. Underlying conditions such as congenital heart disease or metabolic diseases can further confound the clinical picture and, in most instances, make prognosis guarded. Thus, multidisciplinary management including cardiologists, geneticists, and others is needed to develop care plans that are sensitive to both the cardiomyopathy and comorbidities, and ultimately maximize patient outcomes. Therapeutic strategies significantly influence prognosis in pediatric cardiomyopathies, with improved survival rates being achieved by advances in medical and surgical treatment. Pharmacologic therapy, such as the utilization of beta-blockers and angiotensin-converting enzyme inhibitors, has also been shown to improve cardiac function in certain types of cardiomyopathies. Furthermore, device therapy, in the form of implantable cardiac defibrillators, also decreases sudden cardiac death risk among susceptible children. Recent data indicate that earlier intervention and aggressive treatment of heart failure symptoms can result in better prognostic outcomes, with consideration of the emerging field of treatment options. As subsequent research clarifies the biological and clinical subtleties of pediatric cardiomyopathies, reassessment of prognostic markers is imperative to optimize care for this high-risk population.

11.5.2. Potential Complications

Pediatric cardiomyopathies not only present diagnostic and management difficulties but also a range of potential complications that can have a significant impact on patients' health status. Among the important concerns is the risk of implantable cardioverter-defibrillators (ICDs) widely debated in the treatment of life-threatening cardiac arrhythmias in the context of cardiomyopathy. Research indicates that there are unplanned procedures due to device-related complications in a high proportion of children. Specifically, 36% of patients required surgical treatment primarily because of lead-related complications, and this is an indication of the need for proper risk evaluation during selection of ICD in young cardiomyopathy and congenital heart disease subjects (Fetcu et al., 2025). The choice of implantation of such devices must, thus, consider not only the short-term therapeutic benefits but also potential long-term implications of device complications that could cause additional health risks and challenges in the management of this high-risk population. Furthermore, inappropriate ICD shocks can further have significant complications in children. Studies have proven that the overall prevalence of inappropriate shocks is downright scary at a rate of about 13% in children with congenital heart disease receiving such implants. Constant and unexplained shocks can also worsen the anxiety and distress, complicating the overall management of their cardiomyopathy (Fetcu et al., 2025). In addition, patients with some underlying conditions, i.e., those with a history of compromised cardiac function, are particularly vulnerable to these complications. Doctors should have comprehensive talks with families regarding the risk of excessive shocks and psychologic implications, thereby creating informed choices in connection with the application of life-saving devices in the management of cardiomyopathy. In addition to device-related complications, the overall context of pediatric cardiomyopathies is influenced by several psychosocial factors that could complicate medical treatment and outcomes. The integration of digital health technologies has emerged as an area with particular promise for patient surveillance and patient engagement for young patients. However, the evidence identifies several challenges such as data privacy, ethical issues related to consent, and the need for caregiver participation in treatment plans. The conjoining of these technologies must be accomplished carefully, especially since such challenges as digital inequity can hamper such total engagement by marginalized groups. As kids struggle with the medical effects of cardiomyopathy as well as with the complexity that technological interventions pose, practitioners must themselves be sensitive to the threat of complications that involves where healthcare and digital health care intersect.

11.5.3. Importance of Regular Follow-Up Care

Follow-up care on a regular basis is important to ensure that children with cardiomyopathies because this condition is complex, with general implications for their health and development. Complications of cardiomyopathy exist in multiples including heart failure and arrhythmias, which require lifelong monitoring and management. Failure to follow up regularly will mean minor changes in the condition of a child may go unnoticed, exposing the child to the risk of sudden cardiac events. Regular follow-up visits with medical professionals guarantee early detection of complications and enable timely interventions that make a big difference in outcomes. Further, follow-up visits ensure chances for medical teams to adjust treatment plans based on the growth and development of the child's health, a necessity even more in times of rapid growth. Continuous monitoring and treatment are therefore necessary in offering needed care to children with cardiomyopathy in order to efficiently manage it. Apart from the physical health concerns, follow-up care on a regular basis also serves to deal with children with cardiomyopathies' psychological and emotional requirements. Being diagnosed and treated for chronic illnesses can be daunting for children and their families. Regular contact with healthcare providers allows for education and support, reassurance of families, and the resolution of their concerns. Through sustained follow-up, health providers are able to develop close relationships with patients, which result in a facilitative environment where children are assisted to explain their fears and challenges. Such emotional support may lower stress and aid compliance with treatment regimens, which also enhance the quality of life of the child. The integration of psychological support into the clinical follow-up program demonstrates the multidisciplinary nature required for the management of complex health problems such as cardiomyopathies in children. Further, the necessity of follow-up also extends to the realm of prevention health checks and long-term health planning. As put forward by the American College of Cardiology and the American Heart Association, there should be guideline-based management followed for the attainment of optimal health outcomes in those pediatric patients diagnosed with cardiovascular disease (Stout et al., 2018). These suggestions reaffirm the necessity of persistent risk stratification and management of the patient, which are active components of quality follow-up care. This stringent review not only enhances the acute clinical picture but also offers a chance to be proactive in preventing possible complication development once children reach adulthood. Monitoring growth parameters, understanding the impact of cardiomyopathy on daily activities, and adjusting lifestyle counseling are all active components of complete care. Planned follow-up ultimately forms the foundation of an integrated management strategy that increases the long-term pathways to health in children with cardiomyopathies, reflective of its central role within the broader healthcare system (Donna et al., 2019).

SUMMARY

The study of cardiomyopathies in children reveals the complex interaction of clinical, environmental, and genetic variables underlying the disease heterogeneity. The frequency of the familial forms of cardiomyopathy stresses the need for genetic evaluation and counseling because such assessment can guide therapy and provide significant information for families. Particularly, the research indicates that detailed evaluation usually produces more targeted treatment, which in turn results in improved patient outcomes. The historically established male predominance in the majority of cardiomyopathies lends significance to the performance of gender-specific research and therapy modalities because optimal techniques can vary drastically between boys and girls, thereby affecting general treatment protocols in pediatric patients (Şefika et al., 2025). In addition, the addition of newer therapeutic modalities, such as the potential of rituximab in treating associated malignancies, demonstrates that multidisciplinary treatment approaches have potential for enhanced survival rates in these children. The lack of statistically significant differences in event-free survival between various treatment regimens demonstrates that further research must continue to challenge the effectiveness of the addition of new drugs to existing protocols. While the role of rituximab remains to be conclusively established in cardiomyopathy models, indications point to the need for more targeted and innovative therapeutic strategies that directly address the unique requirements of children with cardiac diseases (Şefika et al., 2025). Ongoing issues regarding diagnosing and treating cardiomyopathies in children reinforce the imperative need for more comprehensive and multidisciplinary research programs. Subsequent studies should not only try to demarcate the pathophysiological substrate for each subtype but also seek to close existing gaps in terms of knowing management and outcome. Firm disease-specific criteria of assessment, disease-specific treatment protocols, and active screening systems can play a big role in maximizing healthcare delivery and quality of life in infected children. Continuous education from registries and cohort studies can also advance clinical practice, with the achievement of best-of-care pathways that can limit morbidity and mortality from these multifactorial diseases (Kaski et al., 2024).

The study of cardiomyopathies in children is vital due to the unique presentation and management challenges these conditions present. Cardiomyopathy is a group of diseases that involve the cardiac muscle structure and function, leading to heart failure and dire complications. Diagnostic types of cardiomyopathies in pediatric patients are varied, including dilated, hypertrophic, and restrictive cardiomyopathies. All subtypes share pathophysiologic mechanisms, patient populations, and etiologies that can include genetic syndromes, infections, and metabolic diseases. Moreover, early identification of signs and symptoms also significantly determines prognosis and treatment based on the fact that earlier intervention is able to halt the progression of disease as well as enhance the quality of life. Format reporting in imaging studies becomes increasingly important as a vital factor in the successful management of cardiomyopathies. Advances in technology have enabled the development of consensus report templates that simplify the evaluation process, particularly in pediatric patients. New initiatives have pointed to the benefits of standard reports in cardiovascular imaging that can enhance the quality of communication among healthcare providers and improve decision-making. By providing a more standardized framework for interpreting imaging findings, such as cardiac MR and CT tests, clinicians can determine more precisely the pathophysiology of cardiomyopathy in children and thereby make it feasible to implement appropriate therapy. In the years to come, as the practice evolves, adoption of structured reporting systems will most likely optimize care and improve outcomes for children with cardiomyopathies (Bunck et al., 2019). Treatment-wise, pediatric cardiomyopathies require multi-disciplinary therapy that in most cases involves pediatric cardiologists, surgeons, and other specialists. The model of multi-disciplinary therapy is required because of the high likelihood of complexities relating to each child's individual case, including age, growth rate, and co-morbid medical conditions. The recent advances in surgical techniques, such as those applied in heart transplantation, show the importance of implementing new techniques in the management of advanced cardiomyopathy cases. There are reports from research with favorable outcomes using techniques that seek to minimize complications, such as superior vena cava stenosis during transplantation (Park et al., 2023). The integration of cutting-edge therapies with comprehensive medical management lies at the core of optimizing d outcomes, such that ongoing research and education in the care of pediatric cardiomyopathy remain crucial.

CLOSER LOOK

ARRHYTHMOGENIC RIGHT VENTRICULAR CARDIOMYOPATHY (ARVC)

Arrhythmogenic right ventricular cardiomyopathy (ARVC) is a rare genetic heart muscle disease that affects predominantly the right ventricle. ARVC is characterized by progressive fibro-fatty replacement of the myocardium, with concomitant structural, electrical, and arrhythmogenic changes, and risk of sudden cardiac death, especially in young adults and athletes. ARVC also has a tendency to be inherited in an autosomal dominant pattern and is linked with mutations in genes that code for desmosomal proteins—crucial proteins that offer cell-to-cell adhesion in cardiac tissue. The most commonly affected genes are PKP2 (plakophilin-2), DSP (desmoplakin), and DSG2 (desmoglein-2) (Figure 11.13).

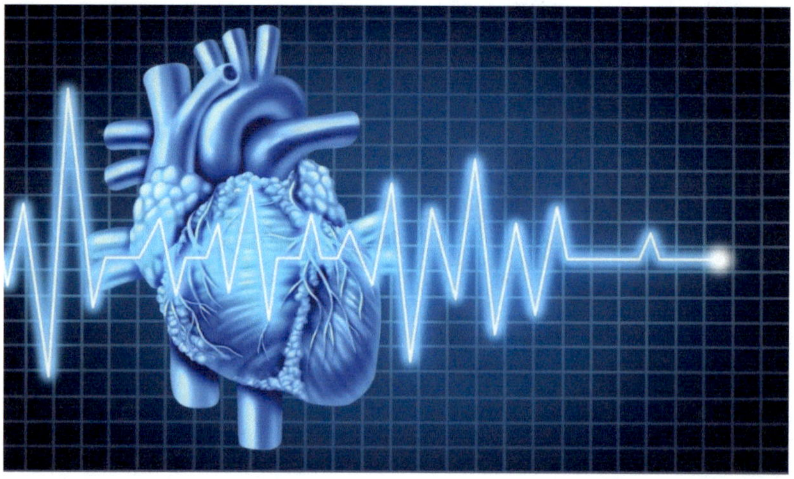

Figure 11.13. Conceptual illustration of the human heart with a superimposed electrocardiographic (ECG) waveform, symbolizing cardiac electrical activity.

Source: https://external-content.duckduckgo.com/iu/?u=https%3A%2F%2Ffamilydoctor.org%2Fwp-content%2Fuploads%2F2006%2F04%2F11840293_l.jpg&f=1&nofb=1&ipt=041e1bb1dbcaad3214b527892b7389a46c398cd1fc54493c59785ab3ec3bcbd5.

The hallmark pathological lesion of ARVC is fibrofatty replacement of the myocardium of the right ventricle, resulting in progressive thinning, dilation, and aneurysm formation. The changes are primarily localized to the "triangle of dysplasia" of the inflow tract of the right ventricle, outflow tract, and apex. With disease advancement, the electrical conduction system of the heart becomes impaired, giving rise to potentially fatal ventricular tachyarrhythmias in the form of palpitations, syncope, or sudden cardiac arrest, particularly during exertion.

Clinically, ARVC typically presents in early adulthood or adolescence but often several years go by before it comes to medical attention. The most frequent initial presentations are syncope or palpitations due to ventricular tachycardia with LBBB morphology. A red flag is family history of sudden cardiac death at under 35 years. Diagnosis is challenging and relies on a blend of clinical presentation, including electrocardiographic findings (e.g., T-wave inversions in leads V1–V3, epsilon waves), imaging studies (with echocardiography or cardiac MRI), arrhythmic symptoms, histopathological evidence from endomyocardial biopsy, and genetic testing.

Management of ARVC is directed towards preventing sudden cardiac death and controlling arrhythmias. Lifestyle modification, particularly the exclusion of competitive and endurance sports, is necessary because excessive exercise will exacerbate the condition. Antiarrhythmic medication, e.g., beta-blockers and amiodarone, can be employed to suppress arrhythmias. In patients with high risk for sudden cardiac death—such as those with sustained ventricular tachycardia or prior syncope—implantable cardioverter-defibrillators (ICDs) form the cornerstone of prophylactic therapy. In well-selected patients, catheter ablation may be used to reduce arrhythmia burden, albeit recurrences are common due to the indolent nature of the disease.

Genetic counseling is indicated for affected families. First-degree relatives of a patient with ARVC should be screened and may require genetic testing. Ongoing research continues to improve the understanding of the molecular substrate of ARVC and to define new therapeutic targets. Although ARVC remains incurable, early diagnosis and appropriate risk stratification have significantly improved outcomes. With strict compliance with medical guidelines and close follow-up, numerous patients with ARVC are able to lead active lives with minimal risk of dangerous cardiac complications.

REFERENCES

1. Aagaard, A., Baggish, A., Ackerman, M., Anderson, J., La Gerche, A., Pelliccia, A., Antzelevitch, C., et al. (2017). International criteria for electrocardiographic interpretation in athletes: Consensus statement. https://core.ac.uk/download/287649657.pdf (accessed on 15th July 2025).
2. Abbate, S., Amodeo, A., Amodeo, A., Amoroso, G., et al. (2021). The frequency of rare and monogenic diseases in pediatric organ transplant recipients in Italy. https://core.ac.uk/download/611911463.pdf (accessed on 15th July 2025).
3. Akyol, Ş., Güzel, T., Özcan, A., Karaman, S., Orhan, M., Üzel, V. H., Özay, M., et al. (2025). Rituximab in pediatric B-cell non-Hodgkin lymphoma: Clinical outcomes and prognostic implications. *Trends in Pediatrics.* https://www.semanticscholar.org/paper/15d993735e79421a6a35fe7719e7d4b96d8d6253 (accessed on 15th July 2025).
4. Alayleh, A., Hollyer, I., Johnstone, T., Khoo, B., Obilo, C., McFarlane, K., Baird, W., et al. (2025). A cadaveric study of the sagittal patellar insertion of the medial patellofemoral ligament in children: Implications for reconstruction. *The American Journal of Sports Medicine, 53*, 826–831. https://www.semanticscholar.org/paper/d55029dffbabd1cb125ca2cd6132a57d67fc49bb (accessed on 15th July 2025).
5. Arbustini, E., Behr, E. R., Carrier, L., Di Toro, A., et al. (2022). Interpretation and actionability of genetic variants in cardiomyopathies: A position statement from the European Society of Cardiology Council on cardiovascular genomics. https://core.ac.uk/download/519718331.pdf (accessed on 15th July 2025).
6. Arnăutu, D., Cozma, D., Lala, I. R., Arnăutu, S., Tomescu, M., & Andor, M. (2024). Risk assessment and personalized treatment options in inherited dilated cardiomyopathies: A narrative review. *Biomedicines, 12.* https://www.semanticscholar.org/paper/f7b347b629ff6ceeff34e2d48959224307725f33 (accessed on 15th July 2025).
7. Barbati, G., DI LENARDA, A., Gigli, M., Merlo, M., et al. (2016). Natural history of dilated cardiomyopathy in children. https://core.ac.uk/download/53748952.pdf (accessed on 15th July 2025).
8. Basso, C., Borjesson, M., Corrado, D., Pelliccia, A., et al. (2017). Risk of sports: Do we need a pre-participation screening for competitive and leisure athletes? https://core.ac.uk/download/85210797.pdf (accessed on 15th July 2025).
9. Berceanu, M., Constantin, A., Donoiu, I., Istrătoaie, D., et al. (2017). Non-compaction cardiomyopathy – Brief review. https://core.ac.uk/download/144553871.pdf (accessed on 15th July 2025).
10. Bhattacharjee, R., Winck, J., & Gozal, D. (2024). The future of big data: Remote monitoring of positive airway pressure treatment for obstructive sleep apnea–insights from adults and implications for pediatric care. *Pediatric Pulmonology, 60.* https://www.semanticscholar.org/paper/48be700d622dcdcd76f788e3ebed73fbc7b74fa7 (accessed on 15th July 2025).
11. Biffi, A., Biffi, A., D'Silva, A., D'Silva, A., Magalski, A., Malhotra, A., Malhotra, A., et al. (2019). Abnormal ECG findings in athletes: Clinical evaluation and considerations. https://core.ac.uk/download/286028675.pdf (accessed on 15th July 2025).

12. Bogle, C., Colan, S. D., Miyamoto, S. D., Choudhry, S., Baez-Hernandez, N., Brickler, M., Feingold, B., et al. (2023). Treatment strategies for cardiomyopathy in children: A scientific statement from the American Heart Association. *Circulation, 148*, 174–195. https://doi.org/10.1161/cir.0000000000001151 (accessed on 15th July 2025).
13. Bonnen, P. E., Carbo, M., Cerbelli, B., D'Amati, G., et al. (2019). Novel compound mutations in the mitochondrial translation elongation factor (TSFM) gene cause severe cardiomyopathy with myocardial fibro-adipose replacement. https://core.ac.uk/download/195777768.pdf (accessed on 15th July 2025).
14. Breinbjerg, A., Mohamed, L., Nielsen, S. Y., Rittig, S., Tullus, K., & Kamperis, K. (2021). Pitfalls in diagnosing urinary tract infection in children below the age of 2: Suprapubic aspiration vs clean-catch urine sampling. *The Journal of Urology, 206*, 1482–1489. https://www.semanticscholar.org/paper/c16eb6abe8152fa50fb538ff68dafb53405ab86e (accessed on 15th July 2025).
15. Bunck, A., Baessler, B., Ritter, C., Kröger, J., Persigehl, T., Pinto, D., Steinmetz, M., et al. (2019). Structured reporting in cross-sectional imaging of the heart: Reporting templates for CMR imaging of cardiomyopathies (myocarditis, dilated cardiomyopathy, hypertrophic cardiomyopathy, arrhythmogenic right ventricular cardiomyopathy and siderosis). *RoFo: Fortschritte auf dem Gebiete der Rontgenstrahlen und der Nuklearmedizin.* https://www.semanticscholar.org/paper/7588e534b7c0a4364c06e2119f22ab0424c32cbf (accessed on 15th July 2025).
16. Caio, G., Volta, U., Sapone, A., Leffler, D. A., De Giorgio, R., Catassi, C., & Fasano, A. (2019). Celiac disease: A comprehensive current review. *BMC Medicine, 17.* https://doi.org/10.1186/s12916-019-1380-z (accessed on 15th July 2025).
17. Chen, Y., Hu, X., Fan, T., Zhou, Y., Yu, C., Ding, J., Yu, J., et al. (2025). Nutritional state correlates to survival and prognosis in children with brain tumor resection. *Journal of Neurophysiology.* https://www.semanticscholar.org/paper/3dae09c2263ac2b4f89d06010938d2f3471fe099 (accessed on 15th July 2025).
18. Computational and Mathematical Methods in Medicine. (2023). Retracted: Clinical characteristics and death risk factors of severe sepsis in children. *Computational and Mathematical Methods in Medicine, 2023.* https://www.semanticscholar.org/paper/36645edf15b36c80d2ce188240427a4e0ead9340 (accessed on 15th July 2025).
19. D'Ascenzi, F., Harmon, K. G., Meyer, T., Orchard, J., & Pieles, G. E. (2024). What is the most appropriate age for the first cardiac screening of athletes? https://core.ac.uk/download/622822844.pdf (accessed on 15th July 2025).
20. Dickson, P. I., Ellinwood, N. M., Esko, J. D., Gordts, P., et al. (2016). Immune-mediated inflammation may contribute to the pathogenesis of cardiovascular disease in mucopolysaccharidosis type I. https://core.ac.uk/download/323078271.pdf (accessed on 15th July 2025).
21. Drastal, M. S., de Ferranti, S., & Gooding, H. (2025). Recent updates on the screening, diagnosis, and management of lipids disorders in children and adolescents. *Current Opinion in Pediatrics.* https://www.semanticscholar.org/paper/e1fc4fb6a4b84a81d622c2b1e6d0e1b37eb9b140 (accessed on 15th July 2025).
22. Ferriero, D. M., Fullerton, H. J., Bernard, T. J., Billinghurst, L., Daniels, S. R., DeBaun, M. R., deVeber, G., et al. (2019). Management of stroke in neonates and children: A scientific

statement from the American Heart Association/American Stroke Association. *Stroke, 50.* https://doi.org/10.1161/str.0000000000000183 (accessed on 15th July 2025).

23. Fetcu, A., Schaeffer, T., Niedermaier, C., Palm, J., Osawa, T., Matsubara, M., Heinisch, P., et al. (2025). Benefits and risks of implantable cardioverter-defibrillators in children and young adults with congenital heart disease, primary electrical disease, or pediatric cardiomyopathy. *European Journal of Cardio-Thoracic Surgery.* https://www.semanticscholar.org/paper/7e361eaf8461b086193521652dfee977a3649e9c (accessed on 15th July 2025).

24. Freixa-Benavente, A., Dolader, P., Gran, F., & Betrián-Blasc, P. (2023). Cardiac catheterization activity in pediatric cardiac transplantation. Can catheterization needs be predicted? *REC: Interventional Cardiology (English Edition).* https://www.semanticscholar.org/paper/f31983791ccdfe91699c28a4fee2b8f0ccea4d48 (accessed on 15th July 2025).

25. Jiang, C., & Zhang, H. (2025). Take the road less traveled: Pulmonary artery banding to rescue the children's failing heart. *Congenital Heart Disease.* https://www.semanticscholar.org/paper/ee725b2b2dd0113b810b4522be7132e99ac96ed3 (accessed on 15th July 2025).

26. Jiménez-Téllez, N., & Greenway, S. C. (2019). Cellular models for human cardiomyopathy: What is the best option? *World Journal of Cardiology, 11*, 221–235. https://doi.org/10.4330/wjc.v11.i10.221 (accessed on 15th July 2025).

27. Kaski, J., Norrish, G., Gimeno Blanes, J. R., Charron, P., Elliott, P., Tavazzi, L., Tendera, M., et al. (2024). Cardiomyopathies in children and adolescents: Etiology, management, and outcomes in the European Society of Cardiology EURObservational Research Programmed Cardiomyopathy and Myocarditis Registry. *European Heart Journal, 45*, 1443–1454. https://www.semanticscholar.org/paper/2793c5d2a69cae22a54626be7c70d2ba689860a1 (accessed on 15th July 2025).

28. Kauk, A., Kungurtseva, A. G., Sokolova, E. S., Pavlinova, E. B., & Dakuko, A. N. (2024). Difficulties in detecting and differential diagnosis of dilated cardiomyopathy in young children. *Meditsinskiy Sovet = Medical Council.* https://www.semanticscholar.org/paper/f667b6127a6741b4605fcad7b480bc5fd077c0e2 (accessed on 15th July 2025).

29. Klein, C. H., Oliveira, G. M. M., Salim, T. R., Soares, D. A., et al. (2019). Fetal and maternal factors are associated with mortality due to circulatory system disorders in children. https://core.ac.uk/download/268291865.pdf (accessed on 15th July 2025).

30. Lee, I. K., Lee, K. H., Han, H. J., Choi, J., Kim, N., & Kim, K. (2025). Different axis approaches for ultrasound-guided centrally inserted central catheterization in children: A systematic review and meta-analysis of randomized controlled trials. *Frontiers in Surgery, 12.* https://www.semanticscholar.org/paper/d74375865bfd78d462abef7871edd9f0d2801440 (accessed on 15th July 2025).

31. Lee, T. M., & Ware, S. M. (2015). Toward personalized medicine: Does genetic diagnosis of pediatric cardiomyopathy influence patient management? https://core.ac.uk/download/84830861.pdf (accessed on 15th July 2025).

32. Llanos, C., Friedman, D., Saxena, A., Izmirly, P., Tseng, C., Dische, R., Abellar, R., et al. (2012). Anatomical and pathological findings in hearts from fetuses and infants with cardiac manifestations of neonatal lupus. *Rheumatology, 51*(6), 1086–1092. https://www.semanticscholar.org/paper/18ee106d7aaef9204e45d2e184bd1fbb154aece5 (accessed on 15th July 2025).

33. Mariucci, E., Bronzetti, G., & Donti, A. (2024). [Sudden cardiac arrest in children and adolescents: Diagnosis, clinical presentation and peculiarities]. *Giornale Italiano di Cardiologia, 25*(9), 640–649. https://www.semanticscholar.org/paper/614feb0dd6897c5ad2dd3410e885eb18d390ec5d (accessed on 15th July 2025).

34. Maron, B. J., Dearani, J. A., Smedira, N. G., Schaff, H. V., Wang, S., Rastegar, H., Ralph-Edwards, A., et al. (2022). Ventricular septal myectomy for obstructive hypertrophic cardiomyopathy (Analysis spanning 60 years of practice): AJC expert panel. *The American Journal of Cardiology, 180*, 124–139. https://doi.org/10.1016/j.amjcard.2022.06.007 (accessed on 15th July 2025).

35. Maron, B. J., Dearani, J. A., Smedira, N. G., Schaff, H. V., Wang, S., Rastegar, H., Ralph-Edwards, A., et al. (2022). Ventricular septal myectomy for obstructive hypertrophic cardiomyopathy (Analysis spanning 60 years of practice): AJC expert panel. *The American Journal of Cardiology, 180*, 124–139. https://doi.org/10.1016/j.amjcard.2022.06.007 (accessed on 15th July 2025).

36. Moeinipour, Y., Moeinipour, A., Alizadeh, B., Raesi, R., & Naghibi, M. (2025). The incidence of heart failure in children with congenital heart disease: A prospective cohort study. *Current Cardiology Reviews.* https://www.semanticscholar.org/paper/8d18325b8bf4c44cdc98c404e1de44857f6a3b6a (accessed on 15th July 2025).

37. Navarro, J., Jeewa, A., Fang, J., Lee, D. S., & Jean-St-Michel, E. (2024). Abstract 4134957: Survival and cardiac recovery in pediatric dilated cardiomyopathy: A long-term cohort study of risk factors, prognosis, and health outcomes followed into adulthood. *Circulation.* https://www.semanticscholar.org/paper/15d0f3f27bbf8e758cd447cd2204af9d5996ca54 (accessed on 15th July 2025).

38. Nguyen, T., Rathakrishnan, A., Bompard, M., She, T., & Chicaiza, H. (2025). Point-of-care ultrasound diagnosis of restrictive cardiomyopathy in a 3-year-old patient. *Pediatric Emergency Care.* https://www.semanticscholar.org/paper/9d4208c79f51df911b6bce09e3c0544d72297016 (accessed on 15th July 2025).

39. Olaosebikan, R. R., Crowgey, E. L., Abdullahi, S., Wudil, B. J., Gambo, S., Ramakrishnaiah, R., Bello, M., et al. (2024). Genetic and clinical determinants of stroke in sickle cell patients: Insights from a Nigerian cohort. *Blood.* https://www.semanticscholar.org/paper/54cb5a9a2deaedf79fdc737ab304206b40acb3f2 (accessed on 15th July 2025).

40. Pan, Y., & Jiao, F. (2025). Addressing functional constipation in children: A call for comprehensive and collaborative management. *World Journal of Gastroenterology, 31.* https://www.semanticscholar.org/paper/093b9d5bd9ff4fa1b8c9455e702ba995d8092b54 (accessed on 15th July 2025).

41. Park, S. U., Song, K., Kim, Y., Kim, I. C., Kim, J. B., Park, N., & Jang, W. (2023). Surgical results of the superior vena cava intimal layer-only suture technique in heart transplantation. *Journal of Chest Surgery, 56*, 322–327. https://www.semanticscholar.org/paper/1a2729070cca805f6a23c62e56e495ad08fa2938 (accessed on 15th July 2025).

42. Roth, G. A., Mensah, G. A., Johnson, C. O., Addolorato, G., Ammirati, E., Baddour, L. M., Barengo, N. C., et al. (2020). Global burden of cardiovascular diseases and risk factors, 1990–2019. *Journal of the American College of Cardiology, 76*, 2982–3021. https://doi.org/10.1016/j.jacc.2020.11.010 (accessed on 15th July 2025).

43. Spaapen, T. O. M., Bohte, A. E., Slieker, M., & Grotenhuis, H. (2024). Cardiac MRI in diagnosis, prognosis, and follow-up of hypertrophic cardiomyopathy in children: Current perspectives.

The British Journal of Radiology, 97, 875–881. https://www.semanticscholar.org/paper/492cdc23a36e2cfe90a9328fcfe44013d8598693 (accessed on 15th July 2025).

44. Stephens, E. H., Dearani, J. A., Guleserian, K. J., Overman, D. M., Tweddell, J. S., Backer, C. L., Romano, J. C., et al. (2020). COVID-19: Crisis management in congenital heart surgery. *The Annals of Thoracic Surgery, 110*, 701–706. https://doi.org/10.1016/j.athoracsur.2020.04.001 (accessed on 15th July 2025).
45. Stout, K., Daniels, C. J., Aboulhosn, J., Bozkurt, B., Broberg, C. S., Colman, J. M., Crumb, S. R., et al. (2018). 2018 AHA/ACC guideline for the management of adults with congenital heart disease: A report of the American College of Cardiology/American Heart Association Task Force on Clinical Practice Guidelines. *Circulation, 139*. https://doi.org/10.1161/cir.0000000000000603 (accessed on 15th July 2025).
46. Suh, D., & Koh, Y. (2011). Assessment of bronchodilator responsiveness after methacholine-induced bronchoconstriction. *Allergy, Asthma & Immunology Research, 3*, 215–216. https://www.semanticscholar.org/paper/8cdbe6af90cecf1d895fdb795c35b7f1d7f1bc73 (accessed on 15th July 2025).
47. Tanwar, S. S., Dwivedi, S., Khan, S., & Sharma, S. (2025). Cardiomyopathies and a brief insight into DOX-induced cardiomyopathy. *The Egyptian Heart Journal, 77*. https://www.semanticscholar.org/paper/4a106bc1178b45f6b4117b832a44eeef7482ebe0 (accessed on 15th July 2025).
48. Yun, J., Shin, J., Lee, H., Kim, D., Choi, I. Y., & Kim, M. (2023). Characteristics and potential challenges of digital-based interventions for children and young people: Scoping review. *Journal of Medical Internet Research, 25*. https://www.semanticscholar.org/paper/2d3279dcf8cddcdbcab7511e03bd506bbc03ce38 (accessed on 15th July 2025).
49. Zaffanello, M., Pietrobelli, A., Zoccante, L., Sacchetto, L., Nosetti, L., Piazza, M., & Piacentini, G. (2024). Insights into pediatric sleep disordered breathing: Exploring risk factors, surgical interventions, and physical and scholastic performance at follow-up. *Children, 11*. https://www.semanticscholar.org/paper/994e458aa42ee18d5a1bf3b98827aa6eefafbf6d (accessed on 15th July 2025).
50. Zeppenfeld, K., Tfelt-Hansen, J., Riva, M., Winkel, B. G., Behr, E. R., Blom, N. A., Charron, P., et al. (2022). 2022 ESC guidelines for the management of patients with ventricular arrhythmias and the prevention of sudden cardiac death. *European Heart Journal, 43*, 3997–4126. https://doi.org/10.1093/eurheartj/ehac262 (accessed on 15th July 2025).
51. Zhang, T., Wu, W., Shu, Y., Weng, H., Weng, M., Zhou, Y., & Wang, X. (2025). The effectiveness of ERCP in managing preoperative complications of choledochal cysts in children and its role in facilitating early surgical intervention. *Frontiers in Pediatrics, 13*. https://www.semanticscholar.org/paper/9513ffa483f16ae9f7b7f9821258f1462efdb188 (accessed on 15th July 2025).
52. Zhao, H., Rong, X., Zhang, Q., Ma, T. T., Yan, H., Zhou, T., & Zhang, Y. (2025). Factors influencing on functional independence outcomes after hospitalization and rehabilitation in children with spinal cord injury. *BMC Pediatrics, 25*. https://www.semanticscholar.org/paper/dda956e7542d306268020527e7357ce82622d76a (accessed on 15th July 2025).

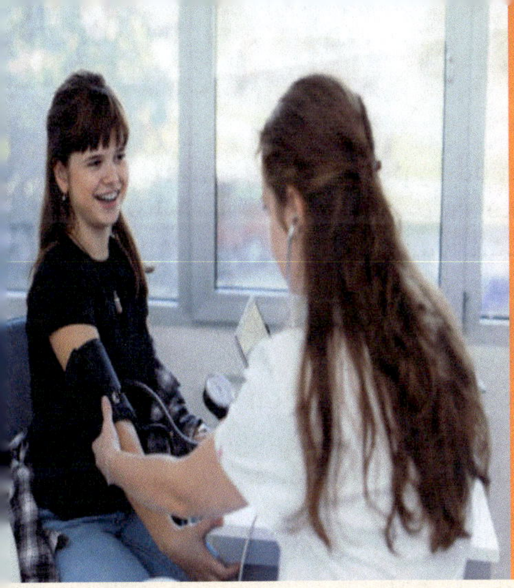

Chapter 12

HYPERTENSION IN CHILDREN AND ADOLESCENTS

Contents

Introduction

Hypertension, or high blood pressure, has traditionally been thought of as a condition prevalent primarily in adults. There is growing evidence that there is an alarming rise in hypertension among children and adolescents. This is significant because hypertension can lead to serious long-term health consequences, including heart disease, stroke, and kidney disease. The definition of hypertension in young people is central to the development of appropriate prevention and management plans. The American Heart Association guidelines for hypertension recommend an aggressive approach in the assessment and management of children's blood pressure, emphasizing early identification and behavioral modifications to reduce cardiovascular risk. As the epidemic of obesity continues, the relationship between obesity and child hypertension indicates all the more imperative a role for focused interventions. The subtleties of childhood hypertension demand a comprehensive process for diagnosis and treatment. As compared with adults, who most commonly have secondary hypertension as a result of disease states other than hypertension itself, childhood hypertension is more likely to be caused by lifestyle factors such as dietary intake and exercise patterns. The ACC/AHA highlight the importance of clinical practice guidelines to direct healthcare providers in evaluation and management of childhood hypertension. These guidelines stress a solid base derived from systematic reviews of the prevailing evidence, with assurances that recommendations are scientific in nature and relevant clinically. As hypertension can have long-term effects on a child's future health, following such guidelines is critical to paving the way to a healthier population in the future. Determination of the determinants of hypertension in youth at the societal and behavioral level is critical to the efficacy of intervention. The epidemic of obesity, diabetes, and sedentary lifestyle has been linked to elevated blood pressure among children and adolescents. These many factors necessitate interdisciplinary collaboration between providers of healthcare, educators, and families in order to create a healthy environment supportive of healthy lifestyle habits. Additionally, public health programs aimed at increasing awareness of hypertension and risk factors among children are necessary. Giving priority to education and preventive interventions, stakeholders can facilitate families to adopt proactive steps in monitoring and controlling blood pressure among children. In summary, managing hypertension in children and adolescents is both difficult and challenging, calling for a customized, multi-aspect approach that will improve the health outcomes of future generations.

Definition of Hypertension

Hypertension definition is the key to proper diagnosis and management, particularly in children and adolescents. Hypertension is characterized by elevated blood pressure levels that, if not corrected, may result in numerous cardiovascular complications in the future. In pediatrics, the hypertension definition is not standardized on all boards but varies based on age, gender, and height percentile.

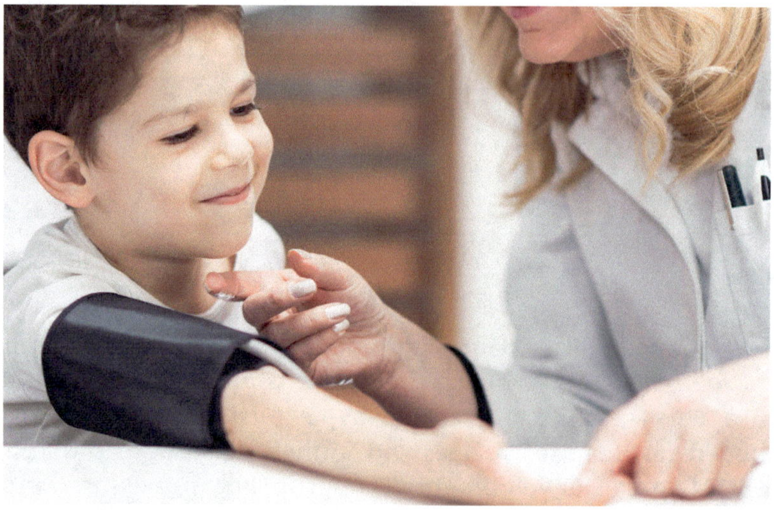

Figure 12.1. Hypertension in children.

Source: https://ae-parenting.s3.ap-south-1.amazonaws.com/2018/04/656352610-H.jpg.

The recent guidelines emphasize the importance of proper steps being taken to measure blood pressure with appropriate methods and age-specific normative values to classify the levels of blood pressure accurately. Since hypertension in children can be different from that in adults, accurate classification is important to determine the treatment options and assess the risk of diseases such as heart diseases and stroke in adult life. Another main consideration in the definition of hypertension is recognition of the phenomenon of masked hypertension, especially reported in some pediatric populations. Masked hypertension describes circumstances where a child's blood pressure is within normal ranges on the day of a clinic visit but is actually elevated in the home or by ambulatory blood pressure monitoring. Masked hypertension is said to have a prevalence as much as 60% in certain groups, for example, patients with chronic kidney disease or obesity, and therefore the office readings taken normally may not accurately represent the true blood pressure profile of such patients. Research has shown that among healthy children with risk factors for hypertension, masked hypertension is present at a rate of about 9%, necessitating individualized screening avenues to identify those at risk and prevent future long-term consequences on health (Tomáš et al., 2023) (Figure 12.1).

The management of pediatric hypertension is also complicated by the realization that no overall agreement on best practice exists, and consequently, this dictates the definitions in clinical guidelines. This is something that the European Society of Cardiology is well aware of and has thus sought to produce a comprehensive Consensus Document specifically for hypertension in children and adolescents. This article talks about some of these areas like clinical evaluation, evaluation of target organ damage, and cause determination of hypertension. It lays stress on the identification of concomitant risk factors, primarily obesity, and recommends lifestyle modification as an integral aspect of treatment. Also, it calls for further research into the establishment of normative blood pressure tables in relation to a multi-ethnic child population and emphasizes the necessity of randomized clinical trials towards enhancing management paradigms of hypertension in children and adolescents (de Simone et al., 2022).

Importance of Addressing Hypertension in Youth

The rising prevalence of hypertension among young people has become a contagious public health problem that needs to be addressed with all due haste. Adolescents with elevated blood pressure are already experiencing dangerous short- and long-term health complications, including cardiovascular disease, obesity, and diabetes. Early life hypertension not only puts one at risk of developing linked chronic diseases in adult life but also raises treatment and management healthcare expenses. Hypertension control in youth is important in reducing future morbidity and mortality rates. Early intervention through lifestyle modifications, such as increased physical activity and improved eating habits, can significantly alter the trajectory of blood pressure values. Recommendations from World Health Organization favor children and adolescents having a minimum of 60 minutes of daily physical activity that is moderate to vigorous, and this is directly associated with the cardiovascular effects on health and blood pressure regulation (Bull et al., 2020). Facilitating the environment of physical activity, thus, can act as a primary preventive measure. Additionally, rising pediatric obesity makes it difficult to combat hypertension among youths. Presently, about 17% of American youth and children suffer from obesity, which is strongly related to their elevated blood pressure rates (Dennis et al., 2017). Additional body mass adds extra load to the cardiovascular system, creating a vicious cycle that threatens both imminent and later development health. Obesity comorbidities must be identified and treated; they are often compounded and can make hypertension worse. Early intervention of remedies on healthy lifestyle changes is necessary to prevent obesity and obesity-related health consequences. This includes promoting healthy nutrition and adequate exercise, which can place adolescents in a favorable position to maintain healthy blood pressure levels. Prevention of the intertwined issues of obesity and hypertension among this group through public health interventions can promote the overall health outcome and quality of life among adolescents. Finally, complete management of hypertension in adolescents should not only encompass medical treatment but should extend to mental and emotional status as well. Psychological stressors such as bullying and school pressure can induce unhealthy coping strategies, including inappropriate diet and inactivity, which worsen hypertension. The need for mental health assistance in the school and community environments has come to the forefront as a means of addressing the root causes of stress and anxiety in young people. The use of programs addressing both physical and emotional health can result in an overall approach to the treatment of hypertension. Due to the multifactorial etiology of youth hypertension, an interdisciplinary team effort by medical caregivers, school staff, and family members is necessary. By placing a premium on physical and mental well-being, within the context of hypertension prevention and control, society can play a pivotal role in furthering the health of forthcoming generations.

12.1. Prevalence of Hypertension in Children and Adolescents

The rising prevalence of hypertension among young people is a public health issue with a multitude of facets that need to be addressed expeditiously. Hypertension, which was once perceived as largely an adult condition, is increasingly being diagnosed among children and teens due to an accumulation of lifestyle factors such as the burgeoning epidemic of obesity and sedentary behavior. This development is alarming, as high blood pressure in youth can lead to early onset cardiovascular disease, propounding long-term health hazards. The recommendations of present research synthesize important details and medical practice, underlining the urgency of a robust system to screen, assess, and manage hypertension among young individuals (Agabiti-Rosei et al., 2016). Improved clinical care and education can significantly contribute to early intervention strategies, eventually lowering the complications of hypertension in later life. The potential of obesity as a cause of significant risk for hypertension in children and adolescents cannot be overstressed. In the country and in states, trends in obesity closely follow rises in hypertension diagnoses, illustrating the critical interrelatedness of the conditions. Whereas the rate of obesity has accelerated during the past few decades, related government policy and public health programming have all too often lagged behind in both size and effectiveness. In establishing the status of current policy responses to obesity, researchers justify an overarching strategy through food guidelines, encouragement of exercise, and school-based education to combat this public health epidemic (Laura et al., 2004). These particular interventions not only cure obesity but are also a preventive strategy against hypertension and its ill health effects in subsequent years. Enhanced research on hypertension has shed further light on the clinical significance of isolated systolic hypertension and the necessity of accurate blood pressure measurement in various environments. New methods for assessing vascular health have been devised, thus leading to more precise detection of hypertension in youth. Out-of-office blood pressure measurement, for instance, is gaining prominence for having knowledge of the true states of blood pressure in children and adolescents. Such methods allow clinicians to more effectively stratify risk and personalize treatment interventions as appropriate (Agabiti-Rosei et al., 2016). As knowledge of the prevalence of hypertensions grows, it supports the development of evidence-based public health policies that strive to promote healthier lifestyle choices among the young, in the hope of decreasing hypertension and overall health outcomes.

12.1.1. Statistical Data on Hypertension Rates

The epidemic increase in the incidence of hypertension in children and adolescents has emerged as a global serious public health problem. Available literature suggests high rates of high blood pressure among this age group, with rates as high as 13.7% for increased blood pressure and 12.9% for hypertension in some groups. For instance, a study involving Lithuanian children and adolescents identified that somebody measures like the neck circumference, mid-upper arm circumference, and wrist circumference have close correlations with such high blood pressure rates. Specifically, the odds ratios after adjustment presented that higher readings are significantly linked with increased risks of hypertension, indicating that there is an urgent need for preventive measures through lifestyle modification and frequent follow-ups to prevent these rising numbers and their effects on long-term cardiovascular consequences (Stankut et al., 2024). Of greater significance, the impact of hypertension extends beyond simply being statistical occurrences; it also encompasses underlying physiology, particularly relating to endothelial function. A comparative study in children with primary arterial hypertension revealed injury to endothelium-dependent vasodilatation responses (Figure 12.2).

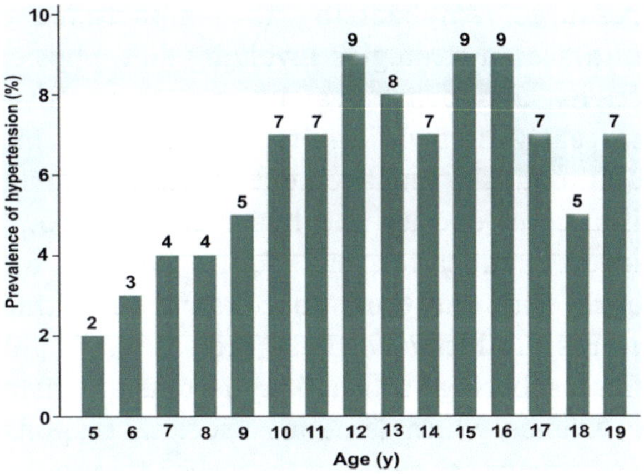

Figure 12.2. Prevalence of hypertension among children and adolescents.

Source: https://media.springernature.com/lw1200/springer-static/image/art%3A10.1007%2Fs12098-021-03686-9/MediaObjects/12098_2021_3686_Fig5_HTML.png.

Out of 52 patients, hypertensive subjects had a substantial reduction in brachial artery flow-mediated dilation, an important indicator of vascular function. This compromised reactivity of the vessels, linking hypertension to potential future cardiovascular events, indicates not just the prevalence of the disorder but also its negative health consequences that may evolve if left uncontrolled. These findings reinforce the importance of early intervention to preserve vascular health in children since the developed arterial health in childhood can have a dramatic influence on future cardiovascular risks (Jukić et al., 2024). In addition, the interaction between obesity and hypertension compounds the public health situation among children and adolescents. With rising prevalence of obesity, risks for the development of hypertension also rise, thus emphasizing integrated planning of obesity prevention that includes blood pressure screening. It has been shown that high body mass index (BMI) in youths is linked to significant increases in both systolic and diastolic blood pressures, emphasizing the importance of multifaceted strategies involving diet, physical activity, and behavioral interventions. Given that early lifestyle habits will carry on into adulthood, the management of the interfacing diseases of obesity and hypertension through targeted education can equip children and youth with the tools to construct healthier futures. Collectively, these facts and insights offer a sobering portrait of hypertensions rising prevalence, which demands a societal response to safeguard the cardiovascular health of future generations.

12.1.2. Demographic Variations in Prevalence

The prevalence of hypertension among children and adolescents reflects significant demographic variation on the basis of a large number of determinants including socioeconomic status, ethnicity, and residence. Research identifies that the prevalence of hypertension is much higher in children belonging to low socioeconomic status, often attributable to inadequate access to health care services, healthy foods, and physical exercise. Furthermore, disparities in the quality of health care can also increase such problems in susceptible groups. These socioeconomic determinants influence not only the development but also the control and treatment outcome of hypertension, pinpointing an important point for public health interventions towards health inequities reduction among young people. It is through the knowledge of these demographic elements that strategic formulation is shaped on how to address the endemicity of hypertension among vulnerable young people. Ethnic and racial disparity are also central in the prevalence of hypertension among youths. Studies have shown that African American youth and children are more likely to have higher hypertension rates than Hispanic or white children and youth. The occurrence is thought to be due to both environmental and lifestyle, as well as genetic, factors, including diet and level of physical activity. In addition, the effect of stress created by socioeconomic challenges and potential discrimination can also contribute to the increased rates in these minority groups. Understanding these variations is crucial not only for the development of intervention strategies but also for facilitating inclusive healthcare practice that takes into consideration the unique issues of different demographic groups (Margaret et al., 2018). Differences in hypertension prevalence have also been identified geographically, with urban locations reporting different rates from rural communities. Urban teenagers may have a higher incidence of hypertension by lifestyle factors, such as being more inactive, having higher intake of processed foods, and being more exposed to psychosocial stressors. Rural kids can also experience difficulties with healthcare access, contributing to a higher underdiagnosis of illnesses such as hypertension. This geographical variation emphasizes the need for targeted public health interventions addressing different lifestyle and environmental determinants influencing hypertension among various populations. By education and access to affordable healthcare, the stakeholders can take steps to minimize the influence of geographical variation and assure better health outcomes for all adolescents and children regardless of where they reside (Rebecca et al., 2016).

12.1.3. Trends Over Recent Years

Hypertension in youths has become a growing concern in recent years with the new trends suggesting an upward trajectory. A 2007 to 2021 data analysis of the Korea National Health and Nutrition Examination Survey indicated ominous trends of overweight and obesity and elevated blood pressure (BP) levels among youth. Specifically, the prevalence of elevated blood pressure was at around 8.22% and hypertension at 10.46% in subjects aged 10–18 years, which reflects a long-term public health concern, particularly in populations that are already experiencing rising obesity rates. While these figures portray a cause for concern, the fact that statistically significant year-to-year differences are not evidenced proves there is a complex interplay of determinants in play on these health indicators, necessitating differential prevention and intervention strategies in this high-risk group (Jeong et al., 2025). Considering longer trends, the evidence of past eras indicates a trend of increase in mean systolic BP among children of Korea, with significant changes being noted between 2007 and 2015. The study revealed a mean increase in systolic BP by 3.9 mm Hg, with a high prevalence of hypertension among the obese subgroup that increased to 27.7% during the observed period. These findings emphasize the extent to which higher body mass index (BMI) is highly associated with elevated blood pressure levels among adolescents. Although the overall trend indicates worsening levels of hypertension, an evident stratification exists regarding risk factors corresponding to different body composition profiles, emphasizing the importance of particular preventive health interventions focused on individual subgroups of children and adolescents (Cho et al., 2020) (Figure 12.3).

Normal BP	<90th percentile
Elevated BP	>90th percentile to <95th percentile OR 120/80 mmHg to <95th percentile (whichever is lower)
Stage 1 HTN	≥95th percentile to <95th percentile + 12 mmHg OR 130/80 to 139/89 mmHg (whichever is lower)
Stage 2 HTN	>95th percentile + 12 mmHg OR ≥ 140/90 mmHg (whichever is lower)
BP: blood pressure; HTN: hypertension	

Figure 12.3. Classification of BP/HTN in children aged between 1 and 13 years. Cutoff values for BP in children <13 years of age using percentiles or absolute values.

Source: https://www.mdpi.com/2227-9067/11/5/518.

The ramifications of the trends are far-reaching and could, if unchecked, signal the beginning of a public health crisis. The increase in hypertension among youth can have serious long-term health effects, including cardiovascular disease that typically appears in later life. Concurrently, the co-morbidity of obesity and hypertension is particularly disturbing, suggesting that future prevention efforts against disease must simultaneously address both conditions. Moreover, awareness of the heterogeneity of hypertension risk factors across the population such as sex and age is expected to facilitate stronger surveillance and prevention. Overall, these reports indicate the need for a multi-dimensional approach to reverse the rising trends in hypertension and underscore the impact of powerful modifiable determinants, such as diet and exercise, to reduce the trends (Cho et al., 2020; Jeong et al., 2025).

12.2. Causes of Hypertension in Youth

The increase in hypertension among the pediatric population has created serious concern in the medical profession. At the top of the list of causes for the rise is high levels of obesity among youth that have been strongly linked to eating patterns such as a diet that is not good and a sedentary lifestyle. These affect an unhealthy weight gain, which poses additional stress to the cardiovascular system, which may affect blood pressure levels. While a leading causative factor remains obesity, it should be indicated that youth-onset hypertension can either be primary or secondary hypertension. Secondary hypertension—caused by identifiable reasons such as renal parenchymal diseases, congenital disorders, and renovascular disease—is particularly more prevalent in children younger than 12 years of age (Chedid et al., 2008). Therefore, a holistic comprehension of these varying causes is essential in order to successfully treat hypertension in the pediatric population. Additionally, adolescence brings with it a myriad of physiological and hormonal changes that predispose an individual to elevated blood pressure levels. During adolescence, children experience growth spurts and hormonal fluctuations, which may influence vascular resistance and cardiovascular health. This transition phase can exacerbate conditions of obesity, leading to increased susceptibility to hypertension. Further, higher degrees of stress, either in terms of academic load, interpersonal relationships, or family dynamics, can also influence blood pressure outcomes at this age level. Cultural and social determinants can also reveal genetic susceptibilities to hypertension, meaning a multi-disciplinary approach is needed to properly understand this disease. Knowledge of these factors will aid healthcare practitioners in identifying at-risk populations and establishing early interventions, fostering improved health outcomes in affected young people (Ellis et al., 2011) (Figure 12.4).

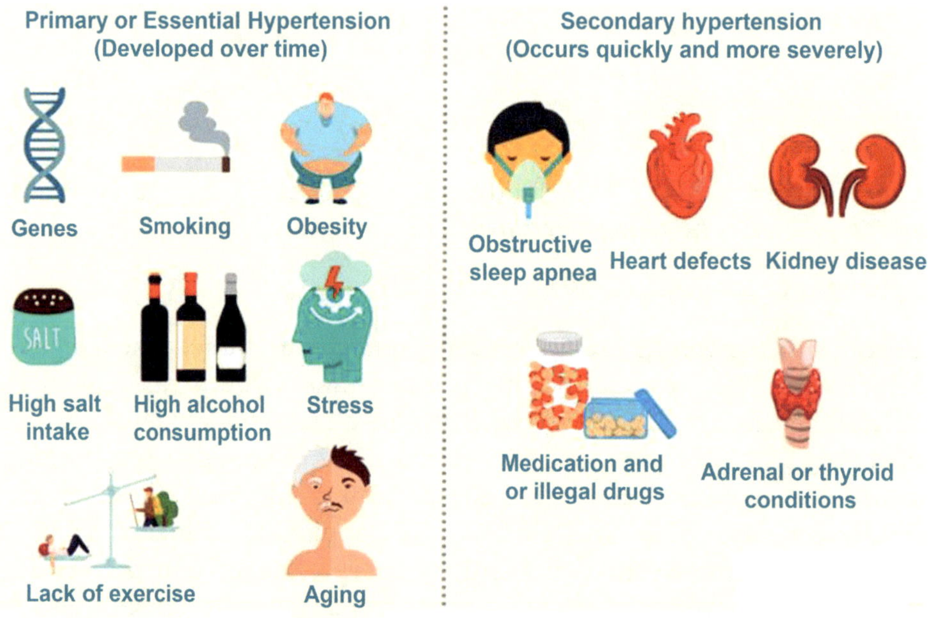

Figure 12.4. Causes of primary hypertension and secondary hypertensions.

Source: https://external-content.duckduckgo.com/iu/?u=https%3A%2F%2Ffaithhearing.com%2Fwp-content%2Fuploads%2F2021%2F07%2Fsingapore-hypertension-causes-primary-essential-secondary-876x657.png&f=1&nofb=1&ipt=23740c1b4dd9bc4e72f04b5b0cff8f406c11e9f3421090108bb2d4bab8a44616.

Lastly, lifestyle issues and technological thrust need to be part of the discussion of hypertension in kids and teens. Sedentary living through excess video game playing and television viewing is responsible for lack of exercise and poor eating habits, all of which result in obesity. Lack of physical exercise combined with the practice of unhealthy snacking can lay the ground for high blood pressure in kids. Furthermore, the risk of drug use, including illegal drugs and prescribed medication, could exacerbate hypertension. As part of a comprehensive public health initiative, pediatricians and health educators must emphasize lifestyle modification, including more exercise and improved dietary intake, to mitigate these risk factors. Through holistic considerations of these lifestyle etiologies, improved prevention and management can be realized for hypertension among pre-school children and adolescents (Chedid et al., 2008).

12.2.1. Genetic Factors and Family History

The role of family history and genetics in the development of hypertension in children and adolescents has been fully acknowledged by physicians. Numerous studies have established that children with a family history of hypertension are at a higher risk of developing elevated blood pressure. This interaction may be due to both genetic predispositions, such as inherited factors that affect vascular resistance and control of blood pressure, and shared family environmental factors.

Furthermore, the involved genes in hypertension are also multifactorial, typically multiple genes, each having a small effect. The genetic susceptibility based on family history can hence be of great significance in determining populations at risk and for the provision of early preventive treatments. These targeted interventions would be successful in minimizing long-term health risk due to hypertension among affected adolescents, resulting in an improved prognosis in the future. Despite the obvious correlation between family history and hypertension, application of parental history as a screening procedure for selecting children at risk has been reported wanting (Figure 12.5).

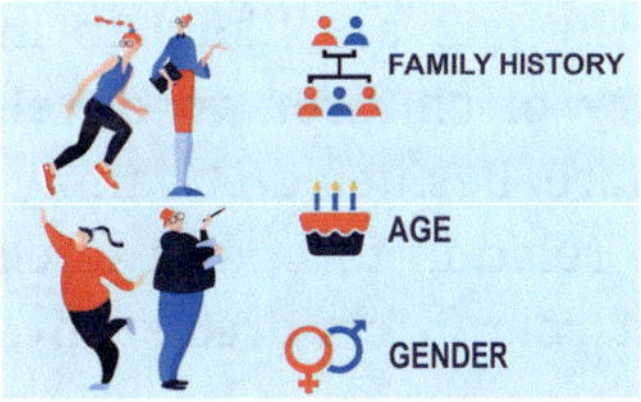

Figure 12.5. Genetic risk factors.

Source: https://external-content.duckduckgo.com/iu/?u=https%3A%2F%2Fmedical.andonline.com%2Fwp-content%2Fuploads%2F2021%2F08%2FJuly-Blog-Images_Risk-Factors-1030x687.jpeg&f=1&nofb=1&ipt=d90beabc6243312e9327877fe349a7d1da42f2b0500bfbca5d6465c4d29da822.

Meta-analysis regarding the utility of a positive family history of hypertension for targeted screening indicated that there was a low sensitivity rate, whereby large numbers of risk children would go undetected in the case where screening were mainly reliant upon family history. This limitation serves to emphasize the need for broader screening tests which are not totally dependent upon familial influences. Also, United States-based cost-effectiveness analyses have indicated that family history-based targeted screening strategies need not always be the most cost-effective approach, as they tend to be more expensive and less effective relative to the universal screening methods. Consequently, healthcare providers are required to advocate comprehensive screening processes involving including genetic factors along with standard measurement of blood pressure for all children. Yet another consideration for the management of hypertension risk in children is genetic susceptibility interacting with environmental influences. Lifestyle, such as diet and exercise, is usually encompassed in the family history and serves to enhance the risk of child development of hypertension as well. For instance, families that consume similar types of diet characterized by elevated sodium and unhealthy fats are likely to increase the susceptibility of children to developing high blood pressure. Besides diet, family values and activities in relation to body exercise can also play a great role in children's physical health practices. In this aspect, a holistic approach to evaluating and addressing hypertension risk is imperative. Methods including the incorporation of genetic factor information, comprehensive family health screening, and education about healthier lifestyles can lead to improved prevention and control of hypertension in children and adolescents and at the same time educate families about the importance of these factors in optimizing overall health.

12.2.2. Lifestyle Factors: Diet and Physical Activity

The lifestyle of adolescents and children is largely responsible for determining their overall well-being, particularly hypertension. Ingestion of highly processed foods, excessive sodium, and intake of sugars significantly increases the blood pressure in adolescents. As there is an increase in the cases of child obesity, there is also an increase in the cases of obesity-related hypertension. Studies have revealed that the development of high blood pressure often begins in childhood, with unhealthy food choices being a major driving force in its development. National Health Surveys have reported a link between obesity and increased rates of hypertension, illustrating how food habits formed throughout these initial years can be capable of impacting cardiovascular health for many years (Jeong et al., 2024) (Figure 12.6).

Besides, the pathogenic mechanism of hypertension in obese children emphasizes the role of nutritional management as a cornerstone strategy for treatment and prevention of hypertension. Physical exercise also plays an extremely vital role in preventing hypertension among children and adolescents. Not only does regular exercise contribute to maintenance of normal body weight, but it also has a role in optimized cardiovascular function as well as in regulation of blood pressure.

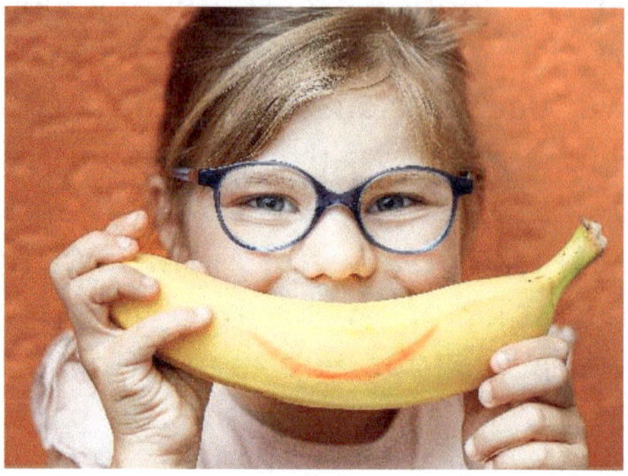

Figure 12.6. Diet factors influencing their overall health, particularly regarding hypertension.

Source: https://www.apa.org/images/kids-health-eating-tile_tcm7-320645.jpg.

Sedentary behavior, such as overexposure to screen time, has also been inextricably linked with obesity, a state that worsens hypertension (Bhagat et al., 2024). Adolescents, more so than other age groups, find it difficult to incorporate exercise into their lifestyle, primarily due to schoolwork and social pressures. Promoting active living through education interventions, public activities, and familial support is thus imperative in changing the decline in physical activity. Establishment of exercise routines during adolescence can be a strong foundation for lifelong health routines, significantly reducing the risk of developing hypertension and other lifestyle diseases. A comprehensive intervention towards lifestyle components of diet and exercise is needed to properly manage hypertension in children and adolescents. Intervention must be aimed at educating the family on nutrition and the importance of balanced diets, along with creating an enabling environment for physical activity. Programmatic interventions focusing on the benefits of balanced diet and exercise can satisfactorily alter the trend of rising incidence of hypertension in young groups. Moreover, measures discouraging use of inappropriate foods and promoting physical activity in young people through schools and communities must be accorded high priority. By encouraging the holistic approach emphasizing healthy life choices, public health initiatives have an important role in averting the epidemic of hypertension among youths and delivering better long-term cardiovascular health outcomes (Bhagat et al., 2024; Jeong et al., 2024).

12.2.3. Environmental Influences: Socioeconomic Status

It is important to know the relationship between socioeconomic status (SES) and hypertension when analyzing the increasing health issue among children and adolescents. SES covers a spectrum of variables, such as income, education level, and occupation, which all impact access to resources that have health effects. Increased SES is most commonly linked with better access to healthcare coverage, nutritional food, and physical activity environments that are all necessary for the maintenance of lower blood pressure levels. Decreased SES, conversely, will raise stress levels, limited access to healthy diet options, and environments that promote an inactive lifestyle, therefore hastening the onset of hypertension in adolescents. The rapid increase of noncommunicable diseases, like hypertension, particularly among low-income communities underscores a need for interventions that will curtail the impact of SES disparities on the health status of adolescents and children (Al-Hazzaa, 2022). Research has established that dietary habits and lifestyle patterns typical of different income groups play a major role in explaining the frequency of hypertension among children. Young people raised in lower SES settings are more likely to consume diets with high amounts of processed foods that have high levels of salt and sugar, leading to obesity and hypertension. Extensive exposure of the unhealthy food products to vulnerable populations by promotion further sustains these eating patterns. Low-income communities also have limited opportunities for safe physical activity and social support for healthy practices, further depressing active living. This cycle develops a self-reinforcing pattern where limited access to resources promoting health continues to limit the choices of children and youths, ultimately resulting in the maintenance of hypertension as well as other related health disorders (Nuryani et al., 2020). It is important to resolve the socioeconomic factors of health to create effective public health policies that will aid in reducing hypertension prevalence among children and youth. Interventions based on the community that address increased food availability, increased access to safe play spaces, and health education can empower families to choose healthier options. Policy aimed at reducing the financial cost of access to healthcare can further promote early detection and treatment of hypertension among youth. Incentivizing collaboration between schools, local authorities, and healthcare agencies can further promote a culture supportive of healthier living. By realizing the profound impact that socioeconomic status has on children's health, stakeholders can implement actions that reduce health inequalities and encourage long-term health for different populations (Al-Hazzaa, 2022).

12.3. Symptoms and Diagnosis

Hypertension identification among children and adolescents is critical to facilitate early detection and appropriate intervention. At times, hypertension signs are subtle or unclear, posing a challenge to both parents and health providers. Headaches, dizziness, and blurred vision are the clinical presentations despite the fact that these may not always be present. In most cases, the high blood pressure readings are found on an incidental basis during regular check-ups or when assessing other areas of concern. This highlighted the importance of routine blood pressure monitoring in the pediatric population, particularly in those at greater risk based on obesity, family history, or concurrent conditions like diabetes. The asymptomatic character of hypertension in this group is meant to reiterate the idea that forward-looking screening is essential for the detection of children who are likely to develop cardiovascular issues in the future. Diagnosis of the condition in children and adolescents requires careful clinical evaluation and the application of adequate criteria for diagnosis. Blood pressure readings must be done over multiple visits to allow for an accurate understanding of the child's baseline blood pressure. Pediatric guidelines have a tendency to classify hypertension based on percentiles to the child's age, sex, and height because direct comparison with adult values will not be accurate.

Such a multifaceted method of diagnosis is needed because normative values in children can vary greatly. Besides, as hypertension in this group can be secondary to some underlying cause, such causes should be identified during diagnosis. Hence, proper evaluation, in the form of history-taking and physical examination, is needed to separate primary hypertension from etiologies such as kidney disease or endocrinopathies, so that modifiable factors are adequately addressed. The addition of family education programs remains at the heart of enhancing overall awareness and management of hypertension in children and adolescents. The need to educate families on signs and symptoms of hypertension and the need for lifestyle modifications in order to prevent long-term health complications is a point of consensus among healthcare providers. Such education can enable the family to recognize hypertension symptoms, enhance compliance with treatment regimens, and encourage home blood pressure monitoring. There is evidence that if parents learn about risk factors and outcomes of hypertension, they are likely to embrace health-promoting behaviors. Such an aggressive approach not only represents an ancillary step towards proper disease management, but also aligns with broader-scale public health efforts to address the rising prevalence of hypertension and other chronic conditions among youths (Marklund et al., 2022; Saletin et al., 2020).

12.3.1. Common Symptoms of Hypertension in Youth

Teen hypertension may develop through a variety of symptoms, but most people who have it will present none. In fact, hypertension has even been called a silent killer because teenagers usually will not exhibit symptoms that are identifiable until the illness has been progressed in level. Repeated headaches, exhaustion, and dizziness are commonly experienced as symptoms that may indicate hypertension.

These symptoms and signs are frequently of another etiology, and diagnosis and management are thus delayed. Early identification is the priority, as untreated hypertension in youth has serious long-term health consequences, including increased susceptibility to cardiovascular morbidity later in life. Accordingly, awareness by parents, teachers, and healthcare providers of such subtle warning signs is necessary for early detection and treatment of this condition in children and adolescents and subsequently better health outcomes and quality of life. In one study evaluating the effectiveness of cardiac screening in young athletes, hypertension was found in approximately 6.2% of those screened (Fox et al., 2023) (Figure 12.7).

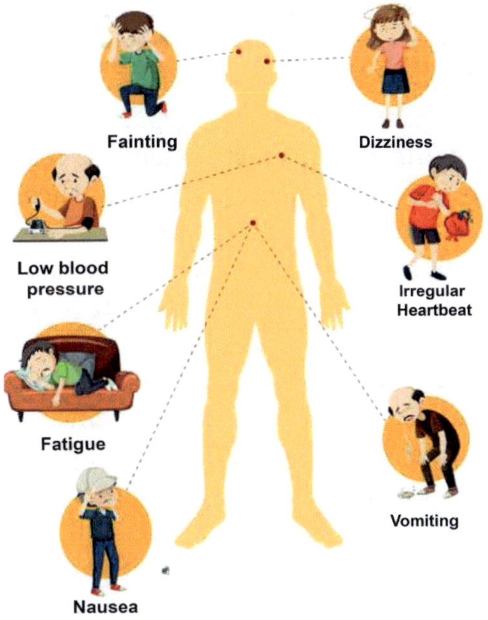

Figure 12.7. Hypertension signs and symptoms.

Source: https://myhealth-redcliffelabs.redcliffelabs.com/media/blog-content/1154/11207440_19871929_11zon-731x1024.jpg.

This frightening statistic highlights the importance of implementing screening programs among children to detect such disorders like hypertension in its initial stage before it gives rise to severe health complications. With the growing number of illnesses like type 2 diabetes among youngsters, the relationship between such illnesses and hypertension becomes evident. For instance, teens with type 2 diabetes have been noted to show increased prevalence of chronic comorbidities such as hypertension and other metabolic syndromes (Mangione et al., 2022). Consequently, it is essential to understand the common presenting symptoms of hypertension in those who are at risk of developing these interlinking ailments. The overlap between diabetes and hypertension renders it vital to have preventive healthcare interventions such as regular screening and awareness of symptoms among adolescent groups. In addition, the relationship between lifestyle factors and high blood pressure in children should not be overemphasized enough. Although obesity, physical inactivity, and poor diets may significantly impact the occurrence of high blood pressure in this group of children, it is important to realize that overweight may, in turn, lead to not only hypertension but also other related illnesses. Besides, increased physical activity level and intake of a balanced diet rich in fruits, vegetables, and whole grains can act as protection against the development of hypertension. Education of adolescents and their families about health may increase awareness about the importance of lifestyle practices and symptom recognition, thereby empowering them to seek early medical care when needed. This multi-disciplinary approach directed at symptom awareness and lifestyle modification is crucial to counteract the rising trend of adolescent and pediatric hypertension.

12.3.2. Diagnostic Criteria and Guidelines

The standards for diagnosing hypertension in children and adolescents have evolved significantly, pointing towards the need for stringent and accurate evaluation procedures. Current recommendations emphasize accurate blood pressure (BP) measurement in diverse settings because sporadic readings would not be representative of a patient's cardiovascular status. Proper technique is required, for example, relaxing the child when being measured and using the appropriate-sized blood pressure cuffs. There are also age, sex, and height percentiles provided in guidelines when measuring BP, allowing for a more personalized method of diagnosing hypertension. By incorporating these enhancements, health professionals can better identify risk youth, eventually avoiding the long-term effects of hypertension (Agabiti-Rosei et al., 2016). With a structured method, treatments will be that much better overall, and health outcomes for the pediatric population will be enhanced. In addition to precise measurement techniques, the detection of risk factors associated with increased blood pressure plays a key role in effective diagnosis. New evidence indicates that the burden of hypertension in children has exceeded 10%, thus becoming a great public health problem (Falkner et al., 2018) (Figure 12.8).

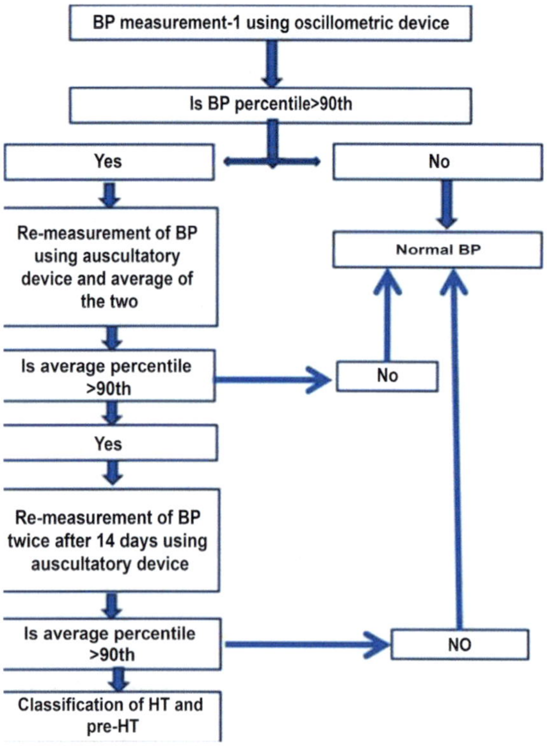

Figure 12.8. Diagnostic algorithm used for HT.

Source: https://www.ceghonline.com/article/S2213-3984%2821%2900140-8/fulltext.

Excess adiposity, eating habits, and psychosocial stressors have been pinpointed as major determinants of BP in adolescents. The guidelines emphasize targeting these risk factors during clinical assessment with importance placed on a broad assessment of each patient's overall wellness. Identification of these risk factors at early stages results in interventions that can make a significant difference in the trajectory of hypertension since these patients are at the entry stage of adult age. Through the production of a more integrated image of hypertension and determinants of risk, practitioners are then in a position to design holistic plans of management that adequately respond to the causation of the condition, rather than its symptomatology. Lastly, the diagnostic guidelines and criteria extend beyond identification into sound treatment practice for managing hypertension. Recommendations have lifestyle modification as the first line of management, with emphasis on the need for children and youth to engage in regular physical activity, follow a low sodium balanced diet, and achieve a healthy weight. To those who do not succeed with these first-line measures, medication may be necessary. Monitoring and follow-up are necessary, with subsequent untreated hypertension having the potential to lead to severe cardiovascular consequences in the future (Agabiti-Rosei et al., 2016). Adhering to these long guidelines will enable medical practitioners to be well equipped with the necessary tools and information needed to combat the growing phenomenon of hypertension among young adults, taking on an active role in preventing impending health disasters.

12.3.3. Importance of Regular Screening

Screening for hypertension in children and adolescents on a routine basis is crucial in the early detection and intervention, reducing ultimately long-term health risk factors for being hypertensive. Hypertension in children is typically asymptomatic and hence leads to delayed diagnosis and treatment. Regular blood pressure measurement at annual health check-ups is recommended by the American Academy of Pediatrics as a method of detecting at-risk individuals. By regular screening of the pediatric population, medical practitioners can monitor changes in blood pressure and implement preventive measures early, addressing potential health complications of obesity, renal disease, or other cardiovascular conditions. Such an early watchfulness is very important in hypertension management since uncontrolled high blood pressure complications such as stroke or heart disease can begin at an early age and extend into adulthood (Madhu et al., 2020). The importance of regular screening for hypertension is underlined by the universal prevalence of the disease among children and adolescents, particularly in high-risk groups. Estimates show that more and more youth are developing hypertension due to excessive weight and sedentary lifestyles. Regular screening makes it possible to identify hypertensive patients, which means they can have timely lifestyle modification and medical treatment if necessary.

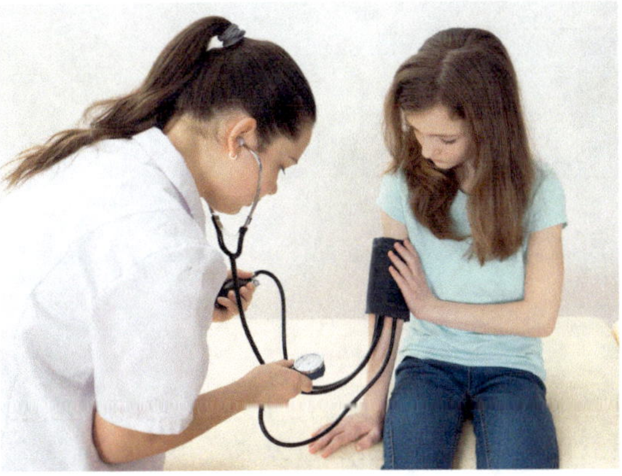

Figure 12.9. Regular screening for hypertension in children and adolescents.

Source: https://www.washingtonpost.com/wp-apps/imrs.php?src=https://arc-anglerfish-washpost-prod-washpost.s3.amazonaws.com/public/GEHVXFQNMUI6NPCT3NRUZKKKFI&w=1200.

Apart from that, educational programs that create awareness of good lifestyles (e.g., consuming a balanced diet and frequent exercise) can be readily integrated into screening processes. These measures not only effectively reverse the short-term effects of high blood pressure but also instill long-term consciousness for good living in the younger generations, which will lead towards a health-conscious future generation (Williams et al., 2018) (Figure 12.9).

Analysis of routine hypertension screening impacts goes beyond individual healthcare advantages. It matters to public health planning as it offers data required by policies to lower hypertension prevalence and ensuing complications in populations. When screenings are performed periodically within schools and community health programs, data obtained may be utilized in assisting in the interpretation of hypertension among teenagers. In addition, such information can guide planning of resources for education programs in lifestyle change, which can reduce the occurrence of hypertension in children significantly. Policymakers need to realize the significance of regular screening in informing effective health interventions, thus creating an environment that involves active management of health among children (Madhu et al., 2020).

12.4. Health Risks Associated with Hypertension

The medical dangers of hypertension in youth extend well beyond the mere elevation of blood pressure measurements. Children with hypertension will often exhibit premature signs of cardiovascular damage, which may manifest in the form of cardiac hypertrophy, or thickening of heart muscle due to the heart needing to work harder. These alterations are significant indicators of potential future health effects. In addition, hypertensive children have also been known to exhibit vascular stiffness and premature atherosclerotic changes, which put them at risk for dangerous cardiovascular events in adulthood. This linkage of childhood hypertension with adult cardiovascular disease centers on the significance of identifying and treating the condition early as recent studies have established that childhood high blood pressure persistently predicts adult hypertension, hence necessitating early intervention of the disease to avoid future effects (Falkner et al., 2018). Besides cardiovascular disease, hypertension imposes severe consequences on the development of cognition in children. Research has revealed that hypertensive children will show impaired cognition, perhaps a result of reduced cerebral perfusion or other vascular alterations in the brain. The impairment will affect learning and interpersonal interactions, leading to a complex interaction between physical and emotional well-being. The psychological distress of having a chronic illness like hypertension will also contribute to stress, exacerbating emotional symptoms and physiological reactions. The negative impacts on mental performance highlight the need for holistic health strategies addressing hypertension in children so that physical and mental well-being are given equal prominence during management and treatment processes (Falkner et al., 2018).

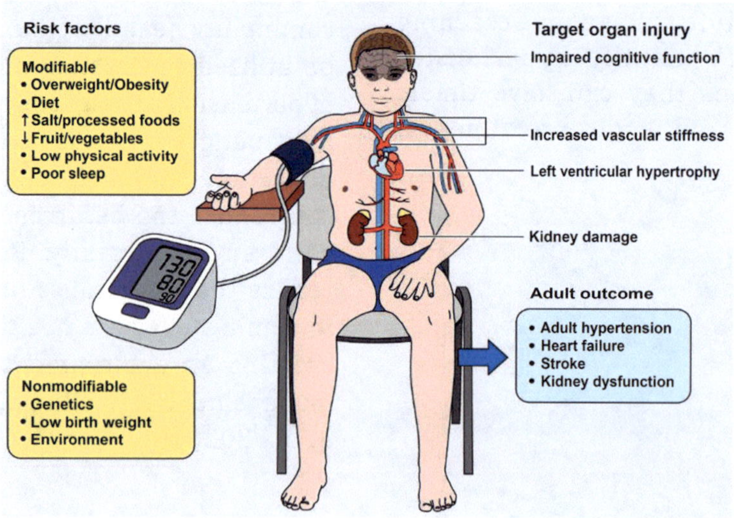

Figure 12.10. Risk factors for high BP in children and adolescents that are modifiable, including improving dietary intake and physical activity, and reducing excess adiposity.

Source: https://www.ahajournals.org/cms/10.1161/HYP.0000000000000228/asset/0ef4f1c6-23e8-40d9-b00f-50180d60468e/assets/graphic/hyp.0000000000000228.fig01.jpg.

The increasing prevalence of hypertension among children and adolescents is quite disturbing, particularly when it occurs in tandem with increased rates of obesity and associated diseases, such as Type II Diabetes Mellitus. This burgeoning epidemic underscores the necessity of treating modifiable risk factors like diet, exercise, and stress management. Childhood obesity is particularly in jeopardy due to the fact that excess weight directly correlates with increased blood pressure. As discussed, the long-term consequence of these interconnected diseases can lead to debilitating comorbidities like cardiovascular disease, renal failure, and blindness—a set of diseases that further intensify as these patients mature into adulthood. Therefore, early identification and targeted interventions are crucial not only in reducing the incidence of hypertension but also in avoiding the endemic lifelong consequences of these chronic diseases (Figure 12.10).

12.4.1. Short-Term Health Implications

The rising prevalence of hypertension among children and adolescents has numerous short-term health consequences that must be addressed with great urgency. Uncontrolled blood pressure can occur in association with a myriad of acute presentations such as headaches, dizziness, and fatigue, which are readily confused with nonspecific complaints. These manifestations also serve as valuable markers of covert cardiovascular stress. In addition, hypertension is likely to lead to short-term complications such as hypertensive crises, in which blood pressure levels become extremely high, necessitating urgent medical attention. It is essential that parents, teachers, and medical providers understand these short-term manifestations so that they can detect and treat likely health crises before they advance to chronic conditions. Apart from direct physiological outcomes, short-term hypertension effects are also likely to include psychological health among youths. The stress of having a chronic disease can induce depression and anxiety, particularly for youths who can struggle with being different from their peers. This psychological stress highlighted by the increased vulnerability to psychosocial stressors can have a significant impact on their overall well-being and quality of life. Young children who are pediatric patients also tend to encounter barriers in social interactions, which can result in social isolation or low self-esteem. Addressing the universal title health effects of hypertension thus calls for interventions that encompass psychological care and also medical attention to render care more comprehensive. The lifestyle determinants and hypertension—and thus the correlation between the two—cannot be stressed enough in regard to short-term health effects. Physical exercise is needed on a regular basis, as it has been found to lower the impact of high blood pressure. For instance, adequate exercise can promote cardiovascular wellness, improve insulin sensitivity, and even trigger favorable body composition changes, as noted in the existing literature (Becque et al., 2007). With the alarming trend towards more sedentary existence among youth, interventions enhancing physical activity participation are urgently required. In addition, healthy food choices education programs can serve as a significant weapon in the prevention and management of hypertension among this patient population, and hence, contribute to better health status in both the long and short terms. As the public health community strives to cope with this severe epidemic, interventions should encompass providing supportive environments that encourage healthy behavior (Agabiti-Rosei et al., 2016).

12.4.2. Long-Term Consequences on Cardiovascular Health

The late consequences of childhood and adolescent hypertension extend to multiple domains of cardiovascular health and warrant rigorous examination and treatment. Elevated blood pressure during growth can lead to the early onset of atherosclerosis—a process in which plaque accumulates within arterial walls. Early arterial stiffening can increase the risk of heart disease and other cardiovascular outcomes substantially across adulthood. Most importantly, hypertension in young individuals is on the rise, making preventive interventions ensuring maximal blood pressure level through lifestyle modification and pharmacological intervention very important. Regular physical activity, according to the amended 2020 WHO guidelines, becomes essential not only in reducing blood pressure but also in preventing the cardiovascular morbidity of uncontrolled hypertension (Bull et al., 2020). Further, the impact of pediatric hypertension reaches beyond physicality of the body but also has implications for mental health. Adolescents with hypertension are stigmatized or socially disadvantaged, resulting in increased stress and anxiety levels. Such psychological stressors further increase cardiovascular risk due to the interplay between psychological and physical health. Studies have revealed that teenagers with chronic stress are more likely to have unhealthy lifestyles, including diet with inadequate nutrition or physical inactivity, which worsens the effects of hypertension. Hence, it is crucial to decipher the complex relationship between mental illness and hypertension to develop efficient strategies that address both holistically, ultimately improving long-term cardiovascular outcomes as defined in recent years' guidelines by the ACC and AHA (Paul et al., 2017) (Figure 12.11).

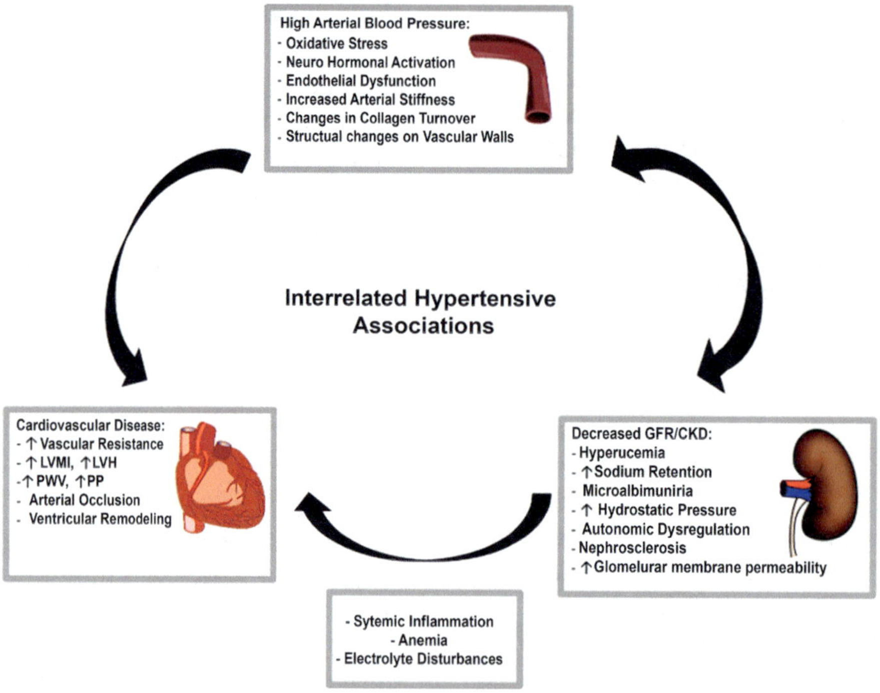

Figure 12.11. Interrelated hypertensive associations.

Source: https://article.imrpress.com/journal/RCM/23/5/10.31083/j.rcm2305166/2153-8174-23-5-166/fig2.jpg.

As increasing attention is directed towards youth hypertension, the current findings identify the need for detection at an early age and intervention. Cumulative effects of hypertension, if left without intervention, will result in precious health inequality as these individuals reach adulthood. Frequent access to health screening for adolescents and children can facilitate early hypertension detection, thereby enabling adequate lifestyle counseling and medical therapy. The combination of lifestyle modification, including increased physical activity and dietary alterations, is associated with significant health benefits, aligning with recommendations put forward by health organizations. Empowerment by prioritizing the initial intervention and conditioning favorable heart-healthy lifestyles will render it possible to decrease long-term cardiovascular risk linked to hypertension among this risk population (Bull et al., 2020; Paul et al., 2017).

12.4.3. Psychological Effects and Quality of Life

The psychological impact of pediatric hypertension on children and adolescents significantly affects their quality of life. With increasing blood pressure, adolescents may experience increased stress, anxiety, and loneliness. These psychological troubles may produce lower levels of social interaction and less activity in activities promoting emotional well-being, which in turn may form a cycle in which both hypertension and poor psychological health exacerbate one another. This communication makes it more difficult to control hypertension, since stressed patients may resort to adverse coping behaviors, aggravating their physical status (Salam et al., 2023). Furthermore, social stigmatization of child high blood pressure may lead to bullying and exclusion, aggravating their mental status, and consequently increasing feelings of incompetence or poor self-esteem. In addition to stress and anxiety, juvenile population hypertension has also been associated with depressive symptoms that significantly impair their quality of life. Studies have indicated that adolescents with chronic illnesses, such as hypertension, are at a higher risk of developing depression compared to those adolescents who do not suffer from similar ailments (Tom et al., 2016). The burden of carrying a chronic disease at a young age may lead to helplessness, usually coupled with a peer lack of knowledge about the disease. This limited knowledge may reinforce isolation further, as infected children cannot relate to their peers or describe their condition, thus perpetuating isolation at the optimal periods of development. In addition, uncontrolled high blood pressure has long-term consequences that build up psychological distress and worsen life satisfaction as these teens transition into adulthood. High blood pressure over time can lead to severe health complications, like cardiovascular disease, which challenge physical health but also create perpetual concern about future health consequences. The psychological load of addressing both physical and mental issues can lead to chronic fatigue, demotivation, and poor academic performance (Salam et al., 2023). Ultimately, the psychological control of hypertension and the development of supportive environments become forefront in increasing the quality of life among the affected youth to face their challenges with hope and resilience.

12.5. Treatment and Management Strategies

Effective management and treatment of hypertension in the young begin with behavior modifications. These are essential, considering the high prevalence of obesity, a strong risk factor for elevated blood pressure in children and adolescents. Control of weight through diet and exercise is most crucial; studies indicate that even modest weight reduction yields impressive blood pressure control benefits. Putting children and adolescents on a regular exercise routine is not only beneficial for weight control but also improves cardiovascular health and overall quality of life. In addition, diet education programs that encourage healthier eating and decreases in sedentary activity can create habits that may reduce hypertension risks over a lifetime. Such early interventions are crucial in that they provide a foundation for a healthier future and thereby address the pediatric obesity case, negatively impacting hypertension levels (Hong, 2024). Apart from lifestyle modification, healthcare providers can also opt for pharmacologic intervention for significant levels of hypertension. For reference, medication should be prescribed when lifestyle modifications are not enough to achieve satisfactory blood pressure control or when hypertension is critical. The most used antihypertensive classes prescribed to pediatric patients are angiotensin-converting enzyme (ACE) inhibitors, calcium channel blockers, and beta-blockers, each one selected based on the specific needs and comorbidities of the patient. Careful monitoring is required because pediatric patients may be differently impacted by drugs compared to adults. In particular, the selection of the drug should always be based on the knowledge of the etiology of the hypertension, whether primary or secondary. The integration of pharmacotherapy as a component of global management increases the likelihood of successful outcomes in the treatment of hypertension in children and adolescents (Herouvi et al., 2023).

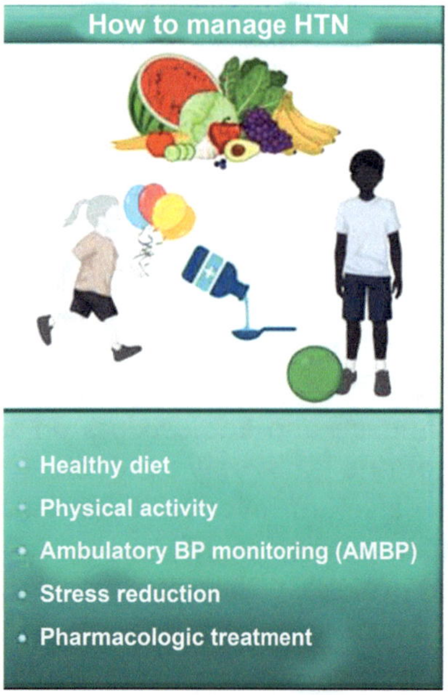

Figure 12.12. The general management of pediatric HTN.

Source: https://www.mdpi.com/children/children-11-00518/article_deploy/html/images/children-11-00518-g004.png.

Lastly, regular monitoring and follow-up are essential components of hypertension management in pediatric populations. Regular measurements of blood pressure and evaluation of lifestyle modifications are essential to assess the effectiveness of treatment regimens and to implement proper adjustments. Secondly, involving parents in education regarding the importance of treatment plan compliance, both lifestyle and pharmacological, provides a supportive environment for adolescents and children. Psychosocial problems like stress and self-esteem should be addressed since they can affect hypertension as well as treatment compliance. Multidisciplinary approaches that incorporate pediatricians, nutritionists, and mental health professionals can provide a balanced approach to managing hypertension. With an encouragement of communication and cooperation among various professions in healthcare, hypertension management can be made more individualized, thus leading to better results in terms of health for the respective children and teenagers (Hong, 2024) (Figure 12.12).

12.5.1. Lifestyle Modifications: Diet and Exercise

Hypertension is now on the increase in children and adolescents and has been blamed on many lifestyle factors, more importantly diet and exercise. Changing to lifestyle can reduce by quite a lot the blood pressure levels and slow the risk of developing cardiovascular diseases., A diet rich in vegetables, fruits, whole grains, and low-fat milk, known as the DASH (Dietary Approaches to Stop Hypertension) diet, can reduce blood pressure effectively. Additionally, sodium intake must be kept low as excess salt directly causes hypertension. In reality, one can encourage improved diets through recommendations to eat a well-balanced diet tailored for the younger population. Hence, modifying eating behavior is essential in preventing hypertension and managing it in children and adolescents, with long-term benefits (Madhu et al., 2020). Exercise also plays a significant role in managing hypertension in youth. Aerobic exercise and strength training are recommended among adolescents in order to control body weight and enhance cardiovascular function. At least 60 minutes of physical activity on a daily basis, which should be moderate to vigorous intensity, is emphasized among children and adolescents by the American College of Cardiology and the American Heart Association. This level of activity not only helps to lower systolic and diastolic blood pressure but also reduces stress, improves mental health, and general wellbeing. Schools and families need to make sure they provide an environment that favors activity through planned sport and recreation and enable children to remain active. Thus, a composite measure involving changes in diet and exercise can be effective in overcoming hypertension (Paul et al., 2017) (Figure 12.13).

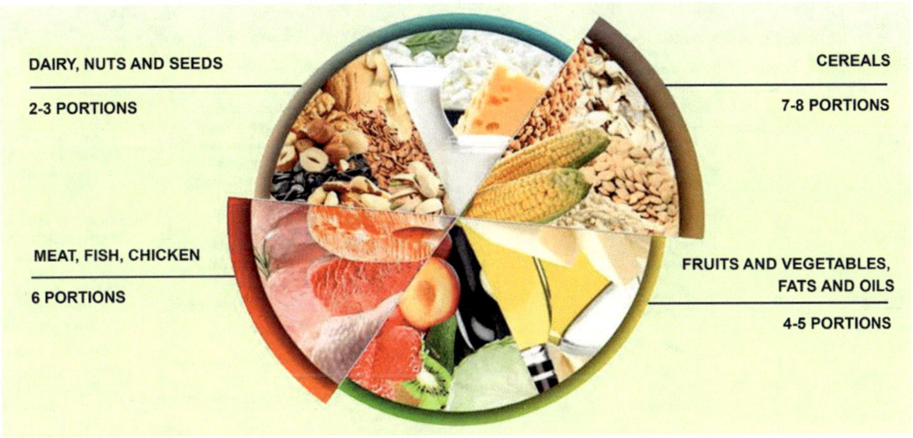

Figure 12.13. Dietary approaches to stop hypertension (DASH) in hypertension.

Source: https://www.dradlingdiabetesclinic.com/image/blogs/dash_CUaLKEO.png.

Moreover, the inclusion of educational content targeting lifestyle changes is critical in maintaining adherence and having success in the management of hypertension. Raising awareness through community interventions among the children and their families can lead to awareness about food related causes and lack of physical activity. Healthy diet and physical activity interventions can equip the young people to become health-aware individuals, hence creating a supportive system that enforces good habits. Monitoring systems and assessment tools can be employed to track developments and stimulate compliance with such changes in lifestyle. By developing a culture of supporting healthy lifestyle, we can significantly reduce the incidences of hypertension among adolescents and young people, consequently minimizing the implications of long-term health hazards (Madhu et al., 2020).

12.5.2. Pharmacological Interventions

Pharmacological treatment of hypertension in children entails a variety of pharmacological strategies to control blood pressure and reduce associated cardiovascular risk. This option to start medication typically arises when interventions like lifestyle change, encompassing diet and exercise, prove to be insufficient. Angiotensin-converting enzyme (ACE) inhibitors and calcium channel blockers are two of the most frequently utilized drugs due to their efficacy and comparative safety profile in the pediatric setting. In evidence, it is shown that effective pharmacologic treatment is able to significantly decrease the incidence of long-term sequelae of untreated hypertension. However, careful consideration is required as treatment regimens must be tailored to meet the requirements of young patients to achieve efficacy and compliance with the regimen given the consideration that children would have a varied response to drugs compared to adults. Pharmacologic therapy for addressing hypertension in the context of comorbid conditions such as obesity and dyslipidemia, which are also common in this group, has received more recent attention. The beta-blockers, for example, may be more suitable for those with concomitant cardiac diseases or chronic stress (Figure 12.14).

Frequently Used Antihypertensive Oral Medications for Treatment of Chronic Pediatric HTN

Medication Class	Agents	Common Pediatric Dose	Contraindications	Adverse Effects
ACEIS	Captopril Enalapril Ramipril Fosinopril Lisinopril	0.1 - 1.5mg / kg 0.08-0.58 mg/kg (max 40 mg) 6mg / (m2) 0.1-0.6 mg/kg (max 40 mg) 0.07-0.6 mg/kg (max 40 mg)	Pregnancy Angioedema Hypersensitivity to ACEIs Concomitant use with Aliskiren (in DM patients)	Common: cough, headache, dizziness, asthenia Severe: hyperkalemia, AKI, angioedema, fetal toxicity
ARBS	Losartan Valsartan Candesartan Olmesartan	0.7-1.4 mg/kg (max 100 mg) 1.3-2.7 mg/kg (max 160 mg) 1-6 yr. 0.2-0.4 mg/kg 20-35 kg: 10-20 mg	Pregnancy Hypersensitivity to ARBS Concomitant use with Aliskiren (in DM patients)	Common: headache, dizziness Severe: hyperkalemia, AKI, fetal toxicity
CCBS	Amlodipine Nifedipine	0.12-0.3 mg (max 10 mg) 0.5 - 1mg / kg	Hypersensitivity to CCBs	Common: flushing, periferia edema, dizziness Severe: angioedema
Beta-blockers	Propanololo Atenolol Metoprolol Carvedilolo	1 mg/kg 1 mg/kg 1-2 mg/kg (max 200 mg) 0.08 - 1.5 mg / kg	Hypersensitivity to beta-blockers Heart blocks (II or III-degree)	Common: bradycardia, hypotension, dizziness, fatigue Severe: skin rash, I-degree AV block
Thiazide diuretics	Furosemide HCTZ Spironolattone	0.5 - 2mg / kg 0.5 - mg / kg 1 mg / kg	Anuria Hypersensitivity to thiazides or other sulfonamide blocks	Common: dizziness, hypokalemia Severe: arrhythmias, cholestatic jaundice, new-onset DM, pancreatitis

Figure 12.14. Pharmacologic treatment of chronic pediatric HTN. Main pharmacologic classes, agents, dosages, contraindications, and side effects.

Source: https://www.mdpi.com/children/children-11-00518/article_deploy/html/images/children-11-00518-g003.png.

Pharmacotherapy can reverse the adverse effects of elevated blood pressure, especially when combined with comprehensive life interventions. Genovesi et al. (2024) continues that non-pharmacological treatment should always precede; nevertheless, in instances where there is a need for pharmacotherapy, one must be careful about potential side effects and drug interactions, particularly since most children with hypertension may also be taking medication for another condition. This is the intricacy that requires a multidisciplinary team comprising pediatricians, dietitians, and specialists. While drug treatment can be crucial to the management of hypertension, its administration must be properly guided through evidence-based interventions. Recent meta-analyses have shown that certain drugs can exacerbate side effects, particularly among adolescents suffering from non-suicidal self-injury (NSSI) and depressive states. Chen et al. (2025) identifies a complicated interaction between pharmacotherapy and mental health outcomes in such a manner that, ironically, the most efficacious treatments may actually increase the frequency of risk-taking behavior in target populations. Practitioners will thus be compelled to weigh the benefits of hypertension treatment against probable psychological impacts, highlighting the need for close monitoring and adjustment of treatment regimens. Lastly, the goal is sustainable management of high blood pressure with drugs while not compromising the overall health of children and adolescents.

12.5.3. Role of Healthcare Providers and Family Support

Optimal control of hypertension in children and adolescents necessitates a multidisciplinary approach by healthcare professionals and families. Healthcare professionals are largely responsible for the early identification and ongoing management of hypertension. This entails regular screening via frequent check-ups as well as the development of individualized plans for intervention based on special risk factors. Additionally, the establishment of a sensitive therapeutic relationship between patients and healthcare professionals enables adherence to treatment guidelines. The connection between the families and healthcare providers forms a basis for awareness of disease implications and hypertension education, in addition to lifestyle modifications. As a direct association exists between childhood obesity and hypertension, as theorized by Jørgensen et al. (2019), treatment aside, prevention care also needs to be augmented by practitioners through lifestyle modification, best achieved with family assistance and support. Family support significantly enhances the control of blood pressure in young patients. Parents and guardians play a major role in creating a health-supportive environment, influencing food intake, the level of exercise, and drug adherence. Empirical findings suggest that teenagers who have healthy family environments exhibit healthier health status and possibly because they are more compliant and motivated. Healthcare professionals can empower families by educating them on the risk of hypertension and the benefits of a healthy lifestyle. Furthermore, family involvement in care, including involvement in goal-setting and decision-making processes, creates a sense of common responsibility towards the condition's management. The efficacy of management interventions is dependent on support systems around children, particularly when the psychosocial determinants of children's health pathways become apparent, as evidenced by Heels et al. (2013). Furthermore, the integration of community resources within support networks serves to boost the impact of healthcare professionals and family participation. Schools, neighborhood groups, and neighborhood health programs provide alternative sources of education and information for the control of hypertension. These support systems are part of an umbrella system that is not only medical in nature but also addresses the emotional and social well-being of the child or adolescent. Educating families about local facilities has the ability to enhance confidence and ability in controlling hypertension. Research highlights that comprehensive approaches involving healthcare practitioners, families, and community support together in a single approach achieve better health outcomes, addressing the growing need to address chronic illness in children and adolescents through comprehensive approaches, as highlighted by Jørgensen et al. (2019). Such interconnection is important in creating sustainable effects on the health of hypertensive children and adolescents.

12.6. Prevention Strategies

Effective prevention strategies for hypertension in children and adolescents are primarily focused on lifestyle modifications with a focus on exercise and proper nutrition. The stimulation of young people into proper exercise can serve to significantly reduce the risk of developing hypertension. Exercise training and physical activity, based on research, are associated with improved cardiovascular health, including reduced risk factors like hypertension and obesity. By establishing physical culture in school and community settings, health professionals have the potential to collaborate with educators and parents to establish environments where children will be encouraged to be active. Further, incorporating structured exercise regimes can be an adjuvant treatment for those already presenting risk factors, promoting long-term health as well as overall well-being (Becque et al., 2007). Nutritional therapy is also essential in order to avoid hypertension in young people. The formation of healthy eating habits that revolve around whole foods, fruits, vegetables, and low-sodium products can help decrease the risk of high blood pressure. Health education must start at a young age in life when a healthy diet that restricts the intake of processed foods and sweetened beverages, both of which are linked with increased blood pressure, will be developed. Effective prevention strategies require collaboration with medical professionals to educate families about nutrition guidelines tailored to children and teenagers, especially those with metabolic risk factors or obesity. The inclusion of these dietary practices not only allows for blood pressure regulation but also achieves healthy growth and development in general, thereby preventing various ailments concurrently (Avci et al., 2011). Also, the role of community involvement in hypertension prevention cannot be overstated. Family-based interventions within lifestyle changes, such as health fairs or local exercise programs, ensure awareness and support of correct behaviors. Schools can implement regular health screenings and education programs that provide valuable information on hypertension risks and prevention, enabling children to make informed healthy lifestyle choices. In addition, comorbid conditions, especially among adolescents taking antipsychotic drugs, should be treated in the customization of prevention interventions. Multidisciplinary management through the coupling of pharmacotherapy and non-pharmacotherapy can treat not only high blood pressure but also possible metabolic syndrome, which suggests that adequate care programs must be developed to accommodate children's and adolescents' special health needs (Avci et al., 2011) (Figure 12.15).

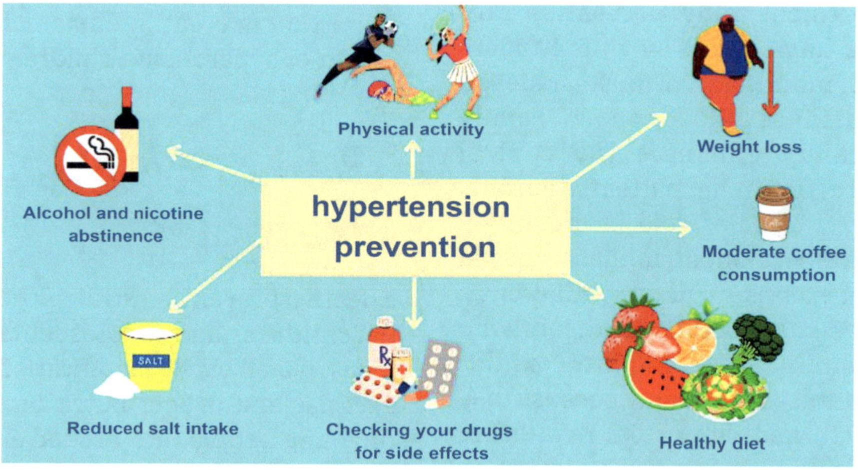

Figure 12.15. Prevention strategies for hypertension in children and adolescents.

Source: https://medconsonline.com/src/Frontend/Files/MediaLibrary/11/hypertension-prevention.png.

12.6.1. Community and School-Based Programs

Interconnection of school and community-level programs is of utmost significance in the prevention of hypertension among children and adolescents. These programs have been designed with the aim of promoting healthier lifestyles and cardiovascular knowledge at an early age. School is the ideal place to bring about such intervention as it is accessible and has a wide, heterogeneous student population. Courses that incorporate physical education, nutrition education, and behavioral health interventions can have a large impact not just on students as individuals but also on families and communities at large. By instilling a culture that encourages healthy behaviors, courses can reduce the rate of hypertension, making long-term health impact a reality in the future trajectory of children and adolescents. It demands community participation in the success of such initiatives, particularly with economically disadvantaged sections who could possess unique health concerns. The Child-Mediated Health Communication (CMHC) model provides an innovative paradigm that allows children to act as messengers for health in the family. By drawing on children's influence and relationships, CMHC interventions can be in a position to drive health practice conversations among caregivers and parents, thereby creating greater understanding and adherence to health principles. This approach acknowledges the massive barriers that tend to complicate traditional health promotion among these groups, including lack of access to healthcare services and cultural misconceptions regarding information on health. Overall, successful community-based interventions need to be responsive to the specific circumstances and needs of the populations with which they will be working, in order that efforts at health promotion have a sense of personal relevance. Investing in programs in schools and communities that work to prevent hypertension is not just good for public health but also derives immense economic gain. Research shows that the nation and states, respectively, could save substantial amounts of money on healthcare if programs for preventing diseases were given high priority to encourage physical activity, improved diet, and smoking cessation among young people. Community-based programs such as these have shown impressive changes in behavior that are associated with long-term health. Through investment in such preventive interventions, the economic burden of healthcare costs arising from hypertension and related complications will be reduced, ultimately enhancing health equity among diverse populations. As communities establish organized programs for promoting healthier environments, joint action by schools and local agencies will be the blueprint for re-writing health outcomes for generations to come.

12.6.2. Education and Awareness Campaigns

Good education and awareness campaigns are central to combating hypertension in children and adolescents. Such campaigns have the purpose of educating families on the danger of elevated blood pressure and promoting healthier ways of living. Through targeting children and their parents, such campaigns are able to create an atmosphere supportive of improved health practice. Interventions based on nutrition education, physical activity frequency, and the significance of frequent health check-ups play a critical role in shaping habits at the young age. As identified through literature, overuse of screens contributes positively to child obesity, which is a direct consequence of hypertension (Saliba et al., 2015). Hence, it is equally crucial that educational programs are interactive and include aspects capable of capturing young people's attention to enable them to be receptive and willing to listen and apply the information presented. The cultural aspects of awareness campaigns cannot be overlooked, particularly when targeting economically-disadvantaged communities. Previous studies have found that traditional health promotion strategies tend to be hindered in reaching such populations by issues such as communication misunderstanding due to language barriers and material incongruence with cultures (DeSorbo et al., 2017). Thus, successful educational interventions must factor in these to achieve a high coverage. Innovative approaches such as involving children as The

Vectors of Health Communication have been successful in reaching parents and caretakers who otherwise fall outside program reach. Leveraging peer pressure and established social networks, the interventions are subsequently able to assist in initiating needed lifestyle changes that reverse hypertension risks as well as other allied chronic diseases. Lastly, education and campaigns must be integrated into public health policy to eradicate hypertension among youth. The campaigns should be multilevel, comprising a mix of community action, policy and funding commitment, and media campaigns to reach as large an audience as possible. School, medical staff, and local organization involvement can ensure maximum impact for these campaigns and ensure maximum potential for health education increase. Promotion of regular health screening and accessibility of physical activity facilities are two necessary components that must be given top priority. Through focused education and community interventions, a healthier generation can be built, hence significantly lowering the prevalence of hypertension and its complications among children and adolescents.

12.6.3. Policy Recommendations for Health Promotion

Rising blood pressure in children and youth necessitates immediate and effective policy response in the domain of health promotion. One of the actions proposed is the creation of comprehensive health education campaigns in schools emphasizing the importance of lifestyle decisions, like nutrition and sport. Such programs can be incorporated into the most recent guidelines supporting a minimum of 60 minutes of at least moderate-to-vigorous intensity physical activity each day, as advocated by the WHO. By establishing an environment that supports healthy diet and physical activity, schools can play a major role in preventing the onset of hypertension among this risk group. As the Global Burden of Disease Study has demonstrated, prevalence of cardiovascular disease is overwhelming, and therefore it is crucial to invest in evidence-based educational interventions for the development of awareness and behavioral change among youth (Gregory et al., 2020). Policymakers should also investigate improving access to healthy food at an affordable price in regions with high prevalence of hypertension. Food deserts (neighborhoods with limited availability of healthy foods) contribute significantly to unhealthy consumption by children and youth, increasing their susceptibility to hypertension and other related complications. Collaboration with local governments and grocery stores can ensure the establishment of farmers' markets and community gardens providing fresh vegetables and fruits. Coupled with nutritional education and culinary skills training, these initiatives can create healthier environments that enable families to make improved nutrition choices. Reducing sedentary behavior, as well as increasing physical activity, is of prime concern in accordance with the WHO guidelines; therefore, policies to ensure healthy food choices need to be complemented by interventions to reduce screen time and promote physical activity (Bull et al., 2020). Furthermore, regulatory actions need to promote the integration of physical activity into children's and adolescents' daily life. This can involve active transport-accommodating policies, for instance, walking or biking to school, and designing safe recreational spaces within communities. Apart from this, organized post-school physical activity can also be used as a countermeasure against sedentary behavior commonly associated with increased screen time and poor diet. Engaging parents and guardians through community programs and workshops can also promote an active lifestyle at home. By focusing on incorporating cost-effective physical activities and dietary education, such policies can greatly reduce the incidence of hypertension, thereby improving the overall health pattern for generations to come (Gregory et al., 2020).

SUMMARY

In summary, it is important to understand the complicated condition that hypertension can pose to the pediatric subgroup of our society. The prevalence of hypertension in today's youth has increased alarmingly, fueled by comorbidities like obesity, lack of exercise, and poor diets. This is important to the long-term cardiovascular futures, as childhood hypertension predisposes one to early development of various comorbidities. The awareness of the necessity of early diagnosis and constant monitoring is vital in that early treatment would prevent the aggravation of hypertension and consequent health issues. Secondly, there is a necessity to implement an aggressive stance by doctors towards family education on the dangers of hypertension and modification of habits necessary to keep such dangers in check. Finally, the relationship between obesity and hypertension cannot be overstressed. Studies have established a strong correlation between hypertension and nonalcoholic fatty liver disease (NAFLD) in children. Of children with NAFLD, an impressive 35.8% presented with elevated blood pressure levels at baseline, and an evident rate of persistence of 21.4% was observed over time (Behling et al., 2014). The findings underscore the need for embracing complementary management strategies that address the two conditions together. Interventions which are specially tailored to cause weight loss and modification of healthy lifestyle can potentially have a significant impact on the outcomes of hypertension in this high-risk population, thus substantiating the importance of an integrated approach. Hence, it is essential that screening for hypertension be incorporated in the process of routine pediatric appointments, particularly in overweight or obese adolescents. Finally, resolution of hypertension in the adolescent is closely related to modifications in obesity treatment and lifestyle. It has been revealed in research that weight reduction not only lowers blood pressure but also restores renal function and circadian rhythm to benefit cardiovascular health (Bruneel et al., 2019). As proved by research, diet modification intervention along with increased physical activity and psychological counseling can lead to tremendous health improvement in obese adolescents. Therefore, public health programs and educational efforts that promote healthy lifestyles from an early age are crucial. Through the promotion of a culture of awareness for health, we may possibly stem the increase in hypertension among children and teens, opening the door to a healthier tomorrow. In the future, a collaborative effort from healthcare professionals, educators, and families is imperative in addressing this emerging public health issue.

Identification of the most significant determinants of hypertension in children and adolescents necessitates an integrated evaluation of its etiology, consequences, and management strategies. Hypertension prevalence in these populations has been of specific interest as early identification and intervention are important for prevention of cardiovascular complications in the future. The underlying causes of increased blood pressure are obesity, genetic syndrome, physical inactivity, and dietary factors. Recent advances in arterial stiffness measurement, particularly through technologies such as pulse-wave velocity (PWV), have also provided significant insights into cardiovascular well-being among youth. Such findings allow health practitioners to approximate the risk of hypertension and then modify interventions, accordingly, once more highlighting the demand for early screening and active intervention among children (Raymond et al., 2015). Hypertension control in children and young people is founded on lifestyle modifications and, in extreme cases, drug therapy. The role of lifestyle modifications, including dietary modification, increased physical activity, and weight management, is the main one since these interventions are capable of lowering blood pressure levels and health status to a great extent. Secondly, clinicians are urged to incorporate guidelines set by health bodies, such as the American Heart Association and the European Society of Cardiology. Both entities have evidence-based recommendations that assist clinicians in recognizing those at risk and putting in place effective treatment programs, toward an overall better management of pediatric hypertension (Elliott et al., 2014). Finally, the implications of uncontrolled hypertension in this group extend beyond existing problems, potentially laying the groundwork for long-term disease into adulthood. It has been found that hypertensive children are more likely to have cardiovascular disease in adulthood, such as heart failure and stroke. It is thus critical for doctors to appreciate the seriousness of the way hypertension must be treated in children and adolescents. Quality of life and long life could be improved by earlier intervention and continuous monitoring of blood pressure in this population. With an active lifestyle approach and implementation of technological innovations in health parameters coupled with rigid clinical protocols, we can potentially avoid the chronic complications of hypertension in young individuals.

CLOSER LOOK

NORMAL VERSUS ELEVATED BP IN NEONATES

Neonatal blood pressure (BP) is a dynamic physiologic assessment that varies with gestational age, postnatal age, birth weight, and general health status. Unlike older children and adults, neonatal BP does not have a generally accepted fixed reference values for both normal and abnormal values. Rather, normative values are typically provided in percentile-based charts, categorized by gestational and postnatal age. Typical neonatal blood pressure is lower than in the adult patient and rises progressively over the initial days and weeks of life as cardiovascular regulatory mechanisms mature and renal function improves.

In term neonates, normal systolic blood pressure is typically in the range of 60 to 80 mmHg, and diastolic is in the range of 30 to 50 mmHg. The MAP typically approximates the gestational age in weeks during the early days of life (e.g., a 40-week neonate will have an MAP of approximately 40 mmHg). Preterm babies have lower blood pressure and rise more slowly. In the initial 72 hours of life, an increase in blood pressure is observed as the neonate adapts to extrauterine circulation through closure of the ductus arteriosus, decreased pulmonary vascular resistance, and increased left ventricular output.

Elevated blood pressure, or neonatal hypertension, is categorized when the blood pressure is consistently higher than the 95th percentile for weight, gestational age, and age. The disease is rather uncommon, occurring in about 0.2% to 3% of neonates in neonatal intensive care units (NICUs), but needs to be approached seriously since it can result in cardiac failure, intraventricular hemorrhage, and permanent vascular damage. A few of the typical etiologies for elevated BP in neonates include renal parenchymal illnesses, renovascular disease (such as umbilical arterial catheter-associated thrombus), bronchopulmonary dysplasia, aortic coarctation, and endocrine disorders such as congenital adrenal hyperplasia.

Clinically, symptomatic neonatal hypertension or asymptomatic hypertension are nonspecifically manifested with indications of irritability, intolerance to feeding, tachypnea, or failure to thrive. End-organ damage, cardiac failure, or seizures may be caused by severe hypertension. The diagnosis is made by repeated and accurate measurement of BP in an optimal environment with oscillometric monitors with appropriate cuff size or invasive monitoring in critically ill patients. Sustained elevation must be confirmed over stress-induced, transient elevation or incorrect technique.

The management of neonatal hypertension is determined by etiology and degree. Mild hypertension might be managed with monitoring only and treatment of the precipitating cause, i.e., pain or fluid overload. Moderate to severe hypertension might be treated with drug therapy using agents like hydralazine, captopril, or labetalol. Careful monitoring of trends in blood pressure and target organ function must be conducted in order to avoid under-treatment or over-treatment.

References

1. Agabiti-Rosei, E., Cruickshank, J. K., Dominiczak, A., Erdine, S., et al. (2016). 2016 European Society of Hypertension guidelines for the management of high blood pressure in children and adolescents. https://core.ac.uk/download/46165193.pdf (accessed on 15th July 2025).
2. Al-Hazzaa, H. (2022). Physical activity research in the Gulf Cooperation Council countries: Progress made but work still to do. *Journal of Physical Activity & Health.* https://www.semanticscholar.org/paper/c2f5727c64bb65c2349590d9de49cd23aad3269f (accessed on 15th July 2025).
3. Avci, A., Tahiroglu, A., & Celik, G. G. (2011). Metabolic and endocrine side effects of atypical antipsychotic drugs in children and adolescents. https://core.ac.uk/download/pdf/27160355.pdf (accessed on 15th July 2025).
4. Becque, M. D., Boreham, C., Corigliano, G., Lee, S., McMahan, C. A., Shea, S., & Thompson, P. D. (2007). Special article: Physical activity, physical fitness, and cardiovascular risk factors in childhood. https://core.ac.uk/download/83049283.pdf (accessed on 15th July 2025).
5. Behling, C., Donithan, M., Hallinan, E. K., Newton, K. P., et al. (2014). Longitudinal assessment of high blood pressure in children with nonalcoholic fatty liver disease. https://core.ac.uk/download/323064808.pdf (accessed on 15th July 2025).
6. Bhagat, A., Mehendale, A., & Muneshwar, K. N. (2024). Study of obesity among adolescents in rural Wardha district. *F1000Research.* https://www.semanticscholar.org/paper/e0cfaa17028136accf8f6a8668a6342b1a89ef92 (accessed on 15th July 2025).
7. Bruneel, E., De Guchtenaere, A., Dejonckheere, S., Everaert, K., et al. (2019). The effect of a multidisciplinary weight loss program on renal circadian rhythm in obese adolescents. [No journal or volume provided].
8. Bull, F., Al-Ansari, S. S., Biddle, S., Borodulin, K., Buman, M. P., Cardon, G., Carty, C., et al. (2020). World Health Organization 2020 guidelines on physical activity and sedentary behavior. *British Journal of Sports Medicine, 54*, 1451–1462. https://doi.org/10.1136/bjsports-2020-102955 (accessed on 15th July 2025).
9. Chedid, A., Hering, A., Losier, A., Welner, A., Stewart, A. F., Tomassoni, A. J., Ewart, A. K., et al. (2008). At the bottom of the differential diagnosis list: Unusual causes of pediatric hypertension. https://core.ac.uk/download/pdf/8335258.pdf (accessed on 15th July 2025).
10. Chen, X., Dong, Y., Ye, M., Wang, X., Yan, J., Yao, Y., Qi, Z., et al. (2025). Comparative efficacy and acceptability of psychotherapeutic, pharmacological, and combination treatments for non-suicidal self-injury in children and adolescents: A systematic review and network meta-analysis. *BMC Psychiatry, 25.* https://www.semanticscholar.org/paper/3ed4d354dd4b314e6b2ab1d7be5b2441799317f6 (accessed on 15th July 2025).
11. Cho, H., & Kim, J. H. (2020). Secular trends in hypertension and elevated blood pressure among Korean children and adolescents in the Korea National Health and Nutrition Examination Survey 2007-2015. *The Journal of Clinical Hypertension, 22*, 590–597. https://www.semanticscholar.org/paper/95eb0136a42b83c81352d105c94a8e5f473cd5a0 (accessed on 15th July 2025).
12. Cho, W., Jung, I., Kim, J., Chae, H., Kim, M., Chung, N., & Suh, B. K. (2015). Two cases of Shwachman-Diamond syndrome in adolescents confirmed by genetic analysis. *Annals of Laboratory Medicine, 35*, 269–271. https://www.semanticscholar.org/paper/

ba1aea356a0f2cfa81bfa1f6ae364f3edad094f7 (accessed on 15th July 2025).

13. De Simone, G., Mancusi, C., Hanssen, H., Genovesi, S., Lurbe, E., Parati, G., Sendžikaitė, S., et al. (2022). Hypertension in children and adolescents. *European Heart Journal.* https://www.semanticscholar.org/paper/5f8d8adf637fb5d0dc8ec81ee83f396e54290a36 (accessed on 15th July 2025).
14. DeSorbo, A., Gerin, W., Hecht, M. F., Hedmann, S., et al. (2017). Child-mediated health communication: A conceptual framework for increasing stroke literacy in hard to reach populations. https://digitalscholarship.unlv.edu/cgi/viewcontent.cgi?article=1437&context=jhdrp (accessed on 15th July 2025).
15. Elliott, P., Anastasakis, A., Borger, M. A., Borggrefe, M., Cecchi, F., Charron, P., Hagège, A., et al. (2014). 2014 ESC guidelines on diagnosis and management of hypertrophic cardiomyopathy. *European Heart Journal, 35*, 2733–2779. https://doi.org/10.1093/eurheartj/ehu284 (accessed on 15th July 2025).
16. Ellis, D., & Miyashita, Y. (2011). Primary hypertension and special aspects of hypertension in older children and adolescents. https://core.ac.uk/download/12213824.pdf (accessed on 15th July 2025).
17. Falkner, B. (2018). The childhood role in development of primary hypertension. https://core.ac.uk/download/213445721.pdf (accessed on 15th July 2025).
18. Fox, N., Fox, N., Farrehi, C., Dikdan, S. J., Hajduczok, A., & Shipon, D. M. (2023). Abstract 18891: Frequency of abnormal cardiac screens in US high school athletes: Analysis of a national cardiac youth registry. *Circulation.* https://www.semanticscholar.org/paper/5fe4c0d0a9a7aafe4b6981dd67ba1e2e5db7b7f9 (accessed on 15th July 2025).
19. Genovesi, S., Vania, A., Caroli, M., Orlando, A., Lieti, G., Parati, G., & Giussani, M. (2024). Non-pharmacological treatment for cardiovascular risk prevention in children and adolescents with obesity. *Nutrients, 16.* https://www.semanticscholar.org/paper/e1dbda44f8036307dece92508360784d975c08b4 (accessed on 15th July 2025).
20. Heels, K., Harkin, N., & Donaghue, K. (2013). Diabetes during adolescence. https://www.semanticscholar.org/paper/365f926892ca4aa719ecbef97235454f707816fc (accessed on 15th July 2025).
21. Herouvi, D., Paltoglou, G., Soldatou, A., Kalpia, C., Karanasios, S., & Karavanaki, K. (2023). Lifestyle and pharmacological interventions and treatment indications for the management of obesity in children and adolescents. *Children, 10.* https://www.semanticscholar.org/paper/6ec5f850918524556c9920e9041a6d483090fd5b (accessed on 15th July 2025).
22. Hong, Y. H. (2024). Suggestions for the management of pediatric obesity in Korea. *Journal of the Korean Medical Association.* https://www.semanticscholar.org/paper/5c73f3b79f2476858410408cf9989402d0c88577 (accessed on 15th July 2025).
23. Jeong, S. I., & Kim, S. H. (2024). Obesity and hypertension in children and adolescents. *Clinical Hypertension, 30.* https://www.semanticscholar.org/paper/545c68fc447abe4db7015679b94d240fe3dfda3d (accessed on 15th July 2025).
24. Jeong, S. I., Kim, H. R., & Kim, S. H. (2025). Different risk factors for elevated blood pressure according to abdominal obesity in overweight children and adolescents. *BMC Pediatrics, 25.* https://www.semanticscholar.org/paper/e10615940c9227b89b4a0d9b3ccbe14fcc1489db (accessed on 15th July 2025).

25. Jørgensen, R., Bruun, J., Kremke, B., Windelborg, B., & Vestergaard, E. (2019). Obesity in children and adolescents: Empowering families through engagement of specialist and municipalities. *International Journal of Integrated Care*. https://www.semanticscholar.org/paper/033eb123b376d9e3c0f3326f7b5c82bfb7832ca7 (accessed on 15th July 2025).

26. Jukić, I., Kos, M., Stupin, A., Mihaljević, Z., Nad, T., Damašek, M., Drenjančević, I., et al. (2024). Flow-mediated dilation of brachial artery in children and adolescents with essential arterial hypertension. *Journal of Hypertension, 42*, e101. https://www.semanticscholar.org/paper/6eec9fbb0d196fe70a3edc238b9053045e774e3a (accessed on 15th July 2025).

27. Kapke, D. R. (2015). Childhood type II diabetes: The risks and complications. https://core.ac.uk/download/58826199.pdf (accessed on 15th July 2025).

28. Kruk, M. E., Gage, A., Arsenault, C., Jordan, K., Leslie, H. H., Roder-DeWan, S., Adeyi, O., et al. (2018). High-quality health systems in the Sustainable Development Goals era: Time for a revolution. *The Lancet Global Health, 6*, e1196–e1252. https://doi.org/10.1016/s2214-109x(18)30386-3 (accessed on 15th July 2025).

29. Madhu, S. V., Chawla, R., Makkar, B. M., Ghosh, S., Saboo, B., & Kalra, S. (2020). RSSDI-ESI clinical practice recommendations for the management of type 2 diabetes mellitus 2020. *Indian Journal of Endocrinology and Metabolism, 24*, 1–1. https://doi.org/10.4103/ijem.ijem_225_20 (accessed on 15th July 2025).

30. Mangione, C., Barry, M., Nicholson, W., Cabana, M., Chelmow, D., Coker, T. R., Davidson, K., et al. (2022). Screening for prediabetes and type 2 diabetes in children and adolescents: US Preventive Services Task Force recommendation statement. *JAMA, 328*(10), 963–967. https://www.semanticscholar.org/paper/2d64e36569909f23aef12879ef74c219370a99b1 (accessed on 15th July 2025).

31. Masters, B., Juliano, C., Levi, J., Cantor, J., Cohen, L., Segal, L. M., & Phillips, R. (2008). Prevention for a healthier California: Investments in disease prevention yield significant savings, stronger communities. https://core.ac.uk/download/71353991.pdf (accessed on 15th July 2025).

32. Neyra Marklund, I., Rullander, A. C., Lindberg, K., & Ringnér, A. (2022). Initial education for families with children diagnosed with type 1 diabetes: Consensus from experts in a Delphi study. *Comprehensive Child and Adolescent Nursing, 45*, 310–319. https://www.semanticscholar.org/paper/b51e6c81f521594317306f95117cae0c49b6eb60 (accessed on 15th July 2025).

33. Nuryani, N., & Paramata, Y. (2020). Associated factors of adolescent's malnutrition in junior high school student. *8*, 9–21. https://www.semanticscholar.org/paper/8bb74cfc3daf72f913fdc44493a4ae01b70a9861 (accessed on 15th July 2025).

34. Roth, G. A., Mensah, G. A., Johnson, C. O., Addolorato, G., Ammirati, E., Baddour, L. M., Barengo, N. C., et al. (2020). Global burden of cardiovascular diseases and risk factors, 1990–2019. *Journal of the American College of Cardiology, 76*, 2982–3021. https://doi.org/10.1016/j.jacc.2020.11.010 (accessed on 15th July 2025).

35. Salam, M. M., Yousuf, R., Salam, M. A., & Haque, M. (2023). Obesity and overweight. *Advances in Human Biology, 13*, 154–156. https://doi.org/10.4103/aihb.aihb_106_22 (accessed on 15th July 2025).

36. Saletin, J., Koopman-Verhoeff, M., Han, G., Barker, D. H., Carskadon, M., Anders, T. F., & Sheinkopf, S. (2020). 1002 Endorsement of sleep problems indexes autism severity in children and adolescents: Evidence from a large community sample. *Sleep, 43*. https://www.semanticscholar.

org/paper/f16d7740d2e4b7cab16826b93ba0627ec7b2a641 (accessed on 15th July 2025).

37. Saliba, M. (2015). Obesity and sedentary behavior in children and their implications in adulthood. https://core.ac.uk/download/46603766.pdf (accessed on 15th July 2025).

38. Seeman, T., Šuláková, T., & Stabouli, S. (2023). Masked hypertension in healthy children and adolescents: Who should be screened? *Current Hypertension Reports, 25*, 231–242. https://www.semanticscholar.org/paper/b2bedbb113ef855841dba24d7bb72fd85a83471e (accessed on 15th July 2025).

39. Segal, L. M., Earls, M. J., Unruh, P. J., Smolarcik, P., & Hearne, S. A. (2004). *F as in Fat: How Obesity Policies Are Failing in America, 2004.* https://core.ac.uk/download/71351404.pdf (accessed on 15th July 2025).

40. Siegel, R. L., Miller, K. D., & Jemal, A. (2016). Cancer statistics, 2016. *CA: A Cancer Journal for Clinicians, 66*, 7–30. https://doi.org/10.3322/caac.21332 (accessed on 15th July 2025).

41. Siegel, R. L., Miller, K. D., Fuchs, H. E., & Jemal, A. (2021). Cancer statistics, 2021. *CA: A Cancer Journal for Clinicians, 71*, 7–33. https://doi.org/10.3322/caac.21654 (accessed on 15th July 2025).

42. Stabouli, S., & Kotsis, V. (2015). Targeted blood pressure screening in children and adolescents: a justifiable option? *Journal of Hypertension, 33*(9), 1977–1978. https://www.semanticscholar.org/paper/ed80b73fcb8ebd9c1587fd2edeed03680f39961e (accessed on 15th July 2025).

43. Stankutė, I., Dulskienė, V., & Kuciene, R. (2024). Associations between neck circumference, mid-upper arm circumference, wrist circumference, and high blood pressure among Lithuanian children and adolescents: A cross-sectional study. *Nutrients, 16.* https://www.semanticscholar.org/paper/3285f3e40e2f9fb463ad86865d76a11ad015c4f3 (accessed on 15th July 2025).

44. Styne, D. M., Arslanian, S., Connor, E. L., Farooqi, I. S., Murad, M. H., Silverstein, J., & Yanovski, J. A. (2017). Pediatric obesity—Assessment, treatment, and prevention: An Endocrine Society clinical practice guideline. *The Journal of Clinical Endocrinology & Metabolism, 102*, 709–757. https://doi.org/10.1210/jc.2016-2573 (accessed on 15th July 2025).

45. Tomás, C., Oliveira, E., Sousa, D. C. F., Chupel, M. U., Furtado, G. E., Rocha, C., Teixeira, A., et al. (2016). Proceedings of the 3rd IPLeiria's International Health Congress. *BMC Health Services Research, 16.* https://doi.org/10.1186/s12913-016-1423-5 (accessed on 15th July 2025).

46. Townsend, R. R., Wilkinson, I. B., Schiffrin, E. L., Avolio, A., Chirinos, J. A., Cockcroft, J. R., Heffernan, K. S., et al. (2015). Recommendations for improving and standardizing vascular research on arterial stiffness. *Hypertension, 66*, 698–722. https://doi.org/10.1161/hyp.0000000000000033 (accessed on 15th July 2025).

47. Whelton, P. K., Carey, R. M., Aronow, W. S., Casey, D. E., Collins, K. J., Dennison Himmelfarb, C., DePalma, S. M., et al. (2017). 2017 ACC/AHA/AAPA/ABC/ACPM/AGS/APhA/ASH/ASPC/NMA/PCNA guideline for the prevention, detection, evaluation, and management of high blood pressure in adults: A report of the American College of Cardiology/American Heart Association Task Force on Clinical Practice Guidelines. *Hypertension, 71.* https://doi.org/10.1161/hyp.0000000000000065 (accessed on 15th July 2025).

48. Williams, B., Mancia, G., Spiering, W., Agabiti Rosei, E., Azizi, M., Burnier, M., Clément, D., et al. (2018). 2018 ESC/ESH guidelines for the management of arterial hypertension. *Journal of Hypertension, 36*, 1953–2041. https://doi.org/10.1097/hjh.0000000000001940 (accessed on 15th July 2025).

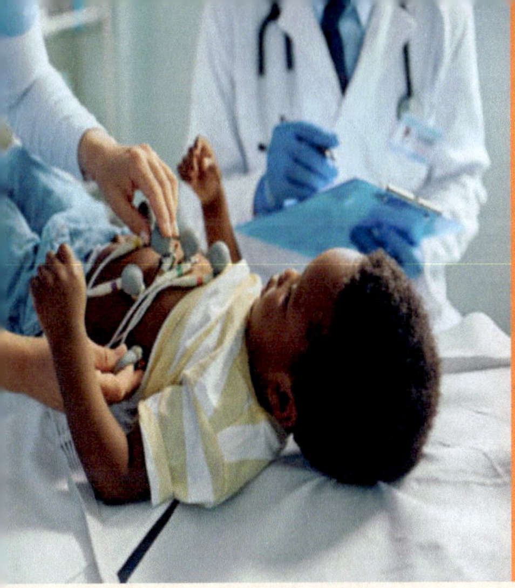

Chapter 13
INTERVENTIONAL PEDIATRIC CARDIOLOGY

Contents

Introduction

The field of interventional pediatric cardiology is a significant advance in the management of congenital and acquired cardiac illness in children. This subspecialty combines diagnostic imaging, catheter-based interventions, and surgical techniques to treat the numerous heart malformations that previously required open-heart surgery. The introduction of less aggressive procedures, though, not only improved the efficacy and safety of child cardiac procedures but also minimized recovery times and hospitalization. Consequently, interventional pediatric cardiology is crucial in providing efficient and timely measures of care that enhance the quality of life for children suffering from cardiac abnormalities, shaping the future of child cardiovascular treatment, ultimately. In the past decade, advancements in technology and technology in interventional pediatric cardiology have provided new therapy modalities. Balloon angioplasty and stenting, amongst others, have been novel catheter-based interventions used to treat conditions like pulmonary stenosis and ductus arteriosus.

Through these new technological advancements, one can provide focused treatment through a minimal invasive technique, thereby lowering patient trauma as well as heart function preservation. Second, the addition of new imaging modalities, such as echocardiography and MRI, has added accuracy to diagnosis and planning of interventions. Thus, continuing innovation in interventional approach is a pledge of dedication towards excellence in the treatment of congenital heart disease so that pediatric patients can be provided with the best treatment (N/A, 2006). Furthermore, the importance of a multidisciplinary approach to interventional pediatric cardiology cannot be overstressed. Multidisciplinary teamwork between pediatric cardiologists, interventional radiologists, anesthesiologists, and skilled nursing staff is essential for successful outcomes. Multidisciplinary teamwork enables seamless communication and simultaneous treatment, crucial in addressing the unique demands of children. The multidisciplinary strategy of interventional pediatric cardiology entails not only advanced technical expertise but also extensive familiarity with the physiological as well as psychological challenges of children and their parents. This comprehensive perspective allows healthcare providers to navigate the treatment complexities mindful of patient-focused care. All these helps highlight the dynamic and evolving nature of interventional pediatric cardiology (N/A, 2007).

Definition of Interventional Pediatric Cardiology

Interventional pediatric cardiology is a branch of pediatric medicine comprising diagnosis and treatment of congenital and acquired cardiac abnormalities in children through minimally invasive procedures. Compared to traditional open-heart surgery, which may involve a long recovery and severe complications, interventional treatments are designed to be less invasive, occasionally using catheter-based procedures. These techniques range from balloon angioplasty, which reopens a patent path through a narrowed artery, to stenting which maintains arteries open. By reducing patient trauma and shortening recovery times, interventional pediatric cardiology is a giant leap ahead in providing care especially tailored to infants, children, and adolescents with serious heart disease. Central to the practice of interventional pediatric cardiology is the integration of advanced imaging technologies with the application of cutting-edge medical devices optimized for small pediatric-specific anatomical structures. Echocardiography, fluoroscopy, and magnetic resonance imaging are all relied upon extensively to navigate interventions both safely and successfully. Moreover, technology advancements have enhanced the understanding of the pediatric patient's unique physiology and pathology such that cardiologists can aim care performance deficiencies with interventions. As highlighted in more recent reviews, including those outlined by specialists within respective fields, the creation of these authoritative clinical decision support guidelines can assist in identifying and prioritizing patient needs, ultimately enhancing clinical outcomes and optimizing treatment avenues for this vulnerable population (Bell et al., 2012) (Figure 13.1).

Furthermore, the interventional pediatric cardiologist's role extends beyond immediate technical intervention, such as long-term management of congenital heart disease as children grow up and the attendant healthcare problems that follow throughout adolescence. Pediatric cardiologists must perform extensive follow-up care observing heart function and taking action when complications, such as arrhythmias or heart failure, occur. As exposure to radiation is bound to be an issue due to the imaging techniques applied in such interventions, experts are rather interested in approaches to minimizing threats while ensuring diagnostic accuracy advantages (Donya et al., 2014). The dynamic landscape of pediatric interventional cardiology hence illustrates the vital process of interaction among innovation, patient safety, and team care, placing it in its significant role in enhancing children's quality of life with cardiac conditions.

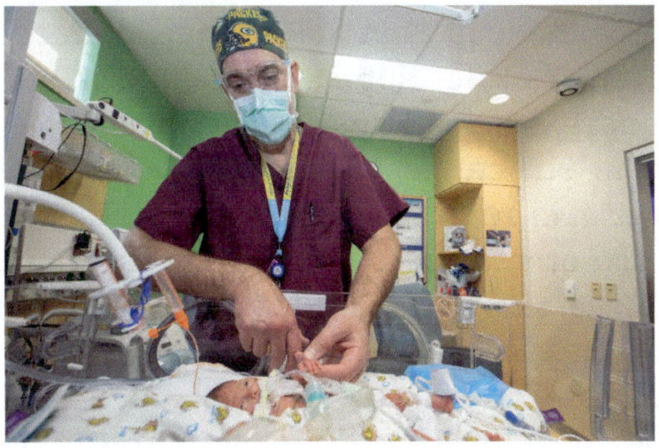

Figure 13.1. Interventional cardiology care.

Source: https://www.hopkinsmedicine.org/-/media/migration/all-childrens-hospital/images/services/heart-institute/heart-stories/interventional-cardiology-2.jpg.

Importance of the Field in Treating Congenital Heart Defects

Interventional pediatric cardiology is of paramount importance in the treatment of congenital heart defects, a collection of malformations significantly impacting the cardiovascular structure and function at birth. These defects can lead to an extensive variety of complications, from heart failure and arrhythmias to growth restriction and developmental impairment in children. The role of the interventional procedures has expanded considerably, with the emphasis directed towards the use of minimally invasive techniques that have drastically improved the outcomes in these patients. Cardiologists can correct or alleviate congenital defects frequently enough using catheter-based techniques without open-heart surgery, with minimal recovery time and body trauma to the patient. Through investigation, it has been proven that early intervention can significantly enhance life expectancy and lifestyle for participating children, and will achieve a greater understanding of how vital the field remains to current pediatric health. Also, the continuous advances in interventional pediatric cardiology are a testament to the changing nature of this clinical discipline. Precise interventions such as balloon angioplasty and stenting have become routine in the treatment of conditions such as coarctation of the aorta (CoA), which, left untreated, has severe long-term implications for health. Current research indicates that treatments developed with insight from computational fluid dynamics can lead to improved hemodynamic outcomes, which directly impacts the patient's quality of life. Doctors are now in a position to define ideal treatment paths through the use of improved imaging and modeling techniques, thereby making interventions more accurate. The character of these practices to change reflects the imperative nature of the role played by interventionist techniques in changing the treatment of congenital heart disease and minimizing its associated morbidity and mortality risks (Feinstein et al., 2010). Finally, new investigation on animal models has extended the boundaries of interventional pediatric cardiology. New advances have introduced novel techniques for causing muscular ventricular septal defects, which promise to provide valuable information on effective therapy. The investigation of such techniques gives greater insight into the way in which defects can be treated or corrected in the clinic and lays the groundwork for new treatments that might not otherwise be considered. This constant interplay between research and clinical application means that pediatric cardiology constantly extends the boundaries of technological and medical advancement. With each advance through intensive testing and examination, each new therapeutic technique broadens the practice's capacity for addressing complex congenital heart disease to an astonishing degree, affirming the position that innovation holds in providing enhanced patient outcomes (Aumann et al., 2008).

Overview of Advancements in Technology and Techniques

The recent technological advances in interventional pediatric cardiology have revolutionized the very face of patient care in CHD. Advances in minimally invasive techniques, such as catheter procedures, have significantly reduced the need for open-heart surgery. These techniques minimize physical trauma, leading to rapid recovery and lesser morbidity in the young population. Imaging and navigation technologies, particularly fluoroscopy and echocardiography, are now standard equipment, allowing cardiologists to perform high-level interventions more precisely. The addition of advanced three-dimensional imaging has further allowed physicians to view congenital abnormalities in greater detail, which in turn enhances pre-procedure planning and outcomes. Such technological advances not only provide a safer experience for the patient but also enhance the efficacy of treatment protocols, providing an overall multi-dimensional solution to tackling pediatric heart ailments in an efficient manner. In addition, the utilization of high-resolution imaging technologies, particularly cardiovascular magnetic resonance (CMR), has been a vital advancement in pediatric cardiology. CMR's ability to yield detailed anatomical and physiological data enables comprehensive assessment of cardiac conditions, which is of the utmost importance in guiding interventional management. This is especially important in the pediatric population, where conventional imaging may prove difficult because of the tiny dimensions and unusual anatomic variability of children. As noted in recent studies, ongoing technological improvements in the area of data acquisition techniques have made possible more advanced imaging protocols tailored for children, which help improve overall care for CHD and acquired heart disease in children. CMR's capability to combine superb 3D anatomy with physiological data offers pediatric cardiologists and congenital heart surgeons a useful perspective, ultimately resulting in more informed clinical choices and improved patient outcomes (Hughes et al., 2011). The development of interventional pediatric cardiology also involves the invention of new devices that have special needs of children. New developments include stents and occluders designed specifically for small-sized vascular structures, which have been found to be crucial in addressing other congenital defects. The use of such personalized devices not only enhances safety during the process but also maximizes the long-term result for children. In addition, improvements in biomaterials have helped develop more biocompatible devices, resulting in fewer complications. As technology moves forward, the combination of sophisticated innovations with conventional methods promises to further improve the quality of treatment given to patients with congenital heart conditions. The convergence of these advances marks a pivotal shift to an era in which outcomes are optimized by precision medicine tailored to the pediatric populations' unique anatomical and physiological requirements (N/A, 1998).

13.1. Historical Background

The historical background of interventional pediatric cardiology is highly inextricably intertwined with technological and surgical advances in medicine. Congenital heart disease has long been difficult since its earliest beginnings, back to early explorations in cardiac anatomy and physiology. Before the 20th century, treatment in children with CHD was largely limited, with most being palliative rather than curative. Pediatric cardiology emerged as a distinct specialty during the mid-20th century with the perception that children with cardiac disease required specialized knowledge different from that for adults. With more sophisticated imaging techniques and a better understanding of cardiac pathophysiology, clinicians began formulating increasingly effective treatments, making it possible for physicians to effectively diagnose CHD and intervene at critical periods in development. This advancement led to the integration of interventional techniques that would revolutionize the management of the condition in children. In the latter half of the 20th century, interventional pediatric cardiology evolved significantly, paralleling advances in catheter-based intervention that revolutionized operating practices. Perhaps most importantly, the introduction of balloon angioplasty in the 1980s was a turning point, allowing minimal invasiveness in the management of stenotic lesions. This paved the way for further advancements, including the stenting techniques and transcatheter closure procedures, which are now a standard practice in the treatment of most congenital abnormalities. These therapies not only reduced the risks associated with open-heart surgery but also improved the outcome in patients through rapid recovery and short hospitalization. With increasing knowledge of CHD physiology, pediatric interventional cardiology turned its focus toward early diagnosis and minimal invasive treatment, which later enhanced the quality of life for children suffering from these severe conditions (Annisa et al., 2025). Advances in state-of-the-art technology have been the main drivers of the evolution of pediatric interventional cardiology. More recent imaging modalities, such as echocardiography and magnetic resonance imaging, have greatly enhanced diagnostic accuracy, allowing for accurate visualization of congenital defects at earlier stages. This has allowed for early intervention, often before the onset of significant morbidity and mortality. Furthermore, continued focus on the optimization of catheter-based interventions has led to better and safer methods of a wide range of cardiac abnormalities. Groundbreaking studies have shown that early intervention, complemented by these advances, significantly improves long-term survival rates and quality of life for children. Nevertheless, existing challenges remain, including the need for rigid training, formalized protocols, and robust clinical models to overcome the multi-faceted approach of pediatric cardiology. As the field advances, long-term studies and healthcare innovation are needed to optimize patient outcomes and counter the growing prevalence of congenital heart disease (Freger et al., 2025).

13.1.1. Evolution of Pediatric Cardiology as a Specialty

The specialty of pediatric cardiology has itself undergone tremendous transformations since its inception and evolved into a distinct specialty dedicated to the cardiovascular health of children and infants. It was initially part of general pediatrics and adult cardiology and had very little specialization and focus on the special needs of pediatric patients. With the advent of imaging technologies and medical interventions during the latter part of the twentieth century, the demand for an expert sector became ever more imperative. The establishment of pediatric cardiology as a specialty area of the medical field not only facilitated the provision of specific training programs but also enhanced research activities aimed at gaining knowledge about congenital heart disease and its treatment. This development, thus, laid the groundwork for innovative treatment modalities that now define the specialty, bridging gaps in care long endemic in young patients. Pediatric cardiology has continued to evolve to incorporate new interventional therapies, which have transformed patient outcomes. Catheter-based interventions allowed the pediatric cardiologist's scope of practice to become more advanced than just diagnosis and medical management, including sophisticated procedures previously the domain of the surgical team. The advances in minimally invasive techniques have provided much value in the form of decreased recovery times and hospital stays for patients. Furthermore, the advances have made patients eligible to be treated for ailments that previously were incompatible with life, therefore revolutionizing paradigms as far as treatment options are concerned. As a result of this evolution, pediatric cardiology has emerged with an established role where innovation and tradition meet, inviting an integrated response to the special cardiological issues of children who require interventional therapy. Multidisciplinary staff and incorporation into pediatric cardiology also helped develop it as a specialty. The interaction of cardiologists with surgeons, radiologists, and nursing staff has become part of delivering maximum benefit to pediatric patients. This model of team ensures continuity of care for the patient, not only time-limited intervention but also extended follow-up and support. Continual education and training have enhanced the merit of interdisciplinary collaboration to improve clinical outcomes. One such manifestation of the teamwork culture is the creation of programs to stimulate research into new approaches and the effectiveness of existing interventions. As pediatric cardiology advances further, these interprofessional teams are bound to continue improving the efficacy of care in a way that the evolving complications in the cardiological care of children are being attended to with new approaches.

13.1.2. Milestones in Interventional Techniques

Evolution of interventional techniques of pediatric cardiology has greatly changed the picture of treatment in congenital and acquired cardiac diseases. Previously, interventions were mostly surgical, often with open-heart surgery involving a high risk, particularly in neonates and infants. The entry of catheter-based techniques was a breakthrough, allowing physicians to have less invasive interventions. These techniques not only minimize trauma but also decrease recovery time, greatly improving clinical outcomes. Furthermore, developments in imaging modalities such as echocardiography and fluoroscopy have enhanced real-time visualization of cardiac structures, enabling effective intervention. These developments not only revolutionized the management of conditions like atrial septal defects and patent ductus arteriosus but also paved the ground for newer methods of therapy that continue to evolve with evolving research and technological advancements (Selvakumari et al., 2025). Artificial intelligence (AI) has emerged as a significant tool towards augmenting diagnostic accuracy and procedural efficacy in pediatric cardiology. Computer vision methods, particularly in image analysis automation, have significantly enhanced the evaluation of cardiac conditions, which are liable to pose challenges within traditional imaging methods. Deep learning techniques using Convolutional Neural Networks (CNN), for instance, have been thoroughly examined and were concluded to outperform traditional methods in segmentation and classification of pediatric cardiac signals and images. These developments are important due to the growing difficulty in getting clear images in pediatric patients, who are not always compliant with imaging studies. As AI integration continues to evolve with clinical practice, it also holds potential for further optimizing existing interventional approaches, further improving patient outcomes as well as enabling more personalized treatment modalities in pediatric cardiac disease management (Selvakumari et al., 2025). Percutaneous retrieval techniques are another significant advancement in the area of interventional pediatric cardiology. Results of a very large study across 17 years highlighted the safety and efficacy of this less invasive technique for the management of fragmented or embolized central venous catheters in children. A high success rate of 92.3% was noted in this study, highlighting the feasibility of successful intervention without resorting to more invasive surgical alternatives. The technique was based largely on femoral vein access and snare retrieval methods, heavily biased in favor of the less traumatic approaches when handling these complications. With 76.9% of the patients being asymptomatic post procedure, the findings suggest percutaneous methods to be chosen over standard surgery in appropriate cases, a landmark in the progression of interventional techniques dedicated to enhancing pediatric cardiac care.

13.1.3. Key Figures and Their Contributions to the Field

The evolution of interventional pediatric cardiology is also shaped by key figures whose careers have contributed to the advancement of innovative techniques and improved patient results. Dr. Norwood is one of such a key figure who has gained wide recognition for his trailblazing work in the treatment of complicated congenital heart disease. His development of the Norwood procedure has shifted surgical treatment of hypoplastic left heart syndrome so that patients now survive who in the past had no hope. His operation is a prime example of what happens when there is a focus to produce change, resulting in dramatic realignment of care for pediatric patients with severe heart disease. These achievements highlight the importance of extensive research and clinical practice in creating pediatric cardiology, providing a legacy that continues to shape current practices in the field. Dr. Greenleaf is another prominent name in interventional pediatric cardiology for his early work in catheter-based interventions. His work has enabled less invasive techniques to combat congenital heart disease, reducing significantly the risks in traditional open-heart surgery. With advancements in procedures such as balloon angioplasty and stent implantation, Dr. Greenleaf has transformed the treatment options available for children with heart defects. These developments not only enhance short-term clinical outcomes but also promote long-term health benefits, allowing patients to lead a higher quality of life. Consequently, Dr. Greenleafs contribution has been the spark for innovation to follow, creating curiosity and inquiry in the new field of interventional methods specifically tailored for children. Lastly, Dr. Lammers impact cannot be understated, as he has been a driving force in promoting multidisciplinary practice in pediatric interventional cardiology. By encouraging teamwork among surgeons, cardiologists, and radiologists, Dr. Lammers has fostered a culture of ensuring holistic care that is individualized to suit the particular needs of children. His initiatives have led to the establishment of centers of excellence for specialized care of the issues entailed in congenital heart disease in children. This collaborative approach emphasizes not only the technicality of intervention but also the psychological, emotional, and developmental needs of children as patients. The efforts of someone like Dr. Lammers promote teamwork and innovativeness in the ongoing pursuit of excellence in the ever-changing practice of interventional pediatric cardiology, ensuring that every patient receives customized and effective treatment (N/A, 2006).

13.2. Common Procedures

In the realm of interventional pediatric cardiology, some interventions are performed with high frequency, primarily to correct congenital cardiac anomalies and other cardiovascular lesions. Cardiac catheterization is one of the most common procedures, which is employed both for diagnostic as well as therapeutic interventions. It is a minimally invasive procedure involving the insertion of a catheter via a blood vessel into the heart. With this method, physicians are able to obtain significant hemodynamic data, visualize the cardiac structures with fluoroscopy, and even carry out procedures such as balloon angioplasty or stenting. The utility of cardiac catheterization renders it a valuable tool in managing pediatric patients, especially when surgery may be more dangerous due to the patient's weight or age. Other than cardiac catheterization, deployment of device closure is another routine intervention in pediatric interventional cardiology. Atrial septal defects (ASDs) and patent ductus arteriosus (PDA) can lead to severe long-term consequences if left untreated. By the use of transcatheter techniques, cardiologists are able to close such defects effectively using closure devices, thus avoiding further heart failure or pulmonary hypertension. The ability to perform such procedures via catheterization minimizes the need for open-heart surgery, ultimately lowering recovery time and hospitalization for child patients. Not only does this method enhance patient outcomes, but it also removes the emotional burden on families through a child's treatment period. Lastly, radiofrequency ablation is a significant procedure applied to heal arrhythmic disorders in child patients. Abnormal cardiac rhythms could lead to serious health complications, and the standard treatment of medication may not always provide the level of control needed. Radiofrequency ablation is a method that uses a catheter to transmit energy to eliminate certain areas of the heart responsible for abnormal rhythms. The method can effectively restore normal sinus rhythm, thereby eliminating the potential for arrhythmia-related complications. As technology and methodology improve, radiofrequency ablation has been increasingly successful, leading to better outcomes for children who are suffering from these potentially lethal illnesses. Incorporation of such procedures as standard practice highlights the importance of refining methodologies in interventional pediatric cardiology, ultimately improving the prognosis for such children.

13.2.1. Balloon Angioplasty

Among pediatric interventional cardiology procedures, balloon angioplasty is a milestone in the treatment of congenital heart conditions, most importantly obstructive lesions. The less invasive procedure has gained prominence with its ability to reverse stenosis in various cardiovascular structures, significantly improving hemodynamics as well as promising long-term effects. Balloon angioplasty is frequently applied in diseases like coarctation of the aorta and stenosis of the pulmonary artery. The balloon dilation of narrowed areas causes immediate relief from occlusive symptoms, often obviating the need for more aggressive operations. Recent figures, as indicated by statistics, have shown the method to be increasingly successful, with astounding success rates seen in pediatric cohorts with congenital malformations (Feinstein et al., 2010). Evidence indicates that balloon angioplasty possesses excellent benefits, both in terms of success in procedure and postoperative recovery, quality of life, and patients. For instance, research into coarctation of the aorta has highlighted that early dilatation using balloons can prevent severe morbidities relating to native coarctation and potentially encompass hypertension and heart failure (Feinstein et al., 2010) (Figure 13.2).

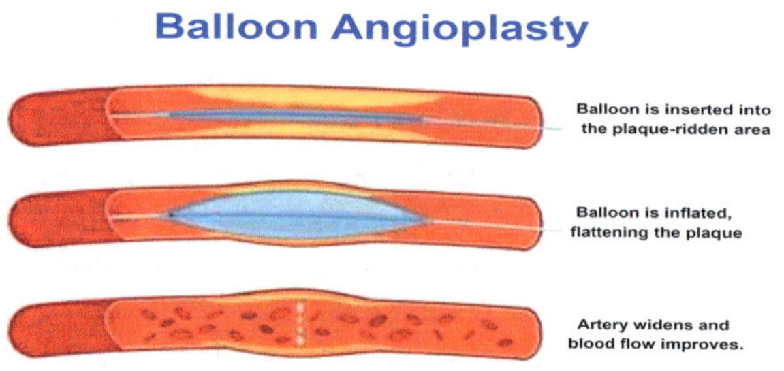

Figure 13.2. Balloon angioplasty.

Source: https://www.practo.com/health-wiki/elephantiasis-causes-symptoms-diagnosis-and-treatment/75/article.

Additionally, advances in imaging and catheter technology have allowed precise navigation and manipulation of devices to enhance safety and effectiveness of the procedure. The minimally invasive balloon angioplasty has little downtime as compared to open surgery, and children can resume their daily activities even earlier, which is one of the primary concerns in the pediatric environment. Although balloon angioplasty is advantageous, there are risks involved, so careful patient selection and follow-up are necessary. Although the procedure works, it may require repeat procedures due to re-stenosis or future complications. Therefore, pediatric cardiology staff must carry out comprehensive preoperative assessment and ongoing patient monitoring post-procedure to identify any developing issues early. The new emergence of interventional procedures such as balloon angioplasty is a continuation of the expanding demand for minimally invasive treatment approaches in the management of congenital heart disease, with promising evidence regarding outcomes and safety (Alvarez-Fuente et al., 2024). The trend not only creates avenues for better management of the patient but also calls for more studies to develop the techniques further and improve their weaknesses in the best possible way.

13.2.2. Stenting in Pediatric Patients

The use of stenting in children is an impressive advancement in pediatric interventional cardiology, addressing functional as well as structural cardiovascular abnormalities. Children typically pose certain specific challenges because of their varying anatomical sizes and developmental states, which necessitate specific devices and techniques. Stenting has also been applied in cases of aortic coarctation, stenotic valves, and other birth heart defects, where traditional surgery may be more risky or less convenient. By employing stents, temporary support structures, treatment professionals can dilate constricted vessels safely, improve circulation, and remove associated symptoms from these children, thereby enhancing their overall quality of life. The efficacy and safety of stenting procedures in younger patients have enhanced over time, particularly with advancements in catheterization procedures and imaging technologies. In line with recent studies, there is a need to set diagnostic reference levels (DRLs) carefully to limit unnecessary exposure to radiation during intervention, particularly in light of the possibility of needing to repeat procedures throughout the life of a patient (Bacher et al., 2019). The technical challenge of procedures, combined with the delicate physiology of pediatric patients, underscores the importance of careful planning and execution. Through close organ dose and effective dose monitoring during stenting, medical practitioners can ensure that the benefits of such interventions far outweigh any potential risks, opening the door to an even greater understanding of pediatric cardiology procedures. Addition of cardiovascular magnetic resonance (CMR) imaging is at the center of enabling stenting procedures and outcomes in children. CMR provides unsurpassed three-dimensional cardiac anatomy and visualization of blood flow, which optimizes procedural decision-making abilities (Hughes et al., 2011). With its progression in use among children, addition of CMR to routine evaluations offers valuable information to enable the delivery of tailored approaches for stenting interventions. The imaging technique assists in assessing congenital heart disease and minimizing radiation exposure compared to traditional imaging modalities. Such a combination of cutting-edge imaging and intervention technology represents a futuristic approach between pediatric cardiology, hopefully resulting in better patient outcomes and long-term follow-up strategies for patients requiring stenting in their care.

13.2.3. Device Closure of Congenital Defects

The development of device closure strategies revolutionized the treatment of congenital heart disease, significantly enhancing the quality of care in pediatric interventional cardiology. Among the various ailments that have been treated using these less invasive techniques, mVSDs stand out due to their historical challenges. Surgical interventions were once perilous and paved the way for new alternatives. Innovative animal model research proves the potential for creating mVSDs to explore new therapeutic options, highlighting the promise of safe closure methods of devices that can be used in beating hearts without extracorporeal circulation and thereby reducing patient morbidity and enhancing recovery periods (Aumann et al., 2008) (Figure 13.3).

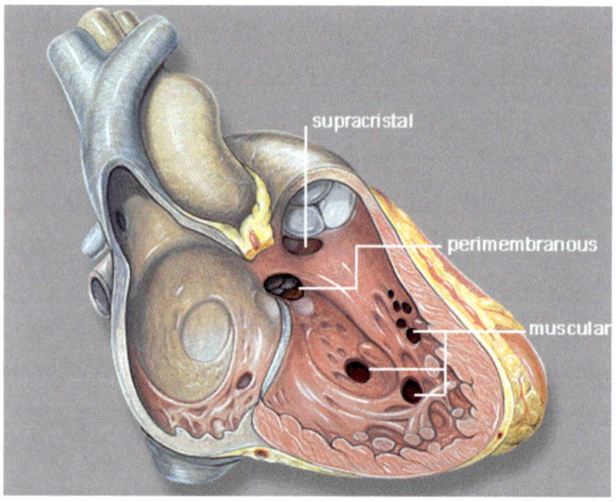

Figure 13.3. Muscular ventricular septal defects (mVSDs).

Source: https://www.healio.com/~/media/learningsites/learntheheart/assets/c/5/d/2/vsd_defects_labelled.gif.

Evolution of such methods not only attempts to circumvent the limitations of open-heart surgery but also opens the doors towards more personalized, patient-specific therapy. Careful preoperative assessment plays a critical role in determining the suitability of device closure for congenital abnormalities. Comprehensive diagnostic modalities like echocardiography, cardiac catheterization, computed tomography, and magnetic resonance imaging play a key role in the evaluation process. These technologies allow doctors to visualize detailed anatomical structures such as atrioventricular valves in conditions such as atrioventricular septal defects. Bedside real-time three-dimensional echocardiography enhances diagnostic accuracy with dynamic images that account for the defects' complexity. These newer imaging techniques guarantee treatment plans to be thoroughly planned to accommodate the unique patient's anatomical shape, thus enhancing more successful outcomes of interventional procedures (Pozza et al., 2003). An aggressive preoperative evaluation not only minimizes device closure morbidity but also generates confidence within the whole healthcare team regarding the interventional strategy chosen. Lastly, the use of device closure for the treatment of congenital defects is representative of the union of technology and pediatric cardiology. This method is one illustration of a paradigm change away from traditional surgery and towards more innovative, less invasive techniques representative of trends in contemporary medicine to improve patient outcomes. With further clinical evidence being accumulated, applications for device closure will likely become even more widespread so that progressively complex lesions can successfully be treated. Through ongoing research and device development, interventional pediatric cardiology holds the promise of remaking the treatment of congenital heart defect, offering a future of increased safety, efficacy, and patient satisfaction. The trajectory of this specialty underscores the imperative for continued innovation and collaboration between clinicians, researchers, and device makers to optimize care in children with congenital heart defect.

13.3. Indications for Intervention

Recognition of the appropriate time for intervention in pediatric cardiology is a careful assessment of specific clinical indicators that predict the requirement for catheter intervention or surgery. Among these indicators, symptomatic congenital heart defects are extremely high; symptomatic infants presenting with cyanosis, exertional dyspnea, or failure to thrive need to be evaluated urgently. Such presentations are most likely to indicate compromised cardiac function, thus requiring an extensive evaluation with advanced imaging techniques. Cardiovascular magnetic resonance (CMR) is particularly valuable at this stage as it provides precise anatomical and physiological details about the child's heart to assist cardiologists in making a well-informed decision regarding intervention. Awareness of the personal anatomy and hemodynamics of every defect is critical, as certain forms of CHD may require urgent treatment, while others can be watched for spontaneous resolution as the child matures, thereby altering the treatment plan based on evolving clinical conditions (Hughes et al., 2011). Certain forms of congenital heart disease are so well defined in terms of indications for intervention that guidelines exist outlining when intervention should be undertaken. For instance, defects with significant left-to-right shunts, i.e., atrial septal defects or ventricular septal defects, can produce pulmonary hypertension and heart failure unless they are repaired. Current guidelines advise surgical closure in such cases where pulmonary blood flow is over a critical ratio to systemic flow, particularly when patients have symptoms or signs of declining function. Additionally, conditions like aortic coarctation require intervention once diagnosed, as they can lead to severe complications and organ dysfunction if corrective measures are delayed. The urgency surrounding these interventions underscores the importance of recognizing specific clinical scenarios where the balance of risks versus benefits may favor prompt corrective action to enhance long-term outcomes for pediatric patients (Arrieta et al., 2013). In the practice of interventional pediatric cardiology, ongoing advances in technique and device continue to decrease the indications for intervention. Transcatheter intervention, such as implantation of transcatheter pulmonary valves, has become an accepted mode of care in children with failing conduits, providing a minimally invasive solution to conventional surgical intervention. Because these valves will have a finite lifespan and need to be replaced, their early correction with more sophisticated devices like the Melody® valve can obviate complications of aging conduits, such as pulmonary stenosis and insufficiency. Such inventions represent a paradigm shift in the perception of the need for early interventions that both extend life as well as improve quality of life in children suffering from congenital heart disease. This technological progress demands ongoing assessment of pointers towards intervention, to identify that contemporary advances are used effectively to maximize patient outcome (Arrieta et al., 2013).

13.3.1. Types of Congenital Heart Defects Requiring Intervention

There are literally hundreds of congenital heart defects (CHDs) that must be treated to mitigate hemodynamic compromise and enhance quality of life. A few of the most common are atrial septal defects (ASDs) and ventricular septal defects (VSDs). ASDs allow oxygen-rich blood from the left atrium to flow into the right atrium, causing volume overload of the right heart and ultimate pulmonary hypertension. VSDs have similar effects by providing an opportunity for the blood to shunt from the higher-pressure left ventricle to the lower-pressure right ventricle, resulting in left-to-right shunting. The two defects, if left uncorrected, can advance to heart failure or fatal arrhythmias. Both defects are usually treated with percutaneous and surgical interventions, such as device closure of ASDs and surgical patching of VSDs, in an attempt to correct these defects and establish normal circulatory dynamics. However, more complex congenital heart disease requires complicated surgery due to its multilateral nature. One such case is tetralogy of Fallot with a combination of four cardiac abnormalities and requires complete surgical repair ideally within the first year of life in order to prevent prolonged cyanosis and growth retardation. Similarly, transposition of the great arteries needs to be treated urgently, usually through atrial septostomy and then arterial switch to correct the inverted aortic and pulmonary artery connection. All these interventions are significant; without urgent treatment, the chances of death are highly enhanced. Procedures such as transcatheter interventions also have emerged, decreasing the need for open-heart surgeries, presenting an alternative that is less invasive to manage such complex conditions while improving patient recovery times and outcomes (Arrieta et al., 2013) (Figure 13.4).

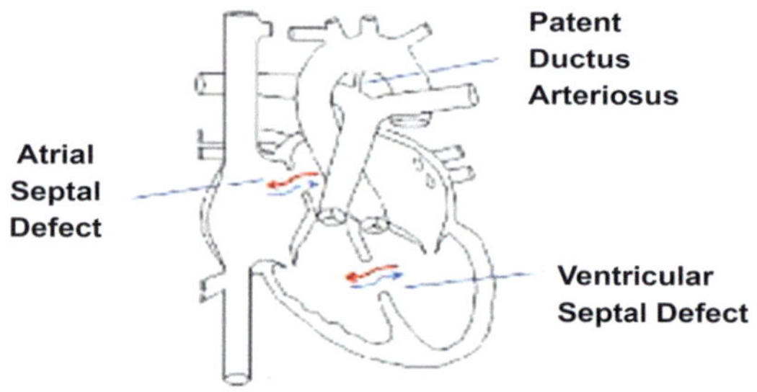

Figure 13.4. Schematics of ASD, VSD, and PDA.

Source: https://www.researchgate.net/figure/Schematics-of-ASD-VSD-and-PDA_fig1_259318609.

The use of advanced imaging technologies has largely changed the diagnosis and management of congenital heart disease. Cardiovascular magnetic resonance (CMR) has emerged as a central tool since it can provide detailed anatomical as well as functional information, particularly in children. As imaging in small children is usually accompanied by many challenges, CMR enables one to perform a non-invasive evaluation for planning the intervention in CHDs. This approach is better than others in delineating complex geometry, thereby assisting cardiac surgeons and pediatric cardiologists in making personalized intervention plans. For example, CMR is utilized in assessing the viability of valvular and outflow conduit conduits prior to surgery, facilitating decision-making and maximizing procedural outcomes (Hughes et al., 2011). As the specialty continues to progress, the position of advanced imaging will be at the forefront of enhancing the effectiveness and precision of interventions in pediatric cardiology practice.

13.3.2. Assessment Criteria for Intervention

In evaluation of interventional pediatric cardiology, it is important to establish robust evaluation criteria for intervention. Not only do they act as a foundation for making sound treatment decisions but as well as a means of guiding clinicians to track patient outcome. Key factors are the complexity and severity of the heart condition, health status of the patients, and the potential for long-term improvement. Of most interest are the newer imaging modalities, which have emerged as potent instruments in this context by enabling accurate characterization of the anatomical and physiological details required for planning interventional treatments. Furthermore, assessment should incorporate multidisciplinary opinion to enable decisions to permit a complete comprehension of the child's requirements and optimize the risk-benefit ratio in proposed interventions. Moreover, in line with the fact that developments in technology are constantly redefining pediatric cardiology, the use of new X-ray imaging systems is a paradigm of the need for revised assessment criteria. New imaging technologies have been shown in recent research to be able to significantly lower the level of radiation exposure without lowering image quality, and this is especially important in pediatrics (Bacher et al., 2015). This reduction in dose not only invites better safety in practice in interventions but also demands great levels of standards in determining the safety and effectiveness of these technologies. Clinicians would need to weigh the advantages of these innovations against any resulting constraints, such as image noise, which can be generated from lower doses of radiation. So, the evaluation standards for identifying the appropriate interventions must shift to include the best available evidence on technological advances along with traditional clinical indicators. Finally, long-term results from interventions must be assessed through a systemic process to quantify the effectiveness of the methodologies employed. For instance, transcatheter pulmonary valve implantation (TPVI) has been proved to be a safe option for conventional surgical procedures, whose primary aim is to circumvent the problems of conduit degeneration and prolong the lifespan of cardiac devices (Arrieta et al., 2013) (Figure 13.5).

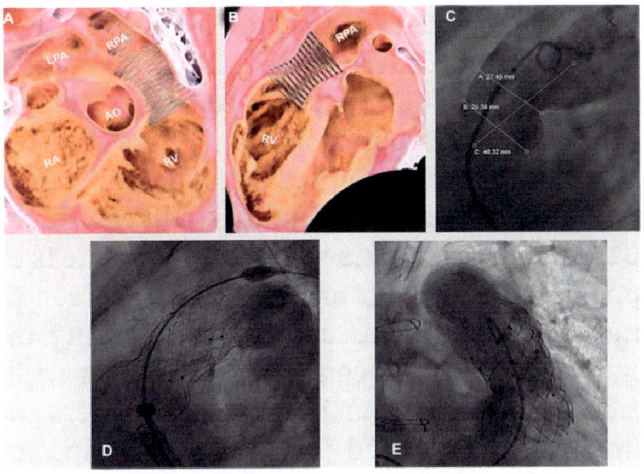

Figure 13.5. Venus P valve implantation. Virtual reality simulation of device implantation based on CT, in right anterior oblique (A) and lateral (B) views. (C) RVOT angiography demonstrating a narrowest diameter of 27.5 mm. (D) A 34 mm × 25 mm Venus P valve was implanted. (E) Final RVOT angiography demonstrated effective device function.

Source: https://www.techscience.com/chd/v19n5/59171/html.

Assessment of the effectiveness of these interventions should be based not just on short-term procedural success but also on long-term sustainability of health outcomes. The evaluation methods must thus be designed to monitor potential complications and the stability of implanted devices so that interventions lead to durable benefits in pediatric patients. Incorporating these elements, the evaluation criteria will significantly enhance the quality of care in interventional pediatric cardiology.

13.3.3. Risks of Non-Intervention

The scenario of interventional pediatric cardiology is dominated by the urgency of correcting congenital heart defects and other cardiovascular abnormalities early on. If intervention is not done, it may appear to be a conservative choice; however, delays or omitted interventions can be devastating. Untreated congenital heart disease in children can often lead to progressive morbidity, which can hinder their physical development, result in worse long-term health, and lower general quality of life. Infants and children are more vulnerable since they are physiologically immature, and if left untreated early on, their disease can very rapidly progress and form life-threatening emergencies. Thus, the refusal to proceed with necessary interventional procedures can have catastrophic results that would have been avoided through early surgical or Cath lab interventions. Besides the immediate medical consequences, the emotional and psychological trauma of non-intervention cannot be overstated. Parents of children with cardiac anomalies endure extended periods of anxiety and suspense. The awareness that a straightforward intervention is able to stave off severe health issues could fuel the feelings of powerlessness on the part of caregivers. For most families, a decision to intervene is a see-saw between potential dangers and strong incentives for improved health benefits. Also, lack of intervention could bring about a cascade effect where the overall development of the child, socialization, and access to a good life is catastrophically impacted. The emotional issues also complicate the decision-making process and highlight the imperative for interdisciplinary intervention by healthcare professionals alongside families to traverse the risk of non-intervention. The enhancement in technology has made more sophisticated methods available in interventional pediatric cardiology, once again highlighting the imperative of urgent treatment. For instance, modern imaging modalities have reduced significantly the radiation dose associated with intervention like coronary angiography, enhancing the safety of interventions. This paradigm shift permits pediatric cardiologists to perform necessary interventions with minimal risk of exposure to the ionizing radiation normally associated with such interventions, as suggested in recent research collating the benefits of newer imaging systems being capable of optimizing diagnostic quality while reducing radiation exposure considerably (Bacher et al., 2015). As intervention technologies progress, the case for non-intervention diminishes, thereby proving active participation in interventional treatment can make a substantial difference in patient outcome in pediatric cardiology. The benefits of early intervention, along with comprehensive knowledge and awareness of procedural risk, ultimately serve to protect and enhance the lives of affected children.

13.4. Patient Evaluation and Preparation

Preparation and evaluation of the patient in interventional pediatric cardiology are necessary for the optimization of clinical outcomes. Comprehensive examination is started by taking a thorough medical history, both family and personal. Such an evaluation assists the practitioner in identifying risk factors and potential comorbidities that affect the success of the procedures. In this case, it is essential to utilize clinical decision support (CDS) resources to enhance the accuracy of diagnostics and therapeutic regimens individual to each child. Through CDS resources, one may establish enhanced understanding of present performance gaps in pediatric cardiology so that health professionals are in a position to cope with specific patient needs more effectively through evidence-based methods and improving the effective utilization of health resources (Bell et al., 2012). Thus, a multidisciplinary team for care involving cardiologists, anesthesiologists, and nursing staff is essential during this stage to deliver comprehensive care. Preparation for intervention does not only involve medical screening but also caters to the psychological and emotional needs of pediatric patients and their families. Various children are anxious about receiving medical interventions, which necessitates procedures that bring comfort and illumination. Preparation of the families and patients includes thorough pre-procedure education on the intervention process, potential outcomes, and post-operative care. Involvement of parents in discussion may alleviate fear and establish a good support mechanism, hence making children less anxious (Drivas et al., 2015). In addition, this pre-procedure time is an opportunity to acquire baseline values of essential vital signs and necessary consent, setting the tone well for the upcoming intervention while fostering trust between healthcare providers and families. Finally, good planning in anticipation of the post-procedure period is all part of the overall patient assessment and preparation process. Complications must be expected and post-operative planning arranged, particularly in a children's hospital where response to intervention can be as varied as for an adult but potentially more unpredictable. Planning of follow-up and visits can play a pivotal role in long-term success and quality of life for the child. Recordation and ongoing assessment of patient response to the intervention are essential in identification of any early signs of complications or requirement for additional intervention. Establishing an orderly follow-up protocol, like education regarding lifestyle change and risk factor control, enhances the holistic vision necessary for patient-centered care in interventional pediatric cardiology (Drivas et al., 2015). Safety is prioritized both for the patient and for families' health literacy and resilience in preparation and follow-up.

13.4.1. Diagnostic Imaging Techniques Used

Accuracy of imaging modalities is of utmost significance in pediatric interventional cardiology for best treatment plan and delivery. Among various modalities, echocardiography remains the gold standard, allowing real-time imaging of cardiac anatomy without any ionizing radiation. The lack of invasiveness of the procedure allows the clinician to assess morphology and function of the heart, particularly in neonates and young children with evolving physiology. Advancements, such as three-dimensional echocardiography, have greatly enhanced visualization and allowed for the performance of in-depth evaluations of complex congenital heart disease. Additionally, it provides necessary information during the conduct of catheter-based procedures, which increases the accuracy of device placement and post-procedure outcomes evaluation. The evolution of echocardiographic technology plays a crucial role in the constant endeavor to improve the management of the child's cardiac apparatus, lowering radiation risk, and ensuring timely interventions. Cardiac magnetic resonance imaging (MRI) has also emerged as another important diagnostic tool in pediatric cardiology, with its excellent soft tissue contrast and lack of ionizing radiation. MRI finds particular application in the evaluation of congenital heart disease and their complications, with outstanding detail in images directing surgical and interventional decisions. Its high-capacity features, including functional testing and contrast perfusion imaging, allow for precise evaluation of not just anatomical resolution but also myocardial function (Figure 13.6).

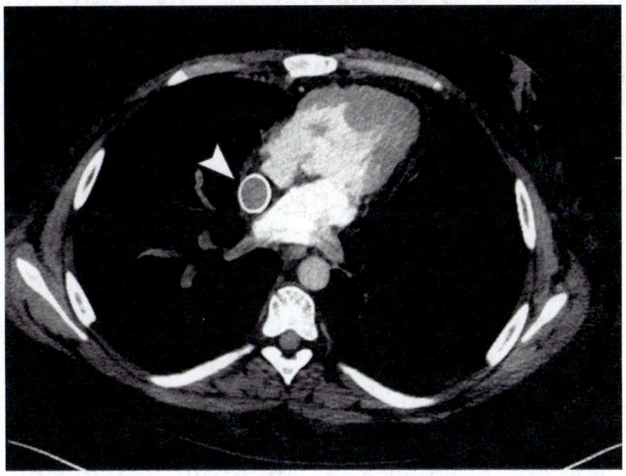

Figure 13.6. Pediatric cardiac CT.

Source: https://ajronline.org/cms/10.2214/AJR.19.22745/asset/images/large/12_19_22745_09b.jpeg.

However, patient compliance has been a problem with MRI, especially among children. Nevertheless, the integration of sedation strategies with accelerated imaging techniques has reduced these problems by making MRI readily accessible for pediatric patients whose cardiac health needs to be monitored closely. Despite advantages from non-invasive imaging modalities, fluoroscopic techniques remain involved in interventional pediatric cardiology, particularly with catheter-based interventions. Fluoroscopy permits real-time imaging of catheter positioning inside the cardiac chamber, critical to successful procedures. New technology in fluoroscopy has reduced exposure to radiation without compromising image quality to any significant extent, rendering it safer for children. A new X-ray imaging technology, for instance, has demonstrated a remarkable 75% reduction in patient dose of radiation without compromising diagnostic quality. The ability to achieve such radiation reduction goes hand-in-hand with the growing emphasis on children's radiation safety, where the risk of cumulative exposure is a serious issue. As these imaging technologies improve with advancements, they have the capability to enhance procedural success safely and effectively in the management of congenital heart disease (Bacher et al., 2015; N/A, 1998).

13.4.2. Pre-Procedural Assessments

Pre-procedure evaluation plays a significant role in interventional pediatric cardiology as it decides the readiness of children for invasive procedures. Thorough assessment through history, physical examination, and diagnostic evaluation forms part of such evaluation. Healthcare providers must consider potential comorbidities, patient-risk factors, and psychosocial issues that could influence procedural outcome. Extensive pre-procedural assessment makes it easier to detect contraindications and allows for individualized planning of anesthetics and procedures specific to the children. This thorough process is conducive to decision-making, allowing for a collective environment among caregivers and families. Pre-procedure preparation not only maintains the safety of the procedure but also the quality of recovery pathways, so pre-procedure evaluation is a characteristic of success in pediatric cardiology interventions. By making systematic pre-procedure assessment a starting point, clinicians are able to reduce risks of interventional procedure complications. Others, for instance the ICPS Contrast Media Usage and Exposure Workgroup, have highlighted identification of and mitigation of risk factors associated with interventional use, that is, contrast media (Indianapolis Coalition for Patient Safety, 2017). Their recommendations emphasize a multidisciplinary approach involving the input of various specialists with expertise to offer an entire view of patient safety. Consensus guidelines are generated from the collaboration that formalizes best practices to optimize interventional outcomes. Addressing potential risks before a procedure allows healthcare providers to anticipate and address undesired effects ahead of time, particularly in fragile pediatric patients who may have unique physiological issues to address. Thus, a good pre-procedural assessment actually contributes significantly to the safety and quality of care provided to children that have cardiac procedures. Pre-procedure interpretation in interventional pediatric cardiology has implications that extend beyond the care of a single patient. The evolution of clinical registries, like New York's revolution in cardiac surgery, underscores the importance of data in driving best practice in pre-surgical evaluation (Cozzens et al., 2012). Clinical registries have facilitated the identification of trends in procedural mortality and complications, enabling health systems to change their approach to patient evaluation and management. By describing differences in outcomes, such registries make institutions review their protocols critically and make changes, accordingly, leading to a culture of quality improvement. Thus, pre-procedure assessment permits systematic changes across pediatric cardiology, prompting ongoing improvement to improve clinical care delivery. Evolving these assessments step by step eventually reflects better patient outcomes, reflecting commitment to excellence in pediatric cardiac interventions.

13.4.3. Family Involvement and Education

Successful engagement of families in the education and care of pediatric patients is at the core of the practice of interventional pediatric cardiology. Family engagement not only improves understanding the complex medical procedures but also the psychological and emotional strength of children and families. Families are heavily involved in the learning process through bringing their own experience and perspective, which can educate healthcare providers to the lessons of treatment. For instance, the incorporation of family anecdotes and wisdom into pediatric residency training programs has been of assistance, evidenced by a study when the curriculum was enriched by the introduction of family voices. By implementing educational interventions involving direct interaction between pediatric residents and families, healthcare providers can foster a more empathetic understanding of patient-specific needs and shared decision-making processes, leading to improved patient outcomes and family satisfaction with care (Pavalagantharajah et al., 2025). Furthermore, collaboration between family providers increases not only the quality of educational content but also empowers families to take on more responsibility for the care of their children's health. There has been evidence to support the fact that families, when engaged in the planning of patient education materials, help ensure that such materials are tailored to respond to their respective needs and interests, thus achieving enhanced comprehension and effectiveness.

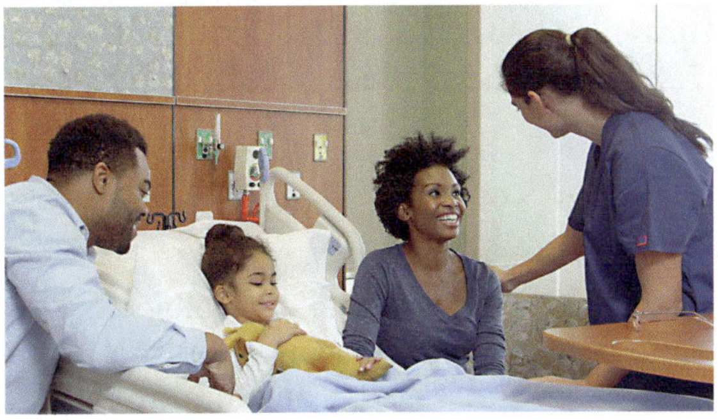

Figure 13.7. Family involvement in the education and care of pediatric patients.

Source: https://external-content.duckduckgo.com/iu/?u=https%3A%2F%2Fwww.ivhouse.com%2Fsites%2Fdefault%2Ffiles%2Finline-images%2Fpatient-parents-nurse-2_134313536.jpg&f=1&nofb=1&ipt=967d7c5403f70eabb9d9808d9a39def982202a3a1f09f5be365467b02d85e8b4.

This type of collaboration is particularly necessary in interventional pediatric cardiology, where interventions can be lengthy and traumatic for patients and families. By using the voices of families in developing these educational materials and tools, as outlined in pediatric oncology commentary, health care providers are empowered to create materials that communicate on a personal level, ultimately leading to enhanced patient understanding and treatment compliance (Reich et al., 2025) (Figure 13.7).

Moreover, if families experience themselves as being members of the medical team, they become more confident in the system, and this has deep repercussions on treatment adherence and health outcomes. The feedback loop from family participants in educational interventions reflects the strong impact of inclusion. By organizing settings in which the voice of families is heard and valued, pediatric cardiology units can generate a collaborative culture of respect. Addressing the educational needs of families via specialized interventions, such as workshops and panels, allows for bi-directional information exchange between clinicians and families. The flow of knowledge in this manner not only facilitates better understanding among families but also arms clinicians with the information that can direct patient care approaches to provide a holistic response to pediatric cardiovascular wellness (Pavalagantharajah et al., 2025).

13.5. Post-Interventional Care

Post-procedure care is an essential part of interventional pediatric cardiology for the recovery of patients. Following procedures such as catheterizations or surgery, the child will likely experience some physiological changes that require observation and management. Complication monitoring, such as bleeding, arrhythmia, or infection, is necessary for the immediate postoperative period. Healthcare professionals use standardized protocols to facilitate effective recovery and minimize hazards, integrating the highest level of evidence-based practice into practice in offering patient care. This is particularly important, as studies have demonstrated that systematized procedures can significantly lower instances of adverse outcomes in children, highlighting the value of specially trained post-interventional procedures in this specialist field. Ideal post-interventional treatment does not end at the recovery ward but also involves ongoing observation and management techniques aimed at addressing both physical and emotional requirements. Children may require additional support as they navigate their recovery, including pain control, feeding support, and emotional support. Family involvement at this point is also equally as crucial, with guardians tasked with keeping an eye on the state of their child and assisting in communicating with health professionals. The adoption of integrative care plans involving parents and clinicians can lead to improved recovery strategies and a better overall experience for patients. Research has shown that family participation largely enhances outcomes, further justifying the necessity of care models in consort in post-interventional pediatric cardiology. Furthermore, adherence to evidence-based recommendations is required to enhance the quality of post-interventional care. For instance, the use of targeted temperature management has emerged as an important means of improving outcomes for pediatric patients with compromised cardiac function after procedures. Practice pattern variations have been seen in facilities for these interventions, highlighting the need for consistent protocols among healthcare systems. By fostering interdisciplinary collaboration among cardiologists, nurses, and allied health professionals, centers can create streamlined workflows that not only promote enhanced patient safety but also eliminate variabilities in care that lead to errors or complications. Establishing such consensus-based recommendations, as with efforts between various healthcare specialties, may go a long way toward enhancing the quality of care delivered during the high-risk post-interventional period of interventional pediatric cardiology (Figure 13.8).

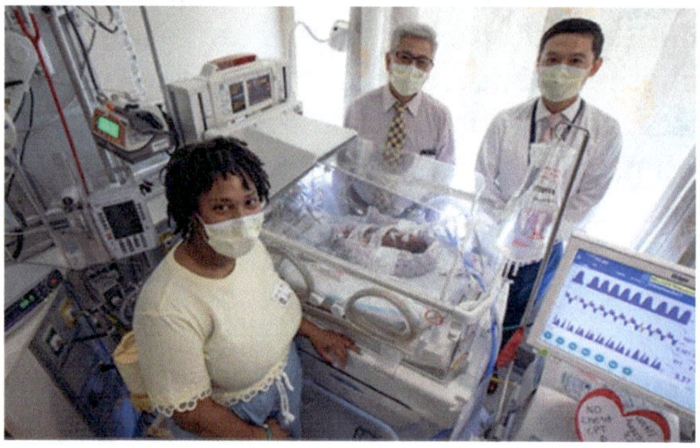

Figure 13.8. Post-interventional care.

Source: https://external-content.duckduckgo.com/iu/?u=https%3A%2F%2Fhealth.ucdavis.edu%2Fmedia-resources%2Fpediatrics%2Fimages%2FMarquee%2Facademic-programs%2Fcardio-556x370.jpg&f=1&nofb=1&ipt=4de3bebfbf06dbba10864075a21175ed145e30e9e97e82a545ea4d8432f9099f.

13.5.1. Monitoring and Follow-Up Protocols

In pediatric interventional cardiology, the role of follow-up and monitoring protocols simply cannot be overstressed. They aim at ensuring continuous safety and health in patients subsequent to repeated invasive interventions. Pediatric patients naturally react differently at a physiological level to interventions, and therefore follow-up tactics must be tailor-made to identify potential complications on an early stage. Effective monitoring not only enables early detection of complications, such as arrhythmias or technical problems, but also enables clinicians to assess the long-term efficacy of interventions. By adhering to strict follow-up regimens, healthcare providers can optimize patient outcomes and enhance quality of care in this subspecialty. The accurate nature of follow-up interventions in pediatric cardiology inevitably intersects with the risks of diagnostic imaging and therapeutic interventions, specifically those involving ionizing radiation. Sophisticated imaging modalities are utilized extensively to evaluate the outcome of cardiac interventions, but as with all modalities, they carry inherent risks, as discussed in the literature (Donya et al., 2014). It is vital that the need for these imaging devices be balanced against harm by clinicians. Follow-up in a structured setting can reduce risks by careful evaluation and modification of imaging approaches to fit individual patient backgrounds. In persistent evaluation, clinicians ensure a judicious approach to follow-up, and a valuable contribution is made to the worldwide success of interventional pediatric cardiology. Besides, patient safety and reduction of the complication rate are contingent on interdisciplinary cooperation by healthcare teams, as seen in the initiatives of the ICPS Contrast Media Usage and Exposure Workgroup (Indianapolis Coalition for Patient Safety, 2017). Such teamwork highlights the significance of extensive protocols for utilizing contrast media, which may be required in subsequent imaging procedures. Through the convergence of insights from diverse groups of healthcare professionals, ranging from radiologists, cardiologists, and nephrologists, monitoring protocols can assimilate best practices that focus on patient safety. Not only does an interdisciplinary methodology increase the quality of follow up examinations, but it also promotes a culture of ongoing quality enhancement in pediatric cardiology, ultimately working towards improved clinical outcomes in the vulnerable population.

13.5.2. Potential Complications and Management

In pediatric cardiology interventions, awareness of potential complications is a critical part of managing patients. Catheter-based interventions, even though they are usually safe, have inherent risks like vascular injury, arrhythmia, and infection. These complications can either be immediate or appear later during the recovery process in the patient, necessitating vigilant monitoring and assessment. For instance, a patient with vascular injury may require surgical correction of the injury. Moreover, arrhythmias, which may be due to electrical instability from a procedure, need close follow-up for ensuring cardiac stability. Identification of such complications early on by clinicians is necessary for restricting their impact, and hence patient education and risk stratification before the procedure are crucial. Interdisciplinary treatment of complications in interventional pediatric cardiology also involves chronic conditions that may arise post-procedure. Long-term conditions like coronary artery complications can occur due to interventions, predominantly in Kawasaki disease patients. The disease, which includes inflammation of the coronary arteries, puts children at dire cardiovascular complications if left untreated. Approximately one-third of untreated Kawasaki patients have coronary aneurysms, leading to potential thrombosis or stenotic lesions, resulting in lifelong cardiac risks for patients transitioning into adult care (Brogan et al., 2020). Continuous surveillance and individualized measures of management are essential to manage such chronic sequelae, emphasizing the incorporation of complete care consisting of both pediatric and adult cardiology models. Novel measures in handling complications have been focused on multidisciplinary measures, such as cardiologists, surgeons, and allied healthcare personnel. This inter-disciplinary approach provides early intervention in cases of complications, resulting in better patient outcomes. For instance, those who have acquired congenital heart disease or arrhythmia can be assisted by a holistic approach of surgical correction and ongoing medical management so their overall health is approached comprehensively. Technology and treatment modality developments are continuously improving the landscape of pediatric interventional cardiology, challenging multidisciplinary care teams to stay abreast of guidelines and practice to optimize care in high-risk patients (N/A, 2006). Finally, commitment to actively managing potential complications is necessary to improve further the quality of life in pediatric patients undergoing cardiac intervention.

13.5.3. Long-Term Outcomes and Quality of Life

Long-term outcomes of children who have been treated with interventional pediatric cardiology procedures show significant improvements in survival and quality of life. Advances in medical technology have enabled cardiologists to repair congenital heart defects more effectively, and with it, children who are afflicted by these defects now enjoy better prognoses. Preterm birth interventions have helped account for the immense rise in children surviving to adulthood, thus longer lives for them to realize to their full potential. Studies have established that children undergoing treatments such as catheterization or surgical corrections are likely to experience not only improved cardiac function but also physical health and emotional well-being improvements. The correlation between medical treatment and favorable life outcomes underlines the importance of these treatments in shaping the course of pediatric patients' lives, further indicating the central position of specialist treatment in the evolving context of pediatric cardiology. Evaluations of quality of life (QoL) in pediatric cardiology patients illustrate the intricate relationship between general well-being and medical interventions. Research has shown that, upon intervention, children are more physically active, have improved psychological well-being, and have greater social interaction. These factors are important because they play a significant role in a child's overall development and social integration. Of particular significance is that these findings highlight the role of ongoing follow-up treatment and psychosocial support to deal with the long-term consequences of congenital cardiac disease. Our interventions for enhancing QoL not only minimize the risk of residual health morbidity but also facilitate children to survive and thrive in daily life. This combined strategy—addressing not just the medical but the psychological and social as well—plays a significant role in promoting the future trajectory of these children. As interventional pediatric cardiology continues to evolve, it is increasingly crucial to focus on longitudinal investigations measuring long-term outcomes and quality of life. The incorporation of clinical decision support systems, according to existing guidelines, can enhance the effectiveness of interventions according to individual needs among children. Alignment of clinical practice with possibilities for betterment allows the healthcare provider to assure optimal care for every child. The utilization of technology and expert knowledge facilitates optimal treatment plans, therefore maximizing long-term health gains and QoL among pediatric cardiology patients. It is through such innovation that we aim to further bridge the difference between survival and thriving, so that children not only live longer, but healthier, more productive lives (Bell et al., 2012; N/A, 1998).

SUMMARY

Overall, pediatric cardiology is a rapidly evolving specialty that demands a comprehensive understanding of both established and emerging therapeutic options. Maturing minimally invasive technologies and sophisticated risk assessment techniques have revolutionized the treatment outcome of congenital heart disease among children. As shown in many studies, including those investigating the causes of complexity in lymphatic disease and interventions, these innovations enhance pediatric cardiac cares safety and efficiency. Implementing evidence-based practices is imperative for formulating centralization of care, which can lead to more specialized care and better patient outcomes. Mostly, the continuous implementation of innovative processes creates a dynamic atmosphere where pediatric cardiology flourishes, enabling children to receive timely care when they suffer from severe cardiac complications. Further, the findings on lymphatic disorders show the complex problems that pediatric cardiologists encounter when treating congenital heart defects. This study illustrates heterogeneity among European centers in treatment strategy and underlines the need for consistency in managing lymphatic complications. By the application of knowledge about prevalence and treatment of chylothorax and protein-losing enteropathy, clinicians can personalize care in ways to minimize risk due to Fontan circulation. Formation of collaborative networks among medical centers can provide opportunities for sharing best practice and successful interventions. Such coordination not only guarantees uniform care but also sets up strong monitoring frameworks for long-term outcomes, which are imperative to the long-term health and quality of life in pediatric patients with complicated cardiac diagnoses. In addition, results from efforts such as the C3PO multicenter registry highlight the need for dynamic risk assessment during pediatric cardiac interventions. By dividing cases into procedural risk and outcome categories, such studies inform clinicians about potential complications and enable patient management to be tailored appropriately. The construction of novel hemodynamic vulnerability scores enables identification of high-risk patients in whom augmented monitoring or other therapies may be therapeutic. As pediatric interventional cardiology progresses day by day, total risk assessment tools integrating with cutting-edge procedures will be the key to enhancing patient safety and overall success rates. Thus, following constant research and liaison is essential in order to drive development and achieve optimum outcomes in future generations for those who are facing congenital heart challengers.

Interventional pediatric cardiology is an extremely specialized field of medicine aimed at diagnosing and managing congenital and acquired heart disease in children through catheter-based interventions. One of the key topics covered is the development of clinical decision support (CDS) systems that enhance the accuracy and efficiency of interventional procedures. The topic addresses the necessity of personalized CDS objectives that tackle unique challenges facing pediatric cardiology. This is accomplished by adopting a conceptual model that blends professional judgment and evidence-based evaluation, ending up in the identification of performance deficits and actionable improvement plans. Implementation of such models can lead to improved patient results, addressing the quality metrics demanded by health care organizations like the U.S. Centers for Medicare and Medicaid Services that incentivize effective CDS intervention in specialty care (Bell et al., 2012). Moreover, the complexity of the conditions treated in interventional pediatric cardiology necessitates an integrated management style to the patient. Hypertrophic cardiomyopathy or congenital heart disease can have different manifestations that not only impact the physical heart but also the psychosocial functioning of the child and his/her family. The argument highlights that the treatment should be appropriate with multidisciplinary collaboration between various specialties of healthcare practitioners to address these multidimensional needs appropriately. Since all conditions need individualized interventions, the importance of continuous communication among experts becomes apparent; discontinuities in care delivery could be mitigated by communication, and the success of overall treatment can be enhanced. Moreover, the application of patient-centered care in interventional cardiology could lead to more well-rounded care plans essential to optimal health outcomes for various populations of patients (Adriaensen et al., 2019). Lastly, as pediatric interventional cardiology advances, the use of new technology and methods in practice remains most important. Developments such as 3D imaging and minimally invasive techniques have transformed the traditional paradigms with less invasive options and shorter recovery periods. But controversies surrounding these technologies place in limelight the necessity for ongoing research and evaluation of their long-term impact on children. Additional professional education and training of practitioners in this field are also needed to be able to adapt to the rapid speed of change in technology and treatment practices. Generally, the cumulative information gathered from the discussion on interventional pediatric cardiology offers a dynamic and intricate approach in the treatment of heart diseases among children that offers a path for on-going improvements in clinical practice and patient experiences (Adriaensen et al., 2019).

CLOSER LOOK

PEDIATRIC CARDIAC CATHETERIZATION LAB SETUP AND SAFETY PROTOCOLS

Pediatric cardiac catheterization is an important diagnostic and interventional method used in the evaluation and treatment of congenital and acquired heart disease in children. The planning of a pediatric cardiac catheterization lab environment is done with close attention to meet the unique anatomical and physiological needs of pediatric patients from neonates to adolescents. The lab environment is comprised of specially designed facilities, well-trained professionals, and strict safety controls to maximize benefits and minimize risk. A typical pediatric cardiac catheterization suite includes a high-resolution biplane fluoroscopy unit for real-time imaging of small cardiac structures in more than one plane with low radiation exposure. The imaging system must include digital subtraction angiography capabilities and pediatric-specific settings to provide the optimal image at lower doses of radiation. The lab also contains hemodynamic monitors, ultrasound machines (intracardiac and transthoracic echocardiography), oxygen and suction systems, anesthesia machines, crash carts, and resuscitation devices. Adjustable lead aprons and radiation shields, including pediatric sizes, are essential for protecting staff and patients from unnecessary exposure.

Pediatric Cath lab staff typically include an interventional pediatric cardiologist, an anesthesiologist, Cath lab nurses with specialty training, radiologic technologists, and an optional perfusionist or pediatric cardiac surgeon for more complex cases. They are educated in technical catheterization skills as well as pediatric life support, including neonatal and pediatric advanced life support (NALS/PALS). Roles are clearly defined and rehearsed with simulation and protocol-based workflow to facilitate coordinated and rapid action during emergencies. Precautions are a routine part of pediatric cardiac catheterization since this patient group is at risk. Safety from radiation is one of the major concerns; the ALARA (ALARA (as low as reasonably achievable)) philosophy is therefore strictly followed. Time, distance, and shielding strategies are used stringently—minimizing the fluoroscopy time, maximizing the distance from the radiation source, and employing adequate shielding on both staff and patients. Dose-monitoring programs are integrated into most modern labs to monitor cumulative radiation dosage.

Practice infection control measures are also of paramount importance. The lab needs to be as sterile as a theatre with sound air filtration systems, aseptic draping, and hand hygiene. Equipment is sterilized and disinfected in accordance with regulatory standards. Intravenous catheters, lines, and access sites are managed with strict aseptic techniques to prevent catheter-associated bloodstream infections. Pre-procedure, as well as informed consent and patient evaluation, include allergy check, coagulation parameters, renal function, and hemodynamic status. Intra-procedural, continuous monitoring of vital signs, oxygen saturation, and ECG is done as well. Anesthesia assistance depends on the age, size, and complexity of the child and is intended for pain control and safety. Post-procedure practice includes monitoring in a specially designed recovery room, observation for complications such as bleeding, arrhythmia, or vascular trauma. Documentation, image archiving, and reporting are completed immediately. Ongoing equipment checks, staff education, and participation in morbidity and mortality meetings also support quality and safety.

REFERENCES

1. Abella, B. S., Lee, B. K., Youn, C. S., Callaway, C. W., Gaieski, D. F., Rittenberger, J. C., Elmer, J., et al. (2018). Variability of extracorporeal cardiopulmonary resuscitation utilization for refractory adult out-of-hospital cardiac arrest: An international survey study. https://core.ac.uk/download/299811647.pdf (accessed on 15th July 2025).
2. Abumehdi, M., Cantinotti, M., Gewillig, M., Hjortdal, V., et al. (2024). Lymphatic disorder management in pediatric patients with congenital heart disease in European pediatric cardiology centers: Current status, disparities, and future considerations. https://core.ac.uk/download/652007659.pdf (accessed on 15th July 2025).
3. Adriaensen, H., Amin, R., Bissler, J., Black, C., Bombardieri, M., Breckenridge, K., Capal, J., et al. (2019). Tuberous sclerosis complex (TSC): Expert recommendations for provision of coordinated care. https://core.ac.uk/download/275574357.pdf (accessed on 15th July 2025).
4. Ait-Ali, L., Andreassi, M. G., Foffa, I., Picano, E., et al. (2025). Cumulative patient effective dose and acute radiation-induced chromosomal DNA damage in children with congenital heart disease. https://core.ac.uk/download/pdf/37831113.pdf (accessed on 15th July 2025).
5. Alvarez-Fuente, M., Amat-Santos, I. J., Ballesteros Tejerizo, F., Betrián Blasco, P., et al. (2024). Registro español de intervencionismo en cardiopatías congénitas. III informe oficial de la ACI-SEC y el GTH-SECPCC (2022). https://core.ac.uk/download/652007352.pdf (accessed on 15th July 2025).
6. Annisa, S. N., Nurlaili, A. I., & Cahyani, I. P. (2025). The role of pediatric cardiology in the management of congenital heart disease: A comprehensive systematic review. *Journal of Advanced Research in Medical and Health Science (ISSN 2208-2425).* https://www.semanticscholar.org/paper/dcf889bed8f678c041812b45d682ae450aed0e25 (accessed on 15th July 2025).
7. Arrieta, R. S., Botrel, T. E. A., Chamié, F., Clark, B., et al. (2013). Transcatheter pulmonary valve implantation: Systematic literature review. https://core.ac.uk/download/37711108.pdf (accessed on 15th July 2025).
8. Aumann, R., Hinterseer, M., Kozlik-Feldmann, R., Lang, D., et al. (2008). Creation of ventricular septal defects on the beating heart in a new pig model. https://core.ac.uk/download/16432659.pdf (accessed on 15th July 2025).
9. Bacher, K., Buytaert, D., De Pooter, J., Drieghe, B., et al. (2015). Novel X-ray imaging technology enables significant patient dose reduction in interventional cardiology while maintaining diagnostic image quality. https://core.ac.uk/download/55848139.pdf (accessed on 15th July 2025).
10. Bacher, K., Buytaert, D., De Wolf, D., Panzer, J., et al. (2019). Local DRLs and automated risk estimation in pediatric interventional cardiology. https://core.ac.uk/download/237012394.pdf (accessed on 15th July 2025).
11. Balzer, D., Quinn, B. P., et al. (2022). Procedural risk in congenital cardiac catheterization (PREDIC3T). https://core.ac.uk/download/515934144.pdf (accessed on 15th July 2025).
12. Beghetti, M., da Cruz, E., Fakler, U., Haas, N. A., et al. (2017). Recommendations from the Association for European Pediatric Cardiology for training in pediatric cardiac intensive care: AEPC's recommendations for European pediatric cardiology trainees–The Working Group on

Pediatric Cardiac Intensive Care. https://core.ac.uk/download/85209479.pdf (accessed on 15th July 2025).

13. Bell, D. S., Damberg, C. L., Schneider, E. C., Timbie, J. W., et al. (2012). A conceptual framework and protocol for defining clinical decision support objectives applicable to medical specialties. https://core.ac.uk/download/323076444.pdf (accessed on 15th July 2025).

14. Bluebond-Langner, M., Brown, K., Butler, A. E., Vemuri, N., et al. (2021). Palliative care for children with complex cardiac conditions: Survey results. https://core.ac.uk/download/477690169.pdf (accessed on 15th July 2025).

15. Brogan, P., Burns, J. C., Cornish, J., Diwakar, V., et al. (2020). Lifetime cardiovascular management of patients with previous Kawasaki disease. https://core.ac.uk/download/323066717.pdf (accessed on 15th July 2025).

16. Cozzens, K., Hannan, E. L., King, S. B., Shah, B., et al. (2012). The New York State Cardiac Registries history, contributions, limitations, and lessons for future efforts to assess and publicly report healthcare outcomes. https://core.ac.uk/download/pdf/82671098.pdf (accessed on 15th July 2025).

17. Dalla Pozza, R., Kozlik-Feldmann, R., Netz, H., Romer, M., et al. (2003). Real-time three-dimensional ultrasound: A valuable new tool in preoperative assessment of complex congenital cardiac disease. https://core.ac.uk/download/46603019.pdf (accessed on 15th July 2025).

18. De Keulenaer, B. L., De Laet, I., De Waele, J., Debergh, D., et al. (2014). Awareness and knowledge of intra-abdominal hypertension and abdominal compartment syndrome: Results of an international survey. https://core.ac.uk/download/55846801.pdf (accessed on 15th July 2025).

19. Donya, M., ElGuindy, A., Firmin, D., Radford, M., et al. (2014). Radiation in medicine: Origins, risks and aspirations. https://core.ac.uk/download/77008838.pdf (accessed on 15th July 2025).

20. Drey, N., Husson, O., May, K., Murray, K., et al. (2019). Ionizing radiation exposure from medical imaging – A review of patient's (un)awareness. https://core.ac.uk/download/266989986.pdf (accessed on 15th July 2025).

21. Drivas, P., Greil, G. F., Mitchell, F. M., Prasad, A., et al. (2015). Cardiovascular magnetic resonance: Diagnostic utility and specific considerations in the pediatric population. https://core.ac.uk/download/83923979.pdf (accessed on 15th July 2025).

22. Drove, B., Gifford, K. L., Gonzalez-Meijome, J. M., Gray, L., et al. (2019). IMI–Industry guidelines and ethical considerations for myopia control report. https://core.ac.uk/download/293867276.pdf (accessed on 15th July 2025).

23. Duman, D., Aykan, H., Ertugrul, I., Ardıçlı, B., Aypar, E., Alehan, D., & Karagöz, T. (2023). Percutaneous transcatheter retrieval of central venous port fragments in pediatric patients: A single-center experience from the pediatric cardiology department. *Journal of Pediatric Hematology/Oncology, 45*, e959–e965. https://www.semanticscholar.org/paper/74a2e19651f46e6dbde08a58e762cadfc10d1ba9 (accessed on 15th July 2025).

24. Feinstein, J. A., LaDisa, J. F., & Taylor, C. A. (2010). Aortic coarctation: Recent developments in experimental and computational methods to assess treatments for this simple condition. https://core.ac.uk/download/213079154.pdf (accessed on 15th July 2025).

25. Freger, S., & Leonardi, M. (2025). Advancements in ultrasound diagnosis of superficial endometriosis: Current challenges and emerging techniques. *Gynecologic and Obstetric Investigation.* https://www.semanticscholar.org/paper/4faf94c4cad0742a23d79333799e431c036c8af0 (accessed on 15th July 2025).

26. Hughes, M. L., Ntsinjana, H. N., & Taylor, A. M. (2011). The role of cardiovascular magnetic resonance in pediatric congenital heart disease. https://core.ac.uk/download/1895946.pdf (accessed on 15th July 2025).

27. Indianapolis Coalition for Patient Safety. (2017). Intravascular iodinated contrast media administration in adults: A patient safety approach. https://core.ac.uk/download/129149083.pdf (accessed on 15th July 2025).

28. Pavalagantharajah, S., Khan, M., Moore, C., Beattie, K., Hunter, A., Bilgic, E., & Babic, B. (2025). An innovative approach to patient and family involvement in postgraduate medical education. *Pediatrics & Child Health.* https://www.semanticscholar.org/paper/543650806315fb2eccc536fe656d33fa914c5cda (accessed on 15th July 2025).

29. Reich, A., Wiener, L., Thompson, A. L., Jones, A. M., Marchetta, A., Parris, K. R., Heidelberg, R. E., et al. (2025). Leveraging the patient and family voice in the development of patient education: Supporting the pediatric oncology experience. *Cancers, 17.* https://www.semanticscholar.org/paper/75ba448459058ff03d8e7f916af701eb65a81403 (accessed on 15th July 2025).

30. Selvakumari, R. S., Punithakumar, K., Selvathi, D., Chrisilla, S., Abinaya, R. S., & Ray, N. (2025). Computerized diagnosis methods for pediatric cardiology: A review. *IEEE Access, 13,* 39192–39213. https://www.semanticscholar.org/paper/9cb742766a8e4a39df661b1e59f4ea512c440840 (accessed on 15th July 2025).

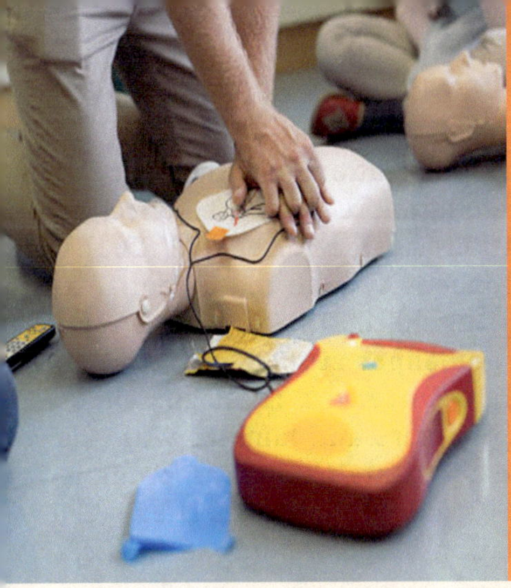

Chapter 14

CARDIAC EMERGENCIES IN CHILDREN

Contents

Introduction

Pediatric cardiac emergencies constitute a significant challenging issue in pediatric care that demands early recognition and treatment. Children have special physiology, which differs significantly from adult physiology, to be appreciated by pediatricians and emergency staff. For instance, due to variations in size and cardiovascular anatomy, children are able to manifest different heart disease differently, thus making them require unique diagnostic and therapeutic approaches. Understanding the intricacies of pathophysiology in cardiology in children is central to achieving maximum outcomes. This foundation enables professionals to identify symptoms that are seemingly innocuous but may be an expression of underlying cardiac distress. On top of this, advanced training and choice models are essential to guarantee that medical personnel are skilled at addressing such emergencies, and therefore, a comprehensive education in medicine specializing in pediatric cardiopathy is necessary. Hypertension and other cardiovascular complications among young age groups are issues that have, in recent years, drawn increasing attention. As documented in contemporary publications, the incidence of hypertension among children and adolescents is increasingly becoming more frequent, reflecting an impending crisis of public health calling for immediate intervention (Agabiti-Rosei et al., 2016). Some of the causes of this rise include obesity, diet, and physical inactivity with the potential to precipitate cardiovascular disorders, including cardiac emergencies. This shifting ground makes early diagnosis and preventive treatment even more important. Proper guidelines at the ready, doctors can not only cure existing cardiac conditions but also prevent future occurrences. These guidelines established through continuing research aim to inform and equip doctors and families with the data they require to counteract the development of serious cardiac events as well as promote healthier lifestyles for youngsters. In order to respond to pediatric cardiac emergencies effectively, inter-layered responses are essential. The incorporation of simulation-based training in medical education among practitioners is an approach that could be utilized. Simulation training allows experts to develop technical skills in pediatric emergency care in simulated, actual environments (Amira et al., 2018). Through simulation technologies, medical personnel can practice their response to simulated high-pressure scenarios that mirror actual cardiac emergencies to become better prepared and confident. These immersive training programs can potentially optimize the quality of patient care in actual emergency conditions and significantly improve outcomes. Developing a culture of continuous education centered on pediatric cardiac well-being will not only prepare clinicians to address current crises but will also foster greater understanding of how, through prevention of cardiac crises in the first place, increased awareness and education will result in better outcomes for children in these desperate cases.

Definition of Cardiac Emergencies

Cardiac emergencies in pediatrics refer to a variety of acute clinical conditions that necessitate immediate intervention in order to avoid morbidity and mortality among children. Cardiac emergencies may manifest as arrhythmias, myocardial infarction, cardiac arrest, and a number of other syndromes. The term also includes the pathophysiologic processes underlying the emergent conditions. For instance, tachycardia or blood pressure changes will reflect serious underlying pathology such as congenital heart disease or acquired illnesses such as myocarditis, and appropriate action should be taken immediately. The understanding of such definitions will help health workers identify and grade cases properly in order to give the timely intervention with appropriate therapeutic interventions that can fundamentally alter clinical outcomes. A specific problem of pediatric cardiovascular emergencies is the rising incidence of hypertension, which has raised much attention in recent decades. Pediatric hypertension, although once underrated, is now more and more regarded as a predictor of adult cardiovascular disease. The most notable characteristics of hypertensive emergencies include not only the elevation of blood pressure but also its immediate potential for end-organ damage. New guidelines for hypertension have illuminated the complexity of pediatric blood pressure measurement, emphasizing the need for accurate out-of-office measurement and understanding of central blood pressure values. This evolving definition challenges clinicians to refine diagnosis and treatment methods in addressing the burden of hypertension and its role in broader cardiovascular problems in children (Agabiti-Rosei et al., 2016). Furthermore, the term cardiac emergencies encompasses instances of secondary conditions, such as adrenal crises, which have the potential to complicate the underlying cardiac conditions in children. These crises normally occur in patients with adrenal insufficiency but their detection is unavoidable in all emergency departments since they can mimic critical cardiac dysfunction. Although glucocorticoid replacement therapy has since recorded favorable results in the majority of patients, adrenal crises still remain a deadly threat, and this underscores the importance of expedited diagnosis and treatment (Falhammar et al., 2019). Understanding the relationship between the conditions and cardiac emergencies allows medical professionals to embrace an integrated management approach, which is paramount to improved survival rates and quality of care in the implicated children.

Importance of Recognizing Cardiac Issues in Children

In pediatrics, the diagnosis of cardiac anomalies in children is very important to avoid the onset of serious consequences. In children, as opposed to adults, symptoms of cardiac diseases may be subtle and easily masquerade as non-pathological states. Early detection of such problems is important because cardiac disease left untreated can generate potentially lethal emergencies. Pediatric healthcare providers should maintain a high suspicion of presenting signs like fatigue, syncope, or unexplained dyspnea that can be manifestations of serious underlying heart disease. Regular screening in high-risk populations coupled with enhanced training for healthcare providers can maximize early intervention and reduce rates of catastrophic cardiac events to a minimum. Anticipatory diagnosis in the identification of potential cardiac distress puts childcare under precautionary care, which guarantees the health and wellbeing of children in general. Moreover, embracing the latest diagnostic technology in child cardiology simplifies the identification of cardiac illnesses that will go undetected on routine tests. Echocardiograms, electrocardiograms, and imaging technologies have revolutionized diagnostics so that it is now possible to comprehensively assess structural and functional defects in the heart of children. Early identification of such abnormalities is necessary because they can become full-blown cardiac emergencies if left unchecked. For instance, conditions like hypertrophic cardiomyopathy or congenital heart disease may be asymptomatic in early childhood but can cause sudden cardiac arrest during physical exertion. Such advancements in technology, along with continuous education, need to be adopted by healthcare personnel in order to effectively diagnose and treat cardiac conditions at an early age. This multi-faceted approach underlines vigilance in ensuring children's cardiac health, leading ultimately to a healthier more resilient pediatric population. Additionally, the psychosocial impact of untreated cardiac disease is not only for the individual child but also for families and communities. In the event of inappropriate diagnosis or treatment of children, there is a greater risk of lifelong disability and early death with resultant emotional and economic cost to families. The consequences of cardiac emergencies underscore the necessity of comprehensive public health measures focused on increasing awareness regarding pediatric cardiac conditions. Communities must be made aware of the warning signs and symptoms of these conditions so that parents and caregivers can approach the condition in time. Education campaigns can make families strong, making them engaged actors in their child's health process. Additionally, understanding the wider ramifications of cardiac conditions in children can promote cooperative action among healthcare professionals, educators, and policy-makers to establish a supportive network that emphasizes early diagnosis and timely treatment, ultimately resulting in healthier child experiences.

14.1. Types of Cardiac Emergencies

Awareness of the causes of cardiac emergencies among children is important to ensure effective and timely management. One such emergency is arrhythmias; a term used for abnormal heart rhythms that can lead to collapse of blood supply to vital organs. They come in the form of bradycardia, an extremely slow heart rate that is fatal, or tachycardia, whereby the heart rate is extremely rapid. Syncope or fainting episodes may occur in pediatric patients, and these can be stressful on the caregivers as well as a sign of underlying pathological conditions. Congenital malformations of the heart are also a significant reason for cardiac emergencies among the younger age groups. Identification and management of the arrhythmias are critical because unmanaged cases lead to severe outcomes like cardiac arrest and permanent neurological damage. Hence, prompt recognition of the symptoms ensures that the appropriate steps are taken towards stabilizing the child and preventing further complications. Another form of cardiac emergency is congestive heart failure (CHF), which can present because of several etiologies such as cardiomyopathy or congenital heart disease. CHF in children can have clinical symptoms like labored respiration, shortness of breath, and failure to feed in infants and hence is not readily identifiable immediately. Younger patients have different physiological reactions from adults, necessitating careful evaluation and early intervention (Figure 14.1).

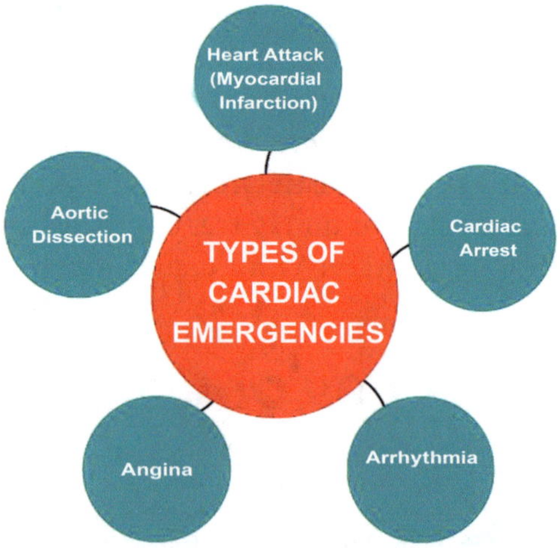

Figure 14.1. Types of cardiac emergencies.

Source: https://linkhospitals.in/blog/cardiac-emergencies:-symptoms-and-types.

CHF therapy often entails diuretics and cardiopulmonary drugs, highlighting the importance of immediate action to prevent deterioration to respiratory failure or shock. Along with this, medical professionals must be cognizant of precipitating causes of CHF, such as infections or fluid overload since children's hearts are generally more susceptible to changes in their physiologic status. Early detection and management of CHF are highly important to improve results in this vulnerable patient population. Lastly, myocardial infarction, although less common in children than adults, remains a severe cardiac emergency and can result from either congenital or acquired heart disease. Kawasaki disease and other diseases have the capability to predispose children to coronary artery abnormalities, leaving them vulnerable to heart attack. Pediatric presentation may also differ significantly from that of adults, with abdominal pain, vomiting, or unexplained malaise being more common than classic chest pain. This distinctive presentation complicates diagnosis, with a high index of suspicion being required in high-risk presentations. The treatment can involve aspirin and supportive management, hence the need for a multidisciplinary team in emergency management. Early detection and management of myocardial infarction among children are crucial, as delay can lead to serious morbidity and mortality, highlighting the importance of education and awareness among caregivers and health providers in the management of such cardiac emergencies (Amira et al., 2018; Thorne-Lyman et al., 2025).

14.1.1. Congenital Heart Defects

Congenital heart defects (CHDs) are a spectrum of heart defects at birth. The defects could lead to severe complications since they usually disrupt the normal flow of blood within the heart and lungs and hence to the body. CHDs are a leading cause of morbidity and mortality in children, for which medical interventions should be initiated in good time. Their complexity varies—mild malformations such as atrial septal defects to the more severe malformations such as hypoplastic left heart syndrome. Due to their potential to lead to serious complications, including heart failure, arrhythmias, and respiratory distress, acute management in the child patient is indicated. Familiarity with the different types of CHD and their importance for emergency treatment is essential for health professionals that are faced with cardiac emergencies in children. The management of infants and children with congenital heart defects typically is by a multidisciplinary team, particularly in acute emergencies. These emergencies can result from some triggers like infections, exertions, or even some trivial activities that exacerbate the underlying cardiac anomalies.

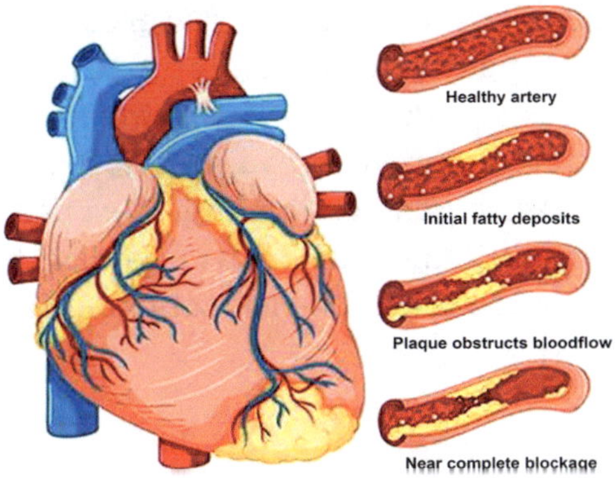

Figure 14.2. Congenital heart disease refers to a range of structural abnormalities in the heart that are present at birth.

Source: https://www.apexhospitals.com/_next/image?url=https%3A%2F%2Fbed.apexhospitals.com%2Fuploads%2FCHD_52ce7787e2.png&w=828&q=75.

In a prospective study of adults with congenital heart disease, a significant number of emergency admissions were related to cardiovascular complications, and arrhythmias and heart failure were among the most frequent of the causative factors (Bauer et al., 2003) (Figure 14.2).

Although adult focus is predominant, this find necessitates observation on an ongoing basis during the life of a patient, starting at birth. Pediatric patients also can experience such emergencies, and their acute care not only involves such immediate stabilization measures but also routine assessment to prevent such events from recurring and to facilitate long-term recovery. Effective intervention strategies for the management of cardiac emergencies in children with congenital heart defects include early identification and proper management of complications. Interventions via surgery are largely the case; for instance, early correction of some malformations can be effective in averting serious health issues during adulthood. Moreover, access to specialized pediatric cardiac services is also a must, especially in low- and middle-income countries, where economic and sociocultural factors can limit the use of otherwise required interventions (Uba et al., 2014). The effect of congenital anomalies in these areas cannot be overemphasized because inappropriate care results in unnecessary death and permanent disability. Therefore, emphasis on the urgency of access to specialist healthcare and urgent surgical treatment is critical in addressing the dangers that congenital heart anomalies present and in optimizing the survival rates of the involved children.

14.1.2. Arrhythmias

The creation of arrhythmias in children poses a significant emergency medical challenge due primarily to the differentials in pediatric and adult physiology. Arrhythmias in childhood can manifest as bradycardia, tachycardia, and atrioventricular block, each having various implications for the management of the patient.

Clinically, it is crucial that clinical practitioners can easily recognize such abnormalities since undiagnosed or uncorrected arrhythmias can lead to significant consequences, such as syncope, heart failure, or even sudden cardiac death. Interestingly, studies show that a majority of emergency presentations of congenital heart disease are composed of arrhythmias, highlighting their position as an emergent condition within pediatric cardiology centers (Bauer et al., 2003) (Figure 14.3).

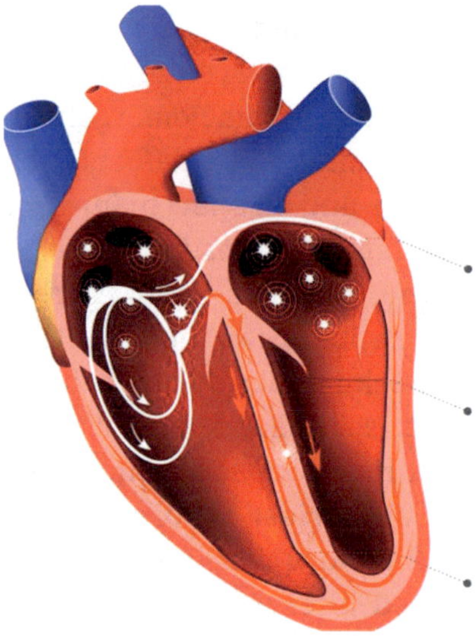

Figure 14.3. Arrhythmias in children.

Source: https://dcmfoundation.org/wp-content/uploads/2018/12/dilated-cardiomyopathy-and-common-arrhythmias.png.

Effective management of arrhythmias in emergencies requires a system process of accurate diagnostics and expeditious therapeutic interventions. At presentation, children with presumed arrhythmias should be urgently evaluated, including electrocardiograms and laboratory studies to determine the cause. The treatment options may be very varied, from medical to invasive treatments, such as catheter ablation or pacemaker insertion. The intricate nature of arrhythmias requires multidisciplinary team management, ensuring that pediatric cardiologists, emergency medicine physicians, and nurses are properly coordinated to deliver effective and timely care. Directing appropriate interventions in cases of arrhythmias is extremely important in improving outcomes and lowering morbidity rates among affected children (Carl et al., 2025). Understanding of the epidemiology and clinical significance of arrhythmias in children extends beyond acute management; it also encompasses prevention and long-term care considerations. As most children with arrhythmias will be accompanied by associated comorbid congenital heart disease or other risk factors, close follow-up during their development is required. Providers need to emphasize individualized care plans that cover not only the immediate events but also subsequent risks of arrhythmia. Educational interventions directed toward families, targeting awareness of warning signs and when to activate the emergency services, are crucial components of total pediatric cardiology. Ultimately, awareness and education on arrhythmias play to produce improved readiness for potential cardiac emergencies among the pediatric population, immediate and long-term health outcomes of these high-risk patients (Bauer et al., 2003).

14.1.3. Myocarditis

Among cardiac emergencies of children, myocarditis is of concern due to its acute course and the multifactorial etiology of the illness. Myocarditis is characterized by inflammation of the myocardium. It is typically secondary to viral infection, autoimmune illnesses, or drug reactions. In children, viral pathogens like enteroviruses and adenoviruses also play a similar role. The clinical presentation can range from nonspecific signs and symptoms of fatigue and palpitations to life-threatening complications like heart failure and arrhythmias. Prompt detection is necessary as late diagnosis can result in cardiogenic shock, which is an acute condition of end-organ underperfusion due to compromised cardiac function. Therefore, an index of suspicion at the clinical level should be high when doctors examine children who come in with unexplained cardiac symptoms to provide timely intervention and commence therapy. Management of myocarditis in children is a wide-ranging one, depending on the cause and the severity of the symptoms. The initial treatment often focuses on stabilizing the patient, which may include optimizing fluid status and administering drug for the support of cardiac function. In cases of severe myocardial damage, particularly in case of symptoms of cardiogenic shock in the child, intensive care treatment may be needed. As noted in literature, comprehensive evaluation and consideration of possible complications (including immune side effects) are significant in cancer patients undergoing treatment who are able to experience myocarditis as a second-line effect (Figure 14.4).

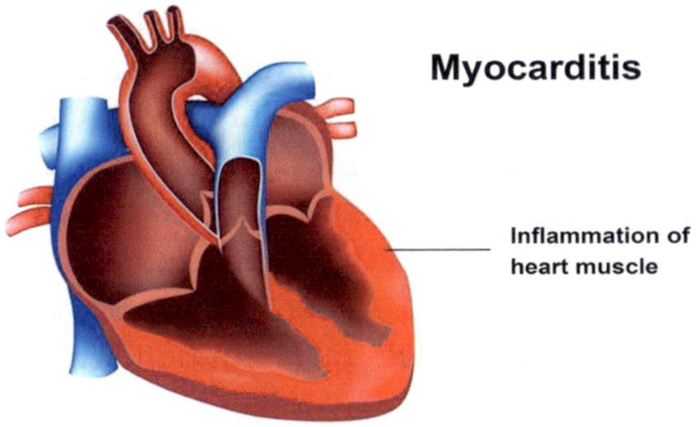

Figure 14.4. Myocarditis.

Source: https://d1edr79mp9g5zc.cloudfront.net/5eb0affe-1991-449b-bfc0-a5a0516548bf/b4bc4b3e-c26e-4d6a-ad35-34fd287d557d/b4bc4b3e-c26e-4d6a-ad35-34fd287d557d_source_v.png.

Immunosuppressive therapy has some basis in certain conditions, particularly when autoimmune mechanisms are the issue. Serial follow-up and monitoring would be necessary to establish the resolution of inflammatory events and change treatment modalities according to such an evaluation. Prognosis of children with myocarditis is variable, depending upon the etiology of inflammation, the degree of myocardial damage, and the timeliness of medical treatment. While a full recovery is possible in some children with suitable treatment, others acquire chronic heart conditions, with serious long-term health effects and sudden cardiac death as a possibility. Cooperation between cardiology and emergency medical knowledge is required, particularly in cases progressing from myocarditis to severe illness like cardiogenic shock. As written by Candini et al. (2020), a systematic therapeutic approach, including identification of the etiology and early initiation of supportive measures, is of paramount importance in reducing the threats of mortality and optimizing outcomes in children. In this regard, appropriate education of healthcare personnel in the recognition and care of myocarditis is called for in the scenario of pediatric cardiac emergencies.

14.2. Symptoms of Cardiac Emergencies in Children

Symptom identification for cardiac emergencies in children is critical to ensure timely intervention and improved prognosis. Relative to adults, pediatric manifestations of cardiac distress may be quite different, at times presenting nonspecifically and easily mislabeled as less serious conditions. Classic presentation is the complaint of sharp or dull chest pain accompanied by other symptoms including shortness of breath and fatigue. Also, children may present with signs of severe distress or anxiety that can further add to the clinical complexity. Unless identified early, the treatment may get delayed, leading to amplified morbidity and even mortality and therefore awareness among health workers and caregivers is essential. This grasp of the unique symptomology of cardiac emergencies will assist in better equipping medical professionals to respond in life-threatening conditions, according to recent literature on pediatric cardiac health. Differential diagnosis of cardiac emergencies among children requires a delicate handling in the presence of concomitant symptoms of other illnesses (Figure 14.5).

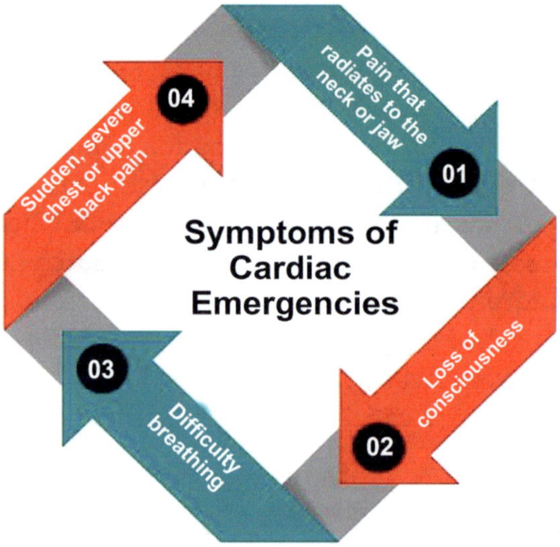

Figure 14.5. Symptoms of a cardiac emergency.

Source: https://linkhospitals.in/blog/cardiac-emergencies:-symptoms-and-types.

For instance, kids can have syncope or near-syncope and it may be confused with exercise-related fatigue or dehydration. Furthermore, palpitations, sometimes confused with being simple evidence of excitement or worry, may herald significant arrhythmic events calling for immediate medical attention. In congenital heart disease, more overt signs like cyanosis (which involves a bluish discoloration) can also manifest as signs of serious underlying conditions. Parents, educators, and healthcare providers must understand these fluctuating and sometimes unobtrusive symptoms since pediatric sudden cardiac events have limited warning signs. Establishing procedures for observing and responding to such symptoms will help enhance the health and safety of children, particularly when in school or competition. Emerging evidence indicates the importance of training and preparedness among those interacting with children in various settings, most importantly school. The American Heart Association advises on handling sudden cardiac arrest (SCA), such as embracing effective communication techniques, joint response protocols, and cardiopulmonary resuscitation (CPR) training. Training and preparedness can enhance response to SCA considerably, with direct results evident in survival rates. A majority of the school nurses reported varying degrees of empowerment and availability of resources to respond to such emergencies, with approximately 44% stating they were adequately empowered in their profession. This disparity serves to highlight the need for uniform training and equipment, such as AEDs, to ensure that personnel dealing with children are competent in recognizing and responding to cardiac emergencies in a timely fashion. These steps enhance individual readiness as well as enhance health and safety culture in schools, as seen in current school health policy reviews.

14.2.1. Chest Pain and Discomfort

Presentation of chest pain and discomfort in children is generally a significant diagnostic challenge, warranting a good knowledge of its potential etiologies. Compared with adults, children present with a broader variety of etiologies. Musculoskeletal chest pain, respiratory tract infections, and gastrointestinal distress are some of the more common etiologies of chest discomfort in children. These non-cardiac etiologies necessitate a long history and physical to rule out major underlying disease. Due to the fact that children have smaller coronary vessels and respond differently than adults physiologically, the assessment of chest pain in children also needs to take into account their unique anatomical and developmental characteristics, which may have a great effect on outcome. Therefore, clinicians must be vigilant, following a methodical process to distinguish between innocent causes of chest pain and those indicating an acute cardiac emergency. The implications of a wrong chest pain diagnosis in children can be severe, as some of these cases may actually be due to cardiac illnesses such as myocarditis or congenital heart disease. While these occurrences are rare, they do emphasize the importance of a strong suspicion, particularly in children with risk factors such as family history of cardiac disease or symptomatology with sinister connotations such as syncope or exertional dyspnea. When evaluating a child presenting with chest pain, prompt consideration must be made for ordering crucial tests, such as electrocardiograms or echocardiograms, to rule out cardiac abnormalities. It is worth remembering that what at first can appear to be non-specific distress can be concealing a serious cardiac event; prompt identification can have a very profound effect on management and outcome (Figure 14.6).

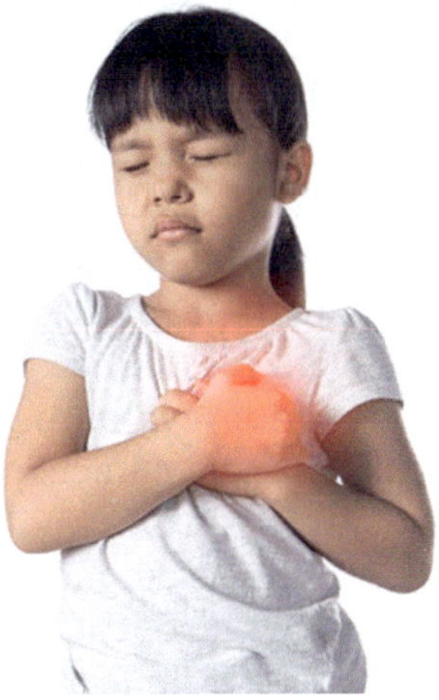

Figure 14.6. Chest pain in pediatric patients.

Source: https://www.medtalks.in/uploads/faqs/faqSquare-Causes_of_Chest_Pain.jpg.

Lastly, designing a multi-disciplinary setting ensures holistic care, leading to better outcomes for pediatric patients with chest pain. An interprofessional education model could be an effective model to address chest pain among kids in emergency settings. Simulation-based training, whereby final-year students from different healthcare professions (e.g., nursing and paramedics) collaborate as a team in managing pediatric emergencies can significantly increase a practitioner's knowledge and management of heart conditions. These findings suggest that interprofessional education enhances skill and role knowledge between various disciplines, providing students with confidence in performing at their best within multidisciplinary teams when responding to cardiac emergencies. Thus, the availability of structured interprofessional training programs will enhance team preparedness and communication in real emergencies, ultimately enhancing patient outcomes. Through continuous education and clinical training, physicians are able to improve their proficiency in the detection and management of chest pain in children, lowering the potential for misdiagnosis and the ability to deliver timely and appropriate care (Alinier et al., 2008; Carl et al., 2025).

14.2.2. Shortness of Breath

Pediatric shortness of breath, or dyspnea, particularly in the presence of cardiac emergencies, is a severe clinical challenge. Unlike adults, children may have atypical presentations of respiratory difficulty, and as such, an accurate diagnosis is challenging. Shortness of breath can be caused by many cardiac conditions, such as cardiomyopathies and congenital heart diseases, among the most frequent causes of heart failure in children. In these cases, the symptomatic expression of dyspnea often follows a child's high levels of activity, which can become problematic during exercise. This is especially significant in infants since their inability to complete feeding might be a sign of cardiac dysfunction, again elucidating the necessity for prompt diagnosis and treatment of such symptoms to avoid lethal sequelae (Grech et al., 2015). In emergent settings, it is important for healthcare providers to recognize the interplay among dyspnea and heart disease. Accurate assessment has to be done to distinguish dyspnea that is secondary to cardiovascular origin versus respiratory etiology. History and physical examination must be complete in combination with the right tests such as chest X-rays and echocardiograms. The occurrence of respiratory distress through impaired cardiac function provides the basis for the development of targeted interventions. Indeed, medication such as angiotensin-converting enzyme inhibitors and diuretics plays an important role in the treatment of heart failure, which consequently unloads shortness of breath symptoms (Grech et al., 2015) (Figure 14.7).

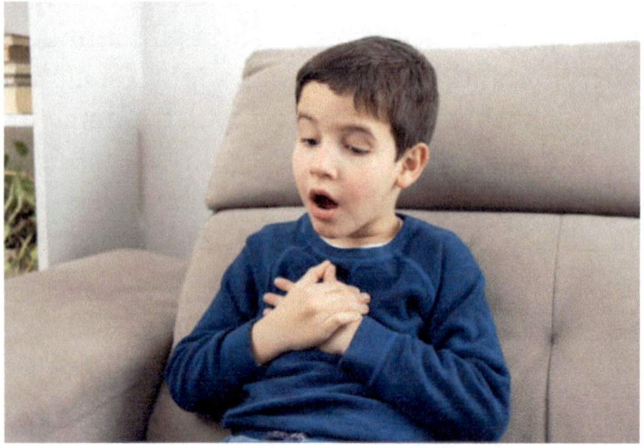

Figure 14.7. Dyspnea in pediatric patients.

Source: https://media.istockphoto.com/id/1682186179/photo/suffering-an-anxiety-attack.jpg?s=612x612&w=0&k=20&c=eBRxgb6tlvv2toxWUYxKTDbrQLrXab-2qPQwbbUjDNk=

These modalities are an expression of how intricate pediatric cardiac treatment is, where intervention done at the right time can go a long way in determining patient outcomes. Further, the role of educational programs in emergency medicine is also realized from the fact that educational programs with innovative teaching methods, like using the flipped classroom model, can enhance the resident's proficiency in recognizing and managing cardiovascular emergencies. It emphasizes active learning and application of knowledge in solving problems through discussion of case studies and interactive inputs, involving a higher level of understanding of causes of symptoms like dyspnea in children. By providing intensive knowledge and reasoning power to healthcare professionals, it enables better responses during acute presentations of cardiac emergencies. Since pediatric cases commonly occur in a special manner, integrating such educational innovations significantly enhances clinical practice and eventually enhances patient care.

14.2.3. Syncope (Fainting)

Syncope, or fainting, is a transient loss of consciousness due to insufficient blood flow to the brain. Diagnosis and treatment of the condition in children come with special difficulties, namely because causes of syncope may be very dissimilar. While some syncope is innocuous, such as vasovagal syncope due to stress or dehydration, other instances can indicate underlying cardiac disease necessitating immediate medical attention. It is essential to know the physiological mechanism and precipitants of syncope because proper diagnosis can lead to appropriate management strategies that prevent recurrence. Pediatricians must be cautious when evaluating attacks of fainting, as risk factors and clinical presentation can differ significantly from adults and can mask pathologies. Syncope diagnosis in children requires a diligent approach, especially in emergency presentations. Clinicians traditionally assess patient history, clinical presentation, and perform full physical examinations to establish the etiology of syncope. Care is especially needed to distinguish syncope with cardiac etiology from non-cardiac etiology. New prohormones, including midregional-pro-A-type natriuretic peptide (MRproANP), have been demonstrated in recent research to be of diagnostic utility in the detection of cardiac syncope in the context of emergency visits. According to evidence, higher plasma levels of MRproANP are able to enhance significantly the detection rates of cardiac syncope among patients with fainting cases. Combining such new biomarker measurements with clinical judgment has the potential to maximize decision-making as well as reduce adverse effects from delayed cardiac diagnosis (Bonsor et al., 2020) (Figure 14.8).

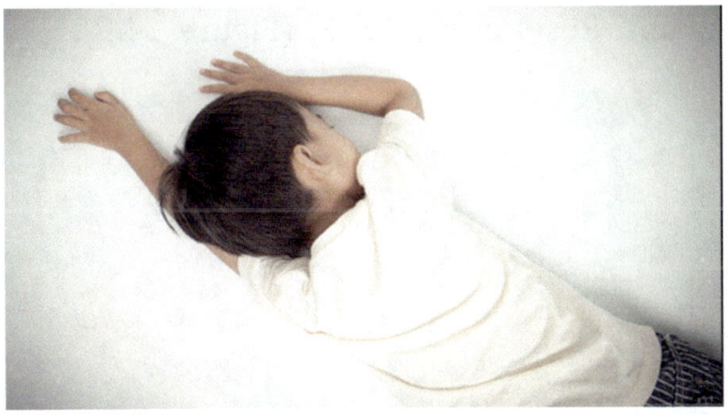

Figure 14.8. Syncope in children.

Source: https://www.hopkinsmedicine.org/-/media/images/health/1_-conditions/heart-and-vascular/syncope-in-children-teaser-image.jpg.

Their inclusion in medical practice can greatly improve the management of syncope in children. For instance, a combination of MRproANP levels and clinical probability assessments proved to be effective for excluding cardiac syncope in children effectively. A combination of an MRproANP level of less than 77 pmol/L with clinical suspicion of less than 20% in an assessment was found to have a remarkable sensitivity and negative predictive value of 99% for diagnosing non-cardiac etiologies. This innovation allows emergency departments to utilize such algorithms to screen patients more effectively, thereby ensuring that those with higher suspicion of cardiac syncope are assessed promptly. Therefore, improved diagnostic precision not just directs immediate management but optimizes long-term outcomes for patients, validating the inherent advantages of timely and precise assessment in syncope (Badertscher et al., 2017).

14.3. Risk Factors for Cardiac Emergencies

Risk factors for pediatric cardiac emergencies are a combination of intrinsic and extrinsic risk factors. Definitive heart defects, such as ventricular septal defect or coarctation of the aorta, significantly increase the likelihood of cardiac events. Structural defects can cause failure of the heart or arrhythmias, which can provoke life-threatening situations to require emergent medical intervention. In addition, comorbid conditions like obesity, diabetes, and hypertension, classically encountered in adults, have now begun to occur in children. Such a trend is a cause of concern about the long-term cardiovascular health of children and calls for preventive measures in early life to neutralize these risks, emphasizing the importance of frequent cardiovascular screening. The other significant factor contributing to cardiac emergencies in children is the increasing rate of physical conditions induced by lifestyle factors. Inadequate exercise and improper diet often lead to obesity, which is fast becoming a significant risk factor for cardiac complications even in younger age groups. The mental illnesses and stress, as anxiety and depression, also have an important role, perhaps manifesting in the form of physical symptoms that can precipitate cardiac events. Environmental factors such as exposure to toxins or secondhand smoking have also been noted to be adverse to cardiovascular health in children. Change of these lifestyle and environmental factors through education and public health interventions can significantly reduce the occurrence of cardiac emergencies.

An indispensable aspect of cardiac emergency risk management in children is the utilization of effective response tactics in community settings such as schools. Widespread education of school personnel and nurses, particularly for sudden cardiac arrest (SCA), is essential. Literature review shows that adequate preparedness, such as resource capacity and coordinated response protocols, significantly affects emergency outcomes (Dahlen et al., 2014). Further, having school programs for automated external defibrillators can enhance the survival rate of children experiencing cardiac events. Additionally, information on risk factors associated with illnesses like severe anemia, as it impacts cardiac function, is very critical, corroborated by research that set the link between low hemoglobin and increased morbidity (Akech et al., 2012). By focusing on individual steps, an overall readiness and response to cardiac emergencies can be easily enhanced.

14.3.1. Family History of Heart Disease

It is vital to appreciate the role of a family history of heart disease in the presentation of cardiac emergencies in children. Hereditary factors are a crucial causative factor in cardiovascular illness, and this highlights the need for active monitoring and management in at-risk groups. Children with a history of heart disease within their families have an inbuilt susceptibility to the development of hypertension and arrhythmias, which may manifest as acute cardiac emergencies. The recognition of these children is facilitated by the evolution of individualized preventive interventions, including lifestyle modification and routine screening, leading to reduced morbidity and mortality from cardiovascular disorders. Secondly, familial aggregation of heart disease increases the importance of family health education on the potential danger and the need for early medical evaluation, creating a culture of prevention and awareness among individuals. Integrating this awareness of family risk factors is essential in the clinical setting because health professionals must be capable of addressing these particular problems. Management is not merely a case of medical treatment but includes engaging the family with care work. By understanding the health history of the family, clinicians can more precisely identify the necessity for interventions like blood pressure monitoring, which has become more vital with the higher incidence of hypertension in children. It is crucial for the surveillance of early signs of cardiovascular stress, which in recent guidelines has been described as having played a part in the youth cardiovascular disease epidemic (Agabiti-Rosei et al., 2016) (Figure 14.9).

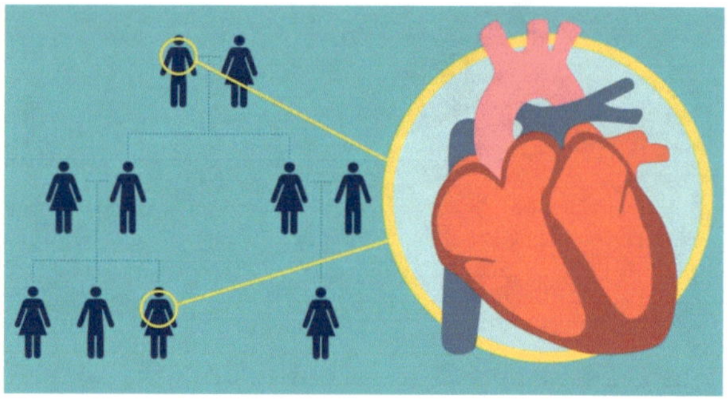

Figure 14.9. Family history of heart disease.

Source: https://www.michiganmedicine.org/sites/default/files/styles/article_main_image/public/blog/UMH_C_GENETICHEART.jpg?h=2d703ee9&itok=qSL8LSp0.

Therefore, recognition of family history of cardiac disease is a significant indicator for health professionals to conduct first-time screening and intervention to match individual risk profiles. Aside from clinical utility, family history of cardiac disease has implications for the psychological and emotional needs of care in children. Parents and other kin of the child may become anxious owing to knowledge that inherited elements can precipitate cardiac emergencies in their children. This anxiety is compounded when presenting with symptoms that simulate cardiac events, creating increased urgency to get the child in for medical assessment. Understanding these dynamics allows healthcare providers to care not just for the child but for the whole family. Furthermore, effective communication about the child's risk factors and preventative measures can significantly lower parental anxiety as well as treatment compliance. As evidenced by studies that investigate transfusion practice morbidity in extreme health conditions, the same strategy can be applied in the case of children who are at risk of cardiac emergencies so that family concerns are taken into account and addressed accordingly (Akech et al., 2012).

14.3.2. Pre-Existing Medical Conditions

Existing medical conditions are a key consideration in the care of cardiac emergencies in children. Children who have medical conditions such as congenital heart disease, asthma, or diabetes present unique challenges to acute care settings. For instance, a child with congenital heart disease may experience decompensation of their underlying condition during a respiratory infection or anaphylactic attack, and this will complicate the clinical situation and necessitate immediate evaluation and management. Identifying these histories of illness is crucial to developing effective treatment strategies that address the immediate crisis along with the underlying medical conditions. Proper identification and care of such conditions are best facilitated by a collaborative approach from healthcare teams, including pediatricians, cardiologists, and emergency medicine physicians, to deliver effective care across the board of pediatric cardiovascular use emergencies. The preconditioned child with cardiac emergencies also highlights the necessity of early detection and treatment. For example, asthma, which is a common respiratory disease among pediatric patients, tends to exacerbate underlying cardiac status during the acute bronchospasm attack. In such instances, early identification of the associated symptoms of respiratory insufficiency and cardiac compromise is important in guaranteeing patient success. Pediatric doctors must be capable of differentiating the heart-related symptoms from the symptoms caused by other diseases, usually mirroring the symptoms of cardiac distress. This extra complexity also indicates the necessity for personalized training and simulation in emergency wards so that the healthcare providers are prepared to handle the multi-factorial nature of cardiac emergencies among children, as evidenced by contemporary advancements in simulation-based training (Amira et al., 2018). Furthermore, the overlap between existing diseases and cardiac emergencies makes the implementation of preventive strategies necessary. For instance, patients with diagnosed risk factors such as obesity or high blood pressure require close monitoring and lifestyle changes to reduce the chances of cardiac events. Education on symptoms and signs of distress among family members is also essential to allow early medical intervention. Also addressing nutritional issues, particularly among children with chronic illness, is a vital aspect of dealing with overall health in crises. As depicted in various research studies, the inclusion of nutritional assessment and interventions can be a significant difference in patient outcomes in acute cardiovascular events (Thorne-Lyman et al., 2025). Thus, an anticipatory approach to treating chronic illnesses not only prepares healthcare professionals to effectively deal with emergencies but also enables greater health and well-being in children.

14.3.3. Lifestyle Factors and Environmental Influences

Cardiac emergency management and prevention in children are significantly influenced by various lifestyle elements and environmental factors that define the overall health and well-being of a child. Eating habits, levels of physical activity, and sleeping patterns are significant components of a child's lifestyle that may complicate or make cardiovascular risks simpler. For instance, overuse of processed fat and sugar can lead to obesity, a confirmed risk factor for hypertension and other cardiovascular diseases in children. Concurrently, the growing popularity of sedentary way of life, especially with increased access to television and other screens, has also been correlated with poor cardiovascular health outcomes, further emphasizing the need to promote better lifestyle options among children and adolescents. Public health interventions that aim at educating families about the proper diet and the necessity of regular exercise can make a groundbreaking difference in the frequency of cardiac emergencies among this risk group. In addition to individual lifestyle choices, the home environment in which children live most of their lives can play a decisive role in their cardiovascular status.

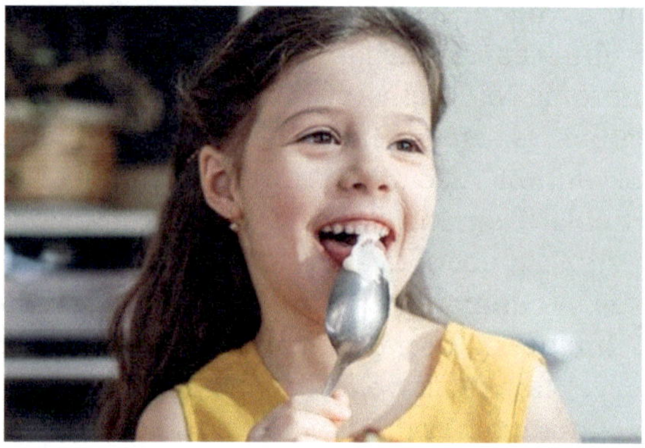

Figure 14.10. Lifestyle changes for kids to prevent heart attacks later in life.

Source: https://images.hindustantimes.com/img/2022/12/10/550x309/child_heart_attack_risk_1670678466089_1670678478969_1670678478969.jpg.

Environmental elements such as exposure to pollution, the presence of open space for recreation, and socioeconomic status have been linked with cardiovascular outcomes. For example, children who have a high level of air pollution exposure in an urban setting might have an increased risk of developing hypertension and other cardiac issues. Moreover, socioeconomic disparities can limit the access to healthy foods and safe space for exercise, further raising the threat of developing diseases that can trigger cardiac emergencies (Figure 14.10).

Managing such environmental factors entails integrated policies intended to offer equitable access to healthcare resources, offer health in the environment, and improve community infrastructure for purposes of promoting healthier lifestyles among children. The interaction between determinants of lifestyle and environmental factors is also worsened by developmental factors responsible for long-term cardiovascular health. Evidence suggests that there may be an association between low birth weight and later cardiovascular disease risk, where genetic and environmental mechanisms become interlinked from the prenatal stage onwards. Inadequate fetal exposures like maternal under-nutrition or stress exposure, coupled with sub-optimal postnatal growth patterns, can lead to the predisposition of children to cardiovascular disease. Attaining these interchanges is significant, as it means interventions aimed at improving maternal health and child nutrition may have a profound effect on preventing future cardiovascular threats. Hence, curing lifestyle and environmental factors holistically can lead to successful prevention against cardiac emergencies in children, leading to a better generation.

14.4. Diagnosis of Cardiac Emergencies

Diagnosis of pediatric cardiac emergencies necessitates a thorough comprehension of the clinical presentation, pathophysiology, and diagnostic tools. Children tend to present with atypical symptoms as compared to adults, and therefore they are not able to diagnose perilous cardiac diseases. Symptoms of primary presentation such as chest pain, syncope, or palpitations can indicate both benign conditions and acute cardiac disorders. The clinical heterogeneity necessitates immediate assessment and integration of a systematic approach into our diagnostic strategy (i.e., the use of heart rate variability or bedside ultrasound). Clinicians also need to be vigilant to assess risk factors such as a family history of cardiomyopathy or arrhythmias since early identification can prevent the risk of life-threatening complications in children with cardiac emergencies. In emergent conditions, an appropriate assessment protocol is essential to diagnose cardiac emergencies in children successfully. A thorough history and a targeted physical examination with the support of diagnostic imaging and laboratory tests are the primary elements of the assessment. Electrocardiograms (ECGs) remain the cornerstone for the diagnosis of arrhythmias, ischemic changes, or other electrical disturbances. Moreover, rapid echocardiography acquisition and interpretation may provide crucial information about structural heart disease, ruling in or ruling out such conditions as cardiomyopathy or congenital heart defect. Having made the diagnosis of the presenting symptom, it would be beneficial for caregivers to have a grounding in advanced cardiac life support (ACLS) procedures to enable rapid intervention, especially in emergencies involving sudden cardiac arrest. This is a procedure that aligns with best practice described in recent literature of the importance of effective communication and preparedness in managing such emergent health crises (Dahlen et al., 2014). Emergent imaging technology has revolutionized the diagnostic protocol of cardiac emergencies in children to facilitate more accurate and timely interventions. Imaging modalities such as cardiac MRI and CT angiography provide accurate data regarding the anatomy and function of the heart and yield valuable information with the potential to influence therapy. In particular, such modalities can elucidate abnormalities such as coronary artery anomalies or aortic dissection that otherwise can be missed in standard evaluation. Assessment of cardiac structure and function, enabled by these imaging technologies, helps in directing clinical decisions regarding additional management or surgical consultation. In addition, inclusion of techniques assessing myocardial perfusion and metabolic function can enhance the global diagnostic sensitivity, thereby simplifying management of childhood cardiac emergencies. Overall, the continuous innovation and coalescence of these diagnostic tools underscore the critical necessity of contemporary approaches to improve outcomes for children with cardiac emergencies (Brém et al., 2020).

14.4.1. Physical Examination and Medical History

The initial step in the management of pediatric cardiac emergencies is a thorough physical examination and careful medical history taking. Clinicians must understand that manifestations of cardiac disease in children can be subtle compared to adults. Key pointers such as heart rate, blood pressure, respiratory rate, and auscultation findings form the pillars of a focused physical examination. For instance, discrepancies in key signs will lead to the detection of underlying pathology (i.e., arterial hypertension), which has been on the rise in adolescents and children. These nuances need to be realized because the pathophysiology of hypertension can contribute significantly to cardiovascular risk profiles. Hence, medical professionals are required to employ well-delineated protocols in measuring and documenting such parameters effectively, ensuring that medical history of each child is documented in a detailed manner to inform future assessment and interventions (Agabiti-

Rosei et al., 2016). In addition to vital signs, a careful history including queries about family history, history of previous cardiac complications, and symptoms like exertional dyspnea or syncope is important. Compiling information on any previous disease or surgeries will enlighten us on likely underlying diseases that may render a child susceptible to cardiac emergencies. Physical inactivity, obesity, and diet are also risk factors which must be considered by pediatric health practitioners as integral parts while evaluating cardiovascular fitness. Current systematic reviews position the significance of putting these risk factors into a strengthened epidemiological context, highlighting the manner in which they contribute to burdening cardiovascular disease among youths. In-depth medical history-taking, thus, not only enhances immediate assessment but is also the building block for preventive health planning directed at protecting against future cardiac risks (Agabiti-Rosei et al., 2016) (Figure 14.11).

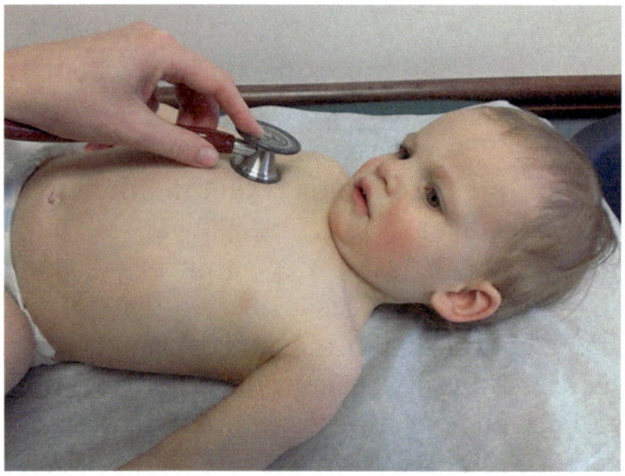

Figure 14.11. Physical exam of child with stethoscope on chest.

Source: https://upload.wikimedia.org/wikipedia/commons/1/10/Physical_exam_of_child_with_stethoscope_on_chest.jpeg.

Finally, while doing physical examination and taking medical history, physicians should remain attentive to the psychosocial aspect of pediatric care. Illness in parents or social stability stressors can significantly affect a child's overall well-being and create cardiovascular stress. In addition, it is necessary to understand that anxiety and emotional distress often present as bodily complaints in order to offer comprehensive care.

Providers are encouraged to incorporate screening tools measuring psychosocial determinants, thereby linking emotional health and physical health. For instance, diseases like hypertension often appear in conjunction with psychosocial stressors, warranting an integrative mode of caring for children patients. By integrating detailed physical examinations with insightful medical histories and psychosocial evaluations, clinicians can develop more tailored, effective interventions for children with cardiac emergencies.

14.4.2. Diagnostic Imaging Techniques

In the scenario of pediatric cardiac emergencies, diagnostic imaging techniques play a crucial role in quickly detecting and assessing causative conditions that threaten the cardiovascular system of a child. Among the numerous modalities employed, echocardiography stands out as the preeminent non-invasive yet extremely valuable imaging technique for evaluating cardiac structures and function. By utilizing sound waves to produce instantaneous images of the heart, echocardiography allows clinicians to delineate abnormalities such as structural defects, valvular disease, and congenital heart disease with a high degree of accuracy. Visualization of hemodynamics and assessment of myocardial function using Doppler imaging make it an even more useful tool in emergency situations where decisions have to be made in a hurry. Another critical imaging technique used in pediatric cardiac emergencies is chest radiography (Figure 14.12).

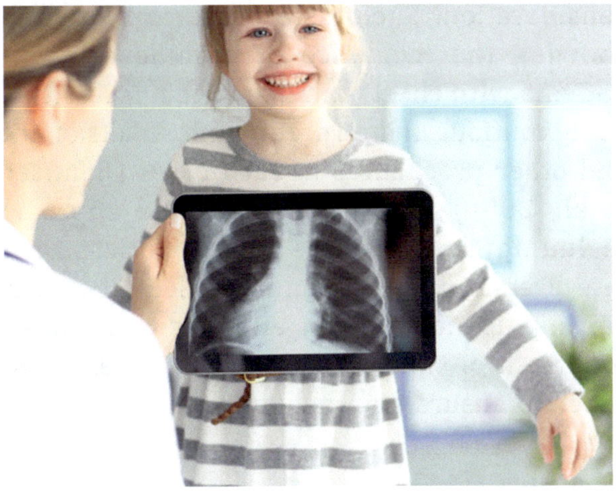

Figure 14.12. Chest X-ray.

Source: https://www.ucsfbenioffchildrens.org/-/media/project/ucsf/ucsf-bch/images/medical-tests/hero/chest-x-ray-708x556-2x.jpg?rev=cacf3513f60f415f8a92d2dc35296379.

Although often considered to be a first-time inquiry, chest X-rays have the potential to provide useful information about the thoracic organs and cardiovascular silhouette. In cases of cardiac failure or other acute conditions, chest X-rays may make evident findings of cardiomegaly, pulmonary edema, or anomalous anatomical structures. In addition, the portability and rapid application of this technique render it particularly useful in emergency situations, where the timeliness of the procedure is important. While it is not providing full information regarding myocardial morphology, its role in arriving at a tentative diagnosis cannot be excluded. Thus, chest radiography serves as a valuable ancillary modality guiding further diagnostic tests and therapeutic management. Magnetic resonance imaging (MRI) has been a sophisticated diagnostic tool for evaluation of intricate pediatric cardiac disorders. Unlike other imaging modalities, MRI offers unambiguous soft tissue contrast with exquisite anatomical detail of the heart and surrounding structures without the need for ionizing radiation. This characteristic renders it particularly useful in children because they are more radiosensitive. MRI is especially useful in the assessment of arrhythmias, myocardial viability, and detection of some congenital abnormalities. Furthermore, the development of MRI protocols tailored to pediatric patients has extended the scope of its application from preoperative planning to postoperative assessment. Therefore, MRI is an efficient complement to more traditional imaging modalities, enhancing the clinician's ability to manage cardiac emergencies effectively and with increased accuracy (N/A, 2000, 2007).

14.4.3. Electrocardiogram (ECG) and Other Tests

In the classification of cardiac emergencies in children, the Electrocardiogram (ECG) features most prominently in diagnosing conditions which could potentially occur acutely. The ECG is a cheap, painless, and non-invasive investigation that measures the electrical activity of the heart, providing very important information about the rhythm, rate, and potential structural abnormalities of the hearts. In young children, arrhythmias like supraventricular tachycardia or bradycardia can occur suddenly, prompting prompt ECG evaluation to determine the requirement for immediate action. Prompt interpretation of ECG findings is crucial, with the risk of adverse outcomes resulting from delay in diagnosis being high where ventricular dysfunction or congenital heart disease may be involved. Secondly, an awareness of the distinctive pediatric ECG presentation, which, in most cases, differs from adult presentation, is required for accurate diagnosis and management protocol of pediatric cardiac emergencies. Along with the ECG, additional laboratory tests can further characterize the clinical presentation of cardiac emergencies. For instance, serum electrolyte level measurement is crucial since imbalances can have cataclysmic impacts on cardiac function. Electrolyte disturbances such as hypocalcemia or hyperkalemia can lead to potentially lethal arrhythmias and hence their rapid detection and correction are essential. Laboratory work, including the concentration of cardiac biomarkers, is equally important for diagnosing myocardial stress or damage. Novel prohormones, including midregional-pro-A-type natriuretic peptide (MRproANP), are presently key markers for conditions such as cardiac syncope, especially in the field of emergency medicine. Evidence indicates that the combination of these biomarkers with clinical assessment can significantly improve diagnostic accuracy, underscoring their suitability in an emergency department environment where rapid decisions take precedence (Badertscher et al., 2017) (Figure 14.13).

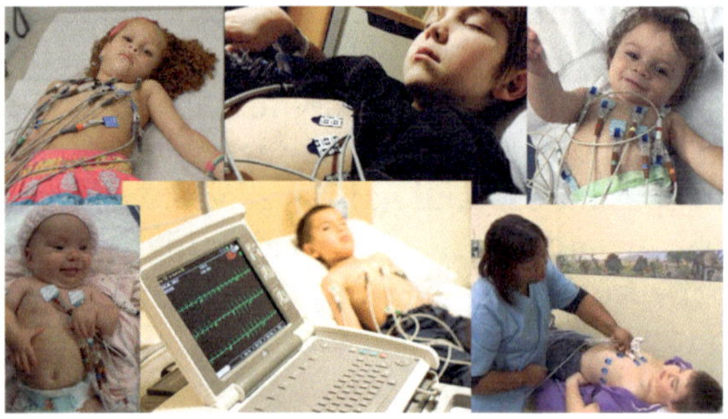

Figure 14.13. Electrocardiogram (ECG) test.

Source: https://i0.wp.com/pemplaybook.org/wp-content/uploads/2018/05/TU_0915_Horeczko_EKG2.png?fit=1200%2C675&ssl=1.

Furthermore, while the ECG and laboratory workup are most important, they should be augmented with good clinical evaluation in order to achieve the highest diagnostic yield and determine the course of treatment. Well-functioning triage within the emergency room will allow children presenting for cardiac symptoms to receive immediate treatment in accordance with their illness severity. For example, patients presenting with chest pain but with a drug abuse background may unveil underlying conditions in need of urgent consideration. Such is the case in one study showing the incidence of cocaine abuse in patients with chest pain due to the necessity of being cautious in interpreting the results of ECG and other procedures in such cases (Bandeeri et al., 2004). Lastly, an integrated approach including appropriate clinical assessment, interpretation of ECG, and detailed laboratory workup is needed for effective and timely treatment of children's cardiac emergencies in order to ensure favorable outcomes.

14.5. Immediate Management of Cardiac Emergencies

Acute management of cardiac emergencies in children is a fundamental aspect of pediatric management that needs immediate and efficient intervention. Cardiac emergencies can manifest as arrhythmias, cardiomyopathies, or myocardial infarctions, which are all fraught with serious risk, particularly for vulnerable groups. Early recognition of signs and symptoms such as chest pain, palpitations, or syncope is crucial, as timely intervention has the potential to limit the severity of outcomes. The initiation of initial life support measures, like cardiopulmonary resuscitation (CPR) and the use of automated external defibrillators (AEDs), is of great importance in early response. These interventions not only address the immediate survival but also prepare the healthcare personnel to deploy advanced cardiovascular life support interventions. Giving appropriate training for emergency responders regarding the detection of pediatric cardiac distress is of greater priority in increasing survival rates among the populace. Furthermore, understanding the underlying pathophysiology can enhance the immediate management of cardiac emergencies. For instance, when encountering a child with chest pain, healthcare providers must consider various etiologies, from congenital heart defects to acquired conditions like myocarditis. The swift administration of appropriate diagnostic tests—including electrocardiograms (ECGs) and echocardiograms—facilitates timely identification of the issue at hand. Also, the patient's clinical history has to be assessed, since disorders like drug abuse may cause cardiac illnesses. Early studies have indicated a significant correlation between drug abuse and cardiac distress among emergency departments, emphasized in research assessing cocaine use among emergency-seeking patients (Bandeeri et al., 2004). Identification of these relationships allows for more individualized and responsive treatment regimens that not only work to stabilize the patient but also strive to prevent relapse. Finally, interdisciplinary collaboration is crucial in the initial treatment of pediatric cardiac emergencies. Pediatric cardiologists, emergency room docs, nurses, and other specialists must work together to ensure an integrated care process. The use of standardized protocols, like those established for the management of acute myocardial infarction in adults, would likely need to be adapted to children due to variation in physiological response and drug requirements. Scheduling emergency department staff with these protocols facilitates a structured response under crisis. Post-event treatment is also important as the psychological impact of a cardiac emergency on children can be drastic. Emotional support and post-discharge follow-up are components of the overall treatment effectiveness and support a comprehensive approach to cardiac emergency care in children, as noted in the health equity and access debate (Thorne-Lyman et al., 2025).

14.5.1. Basic Life Support (BLS) Techniques

It is in pediatric cardiac emergencies that Basic Life Support (BLS) practice constitutes the minimum skills needed in responding to distressed children. BLS entails necessary interventions, such as ensuring an open airway, rescue breaths, and chest compressions. These are vital considerations, particularly in the fact that a child's physiological response is entirely different from that of an adult. For instance, the appropriate compression depth and rate must be established based on age and size to achieve optimum outcome during a cardiac arrest. Training in BLS skills is important, as evidence indicates poor knowledge among clinical personnel with scores indicating a disturbingly low level of comprehension of BLS principles (Basheer et al., 2018). Hence, getting all the healthcare professionals treating children BLS competent can significantly enhance the ability of emergency response and ultimately save lives.

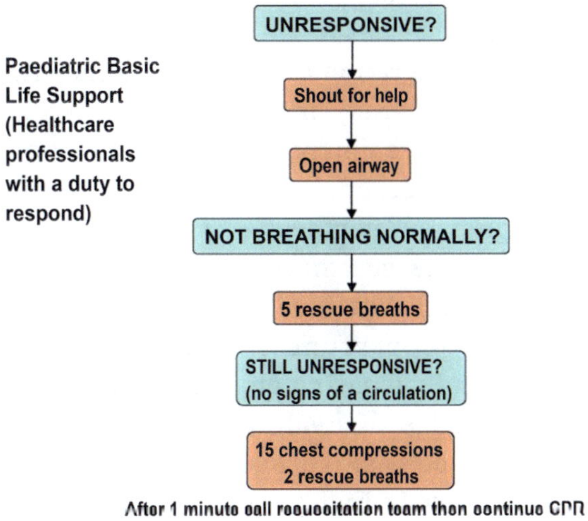

Figure 14.14. Pediatric basic life support algorithm.

Source: https://www.researchgate.net/figure/Paediatric-basic-life-support-algorithm_fig14_7446797.

Apart from this, BLS techniques become more efficient because they are paired with structured training programs for enhancing comfort levels and practical skills among healthcare professionals, particularly in pediatric resuscitation cases. It has been indicated through evidence that resident physicians are less prepared for pediatric emergencies due to receiving fewer trainings and exposures beforehand (Brancati et al., 2003) (Figure 14.14).

Implementing full training courses with the sole purpose of boosting exposure to BLS techniques can significantly enhance the confidence levels of practitioners in their ability. For example, practice training in a simulated environment allows persons to rehearse vital steps such as chest compressions, airway management, and the use of Automated External Defibrillators (AEDs) effectively. The consequences of these courses are time and again demonstrated through higher levels of comfort and knowledge retention, qualities critical to individuals who are responding to cardiac emergencies in the pediatric population. Lastly, the integration of solid BLS skills within pediatric emergency management is urgently needed to ensure timely and sufficient response in cardiac emergencies. Continuous training and heightened alertness of BLS practice not only equip the healthcare providers with the necessary skill but also assist in instilling a culture of preparedness within healthcare institutions. By focusing on enhancing BLS skill and knowledge of healthcare personnel, the probability of positive outcomes in pediatric cardiac arrest is highly increased. With each subsequent assessment pointing out areas for improvement, it becomes ever more crucial to persist in attempts to enhance these essential skills so that every child is provided with the finest possible emergency management when faced with a cardiac dilemma.

14.5.2. Use of Automated External Defibrillators (AEDs)

The integration of automatic external defibrillators (AEDs) into emergency response devices is paramount, particularly in the pediatric population where SCA risk occurs. AEDs have been designed to be user-friendly such that people with minimal training are able to successfully administer lifesaving interventions. The equipment verifies cardiac rhythms and provides audio instructions, which lowers the barrier to successful CPR and defibrillation. In environments such as schools, where children gather and engage in physical training, the presence of AEDs is instrumental. Reports have cited that school nurses have highlighted the importance of organizational readiness in responding to SCA episodes, with many nurses being optimistic regarding their education in the situations regarding AEDs and CPR (Dahlen et al., 2014). Such facilities, supported by timely interventions from bystanders, can considerably enhance survival prospects for children who are experiencing cardiac emergencies. Despite the advanced technology of AEDs and increased availability of the device in public places, there are still a few problems associated with using these devices properly.

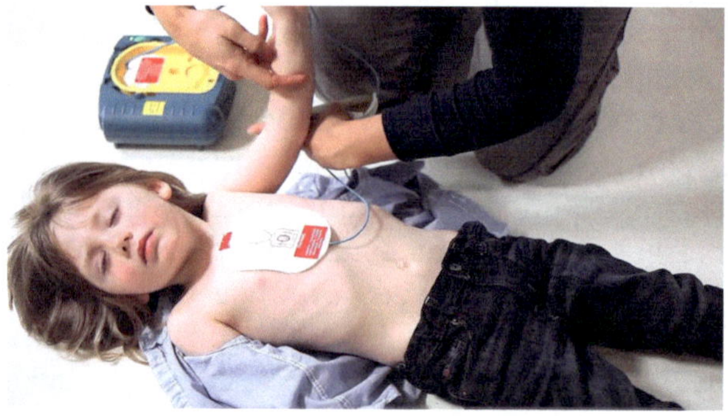

Figure 14.15. Uses of automated external defibrillators (AEDs) in children.

Source: https://first-aid-product.com/blogs/first-aid-product/wp-content/uploads/2015/07/children-automated-external-defibrillation.jpg.

Research indicates that proper training and equipment are not always given evenly to institutions. School nurses often indicate that they are not properly trained to treat SCA, and hence there should be proper training sessions which cover the use of AEDs as well as CPR techniques. Building an effective communication network within schools is essential in order to mobilize during emergencies. In the absence of an organized approach, response times are often slow, and the survival rate is hindered (Dahlen et al., 2014) (Figure 14.15).

For this reason, ongoing education and adequate drills should be afforded top priority to ensure personnel are self-assured in reacting appropriately to cardiac emergencies. The impact of human factors on effective deployment of AEDs cannot be overestimated as the factors contribute heavily to affecting operator performance and consequently patient survival. Studies have shown that while AEDs are easy to use, how and where they are used also determines outcomes. Stress, familiarity with the device, and the environment all play important parts in how well bystanders are able to respond in emergency scenarios. Therefore, it is crucial that research continues in the areas of user modeling and operator studies in an effort to refine the design of AEDs in order to align with the realities on the ground. With the evolving medical landscape, combined efforts must continue to enhance the role of such machines, making them more accessible, user-friendly, and cost-effective, and thereby increasing survival in children with cardiac emergencies.

14.5.3. Emergency Medication Administration

Administration of emergency drugs during pediatric cardiac emergencies is a complicated art requiring a sophisticated grasp of both pharmacology and the subtleties of physiology in children versus adults. In the setting of a cardiac emergency, the clinician needs to quickly evaluate the situation in order to decide on the most appropriate pharmacological intervention. The most commonly used drugs are epinephrine, adenosine, and atropine, each for a specific purpose, such as correcting normal heart rhythm or enhancing perfusion. Dosage is critical; doses of medication in children are usually administered per kilogram of body weight, which necessitates precise estimation of weight during emergencies. Straying from these specific orders might introduce toxicities or ineffective therapy, which may further complicate the child's medical condition and prolong the emergency duration. In addition to doses of medication, routes of administration also play an important part in efficiently coping with emergencies within the cardiac system of children. Intravenous (IV) access is the best, but sometimes finding IV access can be challenging due to smaller veins and restlessness with pediatric patients. Therefore, such routes as intraosseous (IO) access or intramuscular (IM) injections can be employed in cases where IV access cannot be achieved. IO access utilization, for instance, allows the clinician to easily administer life-saving medication in a timely manner, as required in cardiac arrest cases. Emergency practitioners are generally expected to act fast in making medication administration decisions. Proficiency in this skill set can make a tremendous impact on patient outcomes amidst the chaotic environment of pediatric emergencies. Last but not least, open communication among the healthcare team is key to the successful prescription of emergency drugs. The collaborative engagement of pre-hospital care professionals, emergency department members, and specialists ensures that care not only takes place in a timely manner, but is also delivered according to best practice. Research on pre-hospital pain management indicates differences in opinion between patients and healthcare staff on how well treatment would work can prevent optimal care (Iqbal et al., 2013). Therefore, a patient-centered protocol is crucial that facilitates interdisciplinary coordination. Additionally, regular training and simulation can enhance team workflows and make all the providers familiar with pediatric-specific medication guidelines. By doing so, healthcare providers optimize the likelihood of delivering effective care in pediatric critical cardiac emergencies.

14.6. Long-Term Management and Follow-Up

In pediatric cardiac emergency, long-term care and follow-up of the involved children are crucial for maximum health advantage. Effective management begins with an earnest appraisal following the happening of an emergency, where ongoing observation of the cardiac status is essential. These children are likely to require multidisciplinary care through cardiologists, pediatricians, and family guidance to address their physical and psychological demands. Periodic follow-up visits allow healthcare workers to track the improvement of the child, adjust treatment protocols, and easily identify any adverse complications. This surveillance is particularly important since some cardiac ailments can lead to a deterioration of symptoms or unforeseen complications that are not apparent following initial intervention. Additionally, integration of personalized management protocols is also a significant component of long-term care of children who have experienced cardiac emergencies. Personalized treatment can include lifestyle adjustments, such as dietary modification and exercise regimens, which are crucial in recurrence prevention of cardiac events. Continuous family education on the recognition of deteriorating warning signs and adherence to prescribed treatment can greatly enhance the efficacy of the management plan. Given the increased prevalence of hypertension in children, as mentioned in recent literature, its management forms part of the long-term cardiac planning (Agabiti-Rosei et al., 2016). By embarking on the vanguard approach, the medical team is able to effectively reduce risks and improve the quality of life for these patients. Lastly, the role of transitional care to adult care must not be overlooked in the long-term management of pediatric cardiac disease. With aging, their health responsibilities and needs shift and thus a system of organized transition must be followed with training in self-management as well as knowledge of their own cardiac condition. This phase is crucial to reduce risks of poor lapses in care in the daunting phase of late adolescence when the majority of adolescents with chronic medical conditions have a tendency to drop out of health care services. An effective transition helps to ensure ownership towards their health care, thereby promoting adherence to long-term follow-up protocols. Thus, the inclusion of strategies for long-term involvement and education can significantly enhance the overall success for children who have experienced recovery from cardiac emergencies (Brém et al., 2020).

14.6.1. Cardiology Referrals and Ongoing Care

In pediatric cardiology, referral and continuity of care at the appropriate time are crucial to properly address cardiac emergencies. The moment signs of potential cardiac distress, such as chest pain or extreme fatigue, are identified, medical professionals must initiate immediate assessment and refer the patient to a pediatric cardiologist. Early intervention not only helps in accurate diagnosis but also enhances the child's prognosis by introducing optimal management measures, including pharmacotherapy or further diagnostic work-up. The importance of prioritizing early cardiology referrals is emphasized by the need for special knowledge to identify congenital heart disease and acquired cardiac illnesses, which are prevalent among the pediatric population. Thus, the linkage between pediatric cardiology specialists and general practitioners is essential in sustaining care for kids with serious heart diseases, encouraging a unitary care perspective and enhancing the quality of care. Sustained care in pediatric cardiology includes monitoring and management of diagnosed diseases and must be guaranteed through an elaborate framework that includes periodic assessment and education to families. Pediatric cardiac disease patients pose unique challenges for which a multidisciplinary treatment team is optimally equipped. This involves not only cardiologists but also nurses, nutritionists, and psychiatric staff to individualize a complete treatment program. The emphasis on frequent follow-up visits allows therapy modifications as growth and development proceed, which is essential with such a dynamic population. Lastly, parents and caregivers should be adequately educated regarding the indicators of probable regression, which would equip them with the knowledge needed to respond appropriately at moments of crises. This not only instills confidence in the medical system but also allows family members to become participants of their child's care process. The significance of community nursing in providing effective referrals and ongoing care cannot be overstressed, particularly in the context of pediatric cardiovascular health (Figure 14.16).

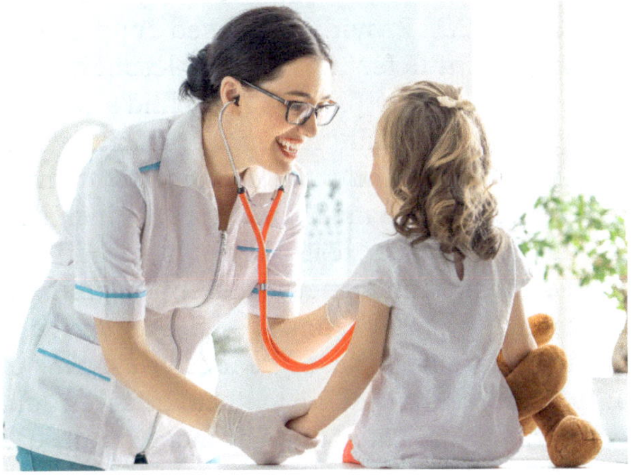

Figure 14.16. Pediatric cardiology referrals.

Source: https://55933-bcmed.s3.amazonaws.com/bcp/images/orlVideoAssets/imgSource/adobestock_227793697.jpeg.

Community nurses are best placed to provide education and support and to bridge specialist and family services. They have an important role in ensuring individualized care plans that address the specific needs of children with heart conditions, especially where the resources are lacking. It is evident from qualitative findings presented in community nursing practice studies that the integration of nurse-driven programs into care planning can enhance the outcomes of pediatric patients with cardiovascular conditions. As written in projects aimed at improving case management models in the community setting, the benefits extend beyond the individual care cases but develop a more robust health system with focus on combined child welfare and chronic heart condition care (Gray et al., 2010). Through promoting interdisciplinary working, community nurses can effectively lead the shifting of the balance of care in direction towards prevention and active management in children's cardiology (Lehigh Valley Health Network, 2018).

14.6.2. Lifestyle Modifications and Education

The growing number of cardiac emergencies in children generates the demand for emphasis on lifestyle modification and educational interventions aimed at cardiovascular risk factor reduction. Lifestyle determinants such as diet, physical inactivity, and being overweight significantly contribute to heart health. As evidence shows, obese children (as characterized by their higher body mass indices) are at risk of hypertension, which contributes to a higher risk of heart disease. The 2020 American Heart Association guidelines recommend to healthcare providers encouraging families to discuss healthy eating and physical activity to promote cardiovascular health. The lifestyle modifications not only are impactful in combating obesity but also are essential preventative methods for hypertension, thus making them an important component of pediatric practice. By educating families of the need to embrace heart-healthy behaviors early on, healthcare professionals can empower a generation of adults in the future who embrace preventive health habits and lower the risk of cardiac crises and long-term complications (Agabiti-Rosei et al., 2016). Apart from diet and physical exercise recommendations, the need for education in prevention and control of cardiac crises among children cannot be overstated. Information on identification of symptoms of cardiac distress is also crucial in allowing intervention on schedule. Parents and guardians must be taught symptoms of cardiac distress, including sudden fainting, shortness of breath, and chest pain. Furthermore, the importance of pre-participation cardiac screening, particularly among child athletes, cannot be overemphasized.

This screening can assist in the identification of occult heart disease that may result in sudden cardiac arrest in children. Interventions aiming to inform young athletes and their families regarding the significance of these screenings, as presented in practices that have been carried out in certain regions of the globe, highlight an active initiative towards heart health that harmonizes with public child health policy targets (Harrington et al., 2013). School- and community-based programs designed to raise awareness of cardiovascular well-being form a critical platform for making lifestyle modifications. These interventions typically consist of educational workshops, fitness competitions, and nutrition workshops with the aim to reach children and their families effectively. Schools are in a strange position to be utilized as areas for the provision of heart-healthy curricula addressing lifestyle choices and health promotion as an interactive and integrated component of the learning process. Working with parents in workshops not only raises awareness but also creates a culture of community that values cardiovascular health and preventive care. These types of initiatives are important not just for supporting individual behavior shift, but for changing social norms around healthy childhood and well-being. Furthermore, expanding the group knowledge of cardiovascular health can equip communities with the knowledge that is required to manage the growing problem of cardiac arrest among children (Agabiti-Rosei et al., 2016).

14.6.3. Psychological Support for Affected Families

The psychological load of children's cardiac emergencies does not just fall on the affected child but also impacts their families considerably. The encouraging support from families is typically disrupted by shock at a child's sudden medical emergency, leading to heightened anxiety and diverse psychological distress. To this end, it has increasingly been understood that psychological treatment for families is a critical component of the holistic treatment strategy. Rather than being limited to the exclusive focus on the medical treatment, the medical professionals must be aware of the many faceted emotional requirements of the families experiencing such calamities. Providing focused support can alleviate painful feelings of helplessness and confusion normally present in a child's cardiac emergency, eventually fostering resilience and strengthening family relationships. Mental health intervention must, therefore, be included in pediatric cardiac care settings to address these evolving familial needs. Parents of children experiencing cardiac emergencies describe a strong preference for comprehensive systems of support beyond the acute medical intervention. Research has indicated that parents typically are bewildered by information and decisions that take place when they are hospitalized with a feeling of isolation and bewilderment regarding their own functions in their child's care. In line with current research, the majority of parents welcome advice from medical professionals for them to manage their child's condition successfully, emphasizing the significance of improved communication and information regarding treatment options and rehabilitation processes (Kendall et al., 2003) (Figure 14.17).

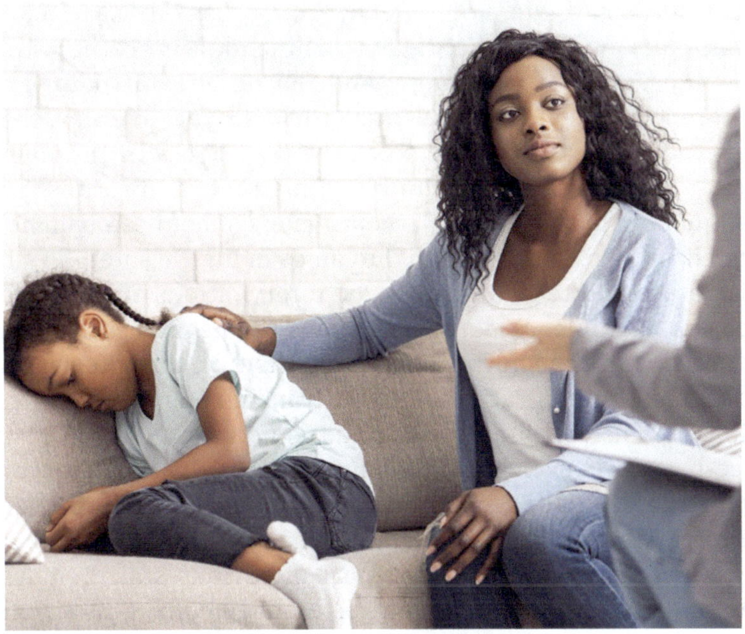

Figure 14.17. Psychological support for affected families.

Source: https://www.namigreaterhouston.org/wp-content/uploads/2020/12/NAMI_Imgs_support-group-02.jpg.

If health workers emphasize the parent's welfare and educate them appropriately, they can empower parents to be actively involved in caring for their child. With this collaboration, the family's knowledge of the disease is increased, positive coping strategies are promoted, and this leads to a favorable prognosis for the child and family. Granting access to psychological assistance to families during and upon hospitalization is critical in fostering long-term resilience. Proper discharge planning should not only include the medical information necessary for continuation of care but also address the emotional needs of the families (Maloney et al., 2008). For example, providing counseling services, support groups, and resources related to the challenges involved in healthcare system navigation significantly enhances the coping ability of families. These interventions can allay distress and permit emotional clarification during a period of turbulence, thereby facilitating families' understanding and being able to cope with the child's condition. Furthermore, implementing family-centered care practices ensures that families are made to feel recognized, heard, and enabled by their own knowledge. Therefore, prioritizing psychological support as a part of care in cardia emergencies not only does good for one's immediate health but also serves as a foundation for ongoing resilience and adaptation based on a child's medical issues.

SUMMARY

In conclusion, the management of cardiac emergencies in children needs to be an interconnected approach with elements of early detection, effective intervention, and comprehensive education programs for caregivers and medical practitioners. The children are not similar in these clinical presentations due to differences in physiology and developmental pathways, and thus most of the generic adult-centered protocols are inadequate. It is imperative that the emergency medical team get familiar with the singular symptoms of cardiac distress in the pediatric patient, which, if overlooked, will lead to serious complications and high mortality rates. The use of continuous training courses and simulation in pediatric emergency management can enhance the preparedness of medical personnel, which, in turn, will diminish outcomes in life-threatening situations. Additionally, a review of current literature shows that customized interventions are of importance in the care of children with diseases. For example, research has shown the negative effects of diseases like severe anemia on children's health and thus how their treatments turn out afterward. Particularly, studies have demonstrated that the administration of blood transfusions can significantly affect recovery, altering both hemoglobin levels considerably after administration (Akech et al., 2012). This puts a high value on evidence-based interventions that enable clinicians to make well-informed decisions regarding intervention strategies. Additionally, recognition of risk factors of undesirable outcomes, including co-morbidities, can inform strategic planning and resource allocation in pediatric emergency departments. Lastly, collaborative action on the part of various stakeholders in pediatric care is needed in an effort to enhance cardiac emergencies management. This involves the development of protocols that focus on timely identification and intervention as well as educating parents about the signs of potential cardiac distress among children. Equipping families with knowledge that enables them to access timely help can bridge the time lag from symptom onset to clinical presentation. Additionally, commitments to research and continuous improvement of treatment modalities will allow healthcare systems to keep pace with the evolving pediatric cardiac emergency environment in a productive way. Just as has been found in complicated condition situations that involve instances of substance abuse, a coherent understanding of factors resulting in them is a requirement for improved patient outcomes in the emergency department (Bandeeri et al., 2004).

Education and awareness are the keys to the management of cardiac emergencies in children, significantly enhancing the success rate of such life-threatening scenarios. A well-informed community shall be capable of recognizing the signs and symptoms of cardiac distress so that help can be obtained in time. For instance, educational intervention for parents, school staff, and caregivers can provide them with knowledge on the warning signs of sudden cardiac arrest (SCA) and how to respond during the occurrence. With awareness creation, education is the first line of defense and can also improve survival rates. The American Heart Association (AHA) emphasizes that effective communication awareness and readiness at the community level is essential to any successful response to SCA incidents, and hence the importance of specially focused educational interventions in school and youth organizations (Dahlen et al., 2014). Moreover, strategically implementing training programs in educational institutions has the potential of increasing the level of readiness among faculty and staff to act in cardiac emergencies. This training commonly includes cardiopulmonary resuscitation (CPR) and automated external defibrillator (AED) use. Making the school personnel proficient in these skills not only prepares them for emergencies but also encourages health-aware culture among students. A recent study found that a significant percentage of school nurses reported to be adequately supported regarding their ability to manage SCA, considering the nice work of training and education centers (Dahlen et al., 2014). However, this must be cascaded to every staff within schools, hence making a general effort in managing cardiac emergencies in children. Furthermore, the significance of educational intervention encompasses also the process of discharge following hospitalization, particularly in the case of children with heart conditions and their families. Communication during discharge is important to enable parents to take care of their child and recognize complications that may arise at home. Evidence indicates that most patients want to receive more information than what they are given, indicating an educational gap. For a family with a child diagnosed with a cardiac condition, it is critical to make educational programs their top priority as it can considerably improve their ability to provide effective care from home and lower the risk of negative consequences when a cardiac problem becomes present. In addressing these needs for information, healthcare professionals can facilitate self-confidence in management by families and therefore healthier health trajectories for their children.

CLOSER LOOK

ACUTE DECOMPENSATED HEART FAILURE (ADHF)

Acute decompensated heart failure (ADHF) is a clinical syndrome characterized by sudden or insidious deterioration of symptoms in new-onset or pre-existing heart failure. It is responsible for a significant rate of hospitalization in the elderly and is associated with high morbidity, mortality, and healthcare costs. ADHF is characterized by an acute exacerbation of either left or right ventricular dysfunction, followed by depressed cardiac output and congestion due to fluid overload (Figure 14.18).

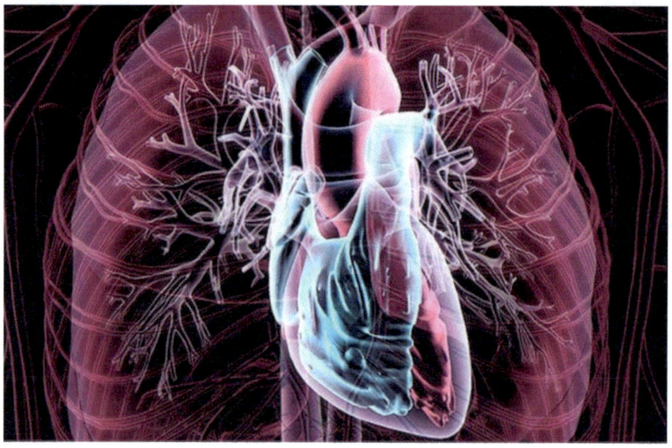

Figure 14.18. Anatomical illustration of the heart and lungs, commonly used to depict cardiopulmonary conditions such as heart failure.

Source: https://www.emra.org/siteassets/emresident/images/articles/2019/04/chf-image.jpg?w=600.

The classic characteristics of ADHF include dyspnea (breathlessness), orthopnea (dyspnea while in the recumbent position), paroxysmal nocturnal dyspnea, weakness, and edema—most commonly in the legs. Other signs include jugular venous distension, pulmonary rales, hepatomegaly, and weight gain due to fluid overload. In severe cases, patients can present with pulmonary edema, hypotension, confusion, or cardiogenic shock.

ADHF is most characteristically precipitated by factors that increase cardiac workload or decrease cardiac output. They include acute myocardial infarction, profound hypertension, arrhythmias (especially atrial fibrillation), failure to take medication or dietary restrictions, infections (like pneumonia), renal failure, and the use of drugs which impair myocardial function or cause fluid overload (like NSAIDs, corticosteroids).

Pathophysiologically, ADHF results from an imbalance between the heart's ability to pump and the body's demand. This results in increased ventricular filling pressures and pulmonary and/or systemic congestion. Stimulation of the sympathetic nervous system and renin-angiotensin-aldosterone system (RAAS) also adds to fluid overload, vasoconstriction, and myocardial stress in a vicious circle that exacerbates cardiac function.

Diagnosis is clinical with support from investigations. Chest X-ray may show pulmonary congestion or cardiomegaly. Electrocardiogram (ECG) can identify ischemia or arrhythmia. Echocardiography checks ejection fraction, chamber size, and valvular disease. Serum measurement of brain natriuretic peptide (BNP) or N-terminal proBNP is useful in diagnosing heart failure and assessing severity. Renal function, electrolytes, and cardiac enzymes are also checked by blood tests.

Management of ADHF is focused on stabilizing the patient, relief of symptoms, and addressing the cause. Hospitalization is usually required. Initial treatment includes supplemental oxygen, noninvasive ventilation if necessary, and diuretics (mainly intravenous loop diuretics like furosemide) to reduce fluid overload. Vasodilators (like nitroglycerin) can be used in hypertensive patients to decrease preload and afterload. Inotropic support with agents like dobutamine or milrinone may be needed with the presence of low-output states or cardiogenic shock.

Long-term care encompasses the maximization of guideline-directed medical therapy (GDMT) for heart failure, such as ACE inhibitors or ARBs, beta-blockers, mineralocorticoid receptor antagonists, and sodium-glucose co-transporter 2 (SGLT2) inhibitors. Lifestyle modification including sodium and fluid limitation, daily weighing, and compliance with medications is significant in an effort to prevent recurrence.

REFERENCES

1. Agabiti-Rosei, E., Cruickshank, J. K., Dominiczak, A., Erdine, S., et al. (2016). 2016 European Society of Hypertension guidelines for the management of high blood pressure in children and adolescents. https://core.ac.uk/download/46165193.pdf (accessed on 15th July 2025).
2. Akech, S., Calis, J., Dalmas, J., Evans, J., Hassall, O., Madjdpour, C., Marcucci, C., et al. (2012). Effectiveness of blood transfusions and risk factors for mortality in children aged from 1 month to 4 years at the Bon Marche Hospital, Bunia, Democratic Republic of Congo. https://core.ac.uk/download/pdf/10674415.pdf (accessed on 15th July 2025).
3. Alinier, G., Harwood, C., Harwood, P., Huish, E., et al. (2008). Development of a programmed to facilitate interprofessional simulation-based training for final year undergraduate healthcare students. https://core.ac.uk/download/109338.pdf (accessed on 15th July 2025).
4. Amira, A., Alsalemi, A., Alsalemi, A., Brindley, P. G., Bensaali, F., Alinier, G., Lansdowne, W., et al. (2018). Extracorporeal membrane oxygenation simulation-based training: Methods, drawbacks and a novel solution. https://core.ac.uk/download/287581746.pdf (accessed on 15th July 2025).
5. Aziz, F., Bachmann, D., Barrie, M., Bubolz, K., et al. (2018). Novel emergency medicine curriculum utilizing self-directed learning and the flipped classroom method: Cardiovascular emergencies small group module. https://core.ac.uk/download/484274721.pdf (accessed on 15th July 2025).
6. Badertscher, P., Boeddinghaus, J., Buser, A., Bustamante, G., et al. (2017). Prohormones in the early diagnosis of cardiac syncope. https://core.ac.uk/download/153368670.pdf (accessed on 15th July 2025).
7. Bandeeri, N., Henry, J. A., Meredith, C., Treacy, M., et al. (2004). The prevalence of cocaine-associated chest pain in a London hospital. https://core.ac.uk/download/5230488.pdf (accessed on 15th July 2025).
8. Basheer, S. V., Hakkim, S., M, S., Majid, S., et al. (2018). Knowledge and attitude of dental students and staffs towards basic life support (BLS). https://media.neliti.com/media/publications/240002-knowledge-and-attitude-of-dental-student-d824c58e.pdf (accessed on 15th July 2025).
9. Bauer, U., Brodherr-Heberlein, S., Fratz, S., Hess, J., et al. (2003). Emergency hospital admissions and three-year survival of adults with and without cardiovascular surgery for congenital cardiac disease. https://core.ac.uk/download/pdf/82597183.pdf (accessed on 15th July 2025).
10. Bonsor, S. J., & Morse, J. (2020). Two eyes, two fingers, two minutes: Making it easier to recognize and manage medical emergencies in dental practice part 2: Algorithms to guide treatment using the M-DEWS2 tool. https://core.ac.uk/download/344890743.pdf (accessed on 15th July 2025).
11. Brancati, D. O., Dobson, J. V., Nagel, R., et al. (2003). Pediatric resuscitation: Evaluation of a clinical curriculum. https://core.ac.uk/download/pdf/85708.pdf (accessed on 15th July 2025).
12. Bree de, A., Britton, A., Gasparrini, A., Oliveira, A., Stang, A., Toprak, A., Trichopoulou, A., et al. (2010). Early influences on cardiovascular and renal development. https://core.ac.uk/download/19185982.pdf (accessed on 15th July 2025).

13. Brém, E., Koyfman, A., & Long, B. J. (2020). Oncologic emergencies: Immune-based cancer therapies and complications. https://core.ac.uk/download/305124082.pdf (accessed on 15th July 2025).

14. Candini, N. A., Indrianto, Y. L., Koentartiwi, D., Suwarnianty, A., et al. (2020). Management of cardiogenic shock in pediatric patients. https://core.ac.uk/download/352916346.pdf (accessed on 15th July 2025).

15. Carl, J. G., & Furukawa, S. (2025). Skylab IMSS checklist application study for emergency medical care. https://core.ac.uk/download/pdf/42887448.pdf (accessed on 15th July 2025).

16. Dahlen, P. (2014). School district assessment for sudden cardiac arrest preparation. https://core.ac.uk/download/162576263.pdf (accessed on 15th July 2025).

17. Daudia, A., Abhay-Gupta, A., Nemer, A. K., Feusi, B., Huang, C., Yueng-Hsiang, C., Nash, C. M., et al. (2011). Etiological profile and treatment outcome of epistaxis at a tertiary care hospital in northwestern Tanzania: A prospective review of 104 cases. https://core.ac.uk/download/pdf/11307803.pdf (accessed on 15th July 2025).

18. Falhammar, H., Rushworth, R. L., & Torpy, D. J. (2019). Adrenal crisis. https://core.ac.uk/download/228075100.pdf (accessed on 15th July 2025).

19. Gray, C. M., James, B., Lauder, W., McCulloch, L., et al. (2010). Developing community nursing practice: Promoting case management and skill enhancement to support shifting the balance of care. https://core.ac.uk/download/110605.pdf (accessed on 15th July 2025).

20. Grech, V. E. (2015). Heart failure in the pediatric age group. https://core.ac.uk/download/83020020.pdf (accessed on 15th July 2025).

21. Harrington, K. (2013). High school and college athletes should be required to undergo pre-participation cardiac screening prior to participation in competitive sports. https://core.ac.uk/download/56325374.pdf (accessed on 15th July 2025).

22. Iqbal, M., Siriwardena, A. N., & Spaight, A. (2013). Patients' and emergency clinicians' perceptions of improving pre-hospital pain management: A qualitative study. https://core.ac.uk/download/5223611.pdf (accessed on 15th July 2025).

23. Kendall, L., Lewin, R. J. P., Parsons, J. M., Sloper, P., et al. (2003). The views of parents concerning the planning of services for rehabilitation of families of children with congenital cardiac disease. https://core.ac.uk/download/55835.pdf (accessed on 15th July 2025).

24. Lehigh Valley Health Network. (2018). *Better Medicine*. https://core.ac.uk/download/267866787.pdf (accessed on 15th July 2025).

25. Maloney, L. R., & Weiss, M. (2008). Patients' perceptions of hospital discharge informational content. https://core.ac.uk/download/213076333.pdf (accessed on 15th July 2025).

26. Strawhun, A. J. (2010). Incorporating new technology into healthcare: An analysis of performance, acceptance, and safety. https://core.ac.uk/download/229272151.pdf (accessed on 15th July 2025).

27. Thorne-Lyman, A., & Webb, P. (2025). Entitlement failure from a food quality perspective: The life and death role of vitamins and minerals in humanitarian crises. https://core.ac.uk/download/pdf/6380030.pdf (accessed on 15th July 2025).

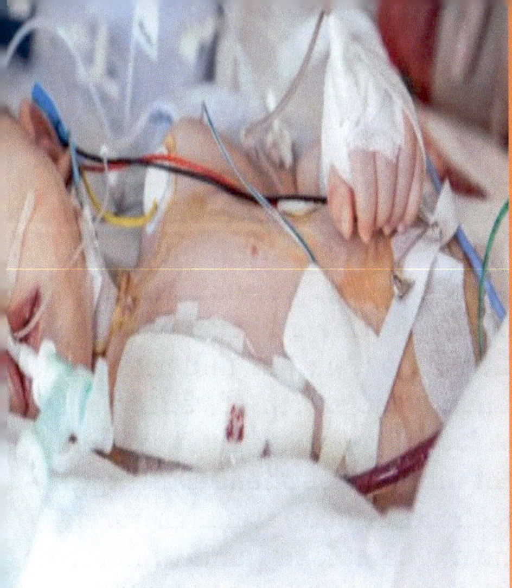

Chapter 15
PEDIATRIC CARDIAC SURGERY

Contents

Introduction

The subspecialty of pediatric cardiac surgery has had dramatic advances in the last few decades, significantly improving outcomes for congenital cardiac malformations and other abnormalities in the heart in children. Pediatric medicine presents special challenges and nuance due to the inherent physiological and anatomical differences between children. The nature of surgical operations involved is complex and requires a deep understanding of cardiac anatomy as well as developmental problems specific to the age of a child. Thus, pediatric cardiac surgery is not just an attempt to correct anatomical defects but also aims at enhancing the quality of life among such children. Effective management in this specialty is multidisciplinary, involving the integration of various medical specializations to optimize preoperative preparation, surgical technique, and postoperative recovery processes. The most significant area of pediatric cardiac surgery is the treatment of surgical complications (e.g., bleeding), and the impact of the latter on the outcome of such patients. Knowledge of the determinants of bleeding among them is vital to the development of proper measures against such complications. Evidence, including surgical procedure and postoperative intervention systematic reviews, has shown that fresh frozen plasma (FFP) has the ability to affect pediatric postoperative blood loss and transfusion demand. Mixed results from more recent studies illustrate its varying effect on FFP priming advantage, particularly commenting on its effect among younger children or those who have lower body weight (Kesumarini et al., 2024). This silent appreciation underlies an individualized approach to each patient's needs, and is used to validate the worth of continuous research and development in surgical techniques. The pediatric cardiac surgery also must contend with less common, but clinically significant, pathologies that present unique treatment challenges. For example, conditions such as cardiac hydatid disease have been described, although rarely, in children. Intracardiac presence of hydatid cysts presents diagnostic complexity and difficulty requiring prompt intervention for the safety and well-being of the patient (Zahri et al., 2024). These cases reemphasize the need for appropriate diagnostic workups and timely intervention modalities in children with cardiac disease. As such, the continued investigation into orphan diseases and their significance enriches the discipline, broadening the totality of what is known about pediatric cardiac disorders and serving to strengthen the importance of interdisciplinarity in striving for the best results for these at-risk patients.

Definition of Pediatric Cardiac Surgery

Pediatric cardiac surgery encompasses a specialized subdiscipline of clinical practice dedicated to the diagnosis and therapy of congenital and acquired heart disease in childhood. The field is directed toward surgical repairs of structural congenital heart defects present at birth or that develop during early childhood. Congenital heart defects can be simple, such as small ventricular septal defects, or complex in nature, requiring multiple surgical repairs. The multidisciplinary nature of pediatric surgery and cardiology involves working together by cardiologists, surgeons, and other doctors to get the best out of their pediatric patients. As defects significantly influence the heart's ability to pump normally, an understanding of the complexities of pediatric cardiac surgery is crucial in the efficacy of treatment and patient care. The intricate anatomy of children's heart surgery requires that the surgeons possess superior skills and experience to surmount the specific anatomical and physiological challenges that the very young present (Figure 15.1).

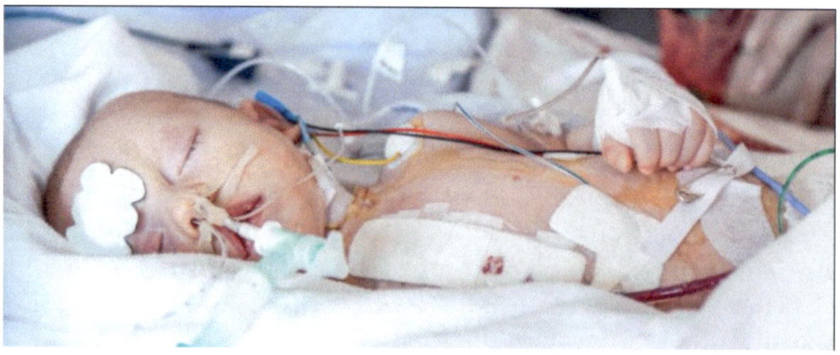

Figure 15.1. Pediatric cardiac surgery.

Source: https://external-content.duckduckgo.com/iu/?u=https%3A%2F%2Fwww.leading-medicine-guide.com%2Fimage%2F90345%2Fkinderchirurgie.jpg&f=1&nofb=1&ipt=1d1ddaaa21b280f692e913e926d80c7aeffeb6fd5ce617299a28d83fa6051d98.

During operation, the surgeon often employs methods modified to meet the increasing physiology and decreased size of child patients. These involve anesthesia management issues, including differential reactions by the immature patient to anesthetic drugs relative to adults. Further, operative treatments can apply less traumatic techniques, such as catheter-based therapies, to reduce trauma and recovery time, thereby enhancing postoperative recovery. The focus on minimizing the physical trauma of surgery is part of a larger effort to improve the quality of life for pediatric patients with heart disease, themselves an increased emphasis on patient care within the specialty. Postoperative care plays an integral role in pediatric cardiac surgery, with monitoring and management extending far beyond the surgery itself. Following cardiac surgery, children often have a complicated postoperative course, necessitating intensive care maneuvers that are particular to meet their needs so that they heal and do not experience complications. Evidence suggests that tight postoperative glycemic control can result in a decrease in pediatric critically ill children's adverse outcomes, supporting the need for having particular strategies to manage their care (Ceriello et al., 2010). Besides, close follow-up of cardiac function, growth, and development offers invaluable feedback in determining the success of surgery over the long term. Holistic care that not only addresses short-term surgical requirements but also assists in the child's overall health trajectory beyond post-surgery years guarantees the significance of employing an integral and multidisciplinary approach in performing pediatric cardiac surgery (N/A, 2003).

Importance of Addressing Congenital Heart Defects

The significance of the treatment of CHDs is underlined by their frequency and ongoing impact on the patient and family it has affected. Congenital heart defects are among the most common types of birth defects, affecting nearly one in 100 live births. Prompt treatment and diagnosis are crucial; if left untreated, these conditions have the potential to generate severe complications and quality of life compromise. The complexities of CHDs necessitate specialized treatment, which can be offered by pediatric cardiac surgery. By treating these defects early, healthcare systems can significantly enhance survival rates and long-term health outcomes for children. In addition, the psychological and emotional tension experienced by the families, primarily as they navigate concerns regarding their child's future well-being, speaks to the necessity of the requirement for comprehensive support networks and services, the emphasis on a highly critical research and intervention area (Burns et al., 2015). Aside from the immediate health condition, addressing congenital heart defects has far-reaching economic implications. The care of CHDs may be extremely expensive – not only for surgery but also for regular medical treatment, therapy, and even a life-long maintenance. With strained healthcare systems trying to keep costs under control, an investment in early diagnosis and pediatric cardiac surgery pays off in the long run as emergency, telemedicine interventions later in life are prevented. Furthermore, preventive interventions, including genetic counseling and screening programs, can be used to minimize the occurrence of CHDs. The recent move at events such as the Eighth World Congress of Pediatric Cardiology and Cardiac Surgery mirrors the collective commitment to enhancing pediatric cardiac care while encouraging sustainable health systems that prioritize CHDs (Ahmad et al., 2023). Furthermore, it is imperative that there be a holistic solution to managing congenital heart defects that covers recognition of special social and psychologic issues challenging patients and families. Scholarship has shown that such experience has a tendency to extend beyond the physical effect of the condition, impacting mental health and social functioning. Patients with CHD and their families are often subject to uncertainty around health, social stigma, and limited resources. Recognizing and attending to these aspects of care is essential to the improvement of a patient's quality of life. Having complete support systems in place that include mental health care and family therapy can minimize the emotional burden of having congenital heart defects to a great extent. The ongoing discussion among healthcare practitioners indicates increasingly heightened sensitivity to these issues, emphasizing the importance of integrated care in managing CHDs (Burns et al., 2015).

15.1. Historical Background

The clinical evolution following pediatric cardiac surgery is marked by great milestones that have transformed the treatment of congenital heart disease. In the early part of the 20th century, surgical operation was highly limited, and the prognosis of individuals suffering from congenital heart defects was often bad. Early surgical attempts at repair using basic methods were fraught with high morbidity and mortality. The pathbreaking surgery by Dr. Alfred Blalock and his colleagues on a cyanotic baby in 1944, successfully creating a shunt to increase pulmonary blood flow, ushered in a new era for cardiac surgery. This pathbreaking work laid the basis for future advances and demonstrated the effectiveness of surgical intervention in the management of congenital heart conditions, ultimately leading to specialized pediatric cardiovascular surgical programs in hospitals around the world. With new developments in the field in the mid-20th century, various surgical approaches evolved that further enhanced the management of children with heart-defective conditions. Significant contributions were provided by prominent leaders such as Dr. Helen Taussig, co-founder of the first pediatric cardiology program, and Dr. F. John Lewis, who introduced methods to repair specific defects like ventricular septal defects. These developments ran parallel with the development of cardiopulmonary bypass in the 1950s that transformed cardiac surgery by allowing surgeons to work on a fixed heart. The improved safety and success of surgical procedures facilitated by this technology led to dramatic improvements in survival rates among children treated with corrections of complex heart malformations, revolutionizing pediatric cardiac expectations and realities.

The association of cardiologists and surgeons during this period laid a firm foundation for the evolution of surgical procedures. Recent advances in pediatric cardiac surgery have also been fueled further by the development of minimally invasive techniques and advanced materials. For example, tissue-engineered treatments such as decellularized heart valve scaffolds show a groundbreaking approach that will replace traditional prosthetic valves without needing pre-implant cell seeding or sophisticated bioreactor conditioning. These achievements not only underscore the promise of regenerative medicine but also respond to the subtlety of age-related and congenital heart valve disease in both children and adults. Although ongoing study will continue to refine and compare these methods, the history of pediatric cardiac surgery sets contemporary breakthroughs against the background of a dazzling record of clinical practice driven by cross-disciplinary innovation and a commitment to improving patient results. An understanding of this historical background is thus essential in plotting future developments in pediatric cardiac surgery (Barth et al., 2017; Gerosa et al., 2015) (Figure 15.2).

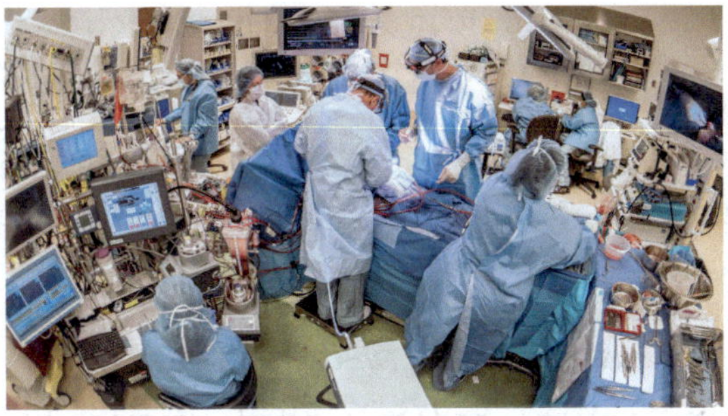

Figure 15.2. The historical evolution of pediatric cardiac surgery.

Source: https://www.facs.org/media/orbjpjmb/recolor24junebull-pediatric-hero1920x1080.jpg?rxy=0.553645833333333333333333,0.337962962962962962962963&rnd=133625201852430000.

15.1.1. Evolution of Pediatric Cardiac Surgery Techniques

The progress of pediatric cardiac surgical techniques over the last few decades is evidence of enormous advances in surgical technique and patient outcomes. Pediatric cardiac operations traditionally were associated with excessive mortality and morbidity, mainly because of the poor comprehension of congenital heart disease and the dearth of surgical instruments available at the time. Mid-20th-century breakthrough work (most famously cardiopulmonary bypass development) revolutionized all surgery, enabling complex repairs that had previously been impossible. This early breakthrough was followed by increasingly complex techniques, including use of minimally invasive approaches and hybrid methods combining catheter-based interventions. As a result, pediatric cardiac surgery has progressed from the rescue operation it once was to one that safely may be performed early in life, having substantially improved survival and quality of life in affected children and infants. Due to the arrival of sophisticated imaging technologies, the success and precision of children's cardiac surgery have also improved. Echocardiography and more recent modalities such as MRI have significantly enhanced preoperative planning and assessment, allowing surgeons to better visualize intricate cardiac anatomy. The evolving intraoperative techniques, such as video-assisted thoracoscopic surgery (VATS), have also decreased surgical trauma and recovery time. Focus on outcomes and patient safety has led to the adoption of evidence-based practices and integrated models of care which consider the long-term implications of congenital heart disease. Training programs have also adopted simulation-based education, enabling surgical teams to hone their skills without compromising patient safety. Here, the integration of technology not only enhances the accuracy of surgery but also prepares upcoming generations of pediatric cardiac surgeons with the competencies to execute intricate procedures. Integration of telemedicine and tele-ultrasound technologies is the latest milestone in the evolution of pediatric cardiac surgery. As has been highlighted in more recent studies, remote support by expert practitioners is capable of making ultrasound evaluation accessible even to non-clinical workers in the acute environment. This distant support and training model demonstrates the potential to enhance access to complex pediatric cardiac care in remote locations. Moreover, it provides the potential for shared diagnosis and treatment plans, with a highly enhanced preoperative assessment and post-operative management. As such revolutionary methods evolve, they reflect the continued dedication to maximizing patient-focused care in pediatric cardiac surgery. The prime goal remains to see that each child with congenital heart disease has timely, efficacious, and empathetic care in order to enhance his or her long-term quality of life.

15.1.2. Key Milestones in Surgical Advancements

Technological innovations have been at the forefront of changing pediatric cardiac surgery, marking significant milestones that have significantly improved the outcomes of surgery. Early procedures in the first decades of the 20th century were often plagued by high mortality due to the limited understanding of pediatric physiology and anatomy. Techniques such as cardiopulmonary bypass have since enabled one to operate extensively on the heart without interfering with the patient's oxygenation. These advances paved the way for more sophisticated procedures, whereby surgeons could manage congenital heart defects with greater precision and assurance. As a result, the mid-20th century witnessed a paradigm shift, where conditions that were once nearly fatal could be treated, further stimulating research and training in the discipline, creating better clinical protocols and outcomes for children with heart defects. The impact of imaging technologies has also been historic in enhancing the efficacy and safety of pediatric cardiac surgery. Developments in echocardiography, particularly fetal echocardiography, have allowed clinicians to diagnose congenital heart diseases prenatally, resulting in early intervention and pregnancy preparations. Current developments in the application of MRI and 3D echocardiography have further accurately improved preoperative planning, allowing better-informed surgical strategies tailored to each patient's unique anatomy. These imaging advances have resulted in decreased intraoperative complications and have provided surgeons with invaluable anatomical data unavailable in the past. Thus, the integration of advanced imaging modalities into routine preoperative practice has immensely improved outcomes and prognoses for infants and children undergoing cardiac surgery. Moreover, pharmacologic therapy advances have ushered in a new era for pediatric cardiac care, transforming pre- and postoperative management at its foundation. Introduction of certain anesthetics, cardioplegic infusions, and novel anticoagulants has made surgery less risky and recovery patterns better. These advancements are vital in addressing the fragile physiology of neonates and infants, whose reaction to medication is very much unlike that of adult children and older individuals. Particularly, as outlined by Feinstein et al. (2022) findings, the development of a complete line of pharmacotherapies has played a pivotal role in the treatment of the unique challenges posed by congenital heart defects, allowing for improved preoperative stabilization and improved postoperative recovery. Such interfacing of surgery with pharmacology has continued to define the nature of pediatric cardiac surgery, with emphasis on a responsive and flexible approach to complex cardiac treatment.

15.1.3. Impact of Historical Figures in the Field

The history of pediatric cardiac surgery has largely been shaped by a line of pioneers whose contributions have transformed the specialty. At the forefront of them is Dr. Alfred Blalock, who, in the 1940s, transformed sophisticated surgery methods for the management of congenital heart diseases. His contributions alongside Dr. Helen Taussig introduced the discovery of the Blalock-Taussig shunt, which helped in the survival of cyanotic congenital heart disease patients. This pioneering work not only laid the groundwork for pediatric cardiac surgery but also highlighted the need for multidisciplinary intervention in medical procedures. The legacy of such figures in the past reaches well beyond their specific contributions; they continue to inspire generations of surgeons and researchers, who push the envelope further with techniques and outcomes for pediatric cardiac surgery. Their legacy reminds us of the important intersection of innovation, collaboration, and striving for improved patient outcomes in this challenging specialty. Continuing the tradition of pioneering surgeons, the growth of specialized centers and innovation has also been influenced by some notable historical figures, particularly in the second half of the 20th century. Personalities such as Dr. C. Walton Lillehei, who embraces direct surgical repair techniques and developed cross-circulation methods, revolutionized the handling of complex pediatric cardiothoracic cases. His contribution to performing open-heart surgery in infants without the use of cardiopulmonary bypass made history. Survival rates have considerably improved for such children who had previously incurable heart issues. The synergy of new technology and technological innovation is a testament to the manner in which these figures have continued to influence the evolution of advanced surgical techniques that enhance patient care in pediatric cardiac surgery, an expression of holistic commitment to pushing the boundaries of what has heretofore been possible. Also, the impact of pioneering work of the past in pediatric cardiac surgery is evident even in postoperative care where advancement has streamlined processes of recovery. For instance, studies show that the employment of closed-loop sampling protocols can dramatically reduce blood loss following surgery in pediatric populations, demonstrating how new techniques are used to optimize ICU care. The application of these methodologies highlights the ongoing influence of those historical figures whose initial work laid the foundation for evidence-based practice. Historical figures lay the foundation, but further research continues in that direction, solving long-standing problems such as the need for fewer hospitalizations and blood transfusions, as justified in research today. This ongoing dialogue of historic innovation with modern surgical practice emphasizes the critical role that historic figures play not only in innovating methods but in contributing to a constant culture of excellence and development in pediatric cardiac surgery (Das et al., 2025; Joubah et al., 2024).

15.2. Surgical Techniques

Surgical techniques within the scope of pediatric cardiac surgery have an overriding function in the outcome of patients. Advanced techniques such as cardiopulmonary bypass are employed to facilitate circulation and oxygenation during corrective procedures. The employment of this technique not only allows for the clear surgical view but also facilitates the surgeon to effect fine repairs or reconstructive procedures on complex congenital heart diseases prevalent among children. By employing specific technology focused on managing circulation and temperature, the delicate physiology of the pediatric patient and the anatomical variations of their heart can be shielded by surgeons. Thus, expertise in such surgical procedures is required for optimization of the efficacy of interventions that repair congenital anomalies. Minimally invasive strategies have recently gained increased attention in pediatric cardiac surgery because they possess several advantages over traditional open-heart methods. Operations such as thoracoscopic cardiac surgery reduce post-operative pain, shorten recovery times, and minimize the risk of scarring. These procedures consist of minimal incisions through which specialized equipment and cameras are inserted, enabling the surgeon to navigate the intricate anatomy of a child's heart with precision. The use of these techniques is advantageous not only to the physical health of the patients by reducing trauma but also to deal with psychological aspects by reducing visibility of scars associated with major surgical procedures. The use of such advanced surgical techniques is a turning point of paramount importance in pediatric cardiac treatment, the focus on overall well-being of the patient and optimal recovery patterns. Moreover, surgery's technology continues to shape the dynamics of pediatric cardiac surgery. Introduction of robotic-assisted surgical systems offers enhanced dexterity, enhanced visualization, and enhanced procedural control during complex procedures. The systems give surgeons the capacity to perform subtle maneuvers with higher accuracy than they can with open methods. In children, where there are often anatomical variations that may pose limited room to maneuver surgical instruments, robotic assistance is an extremely helpful tool. Despite the expense and the need for additional training, the potential for improved outcomes makes the integration of these approaches into practice a very valuable proposition. Improved technology combined with established expertise represents a new era in pediatric cardiac surgery, one which has the potential to give children with cardiovascular problems safer and more efficient solutions.

15.2.1. Open-Heart Surgery

Open-heart surgery is a lifesaver in pediatric cardiac surgery, particularly in children with congenital heart disease (CHD). Cardiopulmonary bypass (CPB) is needed for open-heart surgery, which temporarily replaces the job of the heart and lungs to allow surgeons to operate on a stationary, bloodless heart. During CPB, blood circulation is diverted through a pump that oxygenates and recirculates blood to the body. The procedure, though lifesaving, is associated with a systemic inflammatory response syndrome inducing complications such as low cardiac output syndrome (LCOS), and hence generating the need for new methods to decrease surgical risks. It is important to specify the influence of open-heart surgery on postoperative outcome and long-term outcome since these operative complexities mandate a deep understanding of acute and residual effects in children. Efforts to maximize results in open-heart surgery have been focused on refining technique and use of various adjunctive therapies. Research has indicated the potential benefits of normothermia in CPB, as evidenced by the ongoing Thermic-2 trial, which aims to establish equivalence between hypothermic and normothermic bypass techniques in children undergoing operation for complex congenital heart disease. The trial is attempting to identify the influence control of intraoperative body temperature has on inflammation and organ function and predicts that normothermia will diminish some of the systemic inflammatory reactions triggered by CPB. This evidence can transform perioperative practice, with implications that the approach to body temperature maintenance may be a key component in improving clinical outcomes, including reduced inotropic support and reduced postoperative length of stay (Baos et al., 2015) (Figure 15.3).

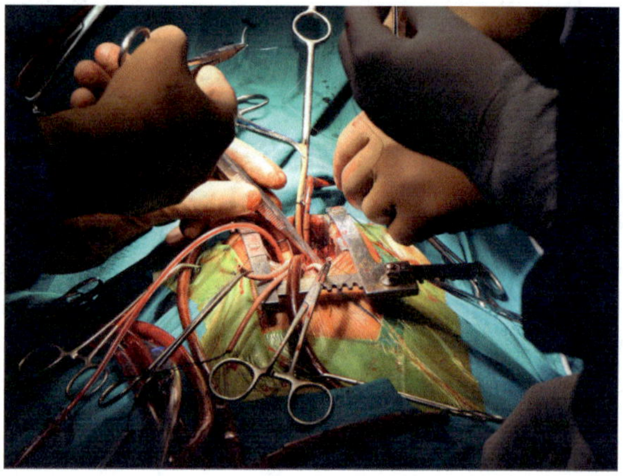

Figure 15.3. Open heart surgery.

Source: https://ellyandjosh.com/wp-content/uploads/2018/07/6.jpg?w=2000&h=1500&crop=1.

Other research studies like the NITRIC trial are studying the administration of nitric oxide during CPB with hypothesis that it will enhance myocardial protection and diminish inflammation. By reducing the risk of LCOS and accelerating recovery, nitric oxide use can improve ventilator-free days—a significant marker for successful recovery among children. These clinical trials illustrate sustained commitment to innovation in pediatric cardiac surgery, highlighting the necessity of strong research in informing and enhancing surgical protocols. As these studies continue, they promise improved outcomes, ultimately culminating in more effective interventions in the treatment of congenital heart disease among infants and children.

15.2.2. Minimally Invasive Procedures

Pediatric cardiac surgery has seen a revolution over the past couple of years with the advent of minimally invasive surgery. Physical trauma from traditional open-heart operations has significantly reduced with these new technologies, which has enhanced the overall patient experience. Minimally invasive procedures, such as thoracoscopic surgery, involve smaller incisions and are often combined with advanced imaging technologies, which allow for subtle movements during a procedure. This advancement is particularly significant for pediatric patients, whose reduced anatomy requires a significant level of finesse and precision by the surgeon.

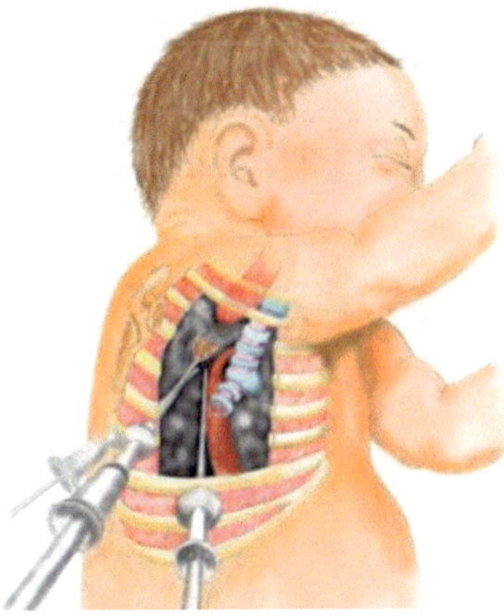

Figure 15.4. Thoracoscopic surgery in children.

Source: https://drsaurabhtiwari.com/wp-content/uploads/2023/06/305.png.

The advantages of such techniques are not only positive for surgical success; they encompass reduced recovery time, less postoperative pain, and lower complications, which are particularly desirable in the handling of children's congenital heart defects (Das et al., 2025). Minimally invasive surgical techniques have been promoted by extensive clinical investigation which highlights their effectiveness in children. The evidence indicates that these operations not only minimize complications but also lower hospital stays significantly, making a better overall healing situation for children. It is discovered in recent research that the level of adoption of such practices in pediatric surgery is unexpectedly high at 75% among doctors (Ranjan et al., 2024) (Figure 15.4).

This widespread acceptance is because of a growing confidence in the safety and effectiveness of such techniques compared to conventional surgical techniques. Moreover, improved preoperative planning aided by advanced imaging and modeling technology assists in ensuring the accuracy of minimally invasive operations so that individual anatomical complexities of congenital heart defects are optimally managed. Despite advantages provided by minimally invasive procedures, difficulties occur in their bulk application. Educating and familiarizing operating room staff with these techniques takes time and resources, including ongoing education and competency testing. Institutional resource variation also impacts availability and application by different healthcare institutions. With hospitals and surgical facilities looking to optimize pediatric cardiac service, integrating these innovative techniques into standard procedures becomes necessary. Stakeholder coordination, through attention to ongoing professional development and collaborative learning initiatives, will continue to advance the efficacy of minimally invasive surgical procedures in pediatric cardiac surgery. With ongoing expansion in the practice, the aforementioned methodologies promise to significantly improve outcomes and quality of life for children afflicted with congenital heart disease (Das et al., 2025; Ranjan et al., 2024).

15.2.3. Catheter-Based Interventions

In the specialty of pediatric cardiology surgery, catheter interventions are now a revolutionary technique in the treatment of congenital cardiac abnormalities. Similar to minimally invasive procedures, these use the anatomic and physiological distinctions between children and adults to enter the heart directly through peripheral vessels. Compared with traditional surgical interventions (which are often accompanied by total thoracotomy) catheter interventions decrease trauma, shorten hospitalization periods, and decrease recovery times. The ability to impact cardiovascular anatomy via catheters has revolutionized therapeutic results in young patients by executing timely interventions for conditions such as atrial septal defects, patent ductus arteriosus, and valvular stenoses. The integration of advanced imaging technologies has significantly enhanced the safety and effectiveness of catheter-based interventions. Fluoroscopy and echocardiography are techniques employed to guide such interventions, allowing pediatric cardiologists to visualize the anatomy of the heart in real time. This precision facilitates targeted interventions, reducing complications and optimizing overall patient safety. With the use of such imaging modalities, operators can quantify the effectiveness of the intervention in real time, optimizing results. The development of new devices, such as transcatheter valves and closure devices, further enhances the potential of catheter-based interventions, underlining the continued evolution of pediatric cardiology (Figure 15.5).

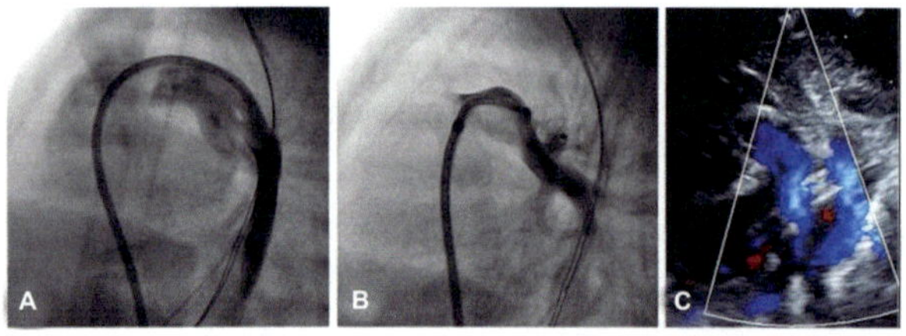

Figure 15.5. Pediatric catheter intervention.

Source: https://media.springernature.com/lw685/springer-static/image/chp%3A10.1007%2F978-3-031-07563-6_40/MediaObjects/486865_1_En_40_Fig27_HTML.jpg.

Collaborative efforts among health organizations have played a crucial role in hastening catheter-based interventions in pediatric cardiovascular surgery. Partnerships and collaborations focused on training have enabled the sharing of best practices and successful innovations. Examples include case studies in which the collaborations facilitate the development of standardized protocols, ultimately making patient care and outcomes better nationwide. As illustrated by a number of projects, the systematic assembly of information regarding catheter-based interventions has allowed for ongoing evaluation and refinement of technique and for the development of standards for success. These common learning cultures play a crucial role in sustaining advancements in pediatric cardiac surgery, so that the most vulnerable patients are given the safest and most advantageous interventions of the era (Acosta et al., 2020; Blumenthal et al., 2006).

15.3. Preoperative Considerations

Preoperative planning in pediatric patients to be operated on for cardiac surgery is paramount in a bid to optimize patient results. There is a need for a detailed history review of the child prior to any surgery. This includes the evaluation of congenital heart defects, related medical conditions, and prior surgical exposures. Operative risk is affected by demographics and comorbidities and therefore needs to be thoroughly analyzed. For instance, syndromic patients may present additional anatomical challenges that must be solved in well-designed manners. The pediatric cardiologists, anesthesiologists, and surgeons form a multidisciplinary team that has discussions which are conducted as a group to create tailored strategies to address the specific patient requirements. This process of detailed evaluation not only increases enhanced surgical planning but also reassures the family, providing a foundation for informed consent as well as shared decision-making. In addition to thorough medical evaluation, preoperative suggestions highlight the significance of preoperative imaging and diagnostic tests. Extremely sensitive imaging techniques, such as echocardiography and MRI, are valuable sources of information about cardiac anatomy and function that direct the surgery. These modalities can uncover underlying lesions that may otherwise have remained undiagnosed, and these could have significant impacts on surgical outcomes. As has been underscored in studies on diverse pediatric populations, systematic reviews point towards the requirement of using the appropriate diagnostic procedures in ascertaining readiness for surgery. Also included in preoperative optimization is the evaluation and management of potential risks of anesthesia from specific heart complications to ensure the child is in the best condition to go under surgery. As testified in documented successful interventions (Blumenthal et al., 2006; Choi et al., 2020), this anticipatory care can decrease postoperative complications and improve overall survival. Finally, psychological and family support systems are included in preoperative management in pediatric patients undergoing cardiac surgery. The psychological impact of surgery on children and families cannot be overlooked as anxiety can complicate the preoperative period and postoperative course. Preoperative counseling visits are an integral part to informally dispel fears and dispel doubts so that families can express their concerns and be educated regarding the surgical procedure. Use of child life specialists may further reassure patients through play therapy and education designed for the age group of the child about the upcoming surgery. Effective communication protocols foster a healthy atmosphere that elicits cooperation from the child and, therefore, optimizes the entire surgical process. With thorough preoperative protocols incorporating medical, psychological, and family considerations, teams for pediatric cardiac surgery can significantly improve preparedness and provide a foundation for successful surgery.

15.3.1. Diagnostic Imaging and Assessments

Diagnosis imaging and assessment in pediatric cardiac surgery are essential for an appropriate plan and execution of operations. A number of modalities, including echocardiography, magnetic resonance imaging (MRI), and computed tomography (CT), provide valuable information regarding the structural and functional characteristics of congenital heart malformations. Echocardiography is used first-line due to its non-invasive nature, ability to offer real-time imaging, and suitability for repeated long-term observation of children and infants. More recent methods, such as three-dimensional echocardiography, enhance imaging and may assist surgeons during pre-operative planning by offering detailed images of complicated heart anatomies. Not only is high-quality imaging needed for diagnosis but also for determining the optimal time and surgical method, thereby having a direct effect on patient outcomes (Figure 15.6).

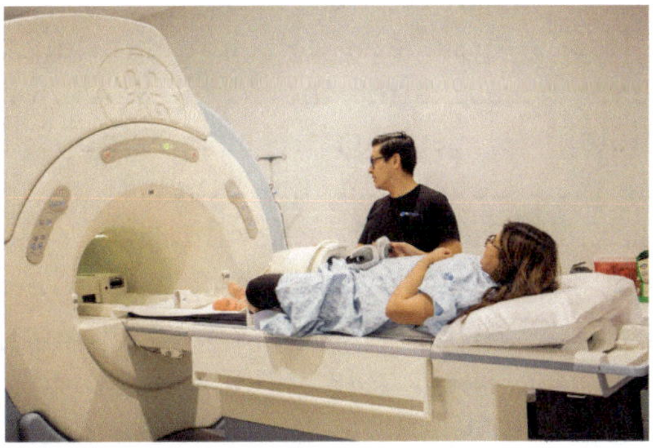

Figure 15.6. Radiologic procedures in children.

Source: https://images.squarespace-cdn.com/content/v1/62cf0df2880df468dd7df097/1657828273019-5AL32CU23MUF8QV8QN1L/IMG_7967.jpg.

Other than echocardiography, MRI and CT scans play crucial roles in the complete assessment of pediatric cardiac disease. MRI with its excellent soft tissue resolution and lack of radiation exposure becomes a vital imaging modality, particularly for the evaluation of vascular structures and myocardial tissue. It can be valuable for the assessment of cardiomyopathies and congenital malformations that have a bearing on surgery. On the other hand, CT scans (which expose the patient to radiation) provide swift cardiovascular imaging of the anatomy of the heart and are particularly useful in emergency presentations or where echocardiographic results are still unclear.

The joint use of the imaging modalities enables clinicians to plan suitable surgical procedures so that the procedure suits the individual anatomy and physiology of the child. In addition, multidisciplinary management of complex patient conditions such as Morquio A syndrome reaffirms the importance of intensive diagnostic evaluation. The storage disease provides a variety of challenges, such as cardiovascular complications that necessitate coordinated imaging to inform surgical planning and perioperative care.

For instance, cardiac disease can manifest with skeletal deformities in affected patients, necessitating thorough evaluation by cardiologists, geneticists, and orthopedists. Guidelines developed by experts in these fields indicate a robust evaluation system, which includes various imaging modalities to address the diverse presentations of Morquio A syndrome. It not only minimizes patient risk during pediatric heart surgery but also improves surgical results through focused interventions (Berger et al., 2014). Thus, effective diagnostic imaging and assessment lie at the core of pediatric cardiac surgery, bridging the diagnosis-therapy gaps (N/A, 2006).

15.3.2. Patient and Family Education

Effective patient and family education is critical in pediatric cardiac surgery because it directly influences outcomes and the patient experience. Families adjusting to the complexity of surgical corrections for congenital heart disease are likely to grapple with a set of feelings, including fear and anxiety. Healthcare providers need to ensure that they deliver clear and concise information about the surgical procedure, risks, and post-operative requirements. Using all manner of education tools, from informative brochures to interactive discussions, healthcare teams can provide all concerned with a solid knowledge of the surgical process.

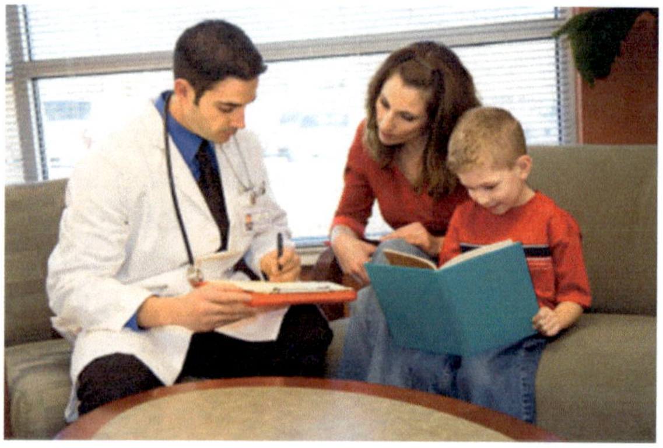

Figure 15.7. Patient and family education.

Source: https://www.pediatricsurgical.com/wp-content/uploads/2013/03/Pediatric-Surgical-Associates.jpg.

This organized process not only helps dispel anxiety but also creates a team atmosphere in which families are empowered to contribute to their child's care. Well-educated families can better provide for their child's requirements, thus leading to improved overall operating room outcomes. Besides that, the educational process should not be limited to just the perioperative period but also to the complete continuum of care. Postoperative recovery in children with cardiology is generally complicated and necessitates ongoing education regarding symptom treatment and identification of signs of complication. For example, parents must be taught how to manage wounds and know when to seek medical assistance, which again supports the need for comprehensive discharge orders and follow-up care plans. This type of longer-term educational system reinforces family confidence and independence and enables them to become proactive participants in their child's recovery (Figure 15.7).

Evidence shows that patient education via an active approach can help in lowering readmission rates and family satisfaction scores. Education of the patient and family, thus, becomes a watershed moment to enhance the quality of care but also to establish trust between families and health workers. Lastly, identifying the heterogeneity of family needs within educational approaches is essential. Differences in health literacy, cultural histories, and individual experiences can have a considerable impact on how families read and interact with health information.

Thus, medical practitioners need to respond to individual family circumstances and needs by tailoring their communication styles. Employing visual resources, clear language, and culturally accurate illustrations can improve understanding among diverse family groups. Moreover, incorporating the utilization of feedback mechanisms after educational sessions can enable providers to find out if their approaches work and where they should make changes. Through the utilization of an individualized model for patient and family education, healthcare teams are able to create an environment that is more inclusive and respects and honors the unique experiences of each family in order to enhance the quality of care offered in pediatric cardiac surgery (Copeland et al., 2019; N/A, 2008).

15.3.3. Risk Assessment and Management

Sound risk assessment and management are crucial aspects in pediatric cardiac surgery, particularly in the assessment of the potential complications of the surgical procedure involved. The unique physiological characteristics of infants and children with congenital cardiac abnormalities, such as their immature systems and varying responses to stress, necessitate thorough understanding of the risks involved for each particular case. Appreciation of the multifactorial nature of these risks allows medical personnel to utilize tailored interventions that minimize complications. For example, systematic monitoring of human factors within the operating room can identify potential threats to patient safety and improve surgical results in this population (Barach et al., 2009). Hence, incorporation of risk assessment procedures into surgical planning becomes imperative to ensure optimal patient safety and successful postoperative recovery. A pivotal area of focus within the management of pediatric cardiac surgical risks is the use of advanced technologies and techniques, such as cardiopulmonary bypass (CPB). The systemic inflammatory response syndrome induced by CPB creates dire threats, including low cardiac output syndrome (LCOS), complicating recovery and leading to augmented morbidity and mortality. To offset these harmful side effects, operating teams have experimented with new practices, such as the administration of nitric oxide during CPB. By evaluating the impact of interventions like this one on ventilator-free days and recovery in general, physicians can rationally offset the risks that come with surgical techniques. This proactive approach not only enhances the short-term outcomes of surgery but also facilitates better long-term survival of children undergoing complex cardiac operations. Additionally, research and clinical trials remain a key aspect in the optimization of risk assessment and management in pediatric cardiac surgery. Explorations of alternative methods and treatments, including in trials the NITRIC study, aim to make clear the best ways of minimizing postoperative complications. In sharing a typical research design, medical professionals can establish risk factors and outcomes associated with alternative interventions, thereby leading to evidence-based practice that maximizes patient safety. Also, such studies facilitate the continued training and evaluation of operating teams and foster a safety culture that cares about the welfare of children. The incorporation of rigorous scholarship into clinical practice not only facilitates the development of further refinement in surgical techniques but also demonstrates the ultimate aim of improving the quality of care for children who are having cardiac surgery.

15.4. Postoperative Care

Postoperative care of children following cardiac surgery is a multifaceted process demanding handling of multifaceted physiological and psychological events unique to children. Postprocedural patients have a diversity of complications like respiratory distress, hemorrhage, and infections following the correction of congenital heart diseases. Effective management during this period is an essential necessity to guarantee their recovery and decrease sequelae. Hence, the medical teams need to sequence multiple care components, including pain management, hemodynamic monitoring, and mobilization that must be performed step by step. Continuous evaluation is feasible and allows early identification of complications such as arrhythmias or ailing organs that must be treated immediately. An organized postoperative care protocol not only prioritizes meticulous monitoring but also enhances the general safety and efficacy of pediatric cardiac surgical results. One of the most significant considerations in postoperative care is the management of blood products. Children are extremely sensitive to hemostatic imbalance-related complications, and these are aggravated by the immature nature of their coagulation pathways as well as inflammation due to CPB and surgery (Karacaer, 2025). Adding to the risk of intraoperative and postoperative bleeding, the children often need allogeneic blood transfusions, necessitating a careful balancing of advantage over risk of transfusion as part of their post-operative treatment protocol. Measures to optimize blood conservation, including preoperative correction of anemia and non-transfusion options, have been beneficial.

These reduce the reliance on blood products, thereby reducing the risk of complications related to transfusion as well as overall patient outcomes. The inclusion of such evidence-based practices highlights the need for regular scrutiny of postoperative care practice in pediatric cardiac surgery. In clinical as well as psychologic terms, the psychologic status of children being operated on for cardiac pathology is a vital aspect of postoperative care. Identification of the emotional needs of such young patients, such as anxiety and fear, should guide the clinical environment and care structures developed in the postoperative area. Providing reassurance and reassurance through the inclusion of family members, child life specialists, and pediatric-trained nursing staff will assist in transitioning the patient from the operating room to recovery significantly. Also, addressing psychological needs will enhance compliance with postoperative instruction, ultimately leading to improved recovery times and reducing the risk for complications. The combined process (unifying physical and emotional care) is critical to establish resilience and promote outcomes for children with cardiac disease as they recover from the complexity of recovery (Ayşe et al., 2025) (Figure 15.8).

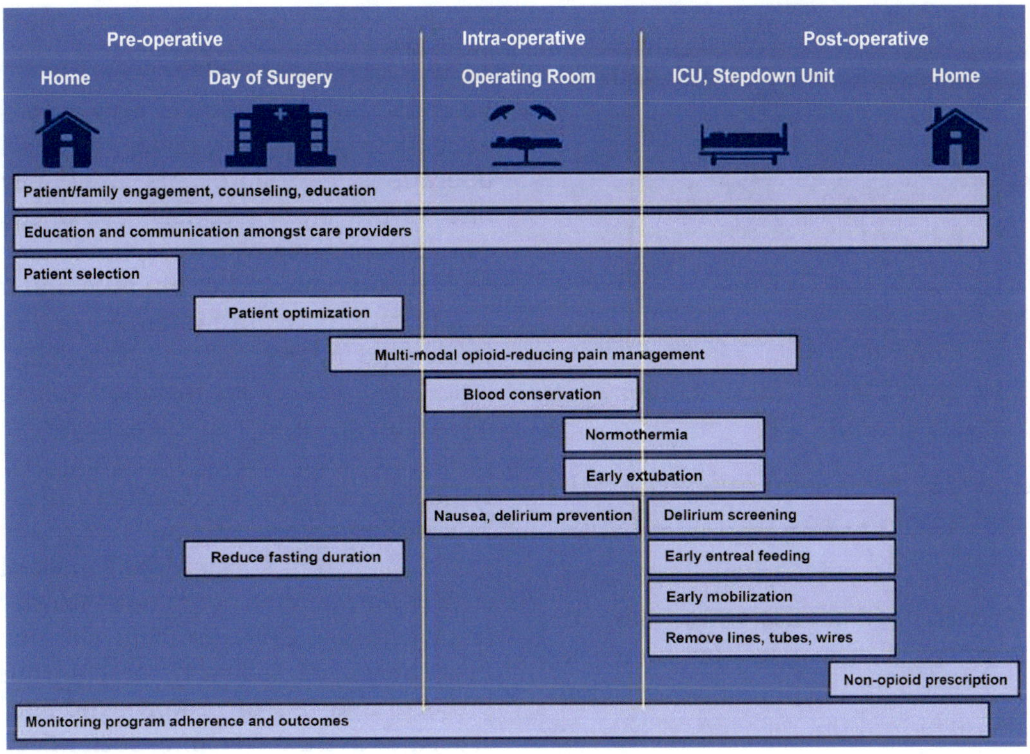

Figure 15.8. Enhanced recovery in pediatric patients after cardiac surgery.

Source: https://www.jtcvs.org/cms/10.1016/j.jtcvs.2021.04.072/asset/425af12d-df79-4fc3-a4ba-64db94740449/main.assets/fx1_lrg.jpg.

15.4.1. Monitoring and Recovery Protocols

Monitoring and recovery strategies are an essential aspect of pediatric cardiac surgery in maximizing patient outcomes, particularly for children with complicated surgeries such as cardiopulmonary bypass (CPB). Inflammatory response as a result of CPB is a causative agent for low cardiac output syndrome (LCOS), which augments mortality and morbidity risk in high-risk groups like infants with congenital heart disease (CHD). Good protocols emphasize close monitoring during surgery, using state-of-the-art technology for monitoring cardiac function and systemic stability. While adopting approaches such as enhanced recovery pathways, an attempt is made to decrease surgical stress and accelerate the recovery process, thus having shorter ICU stay and better ventilator-free days. Early interventions are possible because of close monitoring, which is very important in the first 48 hours post-surgery when the patient is at maximum risk of developing complications. Also, recovery protocols must be made compatible with the special physiological needs of pediatric patients, who typically represent a higher level of complexity in their hemodynamic stability. Recommendations suggest a multidisciplinary approach in which pediatric cardiologists, nurses, and perfusionists work together in order to induce an atmosphere of comprehensive care during the post-operative period. Pain treatment protocols that are rapidly administered—such as early extubation and weaning to intermediate care units—have been shown to decrease hospital stay without any deterioration in safety (Bingold et al., 2013) (Figure 15.9).

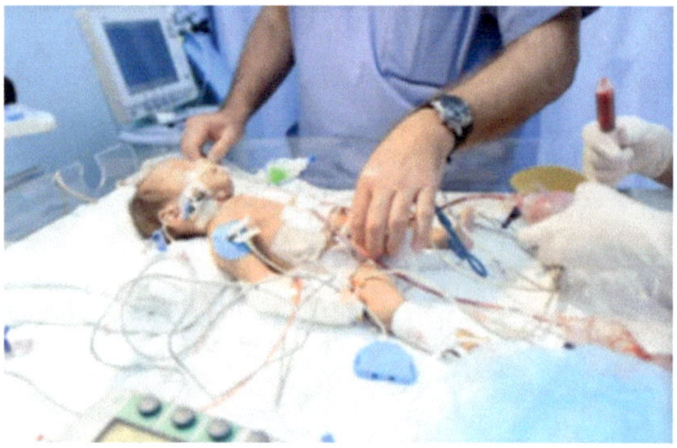

Figure 15.9. Monitoring and recovery of pediatric cardiac surgery.

Source: https://5.imimg.com/data5/GW/SN/DP/SELLER-24597972/pediatric-cardiac-surgery-500x500.png.

However, risk of re-admission to intensive care units remains a cause for concern. Stratification of patients and predictive analytics must be integrated into the recovery pathways in order to classify those at increased risk of post-operative complications so that the surveillance process continues to be proactive and responsive to the needs of each child. The significance of monitoring and the recovery strategy is further attested by clinical trials that look into new approaches to enhancing patient outcomes. For instance, NITRIC trial assesses the application of inhaled nitric oxide during CPB as a method of minimizing inflammatory responses and improving recovery results such as ventilator-free days. This approach embodies the dynamic nature of pediatric cardiac surgery, as it emphasizes the importance of measures that consider shifting evidence. Recovery guidelines are not static; they must shift to encompass emerging evidence and technologies that are better able to assist in patient care. By emphasizing strict monitoring and individualized recovery strategies, healthcare professionals can improve overall post-operative care and improve long-term health in pediatric cardiac surgery patients.

15.4.2. Common Complications and Their Management

Pediatric heart surgery is also beset by a host of complications that can happen during or after operations. Cardiac events after operation are one of the most frequent complications that can present as arrhythmias, infection processes, and thromboembolic phenomena. All these complications require intensive monitoring and immediate intervention to successfully minimize risk. Arrhythmias, for instance, can be induced by ischemic injury or electrolyte imbalances that come about during operation. Management typically involves medication adjustment or, in some cases, pacing on a short-term basis. Additionally, the surgical staff must also watch closely for infection symptoms, which can occur from invasive lines or from sites of surgery. Prevention, in the way of rigorous aseptic protocol and use of prophylactic antibiotics, is crucial to avoid developing such infection. Early detection and treatment can significantly improve surgical outcomes, highlighting the importance of a complete postoperative care strategy.

Complications	Percent
Kidney	44.3
Lung	40.3
Blood	35.9
Cardiovascular	34.4
Gastrointestinal	17.2
Brain	14.2
The need for re- intubation of endotracheal	11.3
Infection	7.8

Figure 15.10. Complications after heart surgery in children with congenital heart disease.

Source: https://www.researchgate.net/figure/Complications-after-heart-surgery-in-children-with-congenital-heart-disease_tbl2_281226092.

Respiratory failure is a common complication of pediatric cardiac surgery, particularly in very young children with underlying pulmonary disease. Mechanical ventilation is often employed to assist these patients, but extubation must be carefully controlled. These variables of lung compliance, airway edema, and patient hemodynamic stability can make this a complex process. Long-term mechanical ventilation carries inherent risks like ventilator-associated pneumonia that necessitate close vigilance and preventive strategies (Figure 15.10).

Furthermore, the use of non-invasive ventilation modalities may add value to the reduction of postoperative respiratory complications. Ongoing monitoring of respiratory status, coupled with targeted intervention, is required for optimizing patient recovery and prevention of morbidity due to respiratory distress following surgery. Complications related to anesthesia are also a significant risk in pediatric cardiac surgery, and a prudent strategy in anesthetic management must hence be adopted. Both anesthetic and perioperative deaths, although rare, remain an issue, as demonstrated by the need for suitable preoperative assessment. Children undergoing cardiac surgery typically have complex medical histories. These underlying challenges may lead to complications that involve severe problems such as cardiac and cerebrovascular events as a result of airway management difficulties or hemodynamic instability (Argo et al., 2019). For interventions such as radiofrequency ablation, complications may be more significant in small patients who are already at increased risk secondary to their developing physiology (Blaufox et al., 2005). Effective communication between surgical, anesthetic, and nursing personnel is thus critical in developing protocols that address not only expected complications but also present a comprehensive approach to patient care during the surgical continuum.

15.4.3. Long-Term Follow-Up and Care

Pediatric cardiac surgery is a type of operation that demands meticulous long-term follow-up and management to ensure the best result in patients. Surgical repair for congenital heart disease is most often the initial approach in managing these intricate lesions; however, it does not stop with the operation. Regular follow-up is necessary in caring for possible complications as well as monitoring the development and growth of the child. Research indicates that long-term follow-up significantly impacts the quality of life in children in such a way that healthcare professionals can manage late complications and optimize health outcomes through particular care strategies. These interventions may include regular imaging modalities and life-style counseling, which together allow an adaptive approach to the patient's deteriorating condition, ultimately resulting in improved survival and quality of life in this high-risk group (Kumar, 2025) (Figure 15.11).

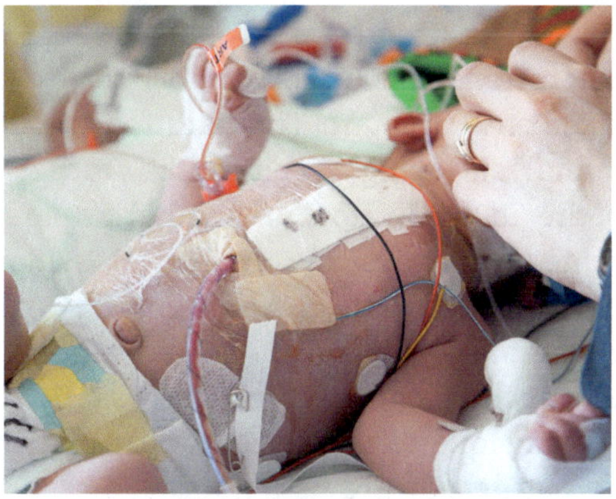

Figure 15.11. Largest randomized trial evaluates steroids for infant heart surgery.

Source: https://corporate.dukehealth.org/sites/default/files/2022-11/Pediatric%20heart%20surgery-505994834_web.jpg.

Apart from physical illness, psychosocial factors are a significant aspect of long-term follow-up for pediatric cardiac surgery. Young patients who have had such surgery are often faced with unique emotional and developmental challenges as they grow up. The impact of these experiences on their existence can lead to anxiety, social isolation, and difficulties with peer relations. Care should therefore be more than physiological monitoring and include mental health assessment and intervention. Development of an interdisciplinarian team composed of cardiologists, psychologists, and social workers could enhance management of the complex needs. Early identification and intervention strategies can build resilience and positive emotional well-being, at the same time enabling the child to be engaged fully in educational and social opportunities, finally facilitating good long-term outcomes (Hessey et al., 2021). Furthermore, heterogeneity of patient response highlights the importance of individualized post-operative care. Given that evidence suggests varying risk for a variety of congenital heart anomalies and surgical procedures, there needs to be individualized care. Age at the time of surgery, genetic considerations, and other comorbidities must be taken into account. The addition of robust data analysis using longitudinal studies can offer the identification of population-specific outcomes and risks and enable an evidence-based approach to individualized care plans. Furthermore, continued improvements in data collection and analysis are essential for uncovering long-term consequences and trends, thus creating a future with improved care. This evidence-based practice not only improves patient safety but also guides innovations in clinical practice, such that pediatric cardiac care advances in sync with new evidence and changing patient needs (Kumar, 2025).

15.5. Ethical Considerations

Ethical concerns are of basic significance in the procedure of pediatric cardiac surgery, impacting choice. Doctors are consistently faced with problems concerning the balance between the potential reward of surgery and the risks to very delicate young patients. Informed consent is a critical problem, particularly in pediatrics, where guardians or parents are faced with significant quantities of complex medical information. The technical nature of surgery increases fear and anxiety in families, and at times raises ethical questions around the choice to utilize aggressive therapy over palliative care. Additionally, the challenge is worsened when considering long-term implications of a child's quality of life and psychosocial development in addition to medical outcomes, making a multidisciplinary team approach necessary to patient management and ethics. A key ethical concern is resource allocation and the equitable distribution of surgical procedures. Pediatric cardiac surgery's growing expense, including preoperative, operative, and postoperative steps, poses ethical concerns with regard to prioritization and allocation of the patients on the basis of medical requirements rather than socioeconomic status or institutional beliefs. Use of extracorporeal cardiopulmonary resuscitation (ECPR) in the operating room also poses other ethical dilemmas, particularly regarding the potential for neurological recovery following post-operative procedures. Research indicates that ECPR can significantly influence patient outcomes, as evidenced by the comparison of survival and neurologic recovery in hospital-based literature (Cavarocchi et al., 2015). Ethical decision-making needs to inform policies such that every pediatric patient has access to equal access to life-saving interventions and surgeries without discrimination or unreasonable hardship. Finally, the need for sustained ethical education and support among healthcare practitioners in pediatric cardiac surgery is fundamental. As medical technology evolves, so do the ethical challenges emanate from novel treatment paradigms. It is essential that healthcare professionals keep abreast of ethical standards through continuous discussion, continuing education programs, and peer-reviewed journals (Copeland et al.,

2019). By fostering an ethical awareness and sensitivity, healthcare practitioners are better equipped to address the multi-faceted problems that surface in pediatric cardiac surgery and continue to enhance patient outcomes. This proactive strategy not only enhances general quality of care but also assists in maintaining the well-being of families confronted with the complexities behind such delicate choices, ultimately aligning professional practice with ethical guidelines in medicine.

15.5.1. Informed Consent in Pediatric Patients

The principle of informed consent is particularly complex when applied to children that have heart surgery, as they do not fully grasp what medical interventions are being conducted and what the risks are. Informed consent is not a laughing matter; it is a serious ethical and legal notion that ensures patients, or in the instance of minors, parents, are appropriately made aware of treatment. This includes the nature of procedure, its benefits, risks, and other treatments. For children, consent comes from the parents or guardians, but the medical professionals must give information in a manner that is clear and understandable. The potential effects, both favorable and unfavorable, must be revealed to allow for an informed decision. Failing to provide proper informed consent can lead to ethical violations and legal sanctions, hence the need for rigid adherence to this principle in pediatric cardiac surgery. In addition, informed consent for pediatric cardiac surgery must be given on an individual basis to address the particular emotional and psychological issues of both young patients and their families. Granted that the nature of surgical intervention is stressful, especially in children suffering from congenital heart disease, the medical practitioner should be empathetic and sensitive while explaining the problem. Family-centered communication may reduce the anxiety of parents and promote trust among the healthcare team. The process becomes highly crucial during high-risk procedures like surgery, where life-altering outcomes are possible. Furthermore, the healthcare professional must be attuned to the level of development of the child, and this can influence how information is presented and received. Visual aid techniques or proper use of terminologies can greatly help in terms of understanding and serve as a basis for successful involvement of the family in the consent process (Figure 15.12).

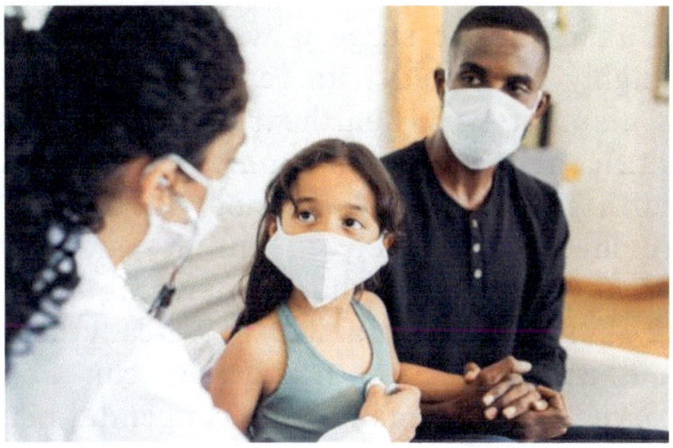

Figure 15.12. Understanding informed consent for pediatric patients.

Source: https://www.medpro.com/image/image_gallery?uuid=342bf854-1414-485a-ba76-8ef52effb36a&groupId=10502&t=1745821623294.

Finally, long-term implications of informed consent extend beyond the immediate postoperative context, particularly in children who might be required to undergo extended medical care. Cardiac diseases often necessitate follow-up treatments, interventions, and lifestyle adjustments as patients progress through age. Health practitioners must, thus, ensure that patients and guardians understand not only the consent for intervention during surgery but also the long-term implications in broad terms on subsequent health management. This extensive information is essential to ensure compliance with treatment plans and overall well-being. Communication of continued care must be included in informed consent proceedings, conceding that pediatric patients develop over the years, and their ability to participate in healthcare decisions grows with age. Consideration of these intricate dimensions of informed consent will eventually enhance the quality of patient care and add ethical soundness to pediatric cardiac surgery.

15.5.2. Resource Allocation and Access to Care

Pediatric cardiac surgery availability to care is highly entangled with resource allocation, as disparity of healthcare facilities can significantly impact outcomes in patients. Health infrastructure in most instances is stretched, particularly in middle- and low-income countries, where operating rooms and skilled staff availability is typically below requirements. These limitations can delay interventions for infants with congenital heart defects, which contribute significantly to infant mortality. Effective resource allocation comes in to counteract these disparities because it enables healthcare providers to set priorities on interventions that yield the best results for patients. Achieving adequate funding, staff, and equipment is not only important for the provision of shorter wait times in surgery but also for improved access to preoperative and postoperative care with resultant gains in patient survival and recovery rates as shown in the NITRIC trial. Economic evaluation of pediatric surgery care also plays a major role in guiding decisions around resource allocation. Systematic review has shown that many pediatric surgeries are very cost-effective, especially in resource-poor settings (Ameh et al., 2016). Procedures such as congenital heart surgery not only improve health outcomes but also provide huge societal benefits, as evidenced by their economic relevance. Policymakers must take into consideration the relevance of such procedures when it comes to resource allocation, especially where health budgets are constrained integrating evidence-based cost-effectiveness analysis in the decision-making process will direct strategic investment into surgical programs yielding the greatest value in health benefits. Following a framework emphasizing economic and clinical outcomes, the healthcare system will enhance the quality of care for children with heart disease while simultaneously making sensible use of limited resources. In addition to official channels of resource allocation, local knowledge and involvement can contribute to expanded access to pediatric cardiac surgery. Public education on congenital heart disease and the importance of early operation can lead to earlier diagnosis and referral and, consequently, a more effective distribution of operating resources. Educational programs that facilitate families to receive medical care when required are essential, particularly for underprivileged populations where health literacy may be low. Also, collaborations between health centers and community organizations can bring about a system that effectively prioritizes the health of children. These community-oriented approaches not only complement formal healthcare systems but also help ensure that critical resources are maximized to support those most in need, ultimately improving outcomes in pediatric cardiac surgery.

15.5.3. Psychological Impact on Families

The pediatric cardiac surgery process often imposes a profound psychological burden on families, particularly when children are discovered to have conditions such as single ventricle disease. While parents cope with the significance of their child's medical condition, the emotional toll is significant. A review of stress in parents with regard to congenital heart disease revealed that nearly half of the parents with children who have single ventricle anatomy experience clinically significant parenting stress. The stress is further added by the factor of illness-related issues of complexity, and it is proposed that families battle more psychological distress than with children who have less complicated heart anomalies. The intricate interaction between medical ambiguity, complexity in treatment, and the demands of suffering children mandate a coordinated care strategy, which addresses not only the medical but also the psychological and emotional demands of family members (Brosig et al., 2018). Given these challenges for families, early intervention programs, such as palliative care, have been shown to be vital in lessening maternal stress. A pilot study looking at the impact of early palliative care for mothers with infant single ventricle diagnoses reports significant benefits. Mothers in this pilot study had extremely high rates of depression and anxiety during pregnancy, and this is the emotional weight that the mother brings with her child's illness. Mothers who were given early palliative care had an extremely high decrease in anxiety when transitioning from prenatal to postnatal. Additionally, there was enhancement in coping mechanisms, indicating that systematic psychosocial care can play an important role in enhancing maternal resilience. These findings underscore the importance of integrating palliative care into the treatment plan of families undergoing pediatric cardiac surgery, thus not only meeting the clinical needs of the child but also the psychological needs of the family (Aiyagari et al., 2018). The emotional impact on families is more than the immediate worry and stress issues; it also extends to family relationships and dynamics. While parents worry their way through the many issues that come with a child's surgery, siblings might feel left out, envious, or bewildered by what's happening. That can cause tension in the family structure, stifling communication and creating an alienated atmosphere. By implementing supportive interventions that would foster family cohesion, healthcare professionals can help families relieve these stresses. Interventions that facilitate open communication, shared experiences, and emotional expression among families can enhance their resilience and enable them to cope. Last but not least, the integration of psychological support into the surgical model of care not only enhances the quality of life of the affected child but also fosters healthier family relationships after pediatric cardiac adversity (Brosig et al., 2018).

SUMMARY

The conclusion of the chapter affirms the imperative need for improved surgical outcomes and techniques for children. As noted during the course of the discussion, the complexity inherent in neonates and infantile children serves to underscore the necessity of specialized cardiac surgery techniques. Evidence from the Neonatal and Pediatric Heart and Renal Outcomes Network (NEPHRON) shows that cardiac surgery-associated acute kidney injury (CS-AKI) in these patients is common, occurring in 67% of neonates treated with the Norwood procedure. This high figure necessitates increased vigilance and novel means to prevent complications, which should lead to improved overall survival. Therefore, it is crucial that practitioners remain current with their surgical skills and procedures such that interventions are closely aligned with the evolving evidence basis for postoperative care and patient outcomes (Bertrandt et al., 2024). Besides, outcomes from nascent pediatric cardiac surgery programs in low-resource settings hold significant potential for improving service delivery to affected populations. Development of sustainable cardiac surgery programs, such as that just initiated in Rwanda, demonstrates that good quality care can be provided in nations that previously relied on foreign referrals or humanitarian missions. With a very low 30-day mortality rate of only 1.9% and an impressive roster of routine operations being successfully performed, these developments augur well for the alleviation of the shortage of pediatric cardiac surgeons and centers, especially in sub-Saharan Africa. The positive impact of local knowledge brings hope towards better surgical results in the future, and similar models could be replicated as blueprints in other under-resourced communities (Ejigu et al., 2024). Overall, the results of the Pediatric Cardiac Surgery discussions emphasize the importance of continuous improvement in operations as well as institutionalizing programs in under-resourced settings. The consciousness of the prevalence of such complications as CS-AKI and the quest for effective interventions are crucial for patient outcomes. The path forward demands unified efforts by seasoned professionals, policymakers, and stakeholders to ensure children in need of cardiac surgery receive optimal care. Such initiatives should be encouraged and reinforced, ultimately guiding the practice towards better survival rates and quality of life in infants with congenital heart defects.

In pediatric cardiac surgery, it is important to understand complications such as acute kidney injury (AKI) in order to improve patient outcomes. Recently, in one study, it was evaluated whether micro-RNA and microvesicle levels can be suitable biomarkers for AKI in pediatric cardiac surgery patients. The researchers discovered that children with AKI had different profiles of these biomarkers than their counterparts. Notably, AKI patients were typically younger and had longer cardiopulmonary bypass durations, suggesting that patient factors and surgical complexity play significant impacts on the risk for developing this fulminant complication. The ability to measure these biomarkers not only better informs us of AKI but possibly can also lead to earlier intervention and personalized management plans for at-risk pediatric patients who are vulnerable, thereby maximizing overall surgical outcomes in the population (JnTala et al., 2018). A second important aspect of pediatric heart surgery is related to the frequency of diagnostic errors that take place in the intensive care unit. A recent survey of pediatric cardiac ICU practitioners in multiple facilities highlighted a sobering suspicion of diagnostic mistakes, with 81% of respondents indicating that these errors harm patients more than five times annually. These statistical findings highlight the necessity of robust diagnostic systems and pinpoint common conditions that are commonly misdiagnosed, such as medication side effects and respiratory illness. Notably, the research isolated systemic failures, like poor care coordination and overburdened clinician workload, as key drivers of these diagnostic mistakes. The findings of this research are most valuable, offering the basis for systemic changes in pediatric cardiac intensive care, thus elevating patient care safety and effectiveness (Aiyagari et al., 2018). In addition, solving both the biomarker identification for AKI and the beliefs in diagnostic error leads to a general sense of acquaintance with the pediatric cardiac surgery issues. By applying new diagnostic technologies and creating a culture of teamwork and effective communication among providers, the pediatric cardiac surgery community can enhance patient safety and quality of care. Tactics such as improving feedback mechanisms and team-based working environments are required to counteract the specified risks of diagnostic error. Moreover, ongoing research into biomarkers can enable proactive patient management, particularly in those at highest risk for developing such complications as AKI, and ultimately this two-pronged approach can result in both improved surgical precision and overall patient outcomes within pediatric cardiac settings. In brief, considering these areas of focus can truly transform pediatric cardiac care and improve the clinical profile for the involved children and families (Aiyagari et al., 2018; JnTala et al., 2018).

CLOSER LOOK

HEART VALVE REPAIR OR REPLACEMENT

Pediatric valve repair or replacement is a critical intervention used for the correction of congenital or acquired valvular heart disease in children. The procedure may involve the aortic, pulmonary, mitral, or tricuspid valves and result in stenosis (narrowing) or regurgitation (leakage), which decreases cardiac function and growth. The decision to repair or replace a valve in children depends on several criteria, including the size and age of the child, the specific valve, the extent of dysfunction, the presence of associated lesions, and long-term implications of the procedure.

Valve repair is generally preferred to replacement in children whenever it is possible. The reparative techniques are created in order to preserve the child's own valve and avoid the problems of prosthetic valves, particularly the lifelong anticoagulation required for patients with mechanical valves. Valve repair can be very effective in mitral or tricuspid regurgitation, where techniques such as annuloplasty (supporting the valve annulus), leaflet resection or augmentation, and chordal reconstruction can restore the valve to competence. In congenital valve stenosis, balloon valvuloplasty in the Cath lab is often the initial therapy of choice, especially for aortic and pulmonary valves. Subsequent surgical correction can be done if balloon dilation is unsuccessful or not feasible because of anatomical complexity.

But replacement of the valve is required when the valve is deformed, calcified extensively, or when repair is not possible to achieve satisfactory function. Valve replacement in children poses some issues with somatic growth—valves made of prosthetic material do not grow along with the child, and reoperations are required as the child advances above the valve. Mechanical valves are durable but require lifelong anticoagulation using warfarin, which has a risk of bleeding and thrombosis and needs regular monitoring. Bioprosthetic valves, which are made from animal tissue, are not anticoagulation-dependent but are less durable and cause more rapid degradation in children.

Homografts (donor human valves) and autografts (using the patient's own pulmonary valve to replace an injured aortic valve, as in the Ross procedure) have been front-runners in recent years for biocompatibility and growth potential. The Ross procedure is particularly valuable for children and infants with aortic valve disease, with good long-term outcome and the added benefit of not needing anticoagulation.

Both the replacement and repair work must be performed with cardiopulmonary bypass and under general anesthesia. Postoperative care in the intensive care unit is most critical, placing emphasis on hemodynamic stability, avoidance of infection, and early detection of complication such as valve dysfunction, arrhythmias, or thromboembolic complication. Long-term follow-up is also required and consists of regular echocardiographic assessment, growth monitoring, and periodic adjustment of anticoagulation.

References

1. Acosta, S., Azuma, N., Bastos Gonçalves, F., Björck, M., et al. (2020). Editor's choice: European Society for Vascular Surgery (ESVS) 2020 clinical practice guidelines on the management of acute limb ischemia. https://core.ac.uk/download/586543271.pdf (accessed on 15th July 2025).
2. Adelson, P. D., Barnhard, S. E., Bobinski, M., Ghetti, S., et al. (2018). Traumatic injury clinical trial evaluating tranexamic acid in children (TIC-TOC): Study protocol for a pilot randomized controlled trial. https://core.ac.uk/download/161772802.pdf (accessed on 15th July 2025).
3. Ahmad, F., Al Halees, Z. Y., Ali, S. K. M., Atallah, S., et al. (2023). Advocacy at the Eighth World Congress of Pediatric Cardiology and Cardiac Surgery. https://core.ac.uk/download/586543271.pdf (accessed on 15th July 2025).
4. Aiyagari, R., Algaze, C. A., Bhat, P. N., Costello, J. M., et al. (2018). Diagnostic errors in pediatric cardiac intensive care. https://core.ac.uk/download/212864670.pdf (accessed on 15th July 2025).
5. Aiyagari, R., Bhat, P., Donohue, J., Fifer, C., et al. (2018). A randomized trial of early palliative care for maternal stress in infants prenatally diagnosed with single-ventricle heart disease. https://core.ac.uk/download/212864275.pdf (accessed on 15th July 2025).
6. Alphonso, N., Beca, J., Blumenthal, A., et al. (2019). Study protocol: NITric oxide during cardiopulmonary bypass to improve recovery in infants with congenital heart defects (NITRIC trial): A randomized controlled trial. https://core.ac.uk/download/228026650.pdf (accessed on 15th July 2025).
7. Ameh, E. A., Farmer, D., Ozgediz, D., Poenaru, D., et al. (2016). Economic analysis of children's surgical care in low- and middle-income countries: A systematic review and analysis. https://core.ac.uk/download/323069938.pdf (accessed on 15th July 2025).
8. Anwar, A., Barach, P., Bhatla, N., Biglino, G., et al. (2018). 3D printing is a transformative technology in congenital heart disease. https://core.ac.uk/download/212858839.pdf (accessed on 15th July 2025).
9. Arcieri, L., Assanta, N., Baggi, R., Di Maurizio, A., et al. (2016). The role of posterior aortopexy in the treatment of left mainstem bronchus compression. https://core.ac.uk/download/74319435.pdf (accessed on 15th July 2025).
10. Argo, A., Buscemi, R., Karch, S. B., Lanzarone, A., Roccuzzo, R., & Zerbo, S. (2019). Perioperative and anesthetic deaths: Toxicological and medico legal aspects. https://core.ac.uk/download/224993621.pdf (accessed on 15th July 2025).
11. Austin, B., Davis, W., Le, D. Q., Ma, J., et al. (2019). Feasibility evaluation of commercially available video conferencing devices to technically direct untrained nonmedical personnel to perform a rapid trauma ultrasound examination. https://core.ac.uk/download/323310769.pdf (accessed on 15th July 2025).
12. Baos, S., Caputo, M., Culliford, L., Ellis, L., et al. (2015). Normothermic versus hypothermic cardiopulmonary bypass in children undergoing open heart surgery (thermic-2): Study protocol for a randomized controlled trial. https://core.ac.uk/download/73981650.pdf (accessed on 15th July 2025).

13. Barach, P., Schraagen, J. M., Smit, M., Ven, J. V., et al. (2009). Teams and cardiac surgery. https://core.ac.uk/download/pdf/11476812.pdf (accessed on 15th July 2025).
14. Barth, P., Briddel, J., Chidekel, A., et al. (2017). Risk factor analysis for 30-day readmission rates of newly tracheostomized children. https://core.ac.uk/download/84904318.pdf (accessed on 15th July 2025).
15. Benson, D. W., Goetsch, M. A., Hidestrand, M., et al. (2016). Impact of *MYH6* variants in hypoplastic left heart syndrome. https://core.ac.uk/download/213078413.pdf (accessed on 15th July 2025).
16. Berger, K. I., Giugliani, R., Harmatz, P., Hendriksz, C., et al. (2014). International guidelines for the management and treatment of Morquio A syndrome. https://core.ac.uk/download/323073271.pdf (accessed on 15th July 2025).
17. Bertrandt, R., Gist, K. M., Hasson, D., Zang, H., Reichle, G., Krawczeski, C. D., Winlaw, D., et al. (2024). Cardiac surgery-associated acute kidney injury in neonates undergoing the Norwood operation: Retrospective analysis of the multicenter Neonatal and Pediatric Heart and Renal Outcomes Network dataset, 2015–2018. *Pediatric Critical Care Medicine, 25*, e246–e257. https://www.semanticscholar.org/paper/3ff885abaaa7cbca8bd52a2c558b2973fd8bcdb4 (accessed on 15th July 2025).
18. Bin Joubah, M., Ismail, A. A., Abdelmohsen, G., Alsofyani, K., Yousef, A. A., Jobah, M. T., Khawaji, A., et al. (2024). Impact of blood sampling methods on blood loss and transfusion after pediatric cardiac surgery: An observational study. *Journal of Cardiothoracic and Vascular Anesthesia*. https://www.semanticscholar.org/paper/4a38b8d94703050972f758753180ef39b1499783 (accessed on 15th July 2025).
19. Bingold, T. M., Huneke, P., Kiessling, A. H., Moritz, A., et al. (2013). Risk factor analysis for fast-track protocol failure. https://core.ac.uk/download/14529228.pdf (accessed on 15th July 2025).
20. Blaufox, A. D. (2005). Catheter ablation of tachyarrhythmias in small children. https://core.ac.uk/download/pdf/86243.pdf (accessed on 15th July 2025).
21. Blumenthal, D., & McCarthy, D. (2006). *Committed to Safety: Ten Case Studies on Reducing Harm to Patients*. https://core.ac.uk/download/71350251.pdf (accessed on 15th July 2025).
22. Bossone, E., Butera, G., Carminati, M., Chessa, M., et al. (2003). Transcatheter closure of atrial septal defect in young children: Results and follow-up. https://core.ac.uk/download/pdf/82458036.pdf (accessed on 15th July 2025).
23. Brosig, C., Kaugars, A. S., & Shields, C. (2018). Stress and quality of life among parents of children with congenital heart disease referred for psychological services. https://core.ac.uk/download/213086845.pdf (accessed on 15th July 2025).
24. Burns, A., Doyle, F., & Hickey, A. (2015). Scoping review of experience of people living with inherited cardiac conditions and congenital heart disease. https://core.ac.uk/download/83917516.pdf (accessed on 15th July 2025).
25. Cavarocchi, N. C., Hirose, H., & Peigh, G. (2015). Saving life and brain with extracorporeal cardiopulmonary resuscitation: A single-center analysis of in-hospital cardiac arrests. https://core.ac.uk/download/83049623.pdf (accessed on 15th July 2025).

26. Ceriello, A., Ceriello, A., Ceriello, A., Chiaretti, A., Rovlias, A., Russo, A., Russo, A., et al. (2010). Control of hyperglycemia in pediatric intensive care (CHiP): Study protocol. https://core.ac.uk/download/20330333.pdf (accessed on 15th July 2025).
27. Cervi, E. (2016). New applications of cardiopulmonary exercise testing and training in pediatric heart disease. https://core.ac.uk/download/76520310.pdf (accessed on 15th July 2025).
28. Choi, J. H., Gordon, J. S., Maynes, E. J., O'Malley, M., et al. (2020). Cardiac interventions in patients with achondroplasia: A systematic review. https://core.ac.uk/download/322850156.pdf (accessed on 15th July 2025).
29. Copeland, L. I. B. T., Duinkerken, M. S. I., Kelsey, J., Gordon, R., et al. (2019). *Jefferson Digital Commons Quarterly Report: October–December 2019*. https://core.ac.uk/download/286097805.pdf (accessed on 15th July 2025).
30. Das, D., & Das, S. (2025). Current trends in pediatric cardiac surgery and their impact on intensive care. *Journal of Pediatric Critical Care*. https://www.semanticscholar.org/paper/0bcb26152036c9f4265988641b270f007b9dd18e (accessed on 15th July 2025).
31. Das, S., & Das, D. (2025). The dawn of a new era in congenital heart surgery: Decadal innovations and future prospects. *International Journal of Scientific Research*. https://www.semanticscholar.org/paper/53197206334383066c856b5e21f74508dc365ae0 (accessed on 15th July 2025).
32. Degtyareva, E., Mwela, B., Kudlay, D., Ovsyannikov, D., Kantemirova, M., Prodeus, A., Kim, A. I., et al. (2024). Immunological screening as infectious complications prediction method in pediatric cardiac surgery. *Pediatric. Journal Named After G.N. Speransky*. https://www.semanticscholar.org/paper/a337f94eb77746d67f732fd5886f6aee562cc92e (accessed on 15th July 2025).
33. Ejigu, Y., Mlambo, V., Neil, K. L., Sime, H., Wong, R., Gatera, M. R., Nyirigira, G., et al. (2024). Short term outcomes of the first pediatric cardiac surgery program in Rwanda. *Journal of Cardiothoracic Surgery, 19*. https://www.semanticscholar.org/paper/dc10edb158c6d37c0d162913afb74670f0bfb752 (accessed on 15th July 2025).
34. Feinstein, Y., Keizman, E., Klugman, D., Koers, A., et al. (2022). The horizon of pediatric cardiac critical care. https://core.ac.uk/download/541130859.pdf (accessed on 15th July 2025).
35. Gerosa, G., & Iop, L. (2015). Guided tissue regeneration in heart valve replacement: From preclinical research to first-in-human trials. https://core.ac.uk/download/53532873.pdf (accessed on 15th July 2025).
36. Hessey, E., Melhem, N., Alobaidi, R., Ulrich, E., Morgan, C. J., Bagshaw, S., & Sinha, M. (2021). Acute kidney injury in critically ill children is not all acute: Lessons over the last 5 years. *Frontiers in Pediatrics, 9*. https://www.semanticscholar.org/paper/e43a959fcc8d7b573a41e3eb880f88bc26b0a363 (accessed on 15th July 2025).
37. Hughes, M. L., Ntsinjana, H. N., & Taylor, A. M. (2011). The role of cardiovascular magnetic resonance in pediatric congenital heart disease. https://core.ac.uk/download/1895946.pdf (accessed on 15th July 2025).
38. JnTala, M., Kumar, T., Lotto, A., Mariani, F., et al. (2018). An observational cohort feasibility study to identify micro vesicle and miRNA biomarkers of acute kidney injury following pediatric cardiac surgery. https://core.ac.uk/download/287585914.pdf (accessed on 15th July 2025).

39. Karacaer, F. (2025). Patient blood management in pediatric cardiac surgery. *Cukurova Anestezi ve Cerrahi Bilimler Dergisi*. https://www.semanticscholar.org/paper/2563ec662147a79f2a80542a1f89b721e708cb8f (accessed on 15th July 2025).

40. Kesumarini, D., Widyastuti, Y., Boom, C. E., Laurentius, A., & Dinarti, L. K. (2024). Postoperative bleeding outcome of fresh frozen plasma primes in pediatric cardiac surgery: A systematic review & meta-analysis. *Perfusion*. https://www.semanticscholar.org/paper/6fec596ecfcfdcbee4fe6d53d10dfd1760b34a3f (accessed on 15th July 2025).

41. Kumar, S. R. (2025). Improving standards in congenital heart surgery using outcomes data and risk stratification. *Seminars in Thoracic and Cardiovascular Surgery. Pediatric Cardiac Surgery Annual, 28*, 138–142. https://www.semanticscholar.org/paper/08efefd41c6932a0956815a46576d592d5d3598d (accessed on 15th July 2025).

42. Mikhailova, A., Ivkin, A. A., & Grigoriev, E. (2024). Diagnostic significance of the near-infrared spectroscopy in the prevention of cerebral injury during surgical correction of congenital heart defects in children. *Complex Issues of Cardiovascular Diseases*. https://www.semanticscholar.org/paper/50c88a592d8f5c535310fc0663ebeddedad365c7 (accessed on 15th July 2025).

43. Ranjan, A., Sahu, S. S., Singh, A. K., Das, K. S., Dubraj, P. N., & Lakra, P. S. (2024). Adoption, outcomes, and healthcare professionals' perceptions of minimally invasive surgical techniques in neonatology and pediatric surgery: A clinical study. *Journal of Pharmacy & Bioallied Sciences, 16*, S2821–S2823. https://www.semanticscholar.org/paper/57a004ce9496bb1258751ec9b7cd8df5c07fb8da (accessed on 15th July 2025).

44. Saraçoğlu, A. G., & Salman, N. (2025). Anesthetic management in pediatric cardiac surgery. *Surgery on Children*. https://www.semanticscholar.org/paper/a33b953df052e40acf0bfce05ee778cb14a6e41f (accessed on 15th July 2025).

45. Zahri, S., Ettagmouti, Y., Zagdan, S., Belhakim, M., Haboub, M., Drighil, A., & Habbal, R. (2024). Pediatric cardiac hydatid cysts: A diagnostic odyssey: A rare case report. *Annals of Medicine and Surgery, 86*, 4776–4779. https://www.semanticscholar.org/paper/b7e72149021bc81a556474ba8e59da73d0b00f84 (accessed on 15th July 2025).

INDEX

C

D

E

F

G

H

O

P

W